Medical Assisting:
Clinical Competencies

Connie Krebs, CMA-C
Barbara A. Wise, BSN, RN, MA(Ed)

Delmar Publishers Inc.™

I(T)P™

Notice to the Reader

Cover Design: Megan DeSantis

Publishing Team:
Associate Editor: Marion Waldman
Developmental Editor: Helen V. Yackel
Project Editor: Megan A. Terry
Production Coordinator: Mary Ellen Black
Art and Design Coordinator: Timothy J. Conners
                    Megan DeSantis

For information write to

Delmar Publishers Inc.
3 Columbia Circle, Box 15015,
Albany, NY 12203–5015

Printed in the United States of America
Published simultaneously in Canada
by Nelson Canada,
a division of The Thomson Corporation

1 2 3 4 5 6 7 8 9 10   XXX   00 99 98 97 96 95 94

Library of Congress Cataloging-in-Publication Data
Krebs, Connie.
      Medical assisting : clinical competencies / Connie Krebs, Barbara
A. Wise. — 1st ed.
        p.   cm.
      Includes bibliographical references and index.
      ISBN 0–8273–4986–6
      1. Medical assistants.   I. Wise, Barbara A.   II. Title.
      [DNLM: 1. Physicians' Assistants. W 21.5 K918m   1994]
R728.8.K74 1994
610.69′53—dc20
DNLM/DLC
for Library of Congress   93-43603
                                        CIP

Table of Contents

Preface   vii
Acknowledgments   ix
A Message to the Learner   x

1
Communications   1

U N I T   1

Verbal and Nonverbal Communication   2

Perception 3 • Body Language 3

U N I T   2

Interacting with Patients and Their Families   4

Right to Privacy 5 • Choice of Treatment 6 • Terminal Illness 6

U N I T   3

Medical Staff Relationships   7

Staff Arrangements 8 • Intraoffice Communication 9 • Career Entry 9 • Employee Evaluation 10

U N I T   4

Essentials in Medical Law and Ethics   10

Licensure Requirements 12 • Ethical Considerations 13 • The Uniform Anatomical Gift Act 14 • Living Will 15 • Legal Considerations 15 • Physician and Patient Rights 18 • Medical Assistant Rights 19 • Negligence 21 • Medical Records 22

2
Personal Behaviors   26

U N I T   1

Nutrition, Exercise, and Rest   26

Nutrition 27 • Exercise 31

U N I T   2

Stress Management   33

Office Stress 37 • Stress and Related Illness 37

U N I T   3

Substance Abuse   39

Alcohol 40 • Drugs 40 • Smoking 45

U N I T   4

Behavior Modification   46

Defense Mechanisms 47 • Mental and Emotional Status Influencing Behaviors 48 • Communicating Emotional States 48

3
Office Environmental Control   50

U N I T   1

Asepsis   50

Handwashing 51

U N I T   2

Disease Transmission   52

Disease Transmission 52 • Disease Prevention 56

U N I T   3

AIDS/Universal Precautions   58

U N I T   4

Care of Instruments   61

UNIT 5

Office Safety and Security   63

> Reception Room 66 · Examination Rooms 67 · Laboratory Area 67

4
Anatomy and Physiology of the Human Body   71

UNIT 1

Anatomical Descriptors and Fundamental Body Structure   71

> Anatomy and Physiology Defined 72 · Language of Medicine 73 · Anatomical Directional Terms 73 · Body Cavities and Organs 74 · The Cell 74 · Passing Molecules Through Cell Membranes 77 · Cellular Division 80 · Homeostasis 81 · Genetic Cellular Change 81 · Tissues 83 · Organs 85 · Systems 85

UNIT 2

The Nervous System   85

> Membrane Excitability 87 · Peripheral Nervous System and Spinal Cord 89 · Central Nervous System 90 · Diagnostic Tests 92 · Diseases and Disorders 94

UNIT 3

The Senses   100

> The Eye and the Sense of Sight 100 · Diseases and Disorders of the Eye 102 · The Ear and the Sense of Hearing 105 · Diseases and Disorders of the Ear 106 · The Nose and the Sense of Smell 107 · Diseases and Disorders of the Nose 107 · The Tongue and the Sense of Taste 108 · Diseases and Disorders of the Mouth and Tongue 108 · The Skin and the Sense of Touch 109

UNIT 4

The Integumentary System   109

> Functions 110 · Structure of the Skin 110 · Skin Color 112 · The Skin as a Diagnostic Testing Site 112 · Diseases and Disorders 112

UNIT 5

The Skeletal System   117

> Bone Structure 118 · Number of Bones 118 · Functions of the Skeleton 118 · Spinal Column 119 · The Skull 120 · The Rib Cage 120 · Long Bones 121 · Bones of the Hands and Feet 121 · The Pelvic Girdle 122 · Joints 122 · Fractures 124 · Amputation 125 · Diagnostic Examinations 125 · Diseases and Disorders 126

UNIT 6

The Muscular System   130

> Muscle Fuel 131 · Functions of Muscle 131 · Muscle Growth 131 · Types of Muscle Tissue 131 · Skeletal Muscle Action 132 · Muscle Tone 132 · Muscle Attachment 133 · Sheaths and Bursae 133 · Major Skeletal Muscles 134 · Muscle Strain and Cramps 135 · Smooth Muscle Action 137 · Disorders and Diseases 138

UNIT 7

The Respiratory System   139

> The Pathway of Oxygen 140 · Respiration 142 · The Lung and the Pleura 143 · The Muscles of Breathing 144 · Diagnostic Examinations 145 · Disorders and Diseases 145

UNIT 8

The Circulatory System   152

> The Heart 153 · The Blood Vessels 158 · The Lymphatic System 162 · The Blood 163 · Cardiovascular Tests 169 · Diseases and Disorders 170 · Angina 171

UNIT 9

The Immune System   177

> Origin of Cells 178 · Organs of the Immune System 178 · Cell Markers 178 · Lymphocytes 179 · Complement System 180 · Cytokines 180 · Natural Killer (NK) Cells 182 · Immune Responses 182 · Immunization 185 · Diseases and Disorders 185

UNIT 10

The Digestive System   197

> The Mouth 199 · The Esophagus 199 · The Stomach 200 · The Small Intestine 202 · The Large Intestine 204 · Diagnostic Examinations 206 · Disorders and Diseases 208

UNIT 11

The Urinary System   215

> The Kidneys 216 · The Ureters 218 · The Urinary Bladder 218 · The Urethra 218 · Dialysis 219 · Kidney Transplant 221 · Diagnostic Examinations 221 · Diseases and Disorders 222

UNIT 12

The Endocrine System   225

> Pituitary Gland 226 · Thyroid Gland 228 · Parathyroid Glands 230 · Adrenal Glands (Suprarenal) 230 · Pancreas 231 · Thymus Gland 231 · Pineal Body 231 · Gonads (Testes and Ovaries) 231 · Interrelationship of the Glands 232 · Diagnostic Examinations 232 · Diseases and Disorders 232

UNIT 13

The Reproductive System 236

Differentiation of Reproductive Organs 237 • Male Reproductive Organs 237 • Diseases and Disorders of the Male Reproductive System 241 • Female Reproductive Organs 244 • Fertilization 250 • Pregnancy 252 • The Birth Process 254 • Contraception 255 • Diagnostic Tests of the Female Reproductive System 255 • Diseases and Disorders of the Female Reproductive System 255 • Malignancy of the Reproductive Organs 259 • Sexually Transmitted Diseases 260 • Transsexualism 263

5
Beginning the Database 266

UNIT 1

Managing Triage 267

UNIT 2

Medical History 270

Patient's Medical History 270

UNIT 3

Mensurations 273

Height and Weight 278 • Head Circumference 284 • Chest Measurement 284

UNIT 4

Vital Signs 285

Temperature 289 • Pulse 302 • Respiration 305 • Temperature–Pulse–Respiration Ratio 307 • Blood Pressure 307

6
Physical Examinations 317

UNIT 1

Head to Toe 319

Preparation of the Examination Room 322 • Preparation of the Patient 322 • Physical Examination Format 322

UNIT 2

Positioning and Draping for Examinations 330

Positioning and Draping Patient 330

UNIT 3

Procedures of the Eye and Ear 336

Eye and Ear Examination 337 • Visual Acuity 339 • Pelli-Robson Contrast Sensitivity Chart 346 • Auditory Acuity 347

UNIT 4

Specialty Examinations 351

The Pap Test and Hormonal Smears 352 • Obstetrics Patients 355 • Pediatric Examinations 358 • Sigmoidoscopy 365

7
Specimen Collection and Laboratory Procedures 369

Guidelines for Lab Safety 370

UNIT 1

The Microscope 372

UNIT 2

Capillary Blood Tests 374

Laboratory Classification and Regulation 374 • Skin Puncture 376 • PKU Test 378 • Hemoglobin and Hematocrit 380 • Blood Glucose Screening 383 • GTT—Glucose Tolerance Test 384 • Blood Count Cell 384

UNIT 3

Venous Blood Tests 396

Venipuncture 396 • Erythrocyte Sedimentation Rate 400

UNIT 4

Urine, Sputum, and Stool Specimens 403

Urine Specimens 406 • Sputum Specimens 415 • Stool Specimens 417

UNIT 5

Bacterial Smears and Cultures 419

Bacteriological Smear 420 • Culturing 420 • Gram Staining 421

8
Diagnostic Tests, X Rays, and Procedures 427

UNIT 1

Diagnostic Tests 427

Skin Tests 428

UNIT 2

Cardiology Procedures 433

Path of Electrical Impulses 436 • Routine Electrocardiograph Leads 437 • Interference 438 Standardization 441 • Stress Tests 444 • Holter Monitoring 444

UNIT 3

Diagnostic Procedures 447

Vital Capacity Tests 447 • Sonographic Studies 448 • MRI—Magnetic Reasonance Imaging 449 • Hemoccult Sensa Tests 451

UNIT 4

Diagnostic X-ray Examinations 452

Radiological Studies 454

9
Surgical Procedures 459

Skin Preparation 463 • Sterile Gloves 463 • Assisting with Procedures 463

10
Medications 473

UNIT 1

Prescription and Nonprescription Medications 473

Commonly Prescribed Medications 474 • Pharmaceutical References 476 • Writing Prescriptions 477 • Recording Medications 483 • Storing Medications 483

UNIT 2

Methods for Administering Medications 483

Administering Medication 483 • Considerations of Drug Action 489

UNIT 3

Injections and Immunizations 490

Injections 490 • Immunizations 497

11
Medical Emergencies 509

UNIT 1

Safety in the Medical Office 509

UNIT 2

Medical Office Emergency Procedures 510

First Aid for Sudden Illness and Injuries 512 • Substance Abuse 524 • Emergency Services 525

UNIT 3

First Aid Care of Accidents and Injuries 526

12
Employment 538

UNIT 1

The Job Search 538

The Resume 539 • The Cover Letter 541 • Classified Advertisements 542 • Public Employment Services 542 • Private Employment Agencies 543 • Other Contacts 543

UNIT 2

Getting the Job and Keeping It 545

Application Forms 545 • The Interview 547 • What Employers Want Most in Employees 548 • The Employee Evaluation or Review 551 • Terminating Employment 552 • Summary 553 • A Final Note 553

Appendix 555
Glossary 573
Index 595

Preface

Medical Assisting: Clinical Competencies provides a current knowledge base, task requirements, and skill development procedures that the clinical medical assistant needs to qualify for entry-level employment in a physician's office, a medical clinic, or any appropriate health care facility.

The content of the text is organized to reflect the various responsibilities of the occupation. To support each of these areas, the authors provide thorough, clearly written, and well-illustrated discussions of the major concepts and tasks associated with achieving competency in each responsibility.

Clinical medical assisting is a most versatile career choice, which is both challenging and rewarding. This text provides you with the areas that are of particular interest to the clinical medical assistant. The first three chapters are concerned with **you,** the learner. Since you are soon going to be in a most stressful environment as the clinical medical assistant, you must first learn how to (1) communicate effectively with others, (2) be aware of personal behaviors that affect yourself and others, and (3) develop a respect for safety and security of yourself and others in the workplace. The chapter on basic anatomy and physiology follows to give essential information containing diseases and disorders. Learning the medical terminology, symptoms, diagnostic tests, and treatments of diseases is of vital importance for precise documentation of data. The chapters that follow provide information in clinical assisting procedures. The last chapter deals with employability information. This is to help you toward your goal of getting and keeping employment in the health care field as a successful clinical medical assistant. In the appendices of this text are many valuable pages of information that you should utilize for your benefit.

The student in a medical assistant program must remember that the geographic location, the type and size of a medical practice, the number and types of employees, and the personal discretion of the physician all tend to affect the role of the medical assistant. The duties performed are largely governed by state and local laws. Also restrictions may be set by physicians as to the types of procedures that can be performed in a particular practice. It is up to you to prove your proficiency and document your worth by becoming a certified medical assistant. This means that you have a basic knowledge of the entry-level skills (knowledge in both administrative and clinical areas). Showing your credentials when searching for employment will prove to be most advantageous.

Throughout the text, the learning required is specified by means of the competency-based unit objectives as well as the terminal performance objectives identified for each procedure. You, the student, must decide to take this profession seriously and do well in your studies. You must remember that the public respect medical professionals for their dedication and service to those in pain and suffering. You have expressed a desire to become a part of this health care team. In order to be successful, you must be both knowledgeable and proficient in your service to others. You will not always be able to rely on your fellow students for answers to questions. You will have to know the information yourself on the job. While you have time and support of the instructor and classmates, you should take advantage of it to learn the subject matter well. Using this text as a reference throughout your career will help you review and regain confidence in your skills.

The content includes all introductory-level areas as identified by the *Essentials and Guidelines of an Accredited Educational Program for the Medical Assistant* as revised in 1991. A plan for providing an externship, as required by the guidelines, is included in the accompanying *Instructor's Guide.*

The text is designed for use as an introduction to medical assisting in a variety of settings

- a structured classroom setting, with the expertise of a qualified instructor;
- for individual instruction of students in programs of diversified training, because much of the content and format are appropriate for self-study;
- for on-the-job training in a physician's office, where the text serves as a resource manual.

Content

Technical advances in equipment and procedures are covered, as well as adherence to infectious disease control, which is necessary to quality health care. The anatomy and physiology content also reflects advances in clinical knowledge, diagnosis, and treatment. Contains information on:

- medical, legal, and ethical concerns facing health care providers today, and their effect on health care delivery; Information on durable power of attorney for health care, Right to Die, Miranda Warning Law, and living wills
- scenarios for medical, legal, and ethical concerns
- new definition from AAMA for medical assistant and new AAMA logo in Appendix
- related health specialty fields information

- section on English grammar in the Appendix
- examples of math applications
- unit on the immune system: includes discussion of allergies, cancer, immunity, lupus erythematosus, chronic fatigue syndrome, rheumatoid arthritis, and AIDS
- interpersonal communications to include sexual harassment and discrimination.
- diseases and disorders, diagnostic tests and treatments in anatomy and physiology chapter. Content on conception, contraception, pregnancy, labor, and delivery.
- discussion of infectious disease control, including utilization of universal precautions in every clinical procedure as appropriate.
- coverage of communicable diseases, medications and surgical instruments.
- coverage of ECG (EKG), history and database information including new history form and examination of the eye and ears
- personal behaviors including second-hand smoke and employability skills information

- laboratory procedure content reflects CLIA recommendations for POL
- immunization tables

Supplements

The *Student Workbook* that accompanies this text provides review questions, vocabulary and skill exercises, forms to complete, puzzles, and other tasks that reinforce the content of the text. The workbook also includes evaluation sheets for measuring performance of the procedures. An *Instructor's Guide* provides answers to the questions in the workbook and guidelines to the instructor for presenting the content.

Use of the text, reinforced by the *Student Workbook* and recommendations from the *Instructor's Guide,* provides for implementation of a complete, competency-based instructional program.

Acknowledgments

John Ross, a very special personal friend, who gave unending encouragement and support as well as computer assistance, photo shooting, and serving as a sounding-board. His contribution and patience was above and beyond all expectations and is gratefully acknowledged.

James C. English, MD, practicing family physician and former instructor in the College of Medicine at The Ohio State University, for reading, identifying, and recommending content to be added or technically updated in Chapter 4, Anatomy and Physiology. His invaluable contribution is truly appreciated.

James B. Soldano, MD, family practice physician who reviewed the content regarding physical examination in Chapter 6.

Jeanne Luddy, retired English teacher, who advised and made contributions to the material on grammar in the Appendix.

Colleen King, RN, of Northwest Family Physicians, who provided in-depth information and assistance with the content on responsibilities involved in the management of a medical practice.

Elaine Glass, MS, RN, OCN, clinical nurse specialist, The Arthur G. James Cancer Hospital and Research Center, who provided technical information and expertise on the immune system and her personal review of the material included in the text.

Diane Hohwald, RN, CNN, educational coordinator of Riverside Outpatient Dialysis Center, for providing information, technical assistance, illustrative materials, and her personal review of the content included in the text.

A special appreciation to the following for permitting the use of their offices as sites for many of the photos in this text:

Andrew J. Pultz, MD, and the staff of Metropolitan Family Practice

George A. Huntress, DO, and the staff of Sullivan Family Medical Center

The physicians and staff of Med-Ohio North

Jack Frost, MD, plastic surgery, Arnold, Maryland

Donna Shea, AS, RMA, CMA, CRT: Medical assisting instructor, National Education Center, San Bernardino, CA

Ruth Darton, CMA; Medical assisting instructor and consultant, National Education Center, San Bernardino, CA

Adrienne L. Carter-Ward, CMA, RMA, EMT; Instructor trainer and medical assisting instructor, National Headquarters NEC, San Bernardino, CA

Carol Hinricher; Medical assisting instructor, Missoula Technical Center, Missoula, MT

Judy Crissip, CMA-AC; Medical assisting instructor and program director, Pinellas Technical Education Centers, St. Petersburg, FL

Sally Emery, RN: Medical assisting instructor, Aristotle Institute, Westerville, OH

Sharon Pass, RMA (AMT); Medical assisting instructor and program director, California Paramedical and Technical College, Riverside, CA

Theresa Bowser; Medical assistant instructor, Bradford School, Columbus, OH

Wilma J. Stoeckle, CMA; Medical assistant instructor, Duff's Business Institute, Pittsburgh, PA

Brenda M. Foster, MS, CMA; Coordinator, Department of Health Related Professions, program director/Medical Assisting, East Tennessee State University, Elizabethton, TN

Linda Scarborough; Instructor, Allied Health Department, Lanier Technical Institute, Oakwood, GA

The authors especially wish to acknowledge and commend the editors and staff of Delmar Publishers Inc. for their encouragement, guidance, recommendations, and expertise during the preparation of this edition. Their assistance during the development of the text was most helpful.

Administrative editor—Marion Waldman

Developmental editor—Helen Yackel

Editorial assistant—Catherine Eads

Dedication

We gratefully acknowledge the support and encouragement of our families, loved ones, and friends throughout the preparation of this edition. We especially recognize the strong friendship and commitment we share for each other, which goes far beyond the pages of this book. Additionally, we wish to make a very special dedication to Lucille Keir, CMA-A, who recently passed away. She was a true inspiration to all in her positive attitude, hard work, and perseverance in spite of her illness. She was a very special person who will be deeply missed. Because of our experiences in employment and teaching, we felt a need for this text and we therefore also wish to dedicate it to you, the reader, for you are the reason it was written.

A Message to the Learner

You are about to begin a new career in the field of health care. You have decided to become a member of the physician's team to help provide for the needs of the people in your community. You will be expected to be knowledgeable, efficient, and capable of assuming a great deal of responsibility in the performance of your duties. As you study this text, keep in mind that you should learn the reasons for performing procedures as well as becoming proficient in carrying them out. Even though you may learn a procedure and go on with other lessons and assignments, you must still keep reviewing lessons and practicing those skills which you have already learned so that you may become expedient and proficient in them. Realize that this is accomplished only by doing procedures over and over again. Knowledge of your subject area will give you confidence. If you have practiced the skills you will need to perform in a medical facility until they are almost second nature to you, then you will have confidence in working with patients.

People go to a physician's office for a variety of reasons. They may desire a general assessment of their health status or they may be injured and need immediate treatment. Often they are very ill and frightened and require assistance with emotional as well as physical problems. The physician must be able to diagnose the reason for their illness or determine the extent of their injury in order to provide the proper treatment or medication. The physician will be better able to concentrate on the needs of the patients if you can be depended upon to carry out your responsibilities. As a medical assistant you will be performing many of the operational tasks necessary for a medical office to function effectively and efficiently as well as assisting the physician to examine and treat the patients.

Purpose of This Text

This text was written to help you acquire the knowledge and skills needed to work successfully in a medical office. Occasionally, the methods of medical practice or policies where you live will differ from those described in the text. This may affect the tasks you perform or the procedural steps of the skills, but the basic information will be the same.

It is important that you understand the reasons for the procedures you will be performing and that you know how to perform them accurately. Remember, you are working with people's lives. Often you cannot correct mistakes once they have been made, so it is very important that you DO NOT make mistakes. Do not be afraid to ask questions when you do not understand.

Keeping Current

Your training will not end when you have completed this text. There is much information that applies to specific kinds of medical practice or is best learned when the specific employment situation arises. In addition, health care methods change whenever a new drug is developed or a different treatment is proved effective. Occasionally, a new finding will completely change the way to deal with an illness or disease. Consider the changes that have occurred due to the virus that causes AIDS. Individuals working in health professions have had to change the way they provide care in order to protect themselves and their patients. Workshops, seminars, technical journals, and your employer will become your means of learning additional skills to stay current.

Organization of Text

The text has been organized into sections, chapters, and units. The basic structure is the unit. Units covering related information are grouped into chapters.

Each unit has important features which specify what you are expected to learn.

Objectives. These identify the knowledge or skill you are to develop by studying the material. Recall the objectives as you read the unit. When you have finished, review the objectives and reread portions of the unit until you can accurately respond to all of them. The workbook that accompanies this text has questions, puzzles, diagrams, and other activities which will help you acquire the knowledge and skills necessary to meet the objectives and later, become successfully employed as a medical assistant.

Words to Know. These are medical terms and related vocabulary words used in the unit. They are listed separately at the beginning of each unit and highlighted in color at the first significant use within the text. You are expected to be able to include the terms in your personal vocabulary. You will find them listed and defined in the Glossary at the back of the text.

Procedures. These are detailed descriptions of skills required of a medical assistant. They list the actions involved, step by step, in a logical sequence. The procedures have been developed from standards of practice that have proven successful. Within each procedure, important points (*Notes*) are emphasized.

The procedures also have specific performance criteria called terminal performance objectives. This type of objective identifies exactly what is required to successfully perform the procedure.

Appendix. The Appendix contains medical abbreviations and the prefixes, suffixes, and Latin and Greek words that make up medical terms. Become familiar with this section as quickly as possible. It will help you to define terminology and to understand the language of medicine. Other useful information is also included in the Appendix such as: converting measurements; weights and measures; symbols; and a chart for stain removal.

Other Titles in Delmar's Leading Medical Assisting Series

- *Administrative Medical Assisting,* 3rd Edition/Fordney, Follis
- *Body Structures and Functions,* 8th Edition/Fong, Scott
- *Computer Literacy for Health Care Professionals*/Anderson
- *Computerized Medical Office Management*/Johnson, Johnson
- *Fundamental Skills for the Clinical Laboratory Professional*/Marshall
- *Human Anatomy and Physiology in Health and Disease,* 3rd Edition/Burke
- *Law, Liability, and Ethics for Medical Office Personnel,* 2nd Edition/Flight
- *Medical Brain Teasers, Puzzles, and Games*/Silverman
- *Medical Terminology for Health Professionals,* 2nd Edition/Ehrlich
- *The Professional Medical Assistant: Clinical Practice*/Lindsey, Rayburn
- *Therapeutic Communications for Allied Health Professionals*/Tamparo, Lindh
- *Understanding Medical Insurance*/Rowell
- Delmar's *Medical Assisting Videos*

C H A P T E R   1
Communications

UNIT 1
Verbal and Nonverbal
Communication

UNIT 2
Interacting with Patients and Their
Families

UNIT 3
Medical Staff Relations

UNIT 4
Essentials in Medical Law and Ethics

One of the most important skills a medical assistant can possess is the art of communicating effectively with others. Both clinical and administrative duties require a constant exchange of written, oral, and nonverbal information.

You must be able to convey messages to many different people and receive vital information in the same manner. You will have daily contact with patients, colleagues, and other professionals, by phone, face to face, or by letter. This chapter deals with both verbal and nonverbal messages. Understanding how one gives and receives these is vital in the exchange of communication.

In dealing with patients and their families, learning to listen and to offer advice in a calm, professional manner will help to reduce unnecessary stress for all concerned. Times of sadness and pain can be extremely difficult for those closely involved. You can be instrumental in providing comfort and compassion to those in need.

Since the medical office is usually a very active place, with many people coming and going, asking questions and making payments or appointments, intraoffice communication can become ragged and ineffective. A harmonious team effort makes for an efficient as well as a pleasant work environment. If an atmosphere of accord and cooperation exists among the staff, patients will sense this during their visits. If an uneasy situation exists, with friction evident, this may add to a patient's apprehensions and anxieties. Working together for the single purpose of providing quality health care to patients in a relaxed and friendly manner will help ease the daily pressures for the members of the medical office team and contribute greatly to their collective effectiveness.

UNIT 1

Verbal and Nonverbal Communication

OBJECTIVES ·······································

Upon completion of the unit you will meet the following terminal performance objectives by verifying knowledge of the facts and principles presented through oral and written communication at a level deemed competent by the instructor or employer.

1. Describe the basic pattern of communication.
2. Give examples of nonverbal communication.
3. Explain how verbal and nonverbal communication can sometimes be misinterpreted.
4. Describe ways that tone and speed of speech can affect the message.
5. Discuss the importance of dress in nonverbal communication.
6. Define *perception* and state its importance in communication.
7. Spell and define, using the glossary at the back of the text, all the words to know in this unit.

WORDS TO KNOW ·······································

articulate	incongruous
conceptualize	intangible
contradict	intuition
distort	perception
empirically	scrupulously

To become effective in the art of communication, it may help to **conceptualize** the communication process, Figure 1–1. The message originates with the sender. The encoded message takes form based upon the sender's reference points (or frames of reference), and off it goes. The message is picked up by the intended receiver, who immediately begins to decode it based on his or her reference points (or frames of reference). In responding (or providing feedback) the whole process is reversed: the original receiver becomes the sender, and the original sender becomes the receiver. In receiving this feedback, the original sender (now the receiver) can assess and evaluate how well the original message was received and interpreted and make any necessary adjustments or clarification.

The whole process seems simple enough, and generally it works well. However, many things can happen to affect the quality of the message or even **distort** it. You must be aware of these potential problems.

Foremost is the issue of reference points. For example, the spoken messages may include terminology familiar to you but unknown to the patient. Therefore, though the message will be heard, it may not be understood. Talking to patients on a level that they can easily understand is a skill requiring quick judgment. You will have to adapt to a vast number of different personalities in conveying information.

Some patients may be hearing- or sight-impaired, developmentally disabled, or non-English-speaking and will therefore require extra understanding. If a patient is in some way handicapped, a family member or friend usually accompanies the person, thereby helping with your task of transmitting necessary information.

Other factors may interfere, such as interruptions or simply the way you feel. These factors must be recognized and dealt with if effective communication is to occur.

The spoken word must be delivered in an **articulate,** clear manner if the intended message is to be received. Correct pronunciation and proper grammar help to convey the meaning. You must also be aware of the rate of the spoken word. Patients need to be spoken to in an unrushed manner so that the information has a chance to register and questions can be asked. Speaking in a pleasant tone of voice is necessary to keep the listener's interest in what you are saying.

Common courtesy is an art which seems to have been lost to some degree. In a professional setting it is essential to be **scrupulously** polite. *Please, Thank you, Excuse me,* and *May I help you?* should be used frequently. In this way the entire health care staff will show respect for others and a sense of caring.

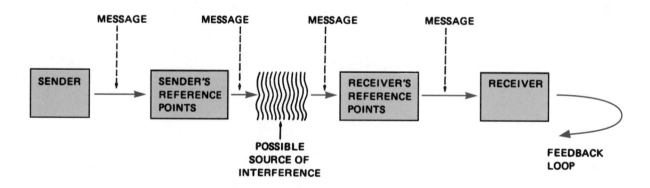

FIGURE 1–1 The communication process

Perception

Perception in the context of communication may be considered as being aware of one's own feelings and the feelings of others. The feelings you have about other people's moods and the way they act are perceptual, nonspoken communication between you. **Intuition** is another term for perception in this sense. Although they cannot be measured **empirically**, these feelings may be strong indeed. Therefore, they must be recognized and reckoned with.

Being perceptive is a skill acquired with experience and practice. Keeping your eyes and ears open to the needs of others and what is going on will help you develop it. Developing the ability to perceive your own needs is a part of perception that will enhance your effectiveness. Planning and thinking ahead will help you develop in this area.

Body Language

The image you project is of utmost importance. Your overall appearance sends out messages to anyone who looks at you. Appropriate dress, uniform, or businesslike attire should be worn. Your professional appearance sends a nonverbal message that you have authority and are in charge.

Proper attire may vary with the medical specialty. For instance, many pediatric practices prefer medical assistants to dress in normal street clothes so as to make young patients feel more at ease. Children sometimes associate a white uniform with an unpleasant hospital visit. Psychiatry and psychology medical office assistants may also be more inclined to wear businesslike dress, for clinical duties are few, if any, and a uniform may not be necessary. Casual wear is considered unprofessional, however, and jeans, sandals, and excessive jewelry are out of the question during working hours. Looking like a professional will not only encourage the respect of others for your profession, but it will help you to feel an integral part of the health care team.

Personal hygiene should be impeccable, because setting a good example for others is a part of your responsibility in the care of others. Daily showering, clean attractive hair, and neatly manicured nails show others that you take pride in yourself and give them a model to pattern themselves after, Figure 1–2.

Another part of your appearance, something **intangible** but very real, is your attitude. Your attitude shows *everyone* who sees you or speaks to you (by telephone or in person) how you feel about your work, others, and yourself. You display your attitude in the way you get along with others and interact with them. The importance of a positive attitude cannot be overemphasized. The many hassles and conflicts that can, and do, arise with patients and colleagues during everyday activity in the busy medical office can be handled much more effectively if you possess and project a positive attitude. Constant complaining only makes situations worse and breeds contempt. Having a good outlook on life carries over into every area and promotes well-being. Pleasant, agreeable working conditions increase

FIGURE 1–2 Pride in appearance

productivity and efficiency besides giving one a sense of satisfaction on the job.

Facial Expression Part of perception is being aware of how others think you feel, or see you. You create this impression partly by your facial expression. It is possible to **contradict** a verbal message by an inappropriate or **incongruous** facial expression. The most common example of a positive, happy facial expression is a smile, Figure 1–3, page 4. This nonverbal signal conveys a positive attitude. Frowning and looking glum only add to other people's troubles. It is especially important to be pleasant and friendly to those seeking medical attention, because their worries concerning their condition are already on their minds. Adding your troubles to theirs is highly inappropriate. A positive attitude and a receptive awareness will show in your facial expression.

Eye contact shows that you are interested in giving and receiving messages of mutual concern and interest. It has been said that the eyes are the windows of the soul. Looking into another's eyes while engaging in conversation permits an open, honest transmission of thoughts and ideas. Looking away while people are talking to you makes them feel that what they are saying is not important. Interest and attention soon disappear, and the intent of your message may be distorted or lost.

FIGURE 1–3   A smile conveys a positive attitude.

Gestures   Still another way of transmitting nonverbal messages is by gesturing. Gestures are body movements that enhance what is being said. You may know people who seemingly could not talk if they had to sit on their hands. Try to follow their example. Using hand and body gestures to accentuate a point can help the receiver understand your meaning.

A handshake is a sign of friendship. Another meaningful body movement is a hug to convey feelings of warmth and affection. A comforting touch helps patients feel that you care and gives them a sense of security and acceptance. Studies have shown that patients who have been touched, by a hand on the shoulder or a hand held, respond significantly better in treatment than those not touched. Patting someone on the back and saying "Good for you" is a positive reinforcer. You might do that in praise of a patient who followed the prescribed treatment of the physician and lost 10 pounds and who needs positive recognition of these achievements to encourage continued compliance. In reinforcing a patient, you should display a positive attitude, facial expression, gestures, and eye contact—all the communication skills so far mentioned. In addition, your tone of voice should be happy and sincere. Patients who believe you are pleased with their progress are more willing to strive to follow future treatment because of the resulting positive feelings.

Another powerful nonverbal communication tool is silence. This method can indeed be most frustrating to the person for whom it is directed. In dealing with patients who exhibit this nonverbal way of communicating, it is best if the inexperienced medical assistant asks for help from a supervisor, a physician, or another staff member who has skill in dealing with this type of situation. Patients who exhibit behavior such as this may have serious underlying problems.

Complete Chapter 1, Unit 1 in the workbook to meet the objectives at the beginning of this unit and therefore achieve competency of this subject matter.

UNIT 2

Interacting with Patients and Their Families

OBJECTIVES ···

Upon completion of the unit you will meet the following terminal performance objectives by verifying knowledge of the facts and principles presented through oral and written communication at a level deemed competent by the instructor or employer.

1. Explain why it is important to develop rapport with patients and their families.
2. Describe means of safeguarding the patient's right to confidentiality.
3. Describe the patient's options in relation to the physician's treatment plan.
4. Describe the stages that follow diagnosis of a terminal illness.
5. Describe your role in dealing with the terminally ill patient.
6. Explain the purpose of the living will.
7. State the purpose of the hospice movement.
8. List the services of the hospice movement.
9. Spell and define, using the glossary at the back of the text, all the words to know in this unit.

WORDS TO KNOW ······································

absurd	inevitable
devastate	marginal
holistic	nonchalant
hostility	terminal
incomprehensible	

The medical profession's first responsibility is to the patient. Thus, you must be able to relate to people of all ages, from tiny infants to senior citizens.

The development and growth of your own personality and interests will help you do so. The ability to converse about a variety of subjects shows an interest in people and makes you interesting to be with. Conversation with patients helps to ease their anxieties and encourages a sense of friendship and trust. At times a patient needs to express pent-up feelings, and you will often be the one who provides this necessary listening service. Sincere empathy will often begin to relieve the inner fears and anxieties of a patient who is experiencing an illness for the first time.

Patients and family members may need to discuss the treatment plan the physician has already discussed with them. Often patients do not hear all of what has been said by the physician because they have been preoccupied with worry about their illness. Their questions may sometimes seem trivial, but to the patient they are real and pressing issues that need immediate attention.

Many patients have never before experienced sickness or injury. They may never have set foot in a health care facility. Having to face strange new surroundings, unfamiliar medical language, and possibly puzzling procedures will add to the patient's apprehensions. The way the patient is treated in these new situations will determine how the patient, and members of the family, accept the diagnosis and prognosis of the patient's condition. Tact and good communication skills will help to promote rapport with all patients and their family members.

Right to Privacy ....

Every patient has a legal right to privacy and confidentiality. Information disclosed to the health care team must be kept in the strictest confidence, and you must be ever mindful of the legal implications in handling patients' records. Information concerning patients may be given to another member of the health care team, such as a laboratory technician or referring physician, only when it pertains directly to the course of treatment. Another medical office may telephone to inquire about a patient's medical history for diagnostic purposes, to confirm symptoms, or to verify a birthdate; patients, in complying with referral appointments or scheduled tests, will have given implied consent for necessary information to be transmitted concerning their condition. In the daily routine, such procedures do not require consent forms to be signed by the patient. If this were not true, very little could be accomplished besides handling forms.

Medical information may be given to parties not concerned in the patient's treatment *only* when the patient has signed a release of information form. Medical insurance forms, for instance, have a section patients must sign to authorize the release of information to insurance companies, Figure 1–4. Only those persons specified by the patient in writing may receive information concerning the patient's condition. Usually the medical facility has a patient information release form, which is completed during the initial visit. Persons to contact in case of emergency are listed there. Inquiries should be made at this time as to who may be informed about the patient's condition. This document should be filed in the patient's chart for future reference. Those of legal age have the right to privacy in all matters of treatment, and even parents may not be given information about a patient's condition unless specific written permission accompanied by the patient's signature is secured.

In the normal course of conversation you may be told personal information that should be kept to yourself, unless doing so would be harmful to the patient. The patient will usually tell you how far the information should go, or whom to tell or not to tell. Emotional stress and other critical data should be relayed to the physician, for it may have some bearing on the condition of the patient. You must use judgment in this important area. A patient who is experiencing domestic problems, for instance, may be asking for help in telling you about them. Patients usually realize that professional persons can put them in touch with assistance and sometimes expect that it will be forthcoming if they merely suggest that help is needed. Tact is required in handling delicate matters of this nature. Patients trust the medical profession to safeguard matters discussed in the privacy of the medical office. Directly asking each patient

FIGURE 1–4 Release of information form (Courtesy of Colwell Systems, Inc.)

RELEASE AND ASSIGNMENT

Date _____

To _____
INSURANCE COMPANY

_____

Group No. _____ Certificate No. _____

I hereby authorize Dr. _____
to release to your company or its representative, any information including the diagnosis and the records of any treatment or examination rendered to me during the period of such Medical or Surgical care.

I also authorize and request your company to pay directly to the above named doctor the amount due me in my pending claim for Basic Medical, Major Medical and/or Surgical treatment or services, by reason of such treatment or services rendered to:

_____
PATIENT

_____
SIGNATURE OF INSURED

_____   _____
WITNESS   ADDRESS

FORM 3340 COLWELL CO., CHAMPAIGN, ILL.

who may receive this confidential information and having appropriate release forms signed will ensure that the patient is aware of what has been done and will also protect you from liability.

Choice of Treatment ....

Advising patients of the choices they have in the treatment of their illnesses is often among your responsibilities. A full explanation of the diagnosis, prognosis, and options in treating the condition are given to the patient by the physician. Some patients, however, have a difficult time in making up their minds and may need additional information and further discussion before deciding to accept a treatment plan, especially when it involves a major event such as elective surgery. There are life-threatening situations in which patients must make these decisions quickly. Often family members must help patients with these difficult decisions.

You play an integral part in reinforcing the physician's orders. You should become proficient in identifying those patients who still seem confused after leaving their conference with the physician. Restating what the physician has already said may be all you need to say to some patients to initiate their compliance. Some patients may have had trouble with the wording used by the physician and look to you to interpret. It is difficult at times to make clear to patients all that is involved in the course of treatment. Great skill in perception is essential for all members of the health care team to ascertain if the approach to treatment is fully understood by the patient. This is a valuable skill which takes time and experience to master.

It is prudent to advise patients to seek a second opinion if they harbor any doubts concerning their condition. It may be that patients disbelieve the diagnosis. Having a second, or even a third, opinion will help them to accept their illness. Many insurance companies encourage patients to seek other opinions before treatment is initiated. This is wise, especially if the patient is troubled about the possible outcome.

In more routine matters patients still may have difficulty in complying with physicians' orders, as in weight reduction, exercising, or taking prescribed medicine. Patients must be given sound reasons for following the advice of the physician even though they already know that it is for their own good. The prescribed treatment plan will most likely change the patient's life-style. The patient who has just been diagnosed as hypertensive may have to cope with several life-style changes, such as losing weight, following a special diet, and giving up cigarettes. If reinforcement and encouragement are not sufficiently provided to the patient by members of the health care team, cooperation may be **marginal.** The risks of not following the physician's advice should be outlined in the simplest terms. Acting **nonchalant** or showing no interest in the patient will not be much help in prompting a patient to follow orders.

The final choice is always the patient's, to accept and follow the outlined plan of treatment or not. Knowing what is best does not always dictate compliance. Motivation is the key. Giving patients realistic suggestions can help them accept a treatment plan that may initially have seemed impossible to follow. Changing behavior will probably be resisted. The patient who experiences setbacks, who does not remember to take medication, who breaks away from the prescribed diet, and the like, will need additional encouragement to get back on track. You can be of particular value in this type of situation. You must always be reinforcing with remarks made to patients concerning the intended goals of treatment. Furthermore, by being a good role model, you subtly reinforce the physician's advice. An assistant who should be, but is not, following a weight-reduction plan will give a negative impression to a patient who has just been told to do so by the physician. A patient who has been instructed by the physician in personal hygiene will be less likely to follow advice if the medical assistant could also well heed the advice.

In conversing with patients you will find that their areas of interest will prompt ideas for encouraging compliance with treatment. One good motivator is the physician's fee for services. Many patients quickly realize that they should follow the physician's advice, for it will certainly be more costly in the long run if they do not.

Terminal Illness ....

Dealing with patients who have been diagnosed as having a **terminal** illness will be a challenging and rewarding experience: challenging because of its difficulty and rewarding because of the knowledge that you are giving supportive care when patients and their families need it most.

Many patients have a hard time accepting the diagnosis. Their initial reaction is to deny it. Indeed, knowing that one's life is about to end is an almost **incomprehensible** fact. Patients wrestling with this new reality claim that the diagnosis is **absurd.** But ignoring the problem cannot provide solace.

As frustration mounts and anger becomes apparent, patients feel isolated, for they see others as the picture of health. Feelings of **hostility** are natural and **inevitable.** Patients in this plight may lash out at anyone with whom they come in contact. Blaming themselves and others becomes a means of dealing with their anger for a time. Questioning becomes a way of venting anger for some. "Why does this have to be?" is the most troublesome question. Following this stage of anger is a period of depression. This is the reaction to the final realization of the course of their illness. Patients in this stage are usually ready to talk about their illness, hoping someone will understand. It is a difficult subject to talk about, but you may be influential in helping them to respond and talk about their fears. Eventually the patient attempts to accept the terminal illness by bargaining, or seeking ways of "buying" more time. This sometimes gives them inner strength to stay a while longer, holding on to see someone be married, wanting to hold the new grandchild, waiting for someone to return from the service. In this stage of bargaining, patients may look for spiritual inspiration. The zest for life is strong and the fight is one not easily given up.

In the final stages of terminal disease, patients come closer to accepting the course of their disease. This is truly a sad time for patients and their families. To know that one may not see the next spring, to know that one will no longer experience the joys and pleasures of loved ones, is **devastating** to the patient. Empathy and genuine compassion may be offered to a patient who is reaching out for comfort. You will be touched deeply, and your fortitude will be challenged to the maximum in interacting with the patient and family members during this most stressful time.

Finally, patients resign themselves to impending death. An inner peace is often evident in patients in this final stage of their illness, and they are willing to make plans for their final days.

Some patients prefer to spare family members the ordeal of prolonging treatment when their physicians reach the decision that death is likely to occur in the near future. The living will is a legal document that allows patients to terminate medical procedures that would sustain their lives if they became unconscious or unable to make further decisions, Figure 1–5, page 8. This document is not recognized in all states in the United States, but is fast becoming a more acceptable way to eliminate continued life-support treatment of the terminally ill patient. With this legal form the patient and family are able to avoid an agonizingly long period in waiting for the inevitable and also keep the cost of health care more realistic and reasonable.

The patient signs this document and a copy is filed with the physician, the attorney, and the family. In assisting patients with this procedure, it would be helpful if you would remind them to make sure that all details have been worked out and that the family has been properly informed and remind them of who is responsible for honoring the document. Patients now know that they have a right to die with dignity and that they have a choice in making their last days of life more meaningful.

For many years a concerned group of individuals has recognized and commiserated with this grief-stricken group of people. These people have formed the hospice movement to provide some health care to those with terminal illness. In recent years the hospice movement has gained strength. Instead of the tiring and impersonal surroundings that are sometimes associated with hospital care, the hospice movement helps the family provide care so that patients can remain in their comfortable, familiar home surroundings during the last days of their lives and be among their family members and friends more conveniently. Support and caring assistance is given to help the family learn to cope with the turbulence of the patients and their illness. Efforts are coordinated with physicians and hospital staffs when necessary to give patients the best possible care.

Patients and their families in this stage of the patient's illness may need more spiritual guidance. The counsel of a minister, priest, or rabbi, may also be found through the hospice movement. **Holistic** care is their purpose. You should refer patients with life-threatening illness to the local hospice movement for consultation.

Society is returning to the idea that there is a human need to share the experiences of birth and death with loved ones. These natural parts of life have been largely removed from our experience for some time now. We have even become uneasy in talking about them. The need for human love in these significant times in our lives is evident in the return to the practice of entering and leaving this world at home.

Complete Chapter 1, Unit 2 in the workbook to help you meet the objectives at the beginning of this unit and therefore achieve competency of this subject matter.

U N I T   3
Medical Staff Relationships

OBJECTIVES ....

Upon completion of the unit you will meet the following terminal performance objectives by verifying knowledge of the facts and principles presented through oral and written communication at a level deemed competent by the instructor or employer.

1. Describe relationships between the medical assistant, the employer, and coworkers.
2. List positive methods for dealing with stress.
3. Describe the reasons for staff meetings.
4. Explain methods of intraoffice communication.
5. State the purpose of an employee evaluation.
6. Discuss the obligations of the employer and the new employee in providing a smooth transition in the work place.
7. Spell and define, using the glossary at the end of the text, all the words to know in this unit.

WORDS TO KNOW ....

evaluation	obligation
externship	perplexing
job descriptions	petty
merit	transition

The medical assistant employed in a medical office or clinic must learn to relate well not only to patients but to other members of the health care team as well. Dealing with day-to-day patient needs can sometimes become overwhelming. Schedules in most medical practices can easily become overbooked; sometimes it seems everyone has an emergency and must be seen by the physician today! Health care employees should be able to shift gears and handle these situations gracefully as well as efficiently. The essential ingredient in running a medical office smoothly is cooperation. When each employee contributes, a good team that works together for quality patient care results.

The field of medicine is by its nature stress-filled. Patients are troubled by an abnormal state of health and are naturally anxious and on edge. Commonly they exhibit their feelings by acting irritable and uncooperative at times. They not only

LIVING-WILL

of _____, Maker

WHEN my attending physician and one other physician decide that:

    (1) I am virtually certain to die in the near future and that I am currently unable to make or communicate my decisions regarding my medical treatment, or

    (2) I am currently unconscious and have a negligible possibility of ever regaining consciousness,

I NOW DIRECT that, under either of these conditions, all medications and medical procedures be withheld or discontinued except for those necessary to provide as complete relief from pain and other suffering as is medically possible. This comfort care should be used as generously as necessary even though it may alter my remaining life span.

THIS LIVING-WILL should be honored by my family, attorney, and physicians as the expression of my legal right to refuse treatment. I am an adult who understands and accept the consequences of its directives. To the extent that it may not be legally enforceable, those who know of its existence should regard themselves as morally bound by it.

SIGNED _____
                                    Maker

I CERTIFY that, on the date shown below, the Maker signed or acknowledged this Living-Will in my presence freely without pressure, that I believe the Maker understands and accepts the consequences of its instructions, that I am eighteen years of age or older, and that I am not related to the Maker by blood or marriage.

Signed _____ _____ _____
             witness' name   witness' address   date

Signed _____ _____ _____
             witness' name   witness' address   date

Prepared and distributed by
Association For Freedom to Die, 490 G Alden Avenue, Columbus 43201

FIGURE 1–5 Living will form (Courtesy of Association for Freedom to Die, Columbus, OH)

expect but demand patience and understanding from medical personnel.

Staff Arrangements

Picture the ideal medical office where patients and medical staff are going about the business at hand in a pleasant, efficient manner. Everyone gets along well with everyone else, patients are smiling and friendly, and every interchange is courteous. The schedule is kept down to the minute, all the filing is caught up, the phone rings only when there is nothing else pressing at the moment, referral reports are all back, and everything runs like clockwork. This picture is unreal. This ideal situation is what every medical practice hopes to achieve, but to bring this model practice into existence would require the perfection of all persons involved. This is, of course, impossible. Nevertheless, each member of the staff has a unique set of values, principles, and standards, and each must respect the others to ensure compatible relationships.

The number of employees varies in the many types of medical practices. Some physicians in private practice employ only one medical assistant to perform both administrative and clinical duties. This is a tremendous responsibility and requires a highly motivated and mature personality. Medical assistants must realize that sometimes long hours and limited benefits may be the result. A good rapport with the employer is necessary to accomplish the objectives of daily patient care. Usually a good friendship develops between physician and medical assistant over time, and working together is an enjoyable learning experience for both. Interest in each patient is easy to cultivate since individual contact is made at each office visit. You may get to know patients even better than the physician because of frequent phone conversation. You will soon become the physician's right hand by supplying important patient information obtained in this manner.

Communication lines must remain open with this one-to-one relationship, as in all employer–employee relationships. If misunderstandings occur, they must be rectified as soon as possible. More complex problems can mushroom if incidental misunderstandings are not cleared up. Solutions to these problems must be worked out together. You will have to be assertive in decisions concerning administrative, clinical, and personal employment matters. Being on one's own as a medical assistant in a private practice has its rewards as well as its disadvantages.

Many physicians in private or group practice find it necessary to employ several medical assistants. Although this can be an enjoyable experience for all members of the staff, a great deal of cooperation and respect for one another is necessary for a harmonious relationship among the staff members to be maintained. Specific **job descriptions** encourage each employee to remain in a particular area and promote efficiency. Overstepping boundaries may cause friction and misunderstandings. At the same time all staff members must be willing to pitch in where help is needed. Again, a positive attitude is needed to create a pleasant work environment.

The physician usually delegates responsibility for office management to one of the employees, most often the one with greatest seniority, qualifications, or both. This frees the physician to attend to patients and also relieves the physician of personnel management. This is a major area of concern, especially in large clinics with many employees, and, as a rule, is an area physicians are not trained to handle. Many of these supervisory or personnel management positions are filled by registered nurses, but they also have little or no specific training in medical office management. Their training centers primarily on the hospital model and direct patient care. Since a trained medical assistant can, in most states, perform most of the procedures that a nurse can, under the supervision of a physician, resentment may arise. You must come to grips with this reality before accepting a position where it may be a source of irritation and discontent.

Many physicians and office managers appreciate the versatility of the medical assistant, respect their initiative and industriousness, and employ them with pride and satisfaction. However, each medical practice has its own unique office policy regarding employees. There are still those physicians who would rather take charge of their own office business affairs.

Working closely with others can have both positive and negative effects. In a large office practice or clinic, when there are many employees, a certain amount of give and take must prevail. Completing assigned tasks is expected so that the work is shared equitably. **Petty** differences should be settled with tact. Sharing enlightening experiences and significant events with other employees is a natural inclination. This is fine if it does not interfere with the patient care. A certain amount of self-discipline and self-control are necessary in a professional setting. Remaining aware of the situation at hand will help you perceive what is appropriate.

Intraoffice Communication

Many physicians hold regular staff meetings that all employees are expected to attend. They are usually held in the medical office either before or after patients have been seen and are announced far enough in advance so that arrangements can be made to attend. At these meetings decisions concerning office policy changes are reached and problems are discussed. This is a time for new ideas to be expressed and exchanged. It also allows all members of the staff to get to know each other.

Some situations between employees may be impossible to iron out. These are usually personality conflicts, and the usual course of action if the situation does not improve is termination of one of the employees, usually the one who is more troublesome or less valuable to the practice. This kind of **perplexing** problem may be discussed during a staff meeting. Personnel managers are often aware of these problems before they are reported, and they are usually handled privately.

Employers sometimes use office meeting time for in-service programs, such as training in cardiopulmonary resuscitation (CPR). Some employers encourage holiday celebrations on occasion to promote better working relationships.

An intraoffice memo is a means of communicating important information to members of the staff, especially between regularly scheduled staff meetings. Each employee is instructed to read the memo and initial it, indicating that the information has been received, and then pass it on to another employee. This helps ensure that all employees are informed. Word of mouth is not a sure way to relay an important announcement for it may get distorted en route.

Some offices and clinics use a bulletin board as a means of intraoffice communication. Notices of educational programs, seminars, or meetings are posted for all members of the staff to read, in an area such as the staff room or eating area. Meetings of the American Association of Medical Assistants should be posted there.

Career Entry

According to recent statistics, there is an increasing need for qualified medical assistants across the nation. Employers in the health care field are recognizing the benefits of employing medical assistants who have had specific training in this most versatile field. This, of course, eliminates the need for extensive and expensive additional training on the job. **Externship** plans are very successful in cooperative programs that provide soon-to-graduate medical assistant students. These students are usually hired at a part-time rate, and the supervisor agrees to allow the instructor to periodically visit the facility and observe the student's performance. (Many programs do not allow the students to be paid.) Other training programs require only that students observe for a certain number of hours to fulfill the program's standards. In either case, the trend is most welcomed after the past practice of hiring assistants without any training in the field, who sought either full-time or part-time employment in the physicians' offices or clinics.

The **transition** from student to medical assistant, at any age, poses certain adjustment considerations to all concerned in the health care setting. Employers have an **obligation** to assist the new employee in feeling accepted in the profession and to give helpful advice with patience. The new employee is obligated to strive to perform skills with both proficiency and efficiency. An effort to get along with others is required of each member of the health care team. A smooth transition by the new member of the team is possible if each employee recognizes the individual worth of each person and the value of each position in fulfilling the health care needs of the patients they serve.

Employee Evaluation........................

In most employment situations, an **evaluation** of work performance is made on an annual basis. This is filed in your record. The initial employment review is usually held after a probationary period of 90 days. In this meeting, you and your employer will discuss your job performance. Most evaluation forms are basically the same, Figure 1–6. They outline the most important qualities and abilities needed for the job and include a section for strengths and weaknesses to be listed. Qualities and abilities are assessed on a point system. High scores will be worthy of praise and recognition, usually in the form of a **merit** raise. Employers are always aware of an employee's behavior. Little goes unnoticed when you share a daily routine. Your attitude shows at all times. Even though the word *attitude* may not be a part of the evaluation, the other categories cover it comprehensively.

Initiative is an important factor. Demonstrating resourcefulness will help you advance in your career. Following office policy is also important. Being on time and being dependable on the job are always pleasing to employers. Absences and tardiness are difficult to tolerate from employees who make it a habit. Another area of extreme importance to employers is the quality and quantity of your work. Performing assigned tasks in a reasonable amount of time, without needing to be reminded, is a valuable trait.

The employee evaluation need not be a threat to the conscientious medical assistant. It is a time when questions about advancement and salary may be openly discussed. If you have lived up to the standards of the job, your performance should receive a favorable review.

Some employers find that annual evaluations motivate employees and keep communication lines open. Others choose not to have official evaluations, but wish employees to discuss whatever is on their mind at any time. For some office personnel this works quite well. For the private practice physician with a single medical assistant this is usually the case.

Complete Chapter 1, Unit 3 in the workbook to help you meet the objectives at the beginning of this unit and therefore achieve competency of this subject matter.

U N I T   4
Essentials in Medical Law and Ethics

OBJECTIVES ....

Upon completion of this unit, you will meet the following terminal performance objectives by verifying knowledge of the facts and principles presented through oral and written communication at a level deemed competent by the instructor or employer.

1. List licensure requirements for physicians.
2. Describe methods of licensure.
3. Define the components of public and private law.
4. Recognize the differences between ethics and law.
5. Identify areas of medical ethics of particular concern to medical assistants.
6. List the five primary elements of the American Association of Medical Assistants code of ethics.
7. List ethical considerations surrounding the life of a fetus.
8. List and define the three categories of medical transplants.
9. Describe a living will.
10. Name four examples of tort law.
11. Describe the three parts of the physician–patient contract.
12. Prepare common consent forms used in medical offices.
13. List instances of legally required disclosure.
14. Describe the conditions for revocation or suspension of a medical license.
15. List rights of the physician and patient regarding medical care.
16. Describe the correct procedure for terminating the physician–patient contract.
17. Give examples of abandonment, professional negligence, sexual harassment, and implied agreement.
18. Describe the precaution that should be observed in giving written instructions to a patient.
19. List the reasons for keeping medical records.
20. Name the six basic principles for preventing unauthorized disclosure of patient information.
21. List six office procedures that cause problems when the physician is involved in a lawsuit.
22. Describe the acceptable method for making changes in medical records.
23. Spell and define, using the glossary at the back of the text, all the words to know in this unit.

```
EMPLOYEE EVALUATION

_____
Employee's name         Position/Title          Date of Review

_____
Department              Supervisor              Date Employed

_____
Type of Review: ____ Probationary ____ Six Month ____ Annual ____*Other

*Explain_____

Date of Last Evaluation _____   Previous Rating _____
_____

Total days absent _____  Total of tardies _____  Total times left early ____
_____

  Place  Appropriate Number for each of the following on the line to the right.

              0  1  2  3  4  5  6  7  8  9  10  11  12  13  14  15  _____
Quantity of Work:  inferior / careless/ does / average/ above / exceptional
Volume and                               just             average
   Consistency                           enough                      _____
_____
Quality of Work: very poor/ fair / good/ acceptable/ excellent/ superior
Accuracy and
   Neatness                                                          _____
_____
Initiative:    lacking/  needs pushing/ adequate/ excellent/ superior
Motivation
                                                                     _____
_____
Judgement:     poor/ unreliable/ limited/ plans well/ reliable/ superior
Planning work,
Make decisions                                                       _____
_____
Adaptability:  poor/ slow / satisfactory/ good/ excellent/ superior
   Adjusts to
   change                                                            _____
_____
Cooperation:   uncooperative/ difficult / cooperative/ excellent/superior
Getting along
   with others                                                       _____
_____
Speed:         slow/ moderate/ average/ above average/ superior
   Rate of
   work                                                              _____
_____
Job Knowledge:  very little/ limited/ adequate/ average/ good/superior
                (almost none)
                                                                     _____
_____
                                                        Total _____

Since last evaluation employee has:        Recommended for pay increas

____ Improved  ___ No change  ___ Regressed    ____ Yes    ____ No

Overall impression of this employee:

____ Unsatisfactory ___ Poor ___ Fair ___Good ___ Excellent ___Exceptional

Comments of strengths/weaknesses:   Supervisor's signature
```

FIGURE 1–6 Employee evaluation form

WORDS TO KNOW ....

abandonment

agent

assault

battery

biennially

breach

chronological

civil

competent

confidentiality

confrontations

criminal

criterion

defamation

deposition

doctrine

emancipated minor

enact

encompass

endorse

enumerate

explicit

express consent

fraudulent

genetic

harmonious

implied consent

insemination

moral

negligence

non compos mentis

obligated

peer

privileged communication

procrastination

reciprocity

res ipsa loquitur

respondeat superior

revoke

senility

statutes

subpoena duces tecum

surrogate

tort

During the past 20 years the numbers of patients bringing lawsuits against physicians has increased dramatically. Medical liability insurance rates have increased so much that physicians in some areas are practicing without liability insurance, although not all states permit this. Laws may be different in different states, but ethical standards are the same in every state. Ethics deals with **moral** choices and rules of conduct. Both the American Medical Association and the American Association of Medical Assistants have codes of ethics.

Our founding fathers saw a need for regulation of the practice of medicine, and in colonial days medical practice acts were in effect for the protection of citizens. These acts were gradually repealed because it was believed the Constitution gave everyone the right to practice medicine. This resulted in a period of time in the nineteenth century when quackery was common. After a Supreme Court decision in 1899 upheld a state's right to establish qualifications for people wishing to practice medicine, all states soon had once again established medical practice acts. Most state **statutes** define two basic elements that constitute the practice of medicine. One is diagnosis and the other is the prescribing of treatment. Only a licensed physician can engage in the diagnosis and prescribing of treatment for the physical condition of human beings. In general terms, medical practice acts define the practice of medicine and establish requirements for licensure and grounds for suspending or **revoking** a license.

Licensure Requirements ....

Licensure requirements are established by each state. A doctor is usually required to:

- be of legal age
- be of good moral character
- have graduated from an approved medical school
- have completed an approved residency program or its equivalent
- be a resident of the state
- have passed the oral and written examinations administered by the board of medical examiners of the state

Physicians who have all of the necessary requirements for licensure may also be licensed by **reciprocity** or **endorsement.** A physician who has been licensed in one state and wishes to move to another state may be granted a license by reciprocity if it is determined that the original licensure requirements are equal to the requirements in the new state. Many physicians take the test administered by the National Board of Medical Examiners at the same time they take their first state test. The high standards of the national board make it possible to obtain a state license by endorsement when the national board examinations have been successfully passed.

Physicians are required to renew their license annually or **biennially.** You should be sure the physician has a record of all continuing education units (CEUs) earned since the previous renewal as this is a requirement in many states. Physicians earn CEUs by attending seminars and scientific meetings as well as university courses. The renewal notice will notify the physician of the number of CEUs necessary to renew the license.

There are some exceptions to the rule requiring a current state license to practice medicine. Any physician is free to administer first aid outside the state of residence.

Physicians in military service must be licensed to practice medicine in their home states. They do not need to be licensed in the state where they are stationed as long as they practice only on the military base.

The state board of medical examiners provides procedures for revocation or suspension of licensure. In some states the board has the power to revoke a license, and in other states a special review committee has this authority.

A physician may lose the license to practice medicine if convicted of a crime, such as murder, rape, violation of narcotic laws, or income tax evasion. A medical license may be revoked for unprofessional conduct. The most usual offenses in this category are betrayal of patient–physician confidence, excessive use of drugs and alcohol, and inappropriate sexual conduct.

A license may be revoked because of proven fraud in the application for a license. In some cases **fraudulent** diplomas are used. Fraud in the filing of claims for services that were not rendered and fraud in the use of unproven treatments are also grounds for revocation of a license.

Physicians who are found to be incompetent to practice because of **senility** or mental incapacity may have their license revoked.

Ethical Considerations ....

Whereas laws concern matters enforced through the court system, ethics deal with what is morally right and wrong. The ethical standards established by a profession are administered by **peer** review, and violation of the standards may result in suspension of membership. The American Medical Association Principles Code of Medical Ethics was revised in 1980 and is reprinted here so that you can see what is expected of a physician.

Physician's Code

Preamble: The medical profession has long subscribed to a body of ethical statements developed primarily for the benefit of the patient. As a member of this profession, a physician must recognize responsibility not only to patients, but also to society, to other health professionals, and to self. The following principles adopted by the American Medical Association are not laws, but standards of conduct which define the essentials of honorable behavior for the physician.

I. A physician shall be dedicated to providing competent medical service with compassion and respect for human dignity.

II. A physician shall deal honestly with patients and colleagues, and strive to expose those physicians deficient in character or competence, or who engage in fraud or deception.

III. A physician shall respect the law and also recognize a responsibility to seek changes in those requirements which are contrary to the best interests of the patient.

IV. A physician shall respect the rights of patients, of colleagues, and of other health professionals, and shall safeguard patient confidence within the constraints of the law.

V. A physician shall continue to study, apply, and advance scientific knowledge, make relevant information available to patients, colleagues, and the public, obtain consultation, and use the talents of other health professionals when indicated.

VI. A physician shall, in the provision of appropriate patient care, except in emergencies, be free to choose whom to serve, with whom to associate, and the environment in which to provide medical services.

VII. A physician shall recognize a responsibility to participate in activities contributing to an improved community.

(Used with permission of the American Medical Association. From the *American Medical Association Principles of Medical Ethics*. Adopted by the AMA House of Delegates, July 1980.)

It must be remembered that the primary objective of the practice of medicine is the welfare of the patient, not the making of a profit. Some offices now notify patients of interest charges on overdue accounts in a brochure introducing the patient to the office practice. The notice of possible interest charge is also included on all billing statements. Some physicians charge for missed appointments and preparing more than one insurance form.

The physician must release patient information when the patient authorizes the release or if the release is required by law. State laws vary regarding release of information. Information that must be reported includes:

- Births and deaths
- Cases of violence, such as gunshot wounds, knifings, and poisonings
- Sexually transmitted diseases
- Suspected cases of child abuse
- Cases of contagious, infectious, or communicable diseases

Medical assistants should check with local authorities for the procedures to be followed in making these reports. They need to be aware also of other required local reports. When a physician moves or retires it is important that the original records be kept until the period for filing of liability suits has expired. A copy of the records is provided to a new physician.

Medical Assistant's Code

As an agent of the physician, you too are governed by ethical standards. The American Association of Medical Assistants code of ethics is in many respects similar to that of the American Medical Association.

CODE OF ETHICS
of the American Association of Medical Assistants

The Code of Ethics of AAMA shall set forth principles of ethical and moral conduct as they relate to the medical profession and the particular practice of medical assisting.

Members of AAMA dedicated to the conscientious pursuit of their profession, and thus desiring to merit the high regard of the entire medical profession and the respect of the general public which they do serve, do pledge themselves to strive always to:

1. render service with full respect for the dignity of humanity;
2. respect confidential information obtained through employment unless legally authorized or required by responsible performance of duty to divulge such information;
3. uphold the honor and high principles of the profession and accept its disciplines;
4. seek to continually improve the knowledge and skills of medical assistants for the benefit of patients and professional colleagues;
5. participate in additional service activities aimed toward improving the health and well-being of the community.

MEDICAL ASSISTANT'S CREED

The creed of the American Association of Medical Assistants reads as follows:

I believe in the principles and purposes of the profession.

I endeavor to be more effective.

I aspire to render greater service.

I protect the confidence entrusted to me.

I am dedicated to the care and well-being of all patients.

I am loyal to my physician-employer.

I am true to the ethics of my profession.

I am strengthened by compassion, courage, and faith.

(Copyright by the American Association of Medical Assistants, Inc. Used with permission.)

You will often find it necessary to make decisions based on the professional nature of your employment. Patients can be extremely insistent at times, but you must be firm in carrying out the expectations of your employer and your profession. A patient may, for instance, demand that you call in a prescription for medication when the physician is not immediately available. You have to stand your ground and say that only the physician can give you the orders to do this. You then carefully record on the chart the request of the patient and how it was taken care of. *Never put yourself in the position of practicing medicine.*

The Federal Drug Administration has established five categories, or "schedules," which classify chemical substances with specific regulations as to their use. The states also have laws that further define the use of drugs. It is important for the medical assistant to understand that only the physician can legally prescribe medications. The medical assistant must understand that certain medications cannot be refilled and that restrictions limit the number of times some medications can be refilled. Some drugs require written prescription to be filled, while others can be called in by telephone.

The United States Department of Justice Drug Enforcement Administration publishes a physician's manual that gives all the information necessary for office personnel to understand the provisions of the Controlled Substances Act. This booklet is furnished on request at no charge.

The Drug Enforcement Administration also publishes a *Pharmacist's Manual*, which lists seven recommendations for physicians about the care and security of prescription pads. These will help reduce the number of forged prescription orders:

1. Treat prescription pads like a personal checkbook.
2. Maintain adequate security for prescription pads.
3. Stock only a minimum number of prescription pads.
4. Keep prescription pads in your possession when you are actively using them.
5. Do not leave prescription pads unattended. When not in use, place them in a locked desk or cabinet.
6. Store surplus prescription pads in a locked drawer or in a safe, appropriate place.
7. Report any prescription pad theft to local pharmacies as well as to the state board of pharmacy.

In the practice of medicine it can be difficult to distinguish between legal and ethical issues. The trend in the United States is to demand good health care as a right for everyone. Not all citizens are willing to finance such a program, however. The present use of diagnostic related groups (DRGs) in determining the payment hospitals will receive for Medicare patients raises both ethical and legal questions. The problem with the system arises when patients may be discharged too early simply because the hospital will not be paid for more than the DRG-allowed number of days. The physician knows the legal responsibility is to the well-being of the patient, but the hospital must have money to stay in business. The physician wants to stay in good standing with the hospital. In a recent decision in California (Wickline versus State of California), a physician was held liable for releasing a patient too early. In fact, the physician had failed to protest the third party's decision to shorten the patient's recommended hospital stay. In this case, the third party payer was a California Medicare agency called Medi Cal.

Insurance companies are presenting more ethical questions to medical care providers when they refuse insurance to individuals who have acquired immune deficiency syndrome (AIDS) and the AIDS-related complex (ARC).

Many ethical considerations surround the life of a fetus, an infant's birth, and the newborn. New technologies allow us to have more control over birth by detecting *in utero* abnormalities. The improved techniques of **artificial insemination** bring before the court system the problems associated with **surrogate** motherhood and paternal responsibility. Many advances have been made in the use of fetal tissue in transplants. Our society must study the ethical and emotional considerations of ending a pregnancy if a serious **genetic** deficiency is found before birth or allowing the infant to be born handicapped. We seem to have more questions than answers at the present time.

The use of transplants has added another series of ethical problems. Medical transplants are divided into three categories:

- Autograft transplantation of a person's own tissue (can also be used to describe transplant between identical twins)
- Homograft transplantation of tissue from one person to another
- Heterograft transplantation of animal tissue to humans

The blood transfusion is the most common transplant. Nearly all the major organs of the body may be transplanted, and research continues to improve these possibilities.

The Uniform Anatomical Gift Act ....

The Uniform Anatomical Gift Act was passed in 1968. By 1978 it was reported that all 50 states had established some system of organ and tissue donor identification once an individual died. Any person of sound mind and legal age may give any part of the body after death for research or transplant. The family may make this decision for the donor if the donor has not done so while living. The time of death must be determined by a physician who will not be involved in the transplant in any way. No money can be exchanged for making an anatomical donation. Many states allow residents to mark and sign a donor card on the back of the driver's license.

Different ethical problems affect the use of organs from living donors. As the technology of transplantation becomes more readily available, the demand for organs will grow. Human organs should never be sold for profit, but our western ethics are not always followed worldwide. In a book titled *Law, Liability, and Ethics for Medical Office Personnel*, Myrtle Flight discusses the medical community's concern over the sale of human organs for transplant. One source has estimated that by the year 2000, most of the poor in India will learn to survive with only one kidney as the result of the common practice of selling kidneys to wealthy foreigners.

Living Will

The health care team will provide a larger percentage of care to geriatric patients as the quality of care extends our life expectancy. It is important that everyone in the office listen to elderly patients and allow them to make decisions regarding a living will, Figure 1–7, page 16. A majority of the states now have laws that define policies on withholding life-sustaining procedures from hopelessly ill patients. The will is signed when the patient is competent and must be witnessed by two individuals. The effect of this will is to protect the wishes of the patient who may become incompetent and thus unable to make rational decisions. The family of the patient and the physician should receive a copy of the document.

Choice in Dying, Inc. now stresses the importance of also completing a durable power of attorney for health care, authorized by either your state's statute or some other legal authority. This allows you to appoint another person (known as your agent) to make health care decisions for you if at any time you become unable to make them yourself. It is strongly advised that an individual appoint an agent, assuming there is someone who can be trusted to make the decisions you would make if you could, and who is willing to act for you in this way, Figure 1–8. It may be helpful to record the wishes of a living will and power of attorney on a video tape so there could be no doubt the patient made the statements regarding care.

A new medical "Miranda warning" law approved by Congress and signed by President Bush gives patients legal options for refusing or accepting treatment if they are incapacitated. The law, which took effect in November 1991, applies to hospitals, hospices, nursing homes, health maintenance organizations (HMOs) and other health care facilities that receive money from Medicare and Medicaid programs. Under the law, patients must receive written information explaining their right-to-die options according to their state laws. The law stipulates that hospitals and other providers must note on medical records whether patients have legal directives on treatment. Providers also must have procedures to ensure they comply with a patient's wishes.

Every medical assistant should be trained to use CPR. An ethical question arises when the elderly patient does not wish to receive CPR in the event of a cardiopulmonary arrest. The courts have held that individuals have the right to make decisions that affect their own deaths.

Legal Considerations

In the United States the laws are divided into the categories of public law and private law. The various branches of public law include criminal law, constitutional law, administrative law, and international law. Criminal law deals with offenses against all citizens. The practice of medicine without a license is an offense under the criminal law. Constitutional law defines the powers of the government and its citizens. Each state has a constitution which defines its powers over matters not covered by the federal government, which are spelled out in the U.S. Constitution. Administrative law is concerned with the powers of government agencies. International law is concerned with agreements and treaties between countries.

The practice of medicine is primarily affected by private or civil, law, specifically by contract law and torts law. The patient–physician relationship is considered a contractual one. A tort is defined as any of a number of actions done by one person or group of persons that cause injury to another. Violations of tort law may be intentional or negligent. The negligent injury, when committed by a physician in the course of professional duties, is commonly referred to as *malpractice*. Intentional torts also result in professional liability suits. Libel and slander are two forms of defamation. Libel refers to written statements, slander to oral remarks. Assault is defined as a deliberate attempt or threat to touch without consent. Another intentional wrong is battery, which is the unauthorized touching of another person. A patient has a right to refuse treatment. Other civil laws govern property ownership, corporations, and inheritance.

The contract between a patient and a physician has three parts. They are the offer, the acceptance, and the consideration. The offer takes place when a competent individual indicates a desire to become a patient. The acceptance takes place when an appointment is given and the physician examines the patient. The consideration is the payment given in exchange for services. When a child is a patient, the parent is expected to pay. A young person is considered to be a minor until reaching full legal age, known as the age of majority. The statutes defining the age of majority vary from state to state. The medical assistant needs to be aware that the rights of minors in medical treatment are changing. More than half of the states allow minors the right to consent to treatment or consultation for pregnancy, contraception, venereal disease, drug abuse, or alcoholism.

An emancipated minor is an individual who is no longer under the care, custody, or supervision of parents. The emancipated minor may be married, in the armed forces, or self-supporting and living apart from parents. An emancipated minor can legally consent to medical care.

An individual who has been judged by the courts to be mentally incompetent must have an appointed guardian. The general legal term for all varieties of mental illness is *non compos mentis*. The guardian is responsible for both the payment of bills and the care of the patient. In this case the parents are not responsible for payment. When a patient–physician contract is entered into, the physician is responsible for the care of that patient until the physician officially withdraws from the case or the patient discharges the physician.

The contract between the patient and the physician may be either implied or written. An express, or written, contract must be entered into if a third party is to be responsible for payment.

Society for the Right to Die

Society for the Right to Die
250 West 57th Street/New York, NY 10107

INSTRUCTIONS
Consult this column for help and guidance.

This declaration sets forth your directions regarding medical treatment.

You have the right to refuse treatment you do not want, and you may request the care you do want.

You may list specific treatment you do not want. For example:
Cardiac resuscitation
Mechanical respiration
Artificial feeding/fluids by tubes
Otherwise, your general statement, top right, will stand for your wishes.

You may want to add instructions for care you do want—for example, pain medication; or that you prefer to die at home if possible.

If you want, you can name someone to see that your wishes are carried out, but you do not have to do this.

Sign and date here in the presence of two adult witnesses, who should also sign.

Living Will Declaration

To My Family, Doctors, and All Those Concerned with My Care

I, _____ , being of sound mind, make this statement as a directive to be followed if I become unable to participate in decisions regarding my medical care.

If I should be in an incurable or irreversible mental or physical condition with no reasonable expectation of recover. I direct my attending physician to withhold or withdraw treatment that merely prolongs my dying. I further direct that treatment be limited to measures to keep me comfortable and to relieve pain.

These directions express my legal right to refuse treatment. Therefore I expect my family, doctors, and everyone concerned with my care to regard themselves as legally and morally bound to act in accord with my wishes, and in so doing to be free of any legal liability for having followed my directions.

I especially do not want: _____

_____

_____

_____

_____

_____

Other instructions/comments: _____

_____

_____

_____

Proxy Designation Clause: Should I become unable to communicate my instructions as stated above, I designate the following person to act in my behalf:

Name _____

Address _____

If the person I have named above is unable to act in my behalf, I authorize the following person to do so:

Name _____

Address _____

Signed: _____ Date: _____

Witness: _____ Witness:_____

Keep the signed original with your personal papers at home. Give signed copies to doctors, family, and proxy. Review your Declaration from time to time; initial and date it to show it still expresses your intent.

FIGURE 1–7 Living will declaration. Choice in Dying makes available legally recognized document forms to residents of states that have enacted right-to-die laws. For people in states that have not enacted right-to-die laws, Choice in Dying supplies Durable Power of Attorney for Health Care forms. (Reprinted by permission of Choice in Dying (formerly Concern for Dying/Society for the Right to Die), 200 Varick Street, New York, New York 10014)

Health Care Proxy

(1) I, _____
hereby appoint _____
(name, home address and telephone number)

as my health care agent to make any and all health care decisions for me, except to the extent that I state otherwise. This proxy shall take effect when and if I become unable to make my own health care decisions.

(2) Optional instructions: I direct my proxy to make health care decisions in accord with my wishes and limitations as stated below, or as he or she otherwise knows. (Attach additional pages if necessary).

_____

(Unless your agent knows your wishes about artificial nutrition and hydration [feeding tubes], your agent will not be allowed to make decisions about artificial nutrition and hydration. See the preceding instructions for samples of language you could use.)

(3) Name of substitue or fill-in proxy if the person I appoint above is unable, unwilling or unavailable to act as my health care agent.

_____
(name, home address and telephone number)

(4) Unless I revoke it, this proxy shall remain in effect indefinitely, or until the date or condition stated below. This proxy shall expire (specific date or conditions, if desired):

_____

(5) Signature _____
Address _____
Date _____

Statement by Witnesses (must be 18 or older)
I declare that the person who signed this document is personally known to me and appears to be of sound mind and acting of his or her own free will. He or she signed (or asked another to sign for him or her) this document in my presence.

Witness 1 _____
Address _____
Witness 2 _____
Address _____

FIGURE 1–8B Durable Power of Attorney for Health Care. (Reprinted by permission of Choice in Dying (formerly Concern for Dying/Society for the Right to Die), 200 Varick Street, New York, New York 10014)

About the Health Care Proxy

This is an important legal form. Before signing this form, you should understand the following facts:

1. This form gives the person you choose as your agent the authority to make all health care decisions for you, except to the extent you say otherwise in this form. "Health care" means any treatment, service or procedure to diagnose or treat your physical or mental condition.

2. Unless you say otherwise, your agent will be allowed to make all health care decisions for you, including decisions to remove or withhold life-sustaining treatment.

3. Unless your agent knows your wishes about artificial nutrition and hydration (nourishment and water provided by a feeding tube), he or she will not be allowed to refuse those measures for you.

4. Your agent will start making decisions for you when doctors decide that you are not able to make health care decisions for yourself.

You may write on this form any information about treatment that you do not desire and/or those treatments that you want to make sure you receive. Your agent must follow your instructions (oral and written) when making decisions for you.

If you want to give your agent written instructions, do so right on the form. For example, you could say:

If I become terminally ill, I do/don't want to receive the following treatments: ....

If I am in a coma or unconscious, with no hope of recovery, then I do/don't want...

If I have brain damage or a brain disease that makes me unable to recognize people or speak and there is no hope that my condition will improve, I do/don't want...

Examples of medical treatments about which you may wish to give your agent special instructions are listed below. This is not a complete list of the treatments about which you may leave instructions.

- artificial respiration
- artificial nutrition and hydration (nourishment and water provided by feeding tube)
- cardiopulmonary resuscitation (CPR)
- antipsychotic medication
- electric shock therapy
- antibiotics
- psychosurgery
- dialysis
- transplantation
- blood transfusions
- abortion
- sterilization

Talk about choosing an agent with your family and/or close friends. You should discuss this form with a doctor or another health care professional, such as a nurse or social worker, before you sign it to make sure that you understand the types of decisions that may be made for you. You may

also wish to give your doctor a signed copy. You do not need a lawyer to fill out this form.

You can choose any adult (over 18), including a family member, or close friend, to be your agent. If you select a doctor as your agent, he or she may have to choose between acting as your agent or as your attending doctor; a physician cannot do both at the same time. Also, if you are a patient or resident of a hospital, nursing home or mental hygiene facility, there are special restrictions about naming someone who works for that facility as your agent. You should ask staff at the facility to explain those restrictions.

You should tell the person you choose that he or she will be your health care agent. You should discuss your health care wishes and this form with your agent. Be sure to give him or her a signed copy. Your agent cannot be sued for health care decisions made in good faith.

Even after you have signed this form, you have the right to make health care decisions for yourself as long as you are able to do so, and treatment cannot be given to you or stopped if you object. You can cancel the control given to your agent by telling him or her or your health care provider orally or in writing.

Filling Out the Proxy Form

Item (1) Write your name and the name, home address and telephone number of the person you are selecting as your agent.

Item (2) If you have special instructions for your agent, you should write them here. Also, if you wish to limit your agent's authority in any way, you should say so here. If you do not state any limitations, your agent will be allowed to make all health care decisions that you could have made, including the decision to consent to or refuse life-sustaining treatment.

Item (3) You may write the name, home address and telephone number of an alternate agent.

Item (4) This form will remain valid indefinitely unless you set an expiration date or condition for its expiration. This section is optional and should be filled in only if you want the health care proxy to expire.

Item (5) You must sign and date the proxy. If you are unable to sign yourself, you may direct someone else to sign in your presence. Be sure to include your address.

Two witnesses at least 18 years of age must sign your proxy. The person who is appointed agent or alternate agent cannot sign as a witness.

New York State Department of Health

Distributed by Concern for Dying
250 West 57th Street, New York, NY 10107

FIGURE 1–8A Durable Power of Attorney for Health Care. (Reprinted by permission of Choice in Dying (formerly Concern for Dying/Society for the Right to Die), 200 Varick Street, New York, New York 10014)

If this agreement is not in writing, it is not possible to press for payment. There are also *implied consent* and *express consent* agreements between patients and physicians. The fact that the patient has come to see the physician implies consent for treatment. The instances when express consent is required are:

- proposed surgery or other invasive treatments, such as cerebrospinal taps
- use of experimental drugs
- use of unusual procedures that may involve high risk

There are exceptions to the rule for surgery. Minor procedures generally involve explanation by the physician and the oral consent of the patient. The notes regarding this conversation need to be entered by the physician in the patient record.

The American Medical Association has developed recommended standardized forms to be used by physicians, Figure 1–9. It will be your responsibility to know what consent forms your employer uses. The physician may wish to develop forms individualized for the practice. It is important that these be **explicit** as to what is to be done. Experiments have been conducted using a tape recorder to keep a record of the information given the patient before a consent form is signed. These were discussions with patients who had to be told they had cancer. Most of these patients had little or no memory of what had been discussed because they were extremely upset by the diagnosis. In some of these cases the patients were certain they were not fully informed, but the replay of the tape proved they had been. The medical assistant should understand that the physician must be legally responsible for obtaining informed consent from a patient. You should not be given that responsibility. Informed consent is necessary to avoid a claim of assault and battery. The law describes this as a threat to make a physical attack on someone and carrying out the attack. You will be expected to prepare consent forms and ideally be present to listen so that you may help determine whether the patient understood before signing the consent form.

If an all-purpose form is used, it is important to cross out the paragraphs that do not apply. You may be asked to sign as a witness. What you say when you ask a patient to sign after the physician has explained the risks is important. A suggested statement is: "If you have no further questions for the doctor and you understand the consent form, will you please sign it?"

If a physician is to treat a patient with unusual or experimental medication, it is best to use a consent-to-treatment form, Figure 1–10. When a physician is to perform a sterilization procedure, it is preferable to have both husband and wife sign a request for sterilization form, Figure 1–11.

Patients have the right to privacy when they are being examined and treated. Many physicians have arrangements with medical facilities to offer training opportunities for medical students or residents, but the patient has the right to refuse to have observers present. Therefore, physicians may protect themselves by having an authority to admit observers form signed, Figure 1–12, page 20.

Information contained in a patient medical record and information exchanged between a physician and a patient are considered to be privileged communications. Every patient has a legal right to privacy and **confidentiality.** Information disclosed to the health care team must be kept in the strictest confidence, and you must be ever mindful of the legal implications of handling patient's records. Information concerning patients may be given to another member of the health care team, such as a laboratory technician or referring physician, only when it pertains directly to the course of treatment. Another medical office may telephone to inquire about a patient's medical history for diagnostic purposes, to confirm symptoms, or to verify birthdate. In complying with referral appointments or scheduled tests, patients will have given implied consent for necessary information to be transmitted concerning their condition.

Medical information may be given to parties not concerned in the patient's treatment only when the patient has signed a release of information form.

A large number of states have privileged communication statutes that have been **enacted** to offer additional protection to the patient. You will find that curious and well-meaning friends and relatives ask about patients and you must remember to give only information that has been authorized by the patient. Each time a patient authorizes release of information the form must state specifically who is to receive what information covering what time period. This authorization must be kept in the medical record.

All health care providers must be aware of any state regulations governing the reporting of human immunodeficiency virus (HIV) test results. At issue is the right of the AIDS patient to confidentiality and the rights of citizens to be protected from accidental exposure to the HIV virus. Such exposure might occur when police, fire, emergency medical personnel, or any medical personnel come into direct contact with the blood or body fluids of a patient whose diagnosis of AIDS is not known to the personnel.

In all 50 states, confirmed cases of AIDS constitute a reportable condition either by statute or administrative regulation.

Physician and Patient Rights ....

Physicians have the right to determine whom they will accept as patients. Physicians who have been in practice for a long time may build up a patient load that is as large as one person can adequately care for. Since a physician must care for all patients accepted, it is not unusual to have to decide to see no new patients. A physician may not, on the other hand, refuse to provide emergency service if assigned to an emergency service, and most physicians will provide emergency service whenever the need exists, since they do not have to continue the patient's treatment. Physicians have the right to decide what types of medicine they wish to practice and where. They have the right to establish their own working hours, to charge for their services, and to take a vacation if they provide names of qualified substitutes to care for their patients while they are unavailable. Physicians have the right to change the location of their office but must notify patients in advance to give them adequate time to make alternative plans for medical care.

FIGURE 1–9 Consent to operation, anesthetics, and other medical services. (Courtesy American Medical Association)

FIGURE 1–10 Consent for treatment. (Courtesy American Medical Association)

Patients have the right to receive care equal to the standards of care in the community as a whole. Patients have the right to choose the physician they wish to receive treatment from. If a patient becomes a member of an HMO, however, the right to choose a physician may be restricted to physicians who are members of the chosen HMO. A patient has the right to accept or reject treatment, and to know when treatment is prescribed whether it has side effects, what the prognosis is, what effect the treatment will have on the body, and any alternatives to treatment.

A physician may choose to withdraw from the care of a patient who does not follow instructions for treatment or follow-up appointments or who leaves a hospital against advice. Withdrawal must be by means of a letter sent by certified mail with return receipt requested as proof the letter was received. The return receipt should be filed in the patient record. The letter may state the reason for the withdrawal and needs to state the date the withdrawal will become effective, Figure 1–13. If the patient needs follow-up, the letter should recommend that the patient make an appointment with another physician. It is appropriate to indicate that a copy of the medical records will be sent to the new physician if the patient sends written authorization to do so. The letter should be signed by the physician.

A patient has a right to change physicians. The patient should notify the physician, but if this does not take place in a written form the physician may send a letter confirming the dismissal. This letter should also be sent by certified mail, return receipt requested, and a copy of the letter and the receipt should be filed in the patient chart.

A physician who has begun care of a patient must carry through until the patient no longer needs treatment or decides to see a different physician, or the physician has withdrawn from care. A physician who has undertaken care of a patient and is then not available to continue that care may be sued for **abandonment** unless coverage by some equally qualified physician is provided for. If a patient is admitted to the hospital and the physician does not see the patient right away to check on condition and order treatment, the physician may be charged with abandonment. If a physician is ill, the office staff must refer patients who need care to other qualified physicians who will care for them.

Physicians are **not obligated** to provide follow-up care when they see a patient for preemployment or insurance examinations or on other occasions when the request comes from someone other than the patient, as when a school athletic department requests assessment of a potential athlete.

Medical Assistant Rights

The medical assistant has the right to be free from sex discrimination. This may involve a man or woman being refused employment because the job is usually filled by someone of the opposite sex. It can involve promotions, paying less for the same work, or being treated as inferior in any way.

Title VII of the Civil Rights Act of 1964 defines sexual harassment as "Unwelcome sexual advances, requests for sexual favors, and other verbal or physical conduct of a sexual nature when submission or rejection of this conduct explicitly or implicitly affects an individual's employment, unreasonably interferes with an individual's work performance or creates an intimidating, hostile or offensive work environment." Sexual harassment can occur in a variety of circumstances. It may include but is not limited to:

FIGURE 1–11 Request for sterilization forms. (Courtesy American Medical Association)

Form E-1
AUTHORITY TO ADMIT OBSERVERS

Patient _____ Place _____

Date _____

I authorize Dr. _____ and the _____

_____ Hospital to permit the presence of such observers as they may deem fit to admit in addition to physicians and hospital personnel, while I am undergoing (operative surgery) (childbirth), examination, and treatment.

Signed _____

Witness _____

FIGURE 1–12 Authority to admit observers. (Courtesy American Medical Association)

FORM A-1

LETTER OF WITHDRAWAL FROM CASE

Dear Mr. _____:

I find it necessary to inform you that I am withdrawing from further professional attendance upon you for the reason that you have persisted in refusing to follow my medical advice and treatment. Since your condition requires medical attention, I suggest that you place yourself under the care of another physician without delay. If you so desire, I shall be available to attend you for a reasonable time after you have received this letter, but in no event for more than five days.

This should give you ample time to select a physician of your choice from the many competent practitioners in this city. With your approval, I will make available to this physician your case history and information regarding the diagnosis and treatment which you have received from me.

Very truly yours,

_____, M.D.

FIGURE 1–13 Letter of withdrawal from case. (Courtesy American Medical Association)

- The victim as well as the harasser may be a woman or a man. The victim does not have to be of the opposite sex.
- The harasser can be the victim's supervisor, an agent of the employer, a supervisor in another area, a coworker, or a nonemployee.
- The victim does not have to be the person harassed but could be anyone affected by the offensive conduct.
- Unlawful sexual harassment may occur without economic injury to or discharge of the victim.
- The victim has a responsibility to establish that the harasser's conduct is unwelcome.

It is in the victim's best interest to directly inform the harasser that the conduct is unwelcome and must stop. Each instance reported to authorities is handled separately and involves a thorough investigation.

Negligence

Torts is the branch of civil law that deals with **breach** of legal duty. Torts **encompass** such wrongs as invasion of privacy, personal injury, malpractice, and slander or libel. The tort of negligence is a primary cause of malpractice suits.

Physicians are expected to be as well trained and to exercise the same degree of skill with the same degree of judgment as other physicians in similar circumstances. These **criteria** are used in determining the standard of care. In lawsuits involving specialists, the standard of care is that practiced nationally rather than that in a given community.

In a case of negligence the patient must establish that he or she was examined by the physician, that the physician did something another physician under similar circumstances would not have done, and that the negligence injured the patient. Testimony of a physician as an expert medical witness is almost always necessary in a case of negligence. In some cases the testimony of an expert witness is not required. In these instances the **doctrine** is *res ipsa loquitur,* or *the thing speaks for itself.* These cases involve such situations as a sponge or instrument left in the patient during surgery, an injury done to the bladder while performing a hysterectomy, and an infection caused by the use of unsterilized instruments. This doctrine has different interpretations in different states.

Physicians are responsible for the actions of their employees. This liability is expressed in the doctrine of *respondeat superior (let the master answer).* This is the law of agency, and you are an agent for the physician. Any individual entering the profession of medical assisting is considered to be accepting a position as a health care professional. If you violate the standard of care, you create the basis for a medical malpractice lawsuit. The physician is responsible for the acts of the medical assistant in the care of patients, and it is reasonable to expect the care to be as professional as the care given by the physician. A medical assistant is not licensed to practice medicine and cannot decide for a patient what care should be given.

After a Roche Laboratories medicolegal seminar, the Los Angeles County Medical Society sent the following directive to its doctors:

When you ask your office assistant to instruct or refill a prescription, you are placing both the assistant and yourself in jeopardy. The physician's aide who directs a pharmacist to fill or refill a prescription becomes guilty of practice of medicine without a license. A physician who directs his assistant to do this places his license in jeopardy by assisting an unlicensed person to practice medicine. The conclusion of this directive is that when you want a pharmacist to fill or refill a prescription, let him or her hear the doctor's own telephone voice, or better, have written orders on a regular prescription blank.

Negligence is not doing something that a reasonable person would do in a given situation. Malpractice is a professional's negligence. Under ordinary circumstances, a medical assistant performing the administrative duties of a receptionist or secretary would be considered a person who could be charged with negligence. A medical assistant performing clinical procedures, such as drawing blood or administering injections, would be considered a professional and charged with malpractice.

Medical assistants who have had special training are expected to perform at a higher standard of care than those with no special knowledge or training.

The medical assistant is not always covered by the physician's insurance, but insurance is available for the protection of medical assistants.

Good Samaritan Act The Good Samaritan Act originated in California in 1959 to protect the physician who gives emergency care from liability for any civil damages. The physician could help in an emergency without fear of being charged with neglect or abandonment for follow-up care. Now all states have Good Samaritan statutes. The statute requires that the emergency care be given to the best ability of the person providing the care. In some states, the statute includes coverage for any health professional or citizen with first aid skills. A Good Samaritan law does not cover physicians if they receive compensation for the emergency care.

An implied agreement is considered to be a legal contract in a medical office. The medical assistant should never make a promise of a cure. You should be certain the patient understands the instructions you give come directly from the physician or from written instruction sheets. When you hand a patient a written instruction sheet you need to be certain the patient can read the instructions. Illiterate people are often reluctant to let anyone know that they cannot follow the directions for use of medications or preparation for a diagnostic test. One indicator of illiteracy might be the patient who becomes a "pest" by asking over and over for office staff to explain the instructions given by the physician. This patient might also ask you to explain a printed instruction sheet as a means of getting you to read it aloud.

The importance of doing everything possible to avoid a medical malpractice suit cannot be overemphasized. Simply being accused has a severe effect on the physician and his or her family, as well as on the community at large. A physician can be ethical, honest, and **competent,** and still be sued for medical malpractice by a single patient who for some reason did not realize the expected result of treatment. The great increase in malpractice cases has caused physicians to order more tests and X rays than are really necessary because they need to protect themselves from the possibility of missing a diagnosis and therefore being sued by the patient. The medical assistant is an extremely important person in the practice of preventive medicine in the medical office. When a friendly, **harmonious** interpersonal relationship is found in the office, the patient is much less likely to feel angry about anything associated with the care received. The well-trained medical assistant will understand the basic skills in good human relations and will then avoid **confrontations** that could lead to lawsuits against the office.

The following is the beginning of a chapter regarding medical office staff written by Melvin Belli, an internationally known attorney:

> A woman once came to me with a complaint that she'd been incorrectly treated by a "dumb doctor."
>
> "How do you know he's dumb?" I asked her.
>
> "Because everybody who works for him is dumb."
>
> It's common for patients to relate a doctor to his or her staff. Therefore, quite often, patient dissatisfaction with an office assistant will put the doctor on a malpractice spot.
>
> (Reproduced with permission from Melvin M. Belli, Sr., and John Carlova. *For Your Malpractice Defense*, Oradell, New Jersey: Medical Economics Company, Inc., 1986.)

The patient who suffers nerve damage as the result of a medical assistant giving an improperly administered injection may sue both medical assistant and physician under this doctrine. You should always inform the physician immediately of any mistakes you have made in the care of a patient so that corrective measures may be taken. You should never attempt to perform a procedure for which you have not been trained. Finally, you should be sure you understand your job responsibilities as outlined in a written procedures manual, which should be periodically updated.

You must be especially careful what you say about a patient within hearing of anyone but the physician or other office personnel. Statements regarding patients may be considered **defamation** of character and a breach of confidentiality. If you should make public the fact that a patient has a venereal disease, for example, this could be damaging to the patient.

You play an important role in preventing negligence by scheduling appointments for careful follow-up, knowing how and where to reach the physician at all times during the day, and making sure that the telephone is adequately covered at all times. The patient who feels well cared for will not be anxious to sue the physician. The patient who can never reach the physician for advice or who has difficulty obtaining an appointment will be much more apt to sue on the grounds of negligence.

The medical assistant should investigate use of an arbitration agreement procedure by contacting your local or state medical society. Not all states have an arbitration statute at the present time but it is well worth investigating as a possible way to settle legal problems without going to court.

Because the incidence of malpractice suits has increased, the medical assistant may need to be involved in preparing materials for court. This may include the professional training and experience of the physician as well as the patient's medical record.

The attorneys may agree to taking the testimony of the physician by **deposition.** A deposition is oral testimony and may be taken in the attorney's office, or the physician's office in the presence of a court reporter.

A medical assistant may also receive a *subpoena duces tecum* (*under penalty you shall bring with you:* usually refers to documents) to appear in court with patient records. This occurs when the physician is not available at the time needed in court.

Statutes of Limitations   A statute of limitations is a law that designates a specific limit of time during which a claim may be filed in malpractice suits or in the collection of bills. Each state is obligated to protect individuals by establishing the statutes that regulate the time period. It is important to research the current law by contacting your state medical association.

Medical Records ....

The medical office staff must understand the importance of maintaining accurate, up-to-date records on all patients. You must have complete records to give adequate care to patients. Your records may be used in research into certain illnesses or forms of treatment, and your records must be complete for protection in case of a lawsuit. A patient record that would meet this criterion would include (1) personal information such as full name, address, occupation, marital status, and insurance carrier; (2) patient's personal and family medical history; (3) all details of physical examinations, laboratory and X-ray findings, diagnoses, and treatments; and (4) consent forms for procedures done and authorization forms for release of medical information. **Procrastination** cannot be tolerated in handling medical records. As legal documents, they are subject to critical inspection at any time.

You should always take a medical history in a private room or ask the patient to complete the information. Make entries on the patient medical record only as requested by the physician. All entries should be factual. All results of findings on a patient should be recorded even if they are normal or negative. Errors on a medical record must be corrected by drawing a single line through incorrect material and adding your initials, the date, and the reason for the change. All prescription refills should be noted along with missed appointments, the reason for the missed appointment, and follow-up. Requests for medical information should be noted along with the information given. Any failure to follow the treatment or advice of the physician should be noted. All notations should be in blue or black ink, as pencil is too easily erased. Standard abbreviations should be used. Upon the death of a patient, a copy of the death certificate should be filed in case of subsequent requests for information. A quality medical record indicates quality medical care.

Medical records are considered the property of the physician who treats the patient. No record should be shown to a patient without the knowledge of the physician, as there may be some reason the patient should not see all of the record.

Each office should have a written policy regarding releasing information from a medical record. This policy must take into consideration local or state statutes. In some states, the legislature has given the patient, his or her physician, or authorized agent the right to examine or copy the medical record. The requirement of confidentiality regarding the medical record is no longer recognized when the patient initiates a malpractice claim against a physician.

Physicians cannot agree on whether patients should be allowed to review their own records. The physician must be careful of personal opinion notes placed in the chart if there is a possibility the patient will be reading it. The following are two examples of patients reading medical records that were not recorded for their viewing:

A female patient was being professionally treated by a young physician when the doctor was suddenly called away from his office and left her medical record open on his desk. The patient read the first sentence: "This woman is a crock." Needless to say, she became very distraught and angry. (From "Personal Comments in Medical Records May Cause Trouble," *Medical World News*, Jan. 12, 1976, 128.)

While waiting to see a physician, a patient had been given her own record. Curious, she took out the notes and read them only to find that the doctor had written on the heading of the page, "Beware, hysterical and manipulative, determined to be unwell." She left immediately. (From "Case Conference: Fain Would I Change That Note," *Journal of Medical Ethics*, 4 [1978] 207–209.)

Any review of the chart by the patient should be done when the physician is present to interpret medical terms or abbreviations. Some physicians give patients a copy of their medical records and believe this reduces any anxiety regarding their health.

The following are six basic principles for preventing unauthorized disclosure of information:

1. When in doubt, err by not disclosing rather than by disclosing. There are exceptions to this principle, but a mistaken refusal to disclose confidential data is, at least, reversible.
2. Remember that the owner of the privilege to keep information confidential is the patient, not the doctor. If the patient is willing to release the data, the physician may not ethically decide to withhold it even 'for the patient's own good.'
3. Apply the concept of confidentiality equally to all patients despite the physician's assessment of their goals, mores and lifestyles. A physician cannot ethically inform an insurer of suspicions that a patient is trying to defraud an insurer.
4. Be familiar with the federal, state and local law plus ordinances, rules, regulations and administrative decrees of various agencies such as public health departments.
5. When required to divulge a confidence, discuss the situation with the patient. When obligations to society conflict with those of the patient, the physician should discuss the conflict with the patient. When legal guidelines are absent or vague, the criteria for decision are the immediacy and degree of danger to either the patient or society.
6. Get written authorization from the patient before divulging information. To meet standard situations such as requests from third parties, have the patient sign a blanket authorization in advance to release pertinent data to specific third parties.

(Reprinted with permission from Leif C. Beck, "Patient Information: When—and When Not—to Divulge," *Patient Care*, April 15, 1972.)

The AMA has several forms for authorization for disclosure. It is a good policy to refuse to answer a telephone question as to whether an individual is a patient. A person coming to the office for information regarding a patient should produce an authorization to disclose information before any is given. It is important to check the specific details authorized to be released and to ask for identification of the individual or organization requesting the information. The signed authorization should be placed in the patient chart with a copy of the information released. According to Myrtle Flight, "when the information requested is disclosed, it must be accompanied by a note forbidding redisclosure" (*Law, Liability, and Ethics for Medical Office Personnel*, 134).

The complete, unaltered medical record is a legal document and is the best defense for a physician who is charged with malpractice. The first step a lawyer will take in a malpractice case against a physician is to obtain a copy of the patient's records and have them examined by an independent physician. The following office procedures have caused problems in malpractice suits:

1. Procrastination in filing lab test results
2. Incomplete medical records
3. Illegible records
4. Unexplained altered medical records
5. Faking or forging a document or signature
6. Loss of records

There are acceptable methods of making changes in medical records. A single line should be drawn through an incorrect entry. An initial of the person making the correction should be written in the margin along with the date the error was discovered. The corrections should appear in the record in **chronological** order.

The contents of a medical record have been **enumerated.** In addition to having complete, up-to-date records you must be aware of the need for keeping these records even after care has ceased or the patient has died. Records should be kept as long as the statute of limitations is in effect on a case history. A few states stipulate the length of time records must be kept. You have a responsibility to see that necessary records are kept for any narcotics used in the office. You also may be responsible for keeping accurate financial records.

Complete Chapter 1, Unit 4 in the workbook to help you meet the objectives at the beginning of this unit and therefore achieve competency of this subject matter.

MEDICAL-LEGAL ETHICAL HIGHLIGHTS

Throughout this chapter you should be mindful of all medical-legal and ethical implications. Listed and below are a few important reminders.

1. Be constantly aware of how you project yourself, verbal and nonverbal messages.
2. Develop and maintain good personal health habits to be alert on the job.
3. Respect the rights of all individuals.
4. Attend all in-service and staff meetings.
5. Follow office policy where employed.

Ms. Right

attends the monthly staff meeting where office policy is reviewed. She is considerate of all coworkers and patients by addressing them with their appropriate titles courteously in a pleasant tone of voice. Her body language exhibits professionalism as her appearance is consistently fresh, neat, and clean without excessive use of makeup, perfume, or jewelry. Patients sense her sincerity because she makes eye contact while speaking to them and she listens carefully when spoken to. She never talks about patients where other patients may overhear her.

Employment outlook: Continuous

Ms. Wrong

rudely calls patients by their first names regardless of their age or status. She does so while alternating cracking her gum, blowing bubbles, sneezing, and coughing. She missed the staff meeting because she was sick, again. Her appearance is untidy, her uniform and "jogging" shoes are obviously dirty. She complains to patients that she's the one who should be seeing the doctor and ignores the patients' questions. She pays no attention to reminders regarding office policy. She talks and laughs about patients where other patients can hear her.

Employment outlook: Termination

REFERENCES

American Association of Medical Assistants. "Law for the Medical Office—1984."

Bates, Richard C. *The Fine Art of Understanding Patients*, 2d ed. Oradell, NJ: Medical Economics, 1972.

Calhoun, James F., and Acocella, Joan Ross, *Psychology of Adjustment and Human Relationships*, 2d ed. New York: Random House, 1983.

Flight, Myrtle. *Law, Liability, and Ethics for Medical Office Personnel*. Albany: Delmar, 1988.

Hasty, Frederick E., III. "Your Most Dangerous Malpractice Gamble." *Medical Economics for Surgeons*. August 20, 1984.

Horsley, Jack E. "Who Can Sue You for Not Rendering Care?" *Medical Economics*. August 20, 1984.

Isele, William. "Legal and Ethical Concerns of the Medical Assistant." *The Professional Medical Assistant*. July–August 1977.

Kinn, Mary E., and Derge, Eleanor. *The Medical Assistant: Administrative and Clinical*, 6th ed. Philadelphia: W. B. Saunders, 1988.

Kubler-Ross, Elizabeth. *On Death and Dying*. New York: MacMillan, 1969.

Lewis, Marti, and Warden, Carol. *Law and Ethics in the Medical Office*. Philadelphia: F. A. Davis, 1983.

Monahan, James S. "How Your Office Staff Can Get You Sued." *Medical Economics*. August 22, 1983.

Physician's Desk Reference. Oradell, NJ: Medical Economics, updated annually.

Physician's Guide to Ohio Law. Ohio State Medical Association, Columbus, 1987.

Purtilo, Ruth. *Health Professional/Patient Interaction*. 2d ed. Philadelphia: W. B. Saunders Co., 1978.

Riker, Audrey Palm, and Riker, Charles. *Me: Understanding Myself and Others*, rev. ed. Peoria, IL: Bennett, 1982.

The Professional Medical Assistant. "Ethics, a Roundtable Discussion." September–October, 1979.

Thompson, Ella M. *Textbook of Basic Nursing*. Philadelphia: J. B. Lippincott, 1973.

U.S. Department of Health and Human Services. *Saying No*. 1981. Alcohol, Drug Abuse, and Mental Health Administration, 5600 Fishers Lane, Rockville, MD 20857.

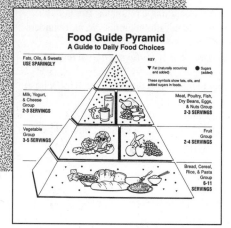

Food Guide Pyramid
A Guide to Daily Food Choices

Fats, Oils, & Sweets
USE SPARINGLY

KEY
▼ Fat (naturally occurring and added)   ● Sugars (added)
These symbols show fats, oils, and added sugars in foods.

Milk, Yogurt, & Cheese Group
2-3 SERVINGS

Meat, Poultry, Fish, Dry Beans, Eggs, & Nuts Group
2-3 SERVINGS

Vegetable Group
3-5 SERVINGS

Fruit Group
2-4 SERVINGS

Bread, Cereal, Rice, & Pasta Group
6-11 SERVINGS

CHAPTER 2
Personal Behaviors

UNIT 1
Nutrition, Exercise, and Rest

UNIT 2
Stress Management

UNIT 3
Substance Abuse

UNIT 4
Behavior Modification

As you gain experience in the field, it will soon become apparent that patients have a tendency to depend on you for advice. The physician prescribes a treatment plan for the patient to follow and usually discusses it with the patient. Almost always the patient's next step is to ask you to explain the details. Therefore, you must have a complete understanding of the policies of the health care facility. Personal opinions should be restrained. This chapter concerns the significance of diet, exercise, and rest and the way personal behavior influences health. The use of habit-forming substances and the benefits of treatment and support groups will be discussed. These areas are vitally important to you personally, as well as to the patients you will serve.

UNIT 1

Nutrition, Exercise, and Rest

OBJECTIVES

Upon completion of this unit, you will meet the following terminal performance objectives by verifying knowledge of the facts and principles presented through oral and written communication at a level deemed competent by the instructor or employer.

1. Explain the significance of diet and exercise to health.
2. Name and discuss the six food groups of the food guide pyramid.
3. Name the fat-soluble vitamins.
4. Name the water-soluble vitamins.
5. Name the essential minerals.
6. Discuss ways to encourage patient compliance in treatment plans.
7. Discuss the importance of sleep and a positive outlook in regard to health.
8. List guidelines for promoting good health.
9. Demonstrate range-of-motion exercises.
10. Demonstrate flexibility exercises.
11. Spell and define, using the glossary at the back of the text, all of the words to know in this unit.

PATIENT EDUCATION

You will notice that this chapter primarily concerns educating the patient on staying well. When educating the patient about the importance of a good diet and proper exercise, you must be supportive and empathetic. If you can gain the patient's confidence, you will be in a better position to help the patient attain certain goals. Whether the patient is dieting, exercising, or working to stop smoking, encourage realistic goals. Offer praise whenever possible no matter how small the accomplishments.

WORDS TO KNOW

anorexia	nutrition
beriberi	positive
calorie	rickets
dietician	ROM
health	scurvy
infirmity	therapeutic

With today's attention to physical fitness, the medical assistant must be well informed to answer the countless inquiries patients make concerning diet and exercise programs. The physician will decide what is best for each patient after all data from the medical history, examination, laboratory findings, and other pertinent information have been evaluated. It is up to you to reinforce the physician's orders and help patients adapt those orders to their particular life-styles.

As you begin to practice skills in communicating information to patients regarding treatment plans and their overall health, it is important for you to have a basic understanding of the meaning of health. **Health** is defined by the World Health Organization as a state of complete physical and mental or social well-being. Health is not merely the absence of disease or **infirmity.** All things conducive to good health are referred to as healthful. Healthful living habits are essential for one to maintain being in good physical condition or in staying physically fit. Fitness, therefore, refers to being in good physical condition or being healthy. There are simple guidelines that can help to keep us in good health, increase vitality, and to even increase life expectancy. Figure 2–1 outlines the suggestions advised for the general population. Those who are in the health care professions are urged to set a good example to those patients for whom we are models.

Nutrition...

Patient education in proper nutrition is one of your many responsibilities. **Nutrition** is defined as the sum of the processes involved in taking in, assimilating, and utilizing nutriments. This includes the processes by which the body uses food for energy, maintenance, and growth.

The Food Guide Pyramid The food guide pyramid was introduced in the spring of 1992 by the U.S. Department of Agriculture. This pyramid concept replaces the "food wheel" and the old basic four food groups that have been used since 1946. The pyramid is divided into six sections; the foods listed in the largest sections are those foods that should be consumed in the greatest quantities. Notice that at the top of the triangle, for example, are fats, oils, and sweets; this indicates that foods such as butter, salad oil, candy, and other sweets should be used sparingly. Explaining the food pyramid to patients will encourage healthful eating habits. Eating sensibly makes people feel better and more energetic. When people feel well they have a more **positive** outlook on life. It is a good idea to post the food guide pyramid shown in Table 2–1 near the scale or on the wall of the examination room. An attractive poster is an even better way to suggest good eating habits. Figure 2–2 illustrates a visual reminder of healthy food choices. You may want to place a note regarding the "other" foods that have only slight nutritional value (fats, oils, and sweets) next to the poster. This reminder may help patients realize the importance of avoiding large amounts of the foods found at the top of the pyramid. Some patients have never been educated in this area of importance. Many pharmaceutical companies offer complimentary instructional materials.

Vitamins and Minerals Vitamins are organic substances found in foods that are essential to good health and growth. Vitamins are called micronutrients. As the name implies, only a trace quantity is required for enzymatic reaction in the body. If the body does not receive adequate vitamins or does not absorb them sufficiently, deficiency diseases may result. The major ones are **rickets, scurvy,** and **beriberi.** Rickets is the result of a deficiency in vitamin D; scurvy, of vitamin C, or ascorbic acid; and beriberi, of vitamin B, or thiamine. Vitamins A, D, E, and K are fat-soluble vitamins. Vitamin C and the B complex vitamins are water-soluble.

TABLE 2–1
The Food Guide Pyramid

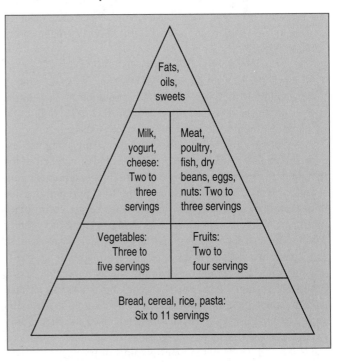

DO:
— exercise regularly
— eat a sensible, well-balanced diet
   include high-fiber, low-fat, cereal and grain foods
— practice health and safety rules at home and work
— include spiritual/emotional nurturing

DON'T:
— smoke or use tobacco
— drink alcohol in excess
— expose skin to sun for prolonged periods
— use drugs or medications unless prescribed for a specific purpose
— overeat or gain too much weight
— expose yourself to unnecessary X rays

FIGURE 2–1 Guidelines for good health

FIGURE 2–2 Eat Your Way to Good Health (Courtesy of the National Cancer Institute)

With a well-balanced diet, there is little likelihood of vitamin-deficiency diseases. Prepared foods display a list of their nutritional values on their labels for consumer information. Vitamins are added to many foods because of their loss in preparation. Patients will be advised by the physician if a vitamin or mineral supplement is necessary.

Minerals are naturally occurring, nonorganic, homogeneous, solid substances. Thirteen are said to be essential to good health. They are supplied by a variety of meats and vegetables. Minerals found to be missing most often from the diet are calcium, iron, and iodine. Metabolic disturbances can be caused by insufficient amounts of zinc, copper, magnesium, and potassium.

The principal micronutrients are listed in Tables 2–2 and 2–3, pages 29–33. Careful study of this chart will give you an understanding of the food sources, the function of each in the body's growth and repair, the effects of deficiency and toxicity, and the dosages recommended for daily intake.

Several servings of Fiber-rich foods (fruits, vegetables, peas and beans, whole-grain cereals) should be included in the daily diet to promote a healthy digestive tract and prevent constipation. Notice that the sections of the food pyramid that list these nutrients are more than half the size of the entire pyramid to show their importance. Encourage patients to modify cooking techniques by using less fats, oils, and sugars (smallest portion of pyramid) and by baking, broiling, boiling, roasting, grilling, poaching, or steaming meats and other foods instead of frying. These modified cooking practices can also help to reduce the amount of calories, cholesterol, sodium, and sugar, as well as saturated and total fat, from the diet. Study the information in Chapter 4 regarding the immune system and foods that aid the body in defense against disease.

Supplements   When patients suffer from loss or lack of appetite or they cannot tolerate a normal diet, it may be necessary for the physician to prescribe a protein-vitamin-mineral food supplement. These food supplements come in the form of a powder or liquid for oral or tube feeding as required by the patient's condition. Patients who might need this type of treatment are the chronically ill, postoperative, underweight, anemic, and **anorexic.** This treatment should be conducted only under the supervision of a physician. Remind patients to take these supplements regularly as directed for their intended affect.

Weight Control   A good weight-control program should contain foods from the food guide pyramid to be nutritionally sound. Eating should be an enjoyable, relaxing experience. But in our fast-food society, people tend to eat more food, with more calories, more often. A **calorie** is a unit of heat, and all food substances have caloric value, Table 2–3, pages 32–33. All of the body's processes burn calories to provide energy and sustain life. If you overeat regularly, the unused calories are stored as fat. If you reduce calorie intake, the fat will be used by the body for energy and you will begin to shed the extra weight. You should make patients aware that they should eat their meals slowly because it takes approximately 20 minutes for the brain to realize that the stomach is full. Those who follow this practice in a relaxed atmosphere eat *less* and digest their food better. It it now recommended that eating several (5 to 6) small meals daily not only allows for better utilization of nutrients by the body for more energy, but is much easier on the digestive tract. This practice also helps in weight control.

A variety of magazines, books, and businesses offer weight-control plans that promise success for each individual. Over-the-counter drugs promise miraculous weight loss in a matter of weeks. You can be influential in helping patients avoid possible health hazards by warning them of the danger in these quick-weight-loss programs. Many people do lose weight in a short time, but they gain it right back as soon as the program ends. Others do permanent damage to their health.

One respected and worthwhile weight-loss program is Weight Watchers. Most people who have reached their weight-loss goals through this program have maintained a satisfactory weight because they have learned how to change their eating habits. Many support groups offer similar programs. Positive reinforcement is one of the keys to their success. Many physicians realize the frustration of trying to reduce and suggest these support groups to patients. You may want to encourage patients who are trying to follow a diet by suggesting low-calorie recipes or cooking techniques. Showing genuine interest in patients' needs will help them reach their goals.

Therapeutic Diets   **Therapeutic** diets are used in the treatment of patients with a specific disease or disorder. So that patients will comply with treatment, these special diets must be presented in a workable manner. The patient's lifestyle and background must be taken into consideration and certain adjustments made on the part of the patient. For the patient to give full cooperation, you must explain acceptable

TABLE 2–2
Principal Micronutrients

Micronutrient	Principal Sources	Functions	Effects of Deficiency and Toxicity	Usual Therapeutic Dosage
Vitamin A	Fish liver oils, liver, egg yolk, butter, cream, vitamin-A-fortified margarine, green leafy or yellow vegetables	Photoceptor mechanism of retina; integrity of epithelia; lysosome stability, glycoprotein synthesis	*Deficiency:* Night blindness, perifollicular hyperkeratosis, xerophthalmia; keratomalacia *Toxicity:* Headache; peeling of skin, hepatosplenomegaly, bone thickening	10,000–20,000 µg (30,000–60,000 IU/day)
Vitamin D	Fortified milk is main dietary source, fish liver oils, butter, egg yolk, liver, ultraviolet irradiation	Calcium and phosphorus absorption, resorption, mineralization, and collagen maturation of bone; tubular reabsorption of phosphorus (?)	*Deficiency:* Rickets (tetany sometimes associated); osteomalacia *Toxicity:* Anorexia; renal failure; metastatic calcification	*Primary Deficiency* 10–40 µg (1400–1600 IU)/day) *Metabolic Deficiency* 1–2 µg/day 1.25–$(OH)_2D_3$ or 1α–$(OH)D_3$
Vitamin E group	Vegetable oil, wheat germ, leafy vegetables, egg yolk, margarine, legumes	Intracellular antioxidant; stability of biologic membranes	*Deficiency:* RBC hemolysis, creatinuria; ceroid deposition in muscle	30–100 mg/day
Vitamin K (activity) Vitamin K_1 (phytonadione) Vitamin K_2 (menaquinone)	Leafy vegetables, pork, liver, vegetable oils, intestinal flora after newborn period	Prothrombin formation; normal blood coagulation	*Deficiency:* Hemorrhage from deficient prothrombin *Toxicity:* Kernicterus	In situations conductive to neonatal hemorrhage, 2–5 mg during labor or daily for 1 wk prior; or 1–2 mg to newborn
Essential fatty acids (linoleic, arachidonic acids)	Vegetable seed oils (corn, sunflower, safflower); margarines blended with vegetable oils	Synthesis of prostaglandins, membrane structure	Growth cessation, dermatosis	Up to 10 g/day
Thiamine (vitamin B_1)	Dried yeast; whole grains; meat (especially pork, liver), enriched cereal products, nuts; legumes; potatoes	Carbohydrate metabolism, central and peripheral nerve cell function, myocardial function	Beriberi; infantile and adult (peripheral neuropathy, cardiac failure; Wernicke-Korsakoff syndrome)	30–100 mg/day
Riboflavin (vitamin B_2)	Milk, cheese, liver, meat, eggs, enriched cereal products	Many aspects of energy and protein metabolism integrity of mucous membranes	Cheilosis; angular stomatitis; corneal vascularization; amblyopia, sebaceous dermatosis	10–30 mg/day
Niacin (nicotinic acid, niacinamide)	Dried yeast, liver, meat, fish, legumes, whole-grain enriched cereal products	Oxidation–reduction reactions, carbohydrate metabolism	Pellagra (dermatosis, glossitis, GI and CNS dysfunction)	Niacinamide 100–1000 mg/day
Vitamin B_6 group (pyridoxine)	Dried yeast, liver, organ meats, whole-grain cereals, fish, legumes	Many aspects of nitrogen metabolism, e.g., transaminations, porphyrin and heme synthesis, tryptophan conversion to niacin. Linoleic acid metabolism	Convulsions in infancy, anemias; neuropathy; seborrhea-like skin lesions Dependency states	25–100 mg/day
Folic acid	Fresh green leafy vegetables, fruit, organ meats, liver, dried yeast	Maturation of RBCs; synthesis of purines and pyrimidines	Pancytoperia; megaloblastosis (especially pregnancy, infancy, malabsorption)	1 mg/day

TABLE 2–2
Principal Micronutrients (continued)

Micronutrient	Principal Sources	Functions	Effects of Deficiency and Toxicity	Usual Therapeutic Dosage
Vitamin B$_{12}$ (cobalamins)	Liver, meats (especially beef, pork, organ meats); eggs; milk & milk products	Maturation of RBCs; neural function; DNA synthesis, related to folate coenzymes; methionine and acetate synthesis	Pernicious anemia; fish tapeworm & vegan anemias; some psychiatric syndromes, nutritional amblyopia Dependency states	In pernicious anemia 50 µg/day IM first 2 wk, 100 µg twice/wk next 2 mo, thereafter 100 µg/mo
Biotin	Liver, kidney, egg yolk, yeast, cauliflower, nuts, legumes	Carboxylation and decarboxylation of oxalocetic acid; amino acid and fatty acid metabolism	Dermatitis, glossitis Dependency states	150–300 µg/day
Vitamin C (ascorbic acid)	Citrus fruits, broccoli, tomatoes, potatoes, cabbage, green peppers	Essential to osteoid tissue; collagen formation; vascular function; tissue respiration and wound healing	Scurvy (hemorrhages, loose teeth, gingivitis)	100–1000 mg/day
Sodium	Wide distribution—beef, pork, sardines, cheese, green olives, corn bread, potato chips, sauerkraut	Acid–base balance; osmotic pressure; pH of blood; muscle contractility; nerve transmission; sodium pumps	*Deficiency:* Hyponatremia *Toxicity:* Hypernatremia; confusion, coma	
Potassium	Wide distribution—whole and skim milk, bananas, prunes, raisins	Muscle activity, nerve transmission, intracellular acid–base balance and water retention	*Deficiency:* Hypokalemia; paralysis, cardiac disturbances *Toxicity:* Hyperkalemia; paralysis, cardiac disturbances	
Calcium	Milk and milk products, meat, fish, eggs, cereal products, beans, fruits, vegetables	Bone and tooth formation; blood coagulation; neuromuscular irritability; muscle contractility; myocardial conduction	*Deficiency:* Hypocalcemia and tetany; neuromuscular hyperexcitability *Toxicity:* Hypercalcemia; GI atony, renal failure; psychosis	10–30 ml 10% calcium gluconate soln IV in 24 h
Phosphorus	Milk, cheese, meat, poultry, fish, cereals, nuts, legumes	Bone and tooth formation, acid–base balance, component of nucleic acids, energy production	*Deficiency:* Irritability; weakness; blood cell disorders; GI tract and renal dysfunction *Toxicity:* Hyperphosphatemia in renal failure	Potassium acid and di-basic phosphate parenteral 600 mg (18.8 mEq)/day
Magnesium	Green leaves, nuts, cereal grains, seafoods	Bone and tooth formation; nerve conduction; muscle contraction; enzyme activation	*Deficiency:* Hypomagnesemia; neuromuscular irritability *Toxicity:* Hypermagnesemia; hypotension, respiratory failure, cardiac disturbances	2–4 ml 50% magnesium sulfate soln/day IM
Iron	Wide distribution (except dairy products)—soybean flour, beef, kidney, liver, beans, clams, peaches Much unavailable (<20% absorbed)	Hemoglobin, myoglobin formation, enzymes	*Deficiency:* Anemia; dysphagia; koilonychia; enteropathy *Toxicity:* Hemochromatosis: cirrhosis; diabetes mellitus; skin pigmentation	Ferrous sulfate or gluconate 300 mg orally t.i.d.

TABLE 2–2
Principal Micronutrients (continued)

Micronutrient	Principal Sources	Functions	Effects of Deficiency and Toxicity	Usual Therapeutic Dosage
Iodine	Seafoods, iodized salt, dairy products Water variable	Thyroxine (T_4) and triiodothyronine (T_3) formation and energy control mechanisms	*Deficiency:* Simple (colloid, endemic) goiter; cretinism; deaf–mutism *Toxicity:* Occasional myxedema	150 µg iodine/day as potassium iodide added to salt 1:10–40,000 ppm
Fluorine	Wide distribution—tea, coffee Fluoridation of water supplies with sodium fluoride 1.0–2.0 ppm	Bone and tooth formation	*Deficiency:* Predisposition to dental caries; osteoporosis (?) *Toxicity:* Fluorosis, mottling, pitting of permanent teeth; exostoses of spine	Sodium fluoride 1.1–2.2 mg/day orally
Zinc	Wide distribution—vegetable sources Much unavailable	Component of enzymes and insulin; wound healing; growth	*Deficiency:* Growth retardation; hypogonadism; hypogeusia; in cirrhosis; acrodermatitis enteropathica	30–150 mg zinc sulfate/day orally
Copper	Wide distribution—organ meat, oysters, nuts, dried legumes, whole-grain cereals	Enzyme component	*Deficiency:* Anemia in malnourished children; Menkes' kinky hair syndrome *Toxicity:* Hepatolenticular degeneration; some biliary cirrhosis (?)	0.3 mg/kg/day copper sulfate, orally
Cobalt	Green leafy vegetables	Part of vitamin B_{12} molecule	*Deficiency:* Anemia in children (?) *Toxicity:* Beer-drinker's cardiomyopathy	20–30 mg/day cobaltous chloride, orally
Chromium	Wide distribution—brewer's yeast	Part of glucose tolerance factor (GTF)	*Deficiency:* Impaired glucose tolerance in malnourished children; some diabetics (?)	

reasons for changes in diets. This area of patient education is vitally important and may take a considerable amount of time. Some physicians refer patients with special dietary needs to a registered dietician (RD). **Dieticians** work closely with other health care team members in therapeutic diet planning.

Exercise

In addition to a well-balanced diet, adequate exercise and sufficient rest are essential to good health. Special diets and exercise programs must be approved for individuals by the physician, who will determine the patient's needs and tolerance from careful examination and medical history. This is done to safeguard the patient from overexertion and stress.

Exercise is defined as physical exertion for improvement of health or correction of physical deformity. The safest form of exercise, and one almost everyone can participate in, is walking, but so many different exercise programs are available that people can choose according to their individual needs and goals. A combination of proper diet and proper exercise brings satisfying results in overall good health.

All of the behaviors which influence health are influenced by one's mental (or social) health and vice versa. A positive outlook is most helpful in coping with life in general. (Refer to Unit 4.) Learning coping and problem-solving skills can help us deal with the everyday stress and the occasional crisis of routine living. Getting sufficient rest is also necessary for good health. Individuals vary in the number of hours of sleep they require. An "average" number is between 6 and 8 hours in a 24-hour period. Sleep is the natural way for the body to rest and restore itself. Adequate rest equips us with strength to

TABLE 2–3
Calorie Chart

Food and Measures	Approximate Calories	Food and Measures	Approximate Calories	Food and Measures	Approximate Calories
Apple, baked, 1 large and 2 tbs sugar	200	syrup, 1/4 cup	200	yogurt, plain, 1 cup	120–160
fresh, 1 large	100	Cocoa, half milk, half-water, 1 cup	150	Mushrooms, 10 large	10
Asparagus, fresh or canned, 5 stalks 5 in. long	15	Cod steak, 1 piece, 3 1/2 by 2 by 1 in.	100	Noodles, cooked, 3/4 cup	75
Avocado, 1/2 4-in. pear	265	Cola soft drinks, 6-oz. bottle	75	Oatmeal, cooked, 3/4 cup	110
Bacon, 2–3 long slices, cooked	100	Collards, 1/2 cup, cooked	50	Oil, corn, cottonseed, olive, peanut, 1 tbs.	100
Banana, 1 medium, 6 in. long	90	Corn, 1/2 cup	70	Olives, green 6 medium	50
Beans, lima, fresh or canned, 1/2 cup	100	Corn flakes, 1 cup	80	ripe, 4–5 medium	50
green or yellow, fresh or canned, 1/2 cup	25	Cracker, graham, 1 square	35	Onions, 3–4 medium	100
canned with pork, 1/2 cup	175	saltine, 2-in. square	15	Orange, 1 medium	80
Beef (cooked), corned, 1 slice 4 by 1 1/2 in. by 1 in.	100	Cream, light, 2 tbs.	65	juice, 1 cup	125
hamburger, 3 oz.	300	heavy, 2 tbs.	120	Parsnip, 7 in. long	100
round, lean, 1 medium slice (2 oz.)	125	whipped, 3 tbs.	100	Peach, fresh, 1 medium	50
sirloin lean, 1 average slice (3 oz.)	250	Custard, 1/2 cup	130	canned in syrup, 2 large halves, 3 tbs. juice	100
tongue, 2 oz.	125	Eggs, medium	75	Peanut butter, 1 tbs.	100
Beets, fresh or canned, 2, 2-in. in diam.	50	Eggplant, 3 slices, 4 in. diam., 1/2 in. thick, raw	50	Peanuts, shelled, 10	50
Bread, corn (1 egg), 1 2-in. square	120	Flour, 1 tbs., unsifted	35	Pear, fresh, 1 medium	50
rye, 1 slice, 1/2 in. thick	70–75	Frankfurter	125	canned in syrup, 3 halves, 3 tbs. juice	100
white, enriched, 1 slice, average	75	Gelatin, fruit flavored, ready to serve, 1/2 cup	85	Peas, canned, 1/2 cup	65
whole wheat, 100%, 1 slice average	75	Grapefruit juice, unsweetened, 1 cup	100	fresh, shelled, 3/4 cup	100
Broccoli, 3 stalks, 5 1/2 in. long	100	Grape juice, 1/2 cup	80	Pepper, green 1 medium	20
Brussels sprouts, 6 sprouts, 1 1/2 in. diam.	50	Griddle cake, 4 in. diam.	75	Pie, apple, 3-in sector	200
Butter, 1 tbs.	95	Halibut, 1 piece, 3 by 1 3/8 by 1 in.	100	mincemeat, 3-in sector	300
Cabbage, cooked, 1/2 cup	40	Ham, lean, 1 slice, 4 1/4 by 4 by 1/2 in.	265	Pineapple, fresh, 1 slice, 3/4 in. thick	50
raw, 1 cup	25	Hominy grits, cooked, 3/4 cup	100	canned, unsweetened, 1 slice, 1/2 in. thick, 1 tbs. juice	50
Cake, angel, 1/10 large cake	155	Ice cream, 1/2 cup	200	juice, unsweetened, 1 cup	135
choc, or vanilla, with icing 2 by 1 1/2 by 2 in.	200	Ice cream soda, fountain size	325	Pork chop, lean, 1 medium	200
cupcake (med.), choc. icing	250	Jellies and jams, 1 rounded tbs.	100	Potato chips, 8–10 large	100
Cantaloupe, 1/2 5 1/2 in. melon	50	Lamb, roast, 1 slice, 3 1/2 by 4 1/2 by 1/8 in.	100	Potato salad with mayonnaise, 1/2 cup	200
Carrot, 4 in. long	25	Lettuce, 2 large leaves	5	Potatoes, mashed, 1/2 cup	100
Cauliflower, 1/4 of head, 4 1/2 in. in diam.	25	Liver, 1 slice, 3 by 3 by 1/2 in.	100	sweet, 1/2 medium	100
Celery, 2 stalks	15	Liverwurst, 2 oz.	130	white, 1 medium	100
Cheese, American cheddar, 1 cube 1 1/8 in. square	110	Macaroni, cooked, 3/4 cup	100	Prunes, dried, 4 medium	100
cottage, 5 tbs.	100	Maple syrup, 1 tbs.	70	Pumpkin, 1/2 cup	50
cream, 2 tbs.	100	Margarine, 1 tbs.	100	Raisins, 1/4 cup	90
Chicken, 1/2 med. broiler	270	Milk, buttermilk, 1 cup	85	Rice, cooked, 3/4 cup	100
Chocolate, milk, sweetened, 1 oz.	140	condensed, 1 1/2 tbs.	100	Rutabagas, 1/2 cup	30
malted milk, fountain size	460	evaporated, 1/2 cup.	160	Salad dressing, French, 1 tbs.	91
		skim, 1 cup	85	mayonnaise, 1 tbs.	100
		whole, 1 cup	170	Salmon, canned, 1/2 cup	100
				Sauerkraut, 1/2 cup	15

TABLE 2–3
Calorie Chart (continued)

Food and Measures	Approximate Calories	Food and Measures	Approximate Calories	Food and Measures	Approximate Calories
Soup, condensed, 11-oz. can, mushroom	360	Tomato juice, 1 cup	60	Alcoholic Beverages beer, 8 oz.	120
tomato	230	Tomatoes, canned, 1/2 cup	25	gin, 1 1/2 oz.	120
vegetable	200	fresh, 1 medium	30	rum, 1 1/2 oz.	150
Spaghetti, cooked, 3/4 cup	100	Tuna fish, canned, 1/4 cup, drained	100	whiskey, 1 1/2 oz.	150
Spinach, cooked, 1/2 cup	20	Turnip, 1, 1 3/4 in. diam.	25	Wines	
Squash, summer, cooked, 1/2 cup	20	Veal roast, 1 slice, 3 by 3 3/4 by 1 1/2 in.	120	champagne, 4 oz.	120
winter, cooked, 1/2 cup	50	Waffle, 6 in. diam.	250	port, 1 oz.	50
Sugar, brown, 1 tbs	50	Wheat flakes, 3/4 cup	100	sherry, 1 oz.	40
granulated, 1 tbs	50			table, red or white, 4 oz.	95
Tapioca, uncooked, 1 tbs	50				

handle various daily situations. People who have trouble sleeping (insomnia) may have either serious physical or emotional (psychological) problems that should be brought to the attention of the physician. Each individual should find outlets to release tension and participate in activities that bring enjoyment and enrichment to his or her life. It is additionally important to practice the virtue of patience and maintain a sense of humor, for it has been said that laughter is the best medicine.

Regular exercise improves circulation and muscle tone and relieves tension. People who have followed an exercise routine regularly report that they experience a better outlook on life, have more energy, and feel healthier. The degree of exertion in any exercise routine will vary with individuals and the physician's advice should be taken.

For patients who cannot engage in strenuous exercise, walking and **ROM** (range-of-motion exercises) are suggested to improve circulation and promote muscle tone, Figure 2–3. These movements help to move each joint through its full range. Patients who have arthritis, bursitis, and other disabilities can be helped by these exercises. Flexibility exercises increase muscle tone and flexibility of the muscles and also relieve tension, Figure 2–4, page 36. You should be familiar with these so that you can teach them to patients.

Complete Chapter 2, Unit 1 in the workbook to help you meet the objectives at the beginning of this unit and therefore achieve competency of this subject matter.

U N I T   2
Stress Management

OBJECTIVES

Upon completion of the unit you will meet the following terminal performance objectives by verifying knowledge of the facts and principles presented through oral and written communication at a level deemed competent by the instructor or employer.

1. Describe the phenomenon of stress and differentiate between "good" stress and "bad" stress.
2. List and describe stress-related illnesses.
3. List positive methods for dealing with stress.
4. Describe type A and type B personalities.
5. List the four basic human physical needs.
6. List the four basic human developmental needs.
7. Describe steps you can take to eliminate unnecessary stress.
8. List mental health resources for referral of patients.
9. Spell and define, using the glossary at the back of the text, all the words to know in this unit.

WORDS TO KNOW

absolute	implement	psychosomatic
absurdity	leisure	receptors
conflict	nurture	rejuvenate
discretion	perspective	respite
exemplify	prioritize	
impending	psychosis	

As you become familiar with patients' symptoms and their diagnoses, it will be evident that a great many illnesses may be ultimately stress-related. Some persons are more stress-prone than others, operating at such a hectic pace and with such compulsiveness or perfectionism that they create many stressful situations for themselves. In general, these persons are referred to as type A personalities. There is a type B personality as well, **exemplified** by a tendency to operate at a slower pace and not to worry as much. These typings are neither **absolute** nor evaluative; that is, one is not better than the other, and most people probably demonstrate characteristics of both types at different times and in differ-

SPINE

CERVICAL

LATERAL FLEXION

ROTATION

FLEXION
EXTENSION
HYPEREXTENSION

TRUNK

LATERAL FLEXION

ROTATION

FLEXION
EXTENSION
HYPEREXTENSION

SHOULDER

ABDUCTION
ADDUCTION

ROTATION:
OUTWARD
INWARD

FLEXION
EXTENSION
HYPEREXTENSION

HIP

ABDUCTION
ADDUCTION

ROTATION:
OUTWARD
INWARD

FLEXION
EXTENSION
HYPEREXTENSION

FIGURE 2-3 Range of Motion (ROM) exercises

FIGURE 2-3   Range of Motion (ROM) exercises (continued)

These exercises are designed to increase the flexibility of the low back extensor ranges and to strengthen the low back flexor muscles. They are to be performed slowly, starting with ten repetitions for each exercise, and increasing gradually to as many as forty or fifty repetitions. These are best performed on a firm, flat surface.

1.   Purpose: To strengthen abdominals. Patient lies on back, with hips and knees bent.

A)   Come to sitting position:

   a) Reaching hands past the knees
   b) With arms folded across chest
   c) With hands clasped behind head

2.   Purpose: To strengthen hip muscles. Patient lies on back, with hips and knees bent.

A)   Roll the pelvis backwards, flattening the low back curve, pinching the buttocks together, raising the tailbone slightly upwards.

3.   Purpose: To stretch the lower back muscles. Patient lies on back, with hips and knees bent.

A)   Stretch the back by pulling the knees to the chest as close as possible. Curve the back by also ducking the head forward.

4.   Purpose: To stretch the lower back and hamstring muscles. Patient sits upright with legs straight.

A)   Keeping the knees straight, bend the head toward the knees to stretch the lower back and hips.

5.   Purpose: To stretch the hip flexor muscles. Patient stands erect.

A)   Place one foot forward. Lean forward on that leg, keeping the other leg straight, the body bent forward so that a good stretch is felt along the front of the hip and thigh.

6.   Purpose: To stretch the lower back and to strengthen the upper leg muscles. Patient stands erect.

A)   Squat down as far as possible and stand up again. Keep feet flat on the floor and curve the back to keep the balance and to stretch the lower back and hip muscles.

FIGURE 2–4   Range of Motion (ROM) exercises

ent situations. For the most part, though, we lean toward one type or the other in our general actions. Although both type A and type B personalities inevitably face stressful situations, the type As probably face them more frequently than the type Bs. Hence, type A personalities should pay particular attention to recognizing stress and learning to deal with its effects.

Basic human survival needs are really few. Physical needs include protection, food, water, and oxygen. Developmental needs are physical, emotional, intellectual, and spiritual **nurturing.** Often materialistic values override real needs to the point of **absurdity.** The quality of personal relationships and meaningful endeavors determine the quality of life more than material things.

A certain amount of stress is necessary to provide motivation. This is "good" stress. The degree of stress that is necessary or helpful varies with the individual. Goals must be set realistically and kept in **perspective.** Reaching goals produces a sense of pride in accomplishment, and these positive feelings reinforce continued personal growth and development. Failure tends to produce feelings of worthlessness and even despair. These negative feelings, if not properly vented, can cause many **psychosomatic** problems. For example, they may lead to aggressive behavior, which is itself stress-producing to the one who displays it as well as to others. Feelings of hostility toward others may lead to difficulty in coping with pressures from change in employment or unemployment, family or personal **conflicts,** and many other problems, usually known only to the individual.

Difficulty in planning the use of time can produce stress. The feeling of being inefficient and unproductive can lead to a vicious cycle of defeat and despair. This negative attitude may encourage dependence on drugs or alcohol to find some pleasure in life and **respite** from feelings of worthlessness. Exaggeration? No. People vary in their coping skills for dealing with stress. Those who have no one to encourage or support them in their lives may have a particularly hard time.

Office Stress

The hectic pace of a medical office practice creates pressure. On some days there may be little time to exchange even a complete sentence with a coworker. Therefore, lunch and rest breaks are essential to your well-being. Time away from the pressures of patient care can give a whole new outlook on a problem. Some offices schedule time for the lunch period between morning and afternoon patients and block the time routinely in the appointment book. This is a good practice. You return to work refreshed and are more productive as a result. Most medical practices have a heavy schedule, and working overtime is a frequent reality. Many find that trading evenings with another employee is a good practice. Since patients do not get sick by appointment, schedules will never run perfectly. Flexibility must be acquired early. A great number of problems stem from the high-pressure nature of the job itself. Realizing this will be of great help in learning to cope well with whatever situation presents itself.

There may be times, however, when you are tired or have a cold or a headache or are worried about a personal problem that things will start to go awry and it seems that everything follows suit. This is the time when every patient who calls has a major health problem or a mistake with their bill or insurance claim.

Taking one thing at a time and completing it before starting something else can ease many tensions. Everyone must learn to help out on days when life itself seems to be a chore. Exchanging common courtesies and being considerate of each other's feelings can also reduce stressful situations. Just knowing that someone cares is what patients need sometimes. You should give this consideration to colleagues as well.

Since you can be the target of patients', and sometimes coworkers', pent-up feelings from time to time, it is clear that your own feelings will need expression, too. Everyone needs to get rid of negative feelings. The bad as well as the good times must be shared; it is human nature to do so. This may lead to feeling overburdened at times, but these emotions must be directed into proper channels. Realizing the difference between the things we can and cannot control is important.

Stress and Related Illness

Stress in itself is a most useful reaction for it is a signal for one to respond to a stimulus. There is both good and bad stress. Good stress is known as *eustress,* such as special events we look forward to and plan for, or even deadlines to meet (when planned). Those things ultimately beneficial and rewarding to us are motivating and energizing. The stress is temporary and useful to us.

All of us are constantly processing various stimuli that aid us in our daily communications and activities. The difficulty in regard to stress occurs when the stressor is chronic (constant) and causes us to be troubled. Because no short-cut or fast relief can resolve the stressor or situation causing the stress, it becomes *distress,* or bad stress. The effects of this chronic stress stay with the affected person, so that a potentially dangerous physical and mental state ensues.

Stress manifests itself in individuals in many ways. The most commonly recognized stress-related illnesses are asthma, headaches (migraines), gastritis, heart disease, insomnia, mental (emotional) illness, and peptic ulcers.

The effect of stress is that the nerve **receptors** send nerve impulses to the brain, where the sympathetic function of the autonomic nervous system reacts by sending a message of **impending** danger to the adrenal glands. These glands pour adrenaline into the circulatory system, as do special nerve cells, to give the body extra strength to deal with the impending threat or danger. The heart beats faster, respirations are increased, and digestion slows down to allow the circulation of adrenaline. As the problem is resolved or removed, the body begins to reorganize impulses. The parasympathetic function sends impulses to slow the previously supercharged body functions back to normal levels. The sympathetic and parasympathetic functions work to create a balance of nerve impulses to regulate the activities of the body.

If one is living under constant stress, the heart and circulatory system, the lungs, and intestinal tract are constantly being literally turned on and off, leaving insufficient time for normal body functioning. The human body, given too much to deal with too often, eventually breaks down and needs repair, as does an automobile run too hard and too long without proper maintenance.

The body reacts to stress by showing various symptoms. Constipation or diarrhea, frequent colds and flu, indigestion, and migraine headaches are a few of the common physical complaints of patients who overtax themselves. Those who seek medical attention for these types of complaints are usually referred to a counseling service, where the cause of the stress may be discovered and eliminated. Once this is accomplished the symptoms usually disappear.

There are, of course, patients whose symptoms have developed over a long period and whose physical problems have progressed into a major illness. These patients need counseling as well as medical supervision and treatment.

Since physicians have become so specialized, there is usually little or no time for counseling during a routine office visit. The general practitioner used to know the whole family and was often the counselor of all members. Some family and general practice physicians still do domestic counseling in a limited manner. You should notice if a patient who has always been pleasant and smiling during previous office visits suddenly demonstrates a change in mood. This patient may begin to complain of headaches or other aches and pains without apparent cause. After the physician's examination and lab reports have been reviewed, if no major cause has been found, the physician may suggest that the patient seek counseling.

In almost every community large or small hospitals, health centers, and clinics offer mental health services. The county medical society will be helpful in referring patients to a physician, psychologist, or psychiatrist if listings are not available in the local phone directory.

Inquiries about mental health services should be treated with **discretion.** Mental illness can be a difficult and delicate problem to deal with, not only for the patient, but for family, close friends, and neighbors. As in all matters of medical records, confidentiality must be carefully maintained.

The family or general practitioner is usually the first professional to have contact with the patient. The referral for appropriate care of the patient will be made by the medical assistant.

Depression

Depression is treated by physicians with both counseling and medication. Some patients may respond well with counseling only, however. Where medication is given, careful supervision of patients is a must. Alerting the physician to any changes that the patient reports by phone is vital in the direction of the patient's therapy.

There are many types of depression. Depression is a predictable reaction to the death of a relative, spouse, or close friend, for example. A person may take some time to overcome this grief, the amount of time varying with the individual. Usually, after a few months, the person should begin to adjust to the loss, however. When normal functioning does not return, assistance is necessary.

Psychosomatic Illness

Psychosomatic illness is not imagined. These patients have very real symptoms. However, the symptoms are usually emotional and not organic in nature. Patients with psychosomatic illness may have deep-rooted guilt feelings, fears, frustrations, hostilities, anxieties, or phobias. The patient may not be conscious of these feelings. The stress-related illnesses described earlier are some of the common physical expressions of psychosomatic illness.

Anxiety

Anxiety is a stress-related condition in which the patient is in a constant state of worry. Those who are constantly feeling apprehension and fear have a variety of physical ailments as a result, which can lead to serious illness if not treated. Concerns over money or sexual dysfunction are common anxieties. Patients with this type of problem usually need a combination of counseling and medication to regain a healthy outlook on life and function productively.

Psychoses

Psychosis is a more profound mental disorder characterized by impairment of normal intellectual and social functioning. These patients usually have either partially or completely withdrawn from reality. Their condition may become so severe that hospitalization is necessary. These patients have severe mood swings, sometimes experience hallucinations, and may not know who they are. Patients may be treated on an out-patient basis, but in the most severe cases patients are hospitalized. Many persons in psychotic states can, with long-term treatment, return to normal functioning. Other psychotic states may be irreversible.

Treatment

Many public service agencies, churches, colleges, businesses, and private organizations offer educational programs in stress management. Most programs deal with methods which can be practiced by individuals in coping with their personal lives. Significant life events, such as major changes in employment or geographic location, marital status, or health create varying levels of stress. Support groups can help; meetings are held to discuss problems or situations which are too complex or difficult to figure out alone. For that matter, a close friend can be a valuable resource. Simply identifying a source of stress may relieve some of it, but some action must usually be taken to relieve most stressful situations. Finding workable solutions to problems may take a considerable amount of time and patience. Counseling can help both in defining problems and in beginning to take definitive action to **implement** changes. Individuals must recognize the importance of **prioritizing** values and standing firm in beliefs while remaining flexible enough to cope with new and challenging situations.

Effective time management involves careful assessment of one's personal routine and deciding how and when to accomplish priorities. Then the primary goal is to eliminate activities that are not worth the time they demand. A good rule to follow is to single out one issue at a time and deal with it thoroughly and appropriately.

Activities that help you relax are a basic necessity. For some, it may be working a jigsaw puzzle, reading, or listening to music; for others, it may be taking a walk after supper, dancing, or gardening. Each person should find an enjoyable **leisure** activity. Something that refreshes the spirit and **rejuvenates** the soul is a must for sound mental and physical health. You also need to give yourself a pat on the back occasionally for doing a good job.

Following a dull pattern of work–eat–sleep–work is not enough. Personal growth and development are rewarding and essential. A hobby or interest is vital to feeling good about yourself. Many find that physical activity is the answer. Regular exercise is not only a good way to relieve tension, it keeps you in shape and stimulates more energy. A daily program of physical activity is an excellent and refreshing outlet.

Many people today participate in exercise groups through community centers, schools, work, private health clubs, or public facilities such as the YMCA/YWCA. Still others follow an individual exercise regimen. Whatever one does to stay physically fit, will have a positive effect in reducing stress.

You may want to place exercise class announcements and other health-related tips on a bulletin board in the reception area or by the scale, or wherever patients have enough time to read and copy the information.

An excellent means of venting one's inner feelings is by associating with your peers. Talking "shop" for a while can be good therapy and can lead to friendships outside the working relationship. Membership in a professional association (AAMA) will provide you with many opportunities. You can make strong friendships and participate in a variety of continuing education programs for personal and professional growth. Membership is encouraged for it adds a new perspective to your career.

Because stress is perceived by each of us differently, a personal evaluation to define the cause of our individual stress is necessary for relieving or eliminating it from our lives. Developing good habits of coping can include quiet "alone" time for reflecting, meditation, daydreaming (and visualization), imaging, or other techniques that help clear the mind and renew the spirit. The old saying, "a healthy mind—a healthy body" is becoming more evident. Maintaining a daily routine of physical and mental exercises to relieve anxiety and tension is a healthy way to cope with stress. A happier healthier life results from successful stress management.

Complete Chapter 2, Unit 2 in the workbook to help you meet the objectives at the beginning of this unit and therefore achieve competency of this subject matter.

UNIT 3
Substance Abuse

OBJECTIVES ....

Upon completion of this unit, you will meet the following terminal performance objectives by verifying knowledge of the facts and principles presented through oral and written communication at a level deemed competent by the instructor or employer.

1. List the most commonly abused major groups of drugs and give an example of each.
2. Explain the effects of the most commonly abused substances.
3. Describe the difference between an alcohol-dependent drinker and alcoholic.
4. Describe research into the causes of alcoholism.
5. Describe ways you can be influential in assisting drug addicts and alcoholics toward rehabilitation.
6. Describe the action that tar, nicotine, and carbon monoxide have on the body.
7. List ways a person can stop smoking.
8. List diseases for which smokers have a higher probability rate.
9. Discuss the effects of secondhand smoke.
10. Discuss the stages of drug or alcohol abuse.
11. List signs of drug or alcohol abuse.
12. List organizations and facilities that assist in the rehabilitation of drug addicts and alcoholics.
13. Spell and define, using the glossary at the back of the text, all of the words to know in this unit.

WORDS TO KNOW ....

acetylcholine	depressant
addiction	detrimental
advantageous	euphoria
Al-Anon	hallucinogen
Al-Ateen	narcolepsy
alcoholic	nicotine
Alcoholics Anonymous	norepinephrine
amphetamine	proclivity
barbiturate	psychedelics
bizarre	stimulant
carbon monoxide	synergism
carboxyhemoglobin	tar
carcinogen	traumatic
cholinergic	veritable

A habit is a pattern of behavior that is acquired over a period of time by repetition. Habits can be either **advantageous** or disadvantageous depending on the effects they have. Many of our habits are so much a part of us that we do not even realize they exist. Changing a behavior that has become a habit is difficult. It takes a great deal of patience and encouragement to repattern personal activities. Teaching good health habits to patients is an important duty of the medical assistant. The entire medical staff must strive to set a good example, for example is the best teacher.

In times of stress one may be temporarily inclined to relieve anxiety or depression by using chemical substances. Even individuals under the supervision of a physician may become dependent. Other persons turn to chemical substances to experiment with the feelings they produce. Often this is a response to peer pressure, which can be strong indeed. Regardless of why persons turn to chemical substances, they need to know that dependency and abuse can follow and that the stakes can be very high.

Unfortunately, the influence of advertising has been to encourage chemical substance use by promoting fast relief, quick weight-loss, instant sleep and wakefulness, and a variety of other "feel-good" promises from the makers of chemical products. Although a substance may well relieve symptoms temporarily, the cause of the problem will still exist. If undetermined or undetected physical or emotional problems are not diagnosed and treated, they may balloon into more complex problems which are, of course, only worsened by the abuse of chemical substances. You can play an important part in recognizing chemical abuse and helping patients take steps toward treatment.

Alcohol ....

Still the nation's number-one drug problem, alcohol is responsible for the destruction of many lives. Its use is commonly accepted by society and to a great degree encouraged. Most persons who drink alcoholic beverages do so moderately, probably because its effects have been learned from either first-hand observation or educational programs. The responsible social drinker can take alcohol or leave it alone.

On the other hand, a person who is dependent on alcohol has a difficult time doing without a drink. An alcohol-dependent drinker will say that cutting down is not a problem, but is then unable to do so. Daily use of alcohol becomes a need and usually leads to increasingly compulsive drinking. Patients who indicate this during conversation or in giving a medical history may be indirectly asking for help with their problem. Privately disclosing this information to the physician may lead to a treatment or counseling program, which may prevent the patient from becoming an alcoholic. An **alcoholic** is a drinker who has become totally dependent on alcohol. All areas of the alcoholic's life are affected by it. It is the number-one priority, and control over drinking is nonexistent. More often than not, the occurrence of a tragedy is the reason the alcoholic seeks treatment, either by court order or sometimes voluntarily in an effort to put a productive life back together.

Alcoholism is now recognized as a disease, as serious as cancer or diabetes, which can be treated. It is a major health problem and recognized as such by the American Medical

Association, American Osteopathic Association, and American Bar Association. Excessive long-term use of alcohol can reduce resistance to infections and eventually lead to cirrhosis of the liver. It can also add complications to other diseases and conditions. In effect, alcohol works to dissolve all tissues with which it comes in contact.

Research efforts continue in the search for the causes of the disease. Many theories have been offered, but none are yet definitive. Current efforts are concentrating on brain chemistry, hereditary traits, and cultural influences. Whereas certain ethnic groups show a **proclivity** to alcoholism, others are virtually free of the disease. Studies in these areas suggest almost evolutionary relationships between habits, value systems, and brain chemistry. Many scientists feel that a combination of factors contribute to alcoholism.

Treatment Alcoholics Anonymous (AA) is a well-known support group for the alcoholic, who must admit to being an alcoholic and be willing to start leading a productive life once again. AA was founded in the mid 1930s to help those who were looked on by society as hopeless degenerates. The program has become extremely successful over the years and has directly and indirectly helped millions to reorder their lives. Other support groups have branched from this initial organization. **Al-Anon** and **Al-Ateen** are for family members or close friends of the alcoholic to help them understand and cope with their loved ones' illness. Many companies maintain alcoholism assistance and rehabilitation programs for employees who are problem drinkers. It has been realized by employers that this practice is not only a service but is a cost-effective alternative to training new personnel.

Drugs

(Refer to Table 2–4, pages 42–44) There was a time when we thought of drugs only in connection with a trip to the drugstore to have a prescription filled, perhaps staying long enough to enjoy something at the soda fountain. Today the meaning has changed, and the term evokes the image of illicit chemical substances available on the street. Most of these are impure, diluted, and extremely addictive, as well as expensive.

Throughout civilized history people have had a desire to soothe the anxieties of life and obtain temporary relief from troubles. But our society, as a whole, is today more than ever before looking for instant gratification. Over-the-counter drugs are practically beyond number. It is a mind-boggling experience to look over a well-stocked drug shelf in a retail store and consider all the substances that can allegedly provide "fast and temporary" relief. In this age of fast food, instant car washes, one-hour dry cleaning, and express lanes, the art of patience has seemingly been lost. Our society has become accepting of drug use as a part of life, even a *way* of life, despite the physical and emotional damage, reflected in the high numbers of drug-related deaths from overdose and accident.

The threat of nuclear war, unemployment, an uncertain economy, and a fast-paced life-style make it difficult for many to deal with the challenges of everyday living. For some people the only way to cope with problems is by resorting to mood-altering drugs. But these drugs alter not only one's mood, but also one's perception of reality, and they are dangerous not only to the user but to others as well. The **euphoric** state they produce exists only in the user's mind.

The reality of drugs in society and the seriousness of their abuse are not going to disappear. A **veritable** smorgasbord of legal and illegal drugs remains widely available and probably always will be. Educating the public to their dangers seems to be the only hope.

You could be most influential in helping someone, a patient or a family member of a patient, recognize the signs of drug abuse so that intervention may be possible. You should always be supportive and understanding. Avoid being judgmental, sarcastic, or accusatory with patients or others seeking your help. The indications of drug abuse are outlined in Figure 2–5.

There are four basic stages of alcohol and drug abuse. In the first stage, one may show no visible signs in outward behavior. Unfortunately, society has taken somewhat an attitude of acceptance in the use of alcohol and drugs, especially in youth. Experimental use is considered normal, and abuse often goes unnoticed until the second stage has begun. In the second stage, use is more frequent and the habit starts. Frequently signs may include a change in the type of friends one associates with and a decline in motivation and performance at school and work. Stage three shows a marked change in one's mood when domestic problems are common. The abuser may exhibit signs of depression and possibly talk of or attempt suicide. The person affected by abuse has an intense preoccupation to seek drugs for daily use. The fourth and last stage requires that the abuser take the drug in increasing amounts just to feel OK. Outward signs of stage four include coughing, frequent sore throats, weight loss, and fatigue. The person may also overdose and have blackouts. To maintain the habit, the person may have begun a life of crime. Deterioration of relationships and family is most evident. Obviously the sooner help is initiated the better in dealing with this situation. Stay firm in your attitudes, explanations, and efforts in seeking help for one who requests it.

The most commonly misused major groups of drugs and medicines in the United States are **depressants, hallucinogens,** narcotics, and **stimulants.** The state of **addiction** stems from periodic or chronic intoxication; that is, from repeated use. The abuser or addict has an overriding desire for the euphoric effect of the substance and will find a means of obtaining it to fulfill that desire. Because of increasing physiological tolerance of the drug, the user gradually must increase the dosage to maintain the desired effects. The user may also mix two or more drugs, including alcohol. This practice, referred to as **synergism,** greatly enhances the intoxicating qualities of each drug into a combined new effect, which can be quite erratic and unpredictable. Though the user may realize the damaging effects of the substance, dependence can become so great that it is quite impossible to stop using the drug without outside intervention and assistance.

Rarely does the drug abuser begin by taking medicine to relieve pain, but more typically to avoid a confrontation with emotional or psychological problems; hence, the addiction is psychological as well as physical. These problems are only made more complex with the addition of mood-altering chemicals.

Depressants Barbiturates, such as Butisol sodium, Donnatal, and Nembutal, to name a few, are used in the treatment of patients who need sedation or for the relief of anxiety. They are also used to induce sleep, and thus are frequently referred to as sleeping pills. They are also known as downers. They vary in strength and action but function by depressing the activity of the central nervous system. This affects the heart rate, respiration, blood pressure, and temperature. Tolerance to the drug is acquired after frequent use over a relatively short period. Psychological effects are similar to those of alcohol and when used with alcohol the danger to the user is great. A person under the influence of barbiturates appears to be intoxicated.

Immediate medical attention must be given in the case of overdose, or death is imminent. For a victim who is still awake, the first step is to induce vomiting.

Hallucinogens Hallucinogens are also referred to as **psychedelics** or sometimes as "mind-expanding" chemicals. Some of the most commonly used street drugs of this type are LSD, or acid, mescaline, and PCP (angel dust). These chemical substances give the user a distorted look at reality. "Taking a trip" refers to the visual hallucinations seen on those short chemical vacations. However, the images may be horrific, and "coming down" may be **traumatic.** Even though dependence does not seem to occur, the danger of hallucinogens is in the **bizarre** behavior that may result, which can cause accidental death to the user and others. In addition, some users experience undesirable "flashbacks" from some hallucinogens, or effects long after the drug was taken.

Marijuana can have hallucinogenic effects on the user. The effects of marijuana are varied, and it can be classified in other drug categories as well. It is also referred to as dope, grass, mary jane, pot, reefer, smoke, and weed. It is one of the oldest and probably most widely used drugs next to alcohol, and it has become more socially acceptable today than ever before. When mixed with other drugs it becomes more powerful and dangerous. Marijuana stimulates the central nervous system and produces a euphoric effect. It also distorts the perception of time and reality and can give rise to feelings of paranoia.

Marijuana may have **detrimental** effects on the respiratory and reproductive systems, and these are being studied. Use in treating nausea in patients undergoing chemotherapy for cancer and use in treating glaucoma have prompted further investigation into potential medical applications.

There is ongoing debate regarding legalization of marijuana. Those who choose to use marijuana are likely to continue whether it is legal or not. There are reports of third-graders (younger) who have already smoked marijuana. Early usage frequently leads to later use of more dangerous drugs.

Narcotics A narcotic is a drug that produces insensibility or stupor. Legally, the term refers to habit-forming drugs, such as opiates: cocaine, heroin, meperidine, and morphine. The lesser narcotics are paregoric, which is used in the treatment of diarrhea and abdominal pain, and codeine, which is a pain reliever. These substances can be obtained legally by a physician's prescription. However, federal, state and local laws prohibit the sale of narcotics for other than medical purposes. These medications are extremely potent and highly addictive. The possibility of overdose is great. Since many physicians store these medications in their offices or clinics, great care must be taken to ensure their security. You have a tremendous responsibility in keeping accurate records of these drugs.

Stimulants The medical uses for stimulants are few. They are used in the treatment of **narcolepsy,** some cases of mental depression and alcoholism, chronic rigidity following encephalitis, and in some cases of obesity. The central nervous system is stimulated by **amphetamines,** which are referred to as uppers or speed. Abusers take speed in pill form to stay awake, to feel more energetic, or to lose weight. Some abusers inject the drug directly into their veins for a faster, more intense reaction. Others "snort" or sniff it to obtain the effects.

Cocaine was used as a local anesthetic many years ago, but today it is rarely used for medical purposes. Its illegal use is nearly epidemic. Songs have been written about it, and fashionable people use it in combination with other drugs for pleasure. Its effects are short-lived, usually about 12 minutes, and the user must constantly increase the dosage to reach the desired state. It is a stimulant that leaves the user depressed after it wears off. Most cocaine addicts must use other drugs to keep them going. The drug leads to frequent upper respiratory and gastrointestinal problems. A nasty side effect suffered by many heavy "snorters" is destruction of the nasal passages. It is an extremely dangerous and expensive addiction.

Heavy use of any stimulant results in physical and psychological dependence. Few deaths are reported from abuse of stimulants, but many result from mixing them with other drugs. Physical ailments and emotional problems are the most evident effects of abusing stimulants.

Over-the-counter diet aids are popular stimulants, which are also abused. Their dangers arise when mixed with other drugs or alcohol. Pregnant women and patients with heart disease or hypertension must be particularly discouraged from using stimulants except under the direct supervision of a physician. This advice should be given to anyone in the use of any stimulant.

Probably the most abused stimulant is caffeine, found in coffee, tea, chocolate, and many cola drinks. Caffeine stimulates the central nervous system and also acts as a diuretic. Moderation is advised in its use. Coffee "jitters," for instance, cause one to feel out of sorts and nervous. Abuse can result in many related physical and emotional problems.

Treatment Comprehensive rehabilitation programs to assist drug abusers are available in a variety of facilities, private and public.

TABLE 2–4
Commonly Abused Substances

Drug	Prescription (Brand Name)	Medical Use	How Administered	Street Name
LSD	None	None	Orally, injected	Acid, cubes, purple haze
Psilocybin, psilocin	None	None	Orally (ingested in natural form)	Magic Mushrooms
Inhalants: Gasoline, airplane glue, paint thinner, dry-cleaning solution	None	None	Sniffed, inhaled	
Nitrous oxide (N$_2$O)	Nitrous oxide	Anesthetic in dentistry	Inhaled	Laughing gas, whippets
Nitrites: Amyl, butyl	Amyl nitrite	Vasodilator	Inhaled, sniffed	Poppers, locker room, rush, snappers
Marijuana, hashish	None	None	Orally, smoked	Pot, grass, reefer, jays, weed, Columbian, hash, hash oil, joint, sinsemilla
Tranquilizers	(Librium, Valium, Tranxene)	Antianxiety, muscle relaxant, sedation	Orally	
Narcotics	(Percodan)	Analgesic	Orally, injection	
	Codeine	Analgesic	Orally, injection	School boy
	Heroin	None	Injection, sniffed	Dreamer, junk, horse, smack, china white, crap, fix H, mother, pearl, stuff, boy, brown
	Morphine	Analgesic	Injection, smoked	
Hallucinogens (drugs that alter one's perception of reality)	PCP, phencyclidine (Sernylan)		Orally, smoked inhaled, snorted, injection	Angel dust, killer weed, supergrass, pearly gates, hog, PeaCe Pill, acid, m&m's
		Veterinary anesthetic		
Mescaline	None	None	Orally, injection	Mesc, cactus, mescal, buttons
Alcohol	ethanol	None	Swallowed in liquid form	Booze, hooch, brew
Depressants (drugs that depress the CNS)				
Chloral hydrate	(Notcec, Somnos)	Hypnotic	Orally	Downer

TABLE 2–4
Commonly Abused Substances

Length of Effects (hrs)	Possible Symptoms of Use	Hazards of Long-Term Use/Overdose	Symptoms of Withdrawal
Variable	Dilated pupils, illusions, mood swings, hallucinations, poor perception of time and distance	Breaks from reality, emotional breakdown, flashback	Not reported
Variable	Poor motor coordination, impaired vision, poor memory and thought processes, abusive and violent behavior	High risk of sudden death; weight loss; and damage to brain, liver, and bone marrow	
	Lightheaded feeling	Death by anoxia, muscle weakness, neuropathy	
Seconds to minutes	Slowed thought process, headache	Anemia, death by anoxia	
2–4	Euphoria, increase in appetite, short-term memory loss, disorientation, loss of interest and motivation, neglect of appearance	Lung damage, possible reproductive system damage, loss of motivation, damage to immune system and heart, interference with psychological maturation, impaired memory perception, psychological dependence	Insomnia, hyperactivity and decreased appetite reported in some individuals
4–8	Drowsiness, confusion, slurred speech, impaired judgment, drunken behavior without odor of alcohol, constricted pupils	Nausea, addiction with severe withdrawal symptoms, loss of appetite, death from overdose, shallow respiration, cold and clammy skin, dilated pupils, weak and rapid pulse, coma	Anxiety, insomnia. tremors, delirium, convulsions, possible death
3–6	Nausea, drowsiness, respiratory depression, constricted pupils, lethargy, euphoria	Addiction with severe from overdose, loss of appetite	Watery eyes, runny nose, loss of appetite, yawning, irritability, panic, chills, sweating, cramps, nausea
3–6			
3–6	Needle marks		
3–6			
Variable	Slurred speech, blurred vision, confusion, aggression, uncoordination, agitation, needle marks	Anxiety, depression, impaired memory and perception, death from accidents/ overdose	Not reported
	Illusions and hallucinations, poor perception of time and distance	Longer, more intense trip episodes, psychosis	
Hours—depends on amount consumed	Impaired muscle coordination, and judgment	Heart and liver damage, death from overdose, death from auto accidents, addiction	Weakness, sweating, hyperreflexia, delirium tremens
5–8	Drowsiness, confusion, slurred speech, impaired judgment, drunken behavior without odor of alcohol, constricted pupils	Nausea, addiction will severe withdrawal symptoms, loss of appetite, death from overdose, shallow respiration, cold and clammy skin, dilated pupils, weak and rapid pulse, coma	Anxiety, insomnia, tremors, delirium, convulsions, possible death

TABLE 2–4

Commonly Abused Substances (continued)

Drug	Prescription (Brand Name)	Medical Use	How Administered	Street Name
Barbiturates	(Butisol, Nembutal,) phenobarbital, (Seconal,) secobarbital	Anesthetic, anticonvulsant, sedation, sleep, epilepsy, heart disease	Orally, injection	Barbs, downers, yellow jackets, red devils, blue devils
Glutehimide	(Doriden)	Sedation, sleep	Orally	
Methaqualone	(Parest, Quaalude, Somnafac)	Sedation, sleep	Orally	
Stimulants (drugs that stimulate the CNS)	cocaine	Local anesthetic	Injection, sniffed, smoked, or snorted orally	Bernice, Big C, blow, Coke, crack, rock, snow, toot, girl, lady, gold dust, snort
Amphetamines	dextroamphetamine (Biphetamine) (Benzedrine)	Hyperkinesis, narcolepsy, weight control	Orally, injection	Speed, uppers, pep, pills, meth, whites, bennies, dexies, speed, black beauties, crank
Phenmatrazine	(Preludin)	Weight control	Orally	lip poppers
Methylphenidate	(Ritalin, Cylert, Didrex)	Hyperkinesis	Orally	Meth crystals
Nicotine		None	Smoked (snuff or chew)	Coffin nail, smoke, butt

Federal government facilities are located in Fort Worth, Texas, and Lexington, Kentucky. These are Public Health Service hospitals that offer treatment to addicts who volunteer for the program of rehabilitation.

Community hospitals and mental health centers provide these services as well. Staffed by psychiatrists, psychologists, counselors, and social workers, treatment centers give the addict the opportunity to receive therapy that can help in getting to the root of the problems leading to the addiction. Support from the health care team is necessary to assist in the return of the addict to a productive and meaningful life. Finally, Alcoholics Anonymous attracts many drug abusers as well as alcohol abusers to its program.

Smoking

According to recent government studies, the risk of premature death due to smoking cigarettes is now the same for men and

INDICATIONS OF DRUG/ALCOHOL ABUSE

- Abrupt change in mood/attitudes
- Sharp decline in attendance/performance at school/work
- Resistance to discipline/rules at home/ school
- Deterioration in relationships
- Sudden unusual temper outbursts
- Increased frequency in borrowing money
- Stealing from others at home, school, or work
- Increased intense secrecy about actions and belongings
- Associating with new friends

FIGURE 2–5 Warning signs of possible drug or alcohol abuse.

TABLE 2–4
Commonly Abused Substances (continued)

Length of Effects (hrs)	Possible Symptoms of Use	Hazards of Long-Term Use/Overdose	Symptoms of Withdrawal
1–16	Needle marks		
4–8			
4–8			
2	Restlessness, anxiety, intense short-term euphoria followed by dysphoria, dilated pupils, increased pulse rate and blood pressure, insomnia, loss of appetite	Intense psychological dependence, sleeplessness and anxiety, lung and nasal passage damage, death from overdose	Apathy, long periods of sleep, irritability, depression, disorientation
2–4	Excess activity, mood swings, irritability, nervousness, needle marks, dilated pupils, increased pulse rate and blood pressure,	Loss of appetite, hallucinations, paranoia, convulsions, coma, agitation, increase in body temperature, death from overdose	Apathy, long periods of sleep, irritability, depression, disorientation
2–4	insomnia, loss of appetite		
2–4			
Variable	Smell of tobacco, stained teeth and fingers, high carbon monoxide levels	Cancers of the lung, throat, mouth, esophagus, heart disease, emphysema, irritation/ diseases of the GI and urinary tract; frequent URI, "smoker's cough"	Irritability, insomnia nervousness

women. The saying, "You've come a long way baby," is unfortunately true. Nicotine dependence, for those smokers who use 20 (or more) cigarettes per day, is responsible for decreasing life expectancy by one-half. There are over 2000 substances that have been identified in tobacco smoke. Of these, the three poisons in tobacco smoke that do the most harm are **tar, nicotine,** and **carbon monoxide**

Tar is the thick, sticky, dark brown or black substance that is carried in inhaling the smoke and deposited in the lungs. Tar is a **carcinogen,** which means that it is capable of producing cancer in tissues with which it comes in contact. Nicotine is believed to be the addictive drug that is absorbed in the lungs and first stimulates and then depresses the nervous system. The stimulation is caused by the release of **norepinephrine** and because nicotine acts similarly like **acetylcholine. Cholinergic** nerves are stimulated by nicotine; and because nerve activity is blocked, depression results. Respiration rate is increased with stimulation of nerve receptors in the carotid arteries to supply more oxygen to the brain. The cardiovascu-

lar system is also stimulated with the release of norepinephrine, which causes an increase in blood flow to the heart and a rise in heart rate and blood pressure.

Nicotine seems to inhibit hunger, raises blood sugar levels slightly, and deadens taste buds in smokers.

Carbon monoxide produces still other dangerous effects. Red blood cells pick up carbon monoxide where it binds together to form **carboxyhemoglobin.** This could be the reason why smokers easily become short of breath with even moderate activity. Smokers have approximately 10% of their blood supply in the form of carboxyhemoglobin, which cannot carry oxygen. This is also a factor in the cause of heart attacks and lower birth weight and survival rate of babies of smoking mothers.

In addition, smokers are more at risk to have cancer of the lungs, larynx, lip, esophagus, and urinary bladder; chronic sinusitis and bronchitis; emphysema; upper respiratory infections (URIs); cardiovascular diseases: coronary artery disease (CAD) and arteriosclerotic heart disease (ASHD); and peptic ulcers.

Even though these facts have been proven and efforts to

discourage smoking in recent years have increased, men and women continue to smoke. The nicotine addiction is difficult for many to overcome. The key to success in the elimination of the smoking habit is first of all becoming thoroughly educated on the facts about smoking. Realizing the health hazards as well as the cost of this habit can be helpful to a smoker in making the decision to stop. Encourage patients, coworkers, family, and friends to consider attending a stop-smoking seminar. Post this information in the waiting room and on the employee's bulletin board. Reward those you know who have stopped smoking by giving them praise and recognition.

Some ways to help the smokers you know to get on the right track to stop their smoking habit are as follows:

1. Keep track of when and why you smoke for at least 2 weeks.
2. Compare a list of reasons why you should and should not stop.
3. Practice not smoking for a period of time (begin with an hour, a morning, a day, etc.)
4. Decide a target date when you are going to give up smoking.
5. Learn deep-breathing relaxation exercises and use at least twice a day when tension becomes apparent. Simply take a deep breath slowly and release slowly, thinking consciously of relaxing. Continue for 5 minutes unless you become dizzy.
6. Find a substitute to replace holding the cigarette.
7. Use nonsugar gums, mints, and mouth sprays to avoid overeating and to help curb the nicotine craving. (Transdermal nicotine patches available by prescription only may help patients break the habit successfully.)
8. Drink plenty of water and eat sensibly. Pay special attention to caloric intake for the first 4 to 8 weeks.
9. Include exercise to relieve tension and restlessness that comes with trying to overcome addiction.
10. Reward yourself with something special with the money saved from not buying cigarettes.

Involuntary smoking and *passive smoking* are terms describing secondhand smoke from active tobacco smokers. It is also called sidestream smoke. Both sidestream and mainstream smoke cause damage to the cells that line the heart and blood vessels. The buildup is a cause of atherosclerosis. Studies have shown that the platelets in the blood of smokers are more likely to clump together abnormally, which can lead to blood clots and the risk of a heart attack. Those exposed to secondhand smoke are not only at higher risk of heart disease and cancer, as are active smokers, they also are more likely to have respiratory illnesses often. Children who are exposed to passive smoke from parents may have poor development and reduced lung function, besides the diseases and disorders already mentioned. Those with chronic respiratory problems are obviously at greatest risk from passive smoke and these individuals certainly should keep from contact to prevent further irritation and difficulty with breathing.

Remind those who smoke to at least think about stopping. Advise them to refrain from smoking around others, especially

FIGURE 2–6 This common symbol is displayed in most public places with the notation "Thank you for not smoking."

children and those with respiratory distress. Smoke-free areas should be encouraged, respected, and applauded by those especially in the health care fields. Figure 2–6 illustrates a commonly posted sign requesting "No Smoking."

In patient education pursuits, make sure that you make them aware that tobacco contains poisons that could be fatal to toddlers if swallowed. All smoking materials should be kept out of the reach of children. Remember, the U.S. Surgeon General's report applies to everyone. **Warning:** The Surgeon General has determined that cigarette smoking is dangerous to your health.

Complete Chapter 2, Unit 3 in the workbook to help you meet the objectives at the beginning of this unit and therefore achieve competency of this subject matter.

U N I T   4
Behavior Modification

OBJECTIVES ....

Upon completion of the unit, you will meet the following terminal performance objectives by verifying knowledge of the facts and principles presented through oral and written communication at a level deemed competent by the instructor or employer.

1. List the commonly used defense mechanisms and give an example of each.
2. Explain what could happen to a person who habitually uses one or more of the defense mechanisms listed in this unit.
3. Discuss why it is necessary to know oneself before one can relate effectively to others.
4. List problem-solving steps and apply them to a particular problem you may have.
5. Explain the importance of one's mental and emotional status in regard to overall health.
6. Spell and define, using the glossary at the back of the text, all the words to know in this unit.

WORDS TO KNOW ....

adjustment	projection
analytical	rationalization
ardently	regression
denial	repression
displacement	stratagem
intellectualization	sublimation
malinger	unobtrusive

We discussed in Unit 1 of this chapter how keeping a positive attitude is of primary importance in our interactions with others. Even though we strive for a good rapport with coworkers, patients, family, and friends, we must realize that we are human beings. Perfection in any relationship, even the best one, is certainly a desirable goal, but rather unrealistic. Understanding ourselves and others is essential in meaningful communications. Often in our daily transactions of conveying and receiving messages, we use certain coping skills to keep ourselves from getting hurt or to protect our image. These complex **stratagems** are called defense mechanisms.

Defense Mechanisms ....

These defenses are largely unconscious acts we use to help us deal with unpleasant and socially unacceptable circumstances or behaviors. They help us make an emotional **adjustment** in everyday situations. Surely we all use various defense mechanisms from time to time. Habitual use, however, can cause one to become somewhat out of touch with reality.

The most commonly used defense mechanisms are repression, displacement, projection, rationalization, intellectualization, sublimation, forms of withdrawal, and malingering.

Repression The most commonly used defense mechanism is **repression**, which is the forcing of unacceptable or painful ideas, feelings, and impulses into the unconscious mind without being aware of it. Certainly, we have all wished something unpleasant would happen to another person when we have experienced feelings of hostility, jealousy, or intense anger from interacting with that person. These feelings do not vanish, but are placed in our unconscious and may surface in dreams or subtle **unobtrusive** behaviors.

Repression, like all of the defense mechanisms, tends to protect us from unwanted messages about ourselves that make us feel bad.

Displacement **Displacement** is the transfer of emotions about one to another. A typical example of displacement for the medical assistant might be as follows: In the course of the day, the medical assistant has many duties to perform for many others, and one patient in particular becomes overly demanding and rude. The medical assistant holds back the strong feelings and deals with the situation professionally. Later in the evening at home,

she feels all the pent-up anger and explodes at a family member. This is also done unconsciously, although sometimes, after the fact, we realize our actions have been displaced from the point where they originated to an innocent, unsuspecting target.

Projection In **projection**, one might blame another unconsciously for one's own inadequacies. An extreme form of projection can lead to hostile, even aggressive behavior if one perceives another to be the cause of the painful feelings. An obese patient may blame a medical assistant for his or her gaining of a few pounds saying that the scales were set up or read incorrectly.

Rationalization With **rationalization**, one justifies behavior with socially acceptable reasons and tends to ignore the real reasons underlying the behavior. This self-discipline unconscious act is relatively harmless. Habitual use of this defense mechanism, as well as all the others discussed in this unit, can become nonproductive or even destructive because they distort reality. A typical rationalization might be, "I dieted very strictly all day; therefore, it's okay to eat a couple of candy bars later in the evening after supper."

Intellectualization **Intellectualization** is still another means of denying socially unacceptable feelings or strong feelings that cannot be easily expressed. With this mechanism, one uses reasoning to avoid confronting emotional conflicts and stressful situations. One might discuss all the facts and provide endless information about how to begin caring for an elderly relative, elaborating on special diets and home health care to avoid dealing with the true feelings of sadness over a relative's illness.

Sublimation **Sublimation** is used unconsciously to express socially unacceptable instinctive drives or impulses in approved and acceptable ways. An example of sublimation might be a 30-year-old frustrated athlete forcing his child to excel in a sport.

Temporary Withdrawal Temporary withdrawal is a defense mechanism in that it is a retreat from facing a painful or difficult situation. This avoidance of something that is unpleasant is another way of protecting ourselves from disagreeable feelings. Watching TV excessively or reading to avoid dealing with an issue are common types of withdrawal.

Putting off issues only makes the situation worse. It produces anxiety and makes the problem more difficult to face the longer the withdrawal goes on.

Malingering Another common defense mechanism is **malingering**. One who malingers deliberately pretends to be sick to avoid dealing with situations that are unpleasant or that cause anxiety. A malingering individual might stay home sick on a day when he or she was to give a presentation, when in fact, that person is as healthy as always, enjoying the time at home.

Denial **Denial** seems to be a commonly used defense mechanism. It is the refusal to admit or acknowledge something so the person does not have to deal with a problem or situation. When one is not accepting of the phases of life that may produce anxiety, as an emotional defense one sometimes uses denial. It is usually seen only in psychosis in adults who have reacted to a traumatic situation of extreme stress.

When one who has been given the diagnosis of a terminal illness does not accept the reality of it and believes that a recovery is certain, that person is going through the denial stage.

Regression

Regression is behaving in ways that are typically characteristic of an earlier developmental level. This usually happens in times of high stress.

A college student consoles herself during final exam week with eating hot fudge sundaes as she did as a child with her mother whenever problems at school piled up.

Indeed, we all use many, perhaps all of these defense mechanisms from time to time. Since they are mostly used without our conscious awareness, they may be relatively harmless. Again, habitual use of defense mechanisms can veil reality and interfere with facing personal issues and crises, as well as with open and honest communication with others.

Problem Solving

In our complex daily lives, we use many coping skills to deal with our difficulties. Defense mechanisms have already been discussed. Another approach to handling interpersonal problems and concerns is to develop problem-solving skills. Taking a step-by-step approach helps one look realistically and logically at a problem. This method encourages **analytical** thinking and confident decision making. Here is an outline of the basic steps in problem solving:

1. Determine just what the problem is and write it down.
   a. Is there a problem chain or a series of events that are contributors?
2. Gather facts and ideas to help you decide what to do about it.
3. Use analytical and creative thinking. (List your decisions and what you think their outcome will be.)
4. Prioritize your decisions and begin testing them one by one until results are satisfactory to you and others concerned.

If results are not pleasing, begin again with step one. Often, step one alone triggers an answer to a problem. Sitting down and writing out what the problem actually is can be most therapeutic. Once you begin to use this skill to think logically about major problems, such as changing employment, relocating geographically, or locating a suitable day care facility, you will begin to think more logically in all matters. Making a habit of this skill will increase your peace of mind and reduce stress because you will deal with problems more efficiently and spend less time and energy worrying about what to do. This skill can be a great stride toward eliminating procrastination.

The medical assistant who concentrates on patient education may want to pass this helpful skill on to patients.

Mental and Emotional Status Influencing Behaviors ....

The medical assistant, in both administrative and clinical capacities, has many opportunities daily to observe patients' mental and emotional states. These observations have a direct influence on the medical assistants' behavior, which in turn directly influences their overall health. We must keep in mind that all medical personnel are patients too. Therefore, all of the information we learn about patients applies to us as well.

As Unit 2 points out, the stress in life can lead to ill health. A true understanding of one's self is the primary key to understanding others.

Learning about ourselves requires us to take a good hard look at who and what we really are. When assessing our "self," our individual presence may come to mind first. This presence comprises both one's physical self (our bodies) and one's self-image (how we view ourselves). Another dimension of self, as termed by psychologists, is the "self as process." This refers to the ongoing process inside us that deals with constant changes, or adjustments, in our lives.

Our response to others is dealt with by our social self. We have many different roles with which we identify **ardently.** Finally, we all have an "ideal self." This is what we picture ourselves to be, the perfect model we have of ourselves.

We are, indeed, complex beings, capable of doing just about anything we choose to. Unfortunately, many of us never come close to realizing our true potential. This may be due to never having to look at ourselves squarely. Sometimes it can be quite difficult and even unpleasant to be honest about ourselves.

A good way to begin a basic assessment of ourselves is by making a list of all the strengths we have, as well as all our weaknesses. This technique can help point out our abilities and qualities and identify areas that need to be changed.

An ideal time to reevaluate yourself and renew your goals and aspirations is annually on your birthday. Many people prefer the traditional New Year's resolution. Knowing yourself will help you become a more complete person and will help you relate to others more effectively.

Communicating Emotional States ....

In Unit 1 of this chapter, we discussed verbal and non-verbal messages. Communication is a complex process in which one must be aware of all facets for complete information exchanges to occur.

The perceptive medical assistant should be able to decide what "feeder questions" to ask a patient to determine whether the look on the patient's face matches the patient's emotional demeanor. The following are feeder questions the medical assistant may use to find out the emotional states of the patients they interview. After greeting the patient with a kind "hello," the assistant may want to ask "What seems to be the problem today?" or "What brings you here to see the doctor today?" or "Can you tell me about the problem you seem to be having?" or "Can we talk about what has been giving you concern that brings you in to see the doctor?"

For a follow-up visit, ask "Are you feeling any better since you were in to see the doctor last?" or "You don't seem to be feeling too well; do you feel any better?" or "Can you tell me how you've been doing since you were here last?"

Hearing patients' answers can provide a general idea of how they feel emotionally. Of course, one can only accomplish this by taking time to find out. That means giving the patients your undivided attention, if only for a few minutes. Unfortunately, many health care professionals lack the skills and perhaps even the concern to establish this rapport, and therefore fail to develop this skill. The medical assistant can be instrumental in pointing out factors that can interfere with a particular treatment approach planned by the physician, Figure 2–7. Patients will likely respond to and comply with the doctor's orders far more readily if the medical assistant imparts a genuine concern for their well-being with each contact.

If a patient seems quieter than usual, for instance, the medical assistant might determine after talking to the patient (with eye contact of course) that he is preoccupied by some problem or matter that he may open up about if interest is shown and the time is taken. If the patient is not allowed to express certain feelings, he may not be attentive enough to listen to the physician's orders, which need to be followed for optimal health benefits. The medical assistant plays an important role in assisting both physician and patient in providing quality health care.

Complete Chapter 2, Unit 4 in the workbook to help you meet the objectives at the beginning of this unit and therefore achieve competency of this subject matter.

1. Travel (business or pleasure)
2. Work schedule (irregular hours)
3. Relocating/moving
4. Lifestyle/cultural influences
5. Economic concerns
6. Comprehension of physician's orders
7. Handicap/mental incompetence

FIGURE 2–7 Factors that can interfere with patient compliance

MEDICAL–LEGAL ETHICAL HIGHLIGHTS

Mrs. Right . . .

keeps the patient education material updated and replenished as necessary. She posts information about meetings and support groups on the bulletin board regularly to keep patients currently informed. She makes an effort to keep attractive displays about nutritional news and advice for patients.

Employment advancement: Excellent

Ms. Wrong . . .

is lazy and doesn't provide any patient education materials. She says that it's not her job.

Employment advancement: None (Probable termination)

REFERENCES

American Cancer Society. *Eating Smart.* 1989.
American Dietetic Association. *Staying Healthy—A Guide for Elder Americans.* 1990.
Kunz, Jeffrey, R. M., ed. *The American Medical Association Family Medical Guide.* New York: Random House, 1987.
Milliken, Mary Elizabeth. *Understanding Human Behavior,* 5th ed. Albany: Delmar, 1993.
Physicians' Desk Reference. Oradell, NJ: Medical Economics, updated annually.
Sehnert, Keith W., M.D. *Stress/Unstress.* Oradell, NJ: Augsburg Publishing House, 1981.
Taber, Clarence W. *Taber's Cyclopedic Medical Dictionary,* 14th ed. Philadelphia: F. A. Davis, 1981.
United States Department of Health and Human Services, Alcohol, Drug Abuse, and Mental Health Administration. *Saying No.* Rockville, MD, 1981.
United States Department of Health and Human Services. *Diet, Nutrition, and Cancer Prevention.* Washington, D.C., 1987.
United States Department of Health and Human Services. *What You Can Do About Drug Use in America.* Publication No. (ADM) 90-1572. Washington, D.C., 1990.
United States Department of Justice, Drug Enforcement Administration. *Drugs of Abuse.* Washington, D.C., 1989.
Webster's New World Dictionary, 100,000 Entry Edition. New York: Penguin, 1971.
Wright, H. Norman. *How to Have a Creative Crisis,* Berkley ed. New York: Berkley Publishing Group, 1987.

C H A P T E R   3
Office Environmental Control

E ach medical facility has the responsibility of providing a safe environment for all who enter the premises. It is up to each individual medical staff employee to be honest and credible. For instance: only *you* will know if an item is **sterile** (or not) before it is used in an invasive procedure; When something is sterile, it is free of all living organisms. You must remove a faulty chair from the office reception area *before* someone gets hurt from falling off of it; only you will know which toys should be washed to prevent other children from contracting the disease of the child who just contaminated (i.e., coughed on) it. Your initiative and follow-through is necessary to maintain surroundings that are as safe as possible for all concerned. Each staff member should take responsibility for this ongoing endeavor. When you see that something needs to be done, *do it.* If you cannot at the instant you see a necessary duty, ask a coworker, or, *immediately* inform your supervisor or physician-employer. Many times a problem can be **averted** by taking early action. Even with the most conscientious staff there may be an occasional accident or mishap for there is no guarantee of perfection in life. Working together as a team can help to create and maintain a pleasant atmosphere, a productive working schedule, and a safer environment for all concerned. This chapter addresses these seriously important areas. You are strongly urged to follow the suggested guidelines outlined within the following pages.

UNIT 1
Asepsis

UNIT 2
Disease Transmission

UNIT 3
AIDS/Universal Precautions

UNIT 4
Care of Instruments

UNIT 5
Office Safety and Security

U N I T   1

Asepsis

OBJECTIVES ···

Upon completion of this unit, you will meet the following terminal performance objectives by verifying knowledge of the facts and principles presented through oral and written communication at a level deemed competent by the instructor or employer and will demonstrate the specific behaviors as iden-

tified in the terminal performance objectives of the procedures, observing all aseptic and safety precautions in accordance with health care standards.

1. Discuss the medical assistant's role and responsibility in environmental control.
2. List potential hazards and problems in a medical facility and the action that should be taken for each.
3. List housekeeping items or supplies that should be on hand for use as necessary.
4. Describe daily routine care of the medical facility.
5. Explain the importance of proper handwashing.
6. Demonstrate the proper procedure for handwashing.

7. List the good habits a medical assistant should practice to reduce disease transmission.
8. Spell and define, using the glossary at the back of the text, all the words to know in this unit.

WORDS TO KNOW ....

asepsis   invasive

averted   microorganisms

biohazardous   pathogens

contaminate   sterile

infections

Part of the daily schedule of any health care provider includes environmental control. Some of the guidelines for maintaining safe environmental control are contained in this unit dealing with **asepsis.** Asepsis is the state of being free from pathogenic organisms. Since all medical facilities are a prime target for pathogenic organisms, it is extremely important that vigilance is upheld. There are many duties that need to be performed on a daily basis. These duties should already be outlined in job descriptions for each employee. If they are not, the supervisor or office manager should assign a daily schedule of necessary duties to help ensure a clean and safe environment for everyone.

Most every business that deals with the public has a contracted cleaning service (often referred to as environmental or custodial services). Even though this may be the case, a well-run facility, especially a medical practice, should be prepared for maintaining the environment as necessary until these services can be secured. There are several housekeeping items which should be available for cleaning up when needed. The following is a list of cleaning supplies and equipment which may be useful: broom, dust pan, vacuum cleaner, mop, bucket, sponges, cleaning solutions, bleach, dust cloths, disposable plastic trash bags, **biohazardous** puncture-proof containers and bags, disposable emesis basins, glass cleaner, and disposable paper towels. A disinfectant spray is also good to keep on hand to disinfect small areas and to help eliminate odors.

A *daily* inspection of the *entire* facility should be performed *before* patients arrive. Surfaces (and door knobs and plates) should be dusted or washed as necessary. Using alcohol or a spray cleaner and paper towels is a quick and easy way to spot clean these areas. Many offices provide children with child-scale furniture and, of course, toys to keep them occupied while waiting to see the doctor. These items should be made of washable materials so that they can be cleaned (washed with soap and water) as necessary (at least daily) to prevent disease transmission to other young patients.

There should be a designated "well" and "sick" waiting area in the reception room. If there is not enough room to separate the patients who are obviously sick and who could possibly **contaminate** others in the reception area, the sick patients should be brought to an examination room immediately upon arrival. This should be explained to others waiting so they will not feel overlooked.

The reception area should provide a neat, comfortable area free of drafts. It should be both well lighted and properly ven-

tilated. The ideal temperature of the facility should be approximately 72° F. Seating should not be placed directly under, over, or beside blowers, heating, or cooling vents. Furniture, lamps, carpet, and so forth should be inspected and cleaned as necessary. Any repairs or replacements should also be made as soon as possible whenever necessary.

All equipment and supplies in the medical facility should be inspected daily and any repairs or replacements should be made or arranged for immediately to keep the schedule flowing smoothly and to avoid any unnecessary accidents or injuries that could be caused from using faulty equipment or supplies. All examination rooms should be cleaned and well stocked daily.

Appropriate reading material (including patient education materials) should be provided in an orderly fashion. A sign stating advice in case of an accident or problem, and to alert those who may be **infectious** should be posted where all patients can see it clearly. The following is an example:

For Your Safety and Health

Please:

1. Report any safety hazard or emergency to the receptionist immediately.

2. Use tissues provided to cover your mouth and nose to catch your coughs and sneezes.

3. Dispose of all waste in the plastic-lined waste can.

4. Tell receptionist if you feel nausea or need to use the restroom.

You should discourage patients from eating or drinking in the reception area. A quick check of the reception area each time you call patients in will alert you to any **potential** hazards. You should empty the trash as necessary because it not only adds clutter and mess, but attracts insects and other pests. If, however, there are any pests or insects found in the facility, they should be eliminated by a professional pest control service immediately.

Clearly post signs showing the location of exits, rest rooms, water fountains, and public phones in your facility.

As you establish a routine for the maintenance of environmental control you will see that it is not as overwhelming as it may now seem. It is much easier to learn good habits than to break bad ones.

Handwashing ....

The first responsibility of all health care providers is to learn to properly wash their hands before beginning the daily routine.

It is also important to repeat this procedure after breaks, lunch, before and after gloving, and handling specimens or any soiled materials or waste. Do not lean into or against sinks, medical supplies, and equipment. Be careful not to touch soiled items or waste with your hands or body or you will contaminate whatever is touched. You must guard against any possible disease transmission to yourself and others at all times. You should avoid touching your hands to your face and mouth. After using tissues you should wash your hands. Practice what you teach patients and cover your mouth and nose with a disposable tissue when you cough or sneeze. This can diminish spreading your germs considerably. If you have a cold or sniffles you should work away from contact with patients and other workers to prevent transmission of your infection. When you are sick and feverish you should stay home until you are fever-free for at least 24 hours.

Since one potential problem in any medical practice is disease transmission, precautions must be taken to reduce this dangerous possibility. **Microorganisms** that are the cause of disease are called **pathogens.** They have certain requirements for growth and multiplication. If one uses steps to prevent or interrupt their growth, disease transmission can be reduced. The requirements of microbial growth are covered in Unit 2 of this chapter. Breaking the infection cycle prevents the spread of disease.

Proper handwashing helps to remove microorganisms from the skin and from finger rings, but minimal jewelry should be worn because it is impossible to eliminate all pathogens from the crevices in them unless the items are autoclaved. Autoclaving is not recommended because it is damaging to most jewelry as well as being highly impractical, and time-consuming.

Many health care professionals use a foamed alcohol product for frequent handwashing. For routine handwashing the foam is applied and spread over the hands for approximately a minute until dry. A surgical scrub can be done with the foam by using a generous application to the hands and forearms for approximately 1½ minutes, and then repeating an application of the foam to the hands for 30 seconds and spreading it over the hands until dry. The foam is an alternative to removing germs from the skin to prevent disease transmission. This method may be the answer for those who have problems with dry skin because this foam is said to be less drying and irritating than some products used to clean the hands.

You should pay special attention to each step of the handwashing procedure shown in the Procedure box. Learning how to perform this essential procedure is a valuable means of preventing disease transmission.

Complete Chapter 3, Unit 1 in the workbook to help you meet the objectives at the beginning of this unit and therefore achieve competency of this subject matter.

U N I T 2
Disease Transmission

OBJECTIVES

Upon completion of this unit, you will meet the following terminal performance objectives by verifying knowledge of the facts and principles presented through oral and written communication at a level deemed competent by the instructor or employer and will demonstrate the specific behaviors as iden-

tified in the terminal performance objectives of the procedures, observing all aseptic and safety precautions in accordance with health care standards.

1. List patient education suggestions to prevent tranmitting disease.
2. Describe methods of controlling the growth of microorganisms.
3. List the growth requirements of microorganisms.
4. Describe the infection cycle of disease transmission.
5. Describe the body's defense against disease.
6. Explain the difference between sanitization and disinfection.
7. Locate and interpret from the communicable disease chart the means of transmission, incubation time, symptoms, and treatment for a given disease.
8. Spell and define, using the glossary in the back of the text, all the words to know in this unit.

WORDS TO KNOW

aerobe	morphology
anaerobes	nits
autotrophs	obligate
bacteria	organic
coma	parasite
confinement	petechial
debilitated	pH
droplet	protozoa
facultative	pruritic
fecal	pustular
flora	resistance
fungi	seizures
heterotrophs	spores
hygiene	susceptible
inorganic	vulnerable
malaise	virulence
microorganism	virus

The medical assistant who has a basic understanding of the pathogens that cause disease will be more careful to use preventive measures. The following basic information should be helpful in gaining a respect for universal precautions in the fight against disease transmission.

Disease Transmission

Microorganisms cannot be seen with the naked eye. Commonly known microorganisms are viruses, bacteria, protozoa, fungi, and parasites. Disease-producing microorganisms are called pathogens.

Bacteria are unicellular microorganisms that vary in their **morphology.** Figure 3–2, page 55, shows the various forms of bacteria. Many different species of bacteria are pathogenic to humans and animals. Some examples: *Escherichia coli* causes

Handwashing

TERMINAL PERFORMANCE OBJECTIVE: Provided with liquid hand soap in a dispenser, cuticle stick, nail brush, paper towels, and waste receptacle, the student will stand at a sink with hot and cold faucets and demonstrate each step in the handwashing procedure as specified in the procedure sheet.

EQUIPMENT: A liquid soap dispenser is desirable. It eliminates the possibility of dropping a bar of soap in the sink or on the floor during the procedure. It is also more economical and more attractive. Bar soap is often wasted as it becomes soft and starts to separate. The water that collects in the soap dish is also a good environment for microorganisms and therefore cancels the effort made in removing them from the hands.

1. Remove all jewelry: rings, bracelets, (wedding rings may be left on but must be scrubbed). **RATIONALE: Jewelry harbors microorganisms.**

2. Stand at sink and turn faucets on using paper towel to avoid direct contact with faucets, Figure 3–1a. Adjust water temperature to moderately warm and discard paper towel. Leave water running at desired temperature. **RATIONALE: The sink and faucets are considered contaminated; water temperature must be properly adjusted because once the procedure is begun, the faucets cannot be touched.**

3. Wet hands and press soap dispenser to obtain approximately 1 teaspoon of soap in palm of one hand. Work soap into lather and distribute soap over both palms and backs of hands in circular motions constantly and vigorously for 2 minutes. Keep hands lower than forearms. **RATIONALE: Circular motion and friction is more effective. Removed soil and water flows into sink not onto arms. Figures 3–1b and 3–1c.**

4. Use nail brush or orange stick to dislodge microorganisms around cuticles and under nails. Figures 3–1d and 3–1e.

5. Rinse well, being careful not to touch inside of sink or faucets during procedure. Figure 3–1f.

6. Rinse hands thoroughly. Leave water running and reach for sufficient paper towels to dry hands completely.

7. Turn off faucet with paper towel and discard in waste container. **RATIONALE: Touching faucet would contaminate clean hands. Figure 3–1g.**

Refer to the patient education section for guidelines that all health care professionals should also follow.

FIGURE 3–1a A dry paper towel should be used to turn the faucet on. (Courtesy of Hegner & Caldwell, *Nursing Assistant: A Nursing Process Approach,* 6th ed. © Albany: Delmar, 1992.)

FIGURE 3–1b Fingertips should be pointed down while washing hands. Use the palm of one hand to clean the back of the other hand. (Courtesy of Hegner & Caldwell, *Nursing Assistant: A Nursing Process Approach,* 6th ed. © Albany: Delmar, 1992.)

FIGURE 3–1c Interlace the fingers to clean between them. (Courtesy of Hegner & Caldwell, *Nursing Assistant: A Nursing Process Approach,* 6th ed. © Albany: Delmar, 1992.)

Handwashing *(continued)*

FIGURE 3–1d Use the blunt end of an orange cuticle stick to clean the nails. (Courtesy of Hegner & Caldwell, *Nursing Assistant: A Nursing Process Approach,* 6th ed. © Albany: Delmar, 1992.)

FIGURE 3–1f Rinse the hands thoroughly with the fingertips down. (Courtesy of Hegner & Caldwell, *Nursing Assistant: A Nursing Process Approach,* 6th ed. © Albany: Delmar, 1992.)

FIGURE 3–1e Another way to clean under the fingernails is to use a hand brush. (Courtesy of Hegner & Caldwell, *Nursing Assistant: A Nursing Process Approach,* 6th ed. © Albany: Delmar, 1992.)

FIGURE 3–1g Use paper towels to dry hands and to turn off water faucets. (Courtesy of Hegner & Caldwell, *Nursing Assistant: A Nursing Process Approach,* 6th ed. © Albany: Delmar, 1992.)

urinary tract infections (among other illnesses) in humans; *Bordetella pertussis* causes whooping cough, which is transmitted by **droplet** infection; and *Vibrio cholerae* causes cholera in humans who ingest contaminated food and water.

Viruses, which are the smallest of the microorganisms, may be viewed only by an electron microscope. Figure 3–3, page 55, shows a magnified view of a virus. Viruses can only reproduce themselves within a host. Commonly known viruses cause herpes, most childhood diseases, the common cold, and influenza.

Protozoa are complex single-celled microorganisms that attach themselves to other organisms, Figure 3–4, page 56. Amebic dysentery, malaria, and trichomonas vaginalis are diseases caused by protozoa.

Fungi are simple parasitic plants (molds) that depend on other life forms for a nutritional source. They reproduce by budding. Multicellular fungi reproduce by spore formation. Approximately 100 fungi are common in humans; however, only 10 of these are pathogenic. Some examples of pathogenic fungus conditions are histoplasmosis caused by *Histoplasma capsulatum,* and tinea pedis (athlete's foot), Figure 3–5.

Parasites are organisms that depend on another living organism for nourishment. An **obligate** parasite is one that depends completely on its host for survival. **Facultative** parasites are able to live independently from their hosts at times. Protozoa, mentioned earlier, are internal parasites for they live within the body of a human or an animal. *External parasites* are those that attach

FIGURE 3–2a–c Bacterial forms: **(a)** *Escherichia coli.* (b) *Haemophilus pertussis.* (c) *Vibrio cholerae.* (Courtesy of Centers for Disease Control, Atlanta, GA)

FIGURE 3–3 Electron micrographs of the various types of herpes simplex virus. (Courtesy of Centers for Disease Control, Atlanta, GA)

themselves on the outside of the body, such as fleas and ticks on animals. Humans are sometimes troubled with the itch mite (scabies), pinworms (Enterobius vermicularis) and hookworms (ancylostomiasis), Figure 3–6. Other microorganisms are helpful and necessary to normal **flora** in humans and animals for they provide a balance in the body and destroy pathogens.

Microorganisms that feed on **organic** matter are called **heterotrophs;** those that feed on **inorganic** matter are called **autotrophs.** Those that need oxygen to grow are called **aerobes,** and those that grow best in the absence of oxygen are called **anaerobes.** Microorganisms grow best at the average body temperature (98.6°F or 37°C). The human body has not only a desirable temperature for microbial growth, but also furnishes darkness and moisture, other growth requirements. In addition, the body has a neutral **pH,** making it a prime target for infection (Figure 3–7). An environment that is too acid or too alkaline will not support microbial growth.

Disease begins when a pathogen finds a body (a host) that offers it the conditions necessary for growth, Figure 3–8, page 58. Microorganisms, in the proper growth environment, can be extremely **virulent,** particularly for **debilitated,** aged, or young **vulnerable** patients. When the microorganism has reached the stage of causing an infection, the patient should take precautions against transmitting it to another. **Confinement** is the best way, but many patients insist on taking their colds and flu to work or play. The next step in the cycle, then, is transmission to another person by way of body openings. The microorganisms leave the host through the discharge of body secretions and make either direct or indirect contact with another host. When a patient with a cold coughs or sneezes, for example, the vapor contains the microorganism that is causing the infection. Someone else may then breathe in that microorganism. This is called *droplet infection* and is a form of indirect contact. Direct

FIGURE 3–4 Intestinal protozoa *Entamoeba coli.* (Courtesy of Centers for Disease Control, Atlanta, GA)

FIGURE 3–5 Ringworm of the foot (tinea pedis). (Courtesy of Centers for Disease Control, Atlanta, GA)

FIGURE 3–6 *Strongyloides*—filariform larvae of hookworm and roundworm. (Courtesy of Centers for Disease Control, Atlanta, GA)

contact is through touch. The growth requirement is then a **susceptible** host, or one whose body **resistance** is low because of poor nutritional habits, or poor hygiene.

Disease Prevention

To prevent the spread of diseases caused by microorganisms it is necessary to provide a defense against them. Becoming aware that the threat of disease is always present will assist you in taking the necessary precautions. Routine cleaning procedures, such as disinfecting room equipment and surfaces, are a means of disease control. Patients should be educated in this area, and it is the responsibility of the medical assistant and the other members of the health care team to see that it is practiced. Refer to Table 3–1, pages 59–60, to learn the common communicable diseases, means of transmission, incubation time, symptoms, and treatment.

Another defense against disease is maintenance of good health through good health habits of proper rest, nutrition, and **hygiene.** Exercise is most helpful in resisting disease because it promotes circulation, encourages nutrition, and reduces stress.

The body also has defense mechanisms. In the respiratory tract are hairlike cilia that filter out invading pathogens. Coughing and sneezing are reflexes to rid the body of invaders. Body secretions, such as tears, sweat, urine, and mucus, also wash pathogens from the body.

The body secretions have a low pH, which discourages bacterial growth. In the digestive tract, hydrochloric acid discourages the growth of pathogens with its low pH.

The methods of preventing disease transmission in the medical practice are many. Sanitization is one that has already been described. *Sanitization* is washing and scrubbing to remove such material as body tissue, blood, or other body fluids. You should wear gloves during this process to protect your hands from any possibility of contamination from the articles which you handle. Gloves also protect your hands from dryness, which may result in chafing and cracking of the skin and possibly lead to infection. Items should be rinsed in cool water, soaked in a detergent solution, usually for 20 minutes, washed thoroughly with a brush, rinsed in warm to hot water to remove the detergent, and dried.

Disinfection is a process by which disease-producing microorganisms are killed. There are many disinfectant solutions in use. The most common are zephirin chloride and chlorophenyl. Disinfectants are used on objects, not patients. They are chemical solutions that must be changed often to ensure their effect. Antiseptics are used in preparing the patient's skin for injection or surgical procedures. The most commonly used are alcohol and Betadine (povidone–iodine).

Disinfectants and antiseptics do not always kill spores, however. **Spores** are thick-walled hard capsules formed by some bacteria when conditions for growth are poor. When the proper growth requirements are present the bacteria break out of the capsule, grow, and multiply to start infection. An example of bacteria that produce spores is *Clostridum tetani,* the cause of tetanus, or lock jaw.

Complete Chapter 3, Unit 2 in the workbook to help you

The medical assistant has a perfect opportunity to instruct patients in the area of basic aseptic technique. During the patients' scheduled appointments it is appropriate to inform patients about proper handwashing and other methods to use at home, especially when one is sick, in preventing the transfer of disease to others. Good personal hygiene practice should be stressed to patients. The following general guidelines are suggested to help decrease the possibility of disease transmission among family members and others who share living, work, or social facilities:

1. Frequent handwashing before and after: especially when taking care of one who is ill, eating, using the toilet, touching soiled objects, or being in direct contact with and body fluids.

2. Encourage daily personal hygiene: shower or bath, dental care, clean clothes and bedding.

3. Always properly wash glasses, dishes, and utensils before reuse (when one is ill with a highly contagious disease, it is best to use disposable items to decrease the possibility of spreading the disease). Remind patients *not* to share their germs by eating, drinking, or smoking after one another.

4. Instruct patients to cough and sneeze into a disposable tissue, use once, and discard in a paper or plastic bag and dispose of properly. (Figure 3–7a and b)

5. Advise patients about the importance of proper ventilation and light (microorganisms do not prosper in a lighted and well-ventilated area).

6. Remind patients to wash hands after touching door knobs, railings, handles, and so on, to avoid the possibility of getting or giving invisible microorganisms.

7. Advise patients to use a commercial disinfectant routinely to clean bathrooms and kitchens (as well as other rooms in the house as necessary) to eliminate germs and discourage insects and rodents that carry disease.

8. Urge sexually active patients of adolescent age and older to use condoms properly to prevent spread of sexually transmitted diseases, AIDS, and hepatitis B (discretion must be used).

9. Remind patients about immunization schedules and urge them to follow them carefully.

As item number 6 advises, all microorganisms are invisible to the naked eye. Therefore, it is easy to forget that they are everywhere. The medical assistant can be most influential in educating others in ways to reduce the threat of disease by following these basic guidelines.

FIGURE 3–7 (A) Patient coughing or sneezing into a tissue to prevent the spread of microorganisms to others. (B) Patient properly discarding used tissue into waste receptacle.

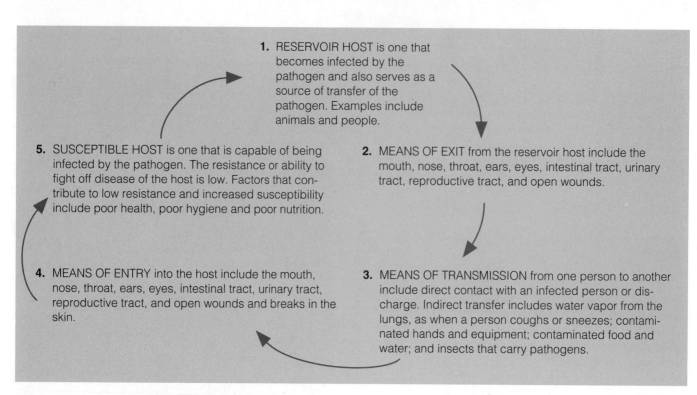

FIGURE 3–8 The infection cycle

meet the objectives at the beginning of this unit and therefore achieve competency of this subject matter.

U N I T   3
AIDS/Universal Precautions

OBJECTIVES

Upon completion of this unit, you will meet the following terminal performance objectives by verifying knowledge of the facts and principles presented through oral and written communication at a level deemed competent by the instructor or employer and will demonstrate the specific behaviors as identified in the terminal performance objectives of the procedures, observing all aseptic and safety precautions in accordance with health care standards.

1. Explain the purpose of compliance with universal precautions.
2. Discuss the recommended universal precautions in regard to human tissue, blood, and body fluids.
3. State the purpose of gloving and other protective barriers in regard to universal precautions.
4. List risks and responsibilities health care workers have regarding themselves and patients.
5. Explain the recommended written statement (and the reason for it) concerning universal precautions that should be in the physician's office laboratory.

6. Spell and define, using the glossary in the back of the text, all the words to know in this unit.

WORDS TO KNOW

bloodborne	perinatal
documentation	obligation
mandatory	resuscitation

The medical assistant who has a basic understanding of the pathogens that cause disease will be more careful to be mindful of preventive measures. The following basic information should be helpful in gaining a respect for universal precautions in the fight against disease transmission.

In addition to giving special regard to patients, health care workers have the responsibility of self-protection. It is recommended that universal blood and body fluid precautions be used for all patients, especially when the infection status of the patient is unknown. Appropriate protection against exposure to blood and body fluids should be routine practice for all health care workers. Gloves should be worn when in contact (direct or indirect) with blood or any body fluids, mucous membranes, or nonintact skin; in handling items or surfaces soiled with blood or body fluid; and when performing venipuncture or any other surgical procedure. After each patient contact, gloves should be changed. If procedures could possibly generate droplets of blood or other body fluids, the health care worker should wear shields to protect the eyes or face in addition to gloves and gown. This will protect the mucous membranes of the eyes, mouth, and nose.

TABLE 3–1
Communicable Diseases

Disease	Means of Transmission	Incubation	Symptoms	Treatment
AIDS (Acquired immunodeficiency syndrome)*	Direct contact: sexual, anal, or vaginal intercourse, sharing IV drug needles, infected mother to child (childbirth), blood to blood (from cuts, scrapes, punctures of skin) Indirect contact: blood transfusions	Onset of AIDS following infection with human immunodeficiency virus (HIV) from 6 months to 10 years +	Early—loss of appetite, weight loss, fever, night sweats, skin rashes, diarrhea, fatigue, poor resistance to infections, swollen lymph nodes Later—cough, fever, shortness of breath, dyspnea, purple blotches on the skin	Research and new developments continue in the search for a cure and a vaccine. Current treatment most commonly used is zidovudine (AZT)
Chickenpox* (Varicellazoster virus)	Direct or indirect contact, droplet, or airborne secretion of infected person	2–3 weeks, usually 13–17 days	Crops of **pruritic** vesicular eruptions on the skin, slight fever and headache, **malaise**	Bed rest, topical antipruritics
Common Colds (Upper respiratory infection—URI)	Direct or indirect contact with infected person	12–72 h (some viruses 2–7 days), usually 24 h	Slight sore throat, watery eyes, runny nose, sneezing, chills, malaise, low-grade fever	Rest, decongestant, mild analgesics, increased fluid intake
Conjunctivitis* (Pink eye)	Direct or indirect contact with discharge from eyes or upper respiratory tract of infected person	Viral: 24 h to days Bacterial: 24–72 h	Redness of eyes, itching, burning of eyes, matted eyelashes	Antibacterial agents, antibiotics, corticosteroids depending on causative agent
Head Lice* (Pediculosis)	Direct contact with infected person; indirect contact, rare	1 wk (**nits,** or eggs, hatch in 1 wk, mature in 2 wks)	Itching of scalp, presence of small light gray lice and nits (eggs) at the base of hairs	Topical use of 1% lindane: shampoo, lotion, or cream (7–10 days); comb nits from hair; launder washable items in hot water with hottest drying cycle, dry–clean or seal in plastic bags nonwashable items (2 wks); Thoroughly vacuum the environment
Haemophilus influenzae Type b Hib (H-flu)*	Direct and indirect contact and droplet infection from respiratory tract	3 days+	URI symptoms, fever, aches, sleepiness, no appetite; as disease progresses, child is irritable and fussy	Antibiotics, increased fluid intake, antipyretics, rest, analgesics
Hepatitis A* (Acute infective hepatitis)	Direct contact or by **fecal**–contaminated food or water	14–50 days, avg. 25–30 days	Slow onset, fever, malaise, loss of appetite, nausea, vomiting, jaundice, weakness, dark urine, whitish stool	Bed rest, increased fluid intake, proper nourishment (no fats or alcohol)
Hepatitis B* (Serum hepatitis)	Contaminated serum in blood transfusion or by use of contaminated needles or instruments	14–50 days	Same as above, of rapid onset, of acute symptoms	Same as above
Herpes Simplex Virus (HSV) (Cold sores, fever blisters)	Direct contact with infected person	2–14 days, usually 4–6 days	Painful blisters on lips, which turn **pustular** and then form crusted scabs; oral lesions are small ulcerated areas	Topical applications of drying medications. Antibiotics for secondary infections
Impetigo	Direct contact with draining sores	2–10 days	Blisterlike lesions (later become crusted), itching	Cleansing of areas with antibacterial soap and water, topical and/or oral antibiotics
Influenza*	Direct and indirect contact and by airborne secretions.	1–3 days	Sudden onset of fever, chills, headache, sore muscles, malaise, (commonly runny nose, sore throat, and cough)	Bed rest, increased fluid intake, antipyretics
Meningitis* (Aseptic)	Direct contact, fecal–oral route, and respiratory secretions	2–21 days	Sudden or gradual fever, intense headache, nausea, vomiting, stiff neck, irritability, sluggishness	Hospitalization, bed rest, increased fluid intake, antipyretics, analgesics

TABLE 3–1
Communicable Diseases (continued)

Disease	Means of Transmission	Incubation	Symptoms	Treatment
Meningitis* (Bacterial) Haemophilus and Meningococcal	Direct contact and droplet infection from respiratory tract	1–10 days, usually 3–4 days	Sudden onset, fever, intense headache, nausea, vomiting; sometimes **petechial** rash, irritability, sluggishness (possible **seizures** and/or **coma**)	Same as above plus antibiotics, by intravenous and/or oral administration
Pinworms (*Enterobius vermicularis*)	Direct transfer of eggs from anus to mouth; indirect contact with eggs in clothing, bedding	3 weeks–3 months	Anal itching, insomnia, irritability	Anthelmintics, initiate scrupulous personal hygiene, shorten fingernails. Launder washable items in hottest or boiled water
Scabies*	Direct contact or indirect contact with infected clothing or bedding	2–6 weeks	Intense itching of small raised areas of skin that contain fluid or tiny burrows under the skin, resembling a line—may be anywhere on the body	Topical scabicide, oral antihistamines, and sabicylates to reduce itching
Strep Throat	Direct contact	1–3 days	Fever, red and sore throat, pus spots on back of throat, tender and swollen glands of neck	Antibiotics, analgesics, antipyretics, increase fluid intake
Scarlet Fever* (Scarlatina) (Streptococcal)	Direct or indirect contact	1–7 days	Same as above, plus strawberry tongue, rash of skin and inside mouth, high fever, nausea, and vomiting	Same as above, plus bed rest

After gloves are removed, hands should be thoroughly washed. If hands or other skin surfaces have been in contact with blood or other body fluids, they should be washed immediately.

At all times, extreme caution must be used by health care workers in handling needles, scalpels, and other sharp instruments to avoid self-injury. To prevent possible self-injury, it is recommended that needles should never be recapped, broken off, or removed from disposable syringes by hand after use. They should be carefully placed in puncture-proof biohazard containers near the area for practical purposes. Reusable needles should be placed in a receptacle (puncture-proof) for sanitization and sterilization.

All infectious waste must be disposed of by placing each contaminated item in its appropriate biohazardous waste container provided by the agency specified by your employer. Any disposable material that has even a trace of human tissue, blood, or other body fluid on it must be considered as infectious and must be treated with extreme caution. Latex gloves must be worn when handling any contaminated item to reduce the possibility of disease transmission, especially human immunodeficiency virus (HIV), acquired immunodeficiency syndrome (AIDS), and hepatitis B virus. The precautions are recommended for all health care professionals by the Centers for Disease Control (CDC) and the U.S. Public Health Service.

It is recommended that disposable mouthpieces, resuscitation bags, or any other ventilation supplies necessary should be used for emergency mouth-to-mouth **resuscitation**. This is a precaution that must be carried out because the health care status of the victim is unknown. This wise practice is meant to protect both patient and health care worker.

Those health care providers who have cuts or skin conditions, such as a dermatitis that has lesions that are either bleeding or seeping, must refrain from direct patient care until the condition clears up because of the risk of direct disease transmission. Caution should also be used in handling equipment and supplies. The infected person should be bandaged and gloved properly to keep the condition contained.

Any female health care provider who is pregnant (or could possibly be pregnant) and works directly with patients whose health status is unknown should be especially cautious. If a female contracts the HIV infection while pregnant, the unborn fetus is at risk of contracting the fatal disease through **perinatal** transmission. Strict precautions must be followed by all health care professionals to reduce the risk of HIV transmissions.

Refer to Chapter 4 Unit 9 for detailed information about AIDS and HIV. *All* patients must be treated as though they are infected. This is a practice that will help prevent you from being careless and possibly contracting one of these deadly diseases. Remember that good habits are easier to learn than breaking bad ones. Keeping ever mindful about these guidelines, you must also remember to treat all patients with respect and compassion regardless of their health status. Treating others as you would like to be treated is a good rule to follow.

New statistics and information concerning AIDS and HIV and other diseases as well appear almost daily. You should keep up with the new findings and post new material in the patient education area. Often in-service presentations are given for employees to keep abreast of current practices and findings. You have an **obligation** to keep current so that you can answer patients' questions intelligently and sufficiently.

Within the procedures in this text are specific reminders of the universal precautions which you should pay special attention to in performing.

Universal precautions must be practiced by all health care providers to be in **compliance** with the standards set by the Occupational Safety and Health Administration (OSHA). Universal precautions have been recommended by the Centers for Disease Control since 1987. They have now become a *federal regulation* and are **mandatory.** Those who do not follow these regulations will be fined. Knowledge of the precautions will not be of use unless the knowledge is put into practice.

The physician's office laboratory (POL), including all personnel, should have a statement in writing that agrees with compliance of OSHA regulations. When employees understand that this is for their protection and the patients they serve, cooperation is achieved. Knowing that these regulations are for the purpose of saving lives makes them far easier to follow. Posting this statement in the lab will hopefully keep members of the staff from becoming careless in performing procedures. The following is an example of how a universal precautions statement should read:

Universal Precautions

All employees in this medical practice must follow universal precautions at all times in performing procedures that may expose them to **bloodborne pathogens** possibly contained in the blood and body fluids from any patient regardless of the patient's health status. All employees must wear protective barriers that are appropriate for the procedure being performed to prevent possible infection. Employees who work with direct patient contact must have HBV vaccine. Any and all accidental needle sticks or other injuries, or contacts with a potentially infectious body fluid must be reported to the physician at once for treatment and **documentation.**

This statement must be signed and dated by the employer. Employees are usually given written guidelines for study and review. Paying strict attention to these precautions may save your life.

Complete Chapter 3, Unit 3 in the workbook to help you meet the objectives at the beginning of this unit and therefore achieve competency of this subject matter.

U N I T 4
Care of Instruments

OBJECTIVES ....

Upon completion of this unit, you will meet the following terminal performance objectives by verifying knowledge of the facts and principles presented through oral and written communication at a level deemed competent by the instructor or employer and will demonstrate the specific behaviors as identified in the terminal performance objectives of the procedures, observing all aseptic and safety precautions in accordance with health care standards.

1. Explain the purpose of sterilization.
2. Discuss the difference between sanitization, disinfection, and sterilization.
3. Explain the reasons for sterilizing all used items, even disposables, before discarding.
4. State the purpose of autoclaving.
5. Discuss the importance of safety when using the autoclave.
6. Demonstrate the proper procedure for wrapping items to be autoclaved.
7. Explain the purpose of using sterilization indicators for autoclaving.
8. Spell and define, using the glossary in the back of the text, all the words to know in this unit.

WORDS TO KNOW ....

autoclave	invasive
biohazardous	sterile
incineration	sterilization

Processing items and instruments for use in procedures that are **invasive** is a vitally important responsibility. When handling any of the instruments or articles that need to be sanitized, disinfected, or prepared for sterilization, you should always wear gloves. This will protect you from becoming contaminated with any possible lingering microorganisms on the item. It will also protect the item from any possible contamination from your hands. Whenever you have a cold or the sniffles, you should glove and mask to avoid disease transmission. Never sneeze or cough on or over any items you are preparing for any procedure. Always follow universal precautions in performing procedures with patient contact.

Since there are microorganisms everywhere, the medical assistant should be ever mindful that pathogens could be present. Practicing proper handwashing and developing good habits is essential in disease control and eliminating the fear of contracting disease.

Something that is free of all living microorganisms and spores is considered **sterile.** *Sterilization* is the process that destroys all forms of living microorganisms. Many types of sterilization techniques are used in medical practice. The most common method is **autoclaving.** However, sharp instruments become dull from sterilizing by this method. Rubber or vinyl articles are damaged by intense heat of autoclaving. An alternative method for these items is to place them in a chemical disinfectant for at least 20 minutes. This disinfectant solution must completely cover the instruments to be effective. The disinfectant must be changed periodically. The number of articles placed in this solution will determine how frequently it must be changed. Obviously, the more you use the solution for sterilizing items, the more often it needs to be changed. If this means of sterilizing instruments is only occasional, changing the solution once a week should be sufficient, Figure 3–9.

Every medical practice should have an autoclave for sterilization of instruments by steam under pressure, which is the only method that guarantees the destruction of spores. The manufacturer's instructions should be followed for the operation and care of the equipment. Instructions are usually printed either on top of the machine or on a tray that pulls out underneath it. It is important that the desired temperature of the sterilizer be maintained for the proper amount of time. Table 3–2 lists the most commonly used articles and the desired times and temperatures for sterilization.

In the process of sterilization the autoclave exerts approximately 15 pounds of steam pressure per square inch at a temperature between 250° and 254°F. The steam flows through the items and destroys all microorganisms and spores, Figure 3–10.

Articles to be autoclaved must be sanitized and then wrapped in a double thickness of paper or muslin. Envelope packaging is manufactured for some instruments such as scissors, Figure 3–11. Figure 3–12, page 64, shows a medical assistant inserting an instrument into an envelope type of packaging in preparation for autoclaving. A section on the paper envelope permits recording the instrument name, the date, and the initials of the person who sterilized it. Sterilization indicators register proper and complete sterilization, Figure 3–13, page 64. Autoclave tape has an indicator stripe that changes color when the proper temperature has been maintained for a long enough time for sterilization to have taken place. The same principle applies to indicators placed inside the wrapped package.

Some offices or medical centers use the autoclaving service of a hospital. In this case, minimum cleaning is all that is necessary, for all items are properly sanitized before autoclaving.

With the identification of the disease AIDS, universal precautions must be taken to eliminate the transmission of this virus. Extreme caution must be practiced whenever the medical assistant, or any member of the health care team, comes into contact with any body fluid. Appropriate barriers, such as latex gloves, goggles, masks, or other protective coverings must be worn when procedures performed on patients could cause possible contamination.

All items, whether disposable or reusable, must be properly autoclaved. The sterilized disposables may then be discarded in proper receptacles without fear of transmitting the AIDS virus. Blood and other body fluid specimens must also be sterilized before discarding.

FIGURE 3–9 Chemical disinfectant solutions are used for aseptic control of sharp instruments (dulled by autoclaving) and other articles damaged by the intense heat of autoclaving. (Courtesy Simmers, *Diversified Health Occupations,* 3rd ed. © Albany: Delmar Publishers, Inc., 1993)

FIGURE 3–10 The (a) incorrect and (b) correct way to place jars of dressings in the sterilizer.

Many companies provide this service for medical facilities with large volumes. They supply containers in various sizes for disposables and schedule periodic pickup of these **biohazardous** items to take back to the company for sterilization before discarding in general city trash dumps.

Any disposable items, such as needles (never recap), scalpels, suture removal forceps and scissors, and the like, must be placed in the container, Figure 3–14, for company sterilization or wrapped and sterilized before discarding in a general trash receptacle.

Another type of sterilization is by flame. This is a method for completely destroying disposable items by **incineration.** Items that will be treated in this way must be properly bagged for the procedure so that anyone handling the contaminated articles will not be affected.

TABLE 3–2
Sterilization Times and Temperatures

Articles	Time 250° to 254° (121° to 123°C)
Glassware. empty. inverted	15 minutes
Instruments. metal in covered or open tray. padded or unpadded	
Needles. unwrapped	
Syringes. unassembled. unwrapped	
Flasked solutions. 75–250 mL	
Instruments. metal combined with other materials in covered and/or padded tray	20 minutes
Instruments wrapped in double-thickness muslin	
Rubber gloves. catheters. drains. tubing, etc. unwrapped or wrapped in muslin or paper	
Dressings. wrapped in paper or muslin—small packs only	
Flasked solutions, 500–1000 mL	
Needles. individually packaged in glass tubes or paper	
Syringes. unassembled. individually packed in muslin or paper	30 minutes
Sutures. silk, cotton, or nylon. wrapped in paper or muslin	
Treatment trays. wrapped in muslin or paper	

FIGURE 3–11   Envelope-type packaging for autoclaving.

Still another method of sterilization is the *dry heat oven*. Instruments with sharp blades, such as scissors or scalpels, are sometimes sterilized in this way. It is not the most desirable sterilization method, because it is time-consuming. The process takes 1 to 2 hours at a temperature of 350°F, depending on the article. It is *not* a way to sterilize items made of rubber. For rubber articles, thorough washing and rinsing is the first step in preparing them for reuse. They must be completely dry before being placed in a disinfectant for chemical sterilization. Spores may still be a threat with this method. Finally, in every medical practice the policy of the establishment must be followed.

Complete Chapter 3, Unit 4 in the workbook to help you meet the objectives at the beginning of this unit and therefore achieve competency of this subject matter.

U N I T   5
Office Safety and Security

Patients who are very ill should not be left in the waiting room but placed in an examination room where they can be made more comfortable.

OBJECTIVES ••

Upon completion of the unit, you will meet the following terminal performance objectives by verifying knowledge of the facts and principles presented through oral and written communication at a level deemed competent by the instructor or employer.

1. List the appropriate drugs, supplies, and equipment for an emergency tray.

FIGURE 3–12 Placing an instrument into an envelope package for autoclaving

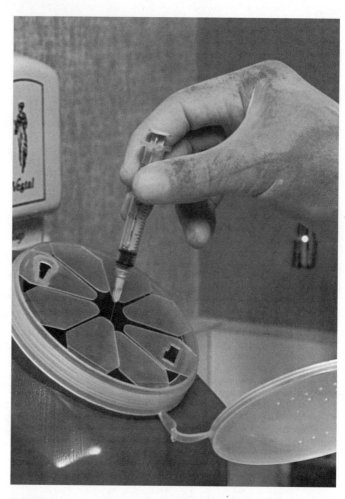

FIGURE 3–14 Discard the entire disposable syringe with used needle intact in the biohazardous sharps container.

A

B

FIGURE 3–13 Package of towels (a) before and (b) after autoclaving. Note that the sterilized package has diagonal lines on the tape, a positive sign that autoclaving has been done correctly.

2. Know what telephone numbers should be posted near each telephone.
3. Know the procedures for handling narcotic drugs in the office.
4. Know which emergencies require special evaluation procedures.
5. Identify special needs of a laboratory for safety of personnel.
6. Describe the two general kinds of emergencies that may be encountered in a medical office.
7. List examples of accidents that may take place in the office.
8. List examples of accidents that may take place outside of the office.
9. Describe illnesses that may be emergency situations.
10. Prepare a sample accident report form.
11. Describe where accident reports should be kept.
12. Spell and define, using the glossary at the back of the text, all the words to know in this unit.

Wrap Items for Autoclave

PURPOSE: To wrap items to be autoclaved so that they will be protected from contamination after the sterilization process is completed for storage and handling.

EQUIPMENT: muslin, autoclave paper, disposable paper bags, or envelopes; autoclave tape; items to be sterilized or autoclaved; sterilization indicator; pen.

TERMINAL PERFORMANCE OBJECTIVE: Provided with several items, to be autoclaved or sterilized, the student will wrap each in autoclave paper or muslin, in preparation for the sterilization process. Each item must be wrapped neatly and snugly but not too tightly; the instructor and student will jointly determine if each wrapped item is suitable for autoclaving.

After the paper wrapping procedure is demonstrated and checked, the paper should be removed from each item and discarded. The above-stated procedure will be repeated using muslin cloth (*Note:* When the muslin cloth wrapping procedure is completed, the muslin cloth is retained).

1. Wash hands and assemble all necessary items. *Note:* Work in a clean area where there is sufficient work space.
2. Check items for flaws and to make sure that they function properly. *Note:* Items must be sanitized before wrapping for autoclave process. **RATIONALE: Instru-**ments must be working properly and materials in useable condition.
3. Wrap item(s) in desired wrap so that there is a double thickness of protection. Make sure that there is no opening and seal with autoclave tape. Wrap item(s) snugly but not too tightly, Figure 3–15. **RATIONALE: Double thickness and complete enclosure prevent pathogenic entry.**

Note: For envelope wrap, place item into envelope, seal, and label. Items suitable for envelope wrap include but are not limited to forceps, hemostats, needle holders, and towel clamps. All hinged instruments must be autoclaved open. **RATIONALE: Sterilizing process must reach all parts of the instruments.**

Place spinal needles (small items) in glass test tube with cotton or gauze padding at bottom. Wrap autoclave tape around top to seal, with a pull tab for ease in opening. Label contents on a piece of tape secured to glass.

4. Make a tab for ease in opening wrapped packages after autoclaving by taping 1 to 2 in. of tape to itself at edge of package.
5. Label contents, write date and your initials on tape. *Note:* Refer to Table 3–2 for proper time and temperature for items to be autoclaved.
6. Return all items to proper storage area when finished.

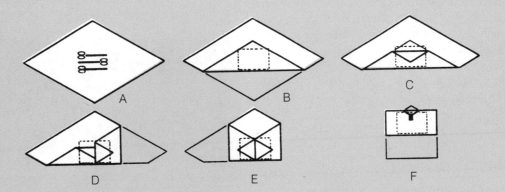

FIGURE 3–15 To wrap instruments for autoclaving: (a) place items in center of wrap, (b) fold the material up from the bottom, (c) double back a small corner, (d) fold the right and then (e) left edges in, again leaving corners doubled back, (f) fold the pack up from the bottom and secure with pressure-sensitive tape.

activated	eyewash
alleged	grille
anaphylactic shock	hyperventilation
antihistamine	hypoglycemic
asphyxiation	hypothermia
attenuated	illicit
concealed	inoculating loops
contaminated	preliminary
diabetic	procurement
disposition	rapport
emetic	sharps
epilepsy	snap locks
ergonomics	volatile
evacuation	

The medical office must be run as a business whether it is a solo practice or a large number of physicians operating as a corporation. Every business is responsible for the safety of those who enter the premises. The medical assistant is part of the team responsible for recognizing any safety hazards, helping to eliminate them, and warning patients of any dangers.

Ergonomics is the scientific discipline devoted to the study and analysis of human work, especially as it is affected by individual anatomy, psychology, and other human factors. The workplace should be a safe environment where one can effectively and efficiently perform required duties. Since all of the factors listed above affect each of us in the daily performance of our jobs they are of extreme importance. Physical safety is of primary importance and is discussed further in the text. Getting along well with others is critical and is necessary for a good atmosphere to be maintained. People work far better when they feel good about themselves and others. If and when a conflict should arise, it should be taken care of as soon as possible to protect the harmonious environment and thus maintain a good **rapport** for a healthy workplace. All of us want to feel useful and needed. Giving each other support and reassurance helps to build good work relationships, and helps feed a spirit of teamwork, as we are all members of the health care team.

Reception Room ································

The medical assistant should conduct a visual check of the reception area daily to be sure the furniture is clean and in good repair. All electrical cords should be checked routinely for frayed wires and should be removed immediately if defective. Children's toys or books should be off the floor when not in use. All toys should be washable and made of safe materials. It is common practice to display a "no smoking" sign in the office. Smoking is a health hazard and fire can result from

careless smoking. Any type of smoking can cause a patient with asthma or other respiratory conditions to have serious breathing problems.

Care should be taken to make the reception area accident-proof. An injury in the office can result in a patient's demanding that the physician pay for the **alleged** pain and suffering. If anyone should be injured in the waiting room, no matter how slightly, the medical assistant must be sure the individual is examined by the physician.

Never leave a file drawer open at floor level when you are away from the file cabinet. There is danger of tripping over such an obstacle. In a vertical file cabinet if you pull out more than one drawer at a time you may cause the cabinet to tip forward and cause injury. Cupboard doors left open are a hazard.

Be sure to unplug appliances such as coffee makers and sterilizers at the end of the day because they are a fire hazard if allowed to boil dry.

Your office should have a well-planned procedure and route for **evacuation** in the event a fire should occur in the office building. Evacuation routes marked with arrows that outline the path for safe exit should be posted in all areas of the facility. Smoke detectors should be installed and batteries checked monthly to evaluate their effectiveness. Fire extinguishers that are effective in putting out fires of all types of burning materials should be mounted on the walls near an exit. A sufficient number of extinguishers for the amount of space must be considered. These should be checked by the fire department annually. Replacement of them must be done as necessary. All office personnel should know the location of fire extinguishers and how to use them, Figure 3–16. All personnel should know the location of the nearest fire escape. Battery-powered lights should be available to use in the event of a power failure.

All office personnel should know the procedure to use during a tornado, severe storm or any natural disaster. The safest area of the building should be identified. Your local disaster service can assist you in identifying the safest location.

FIGURE 3–16 Know the location of fire extinguishers and how to use them. (Courtesy of American LaFrance)

The reception desk should be placed so that the medical assistant can have a clear view of the waiting room, but it should not be in the waiting room. It is generally advisable to have a window, which can be closed for privacy (and security) when you are engaged in telephone conversation or interviewing a patient.

Police officials now inform us that if your business office is accessible to the general public through the waiting room, the office entrance window should be covered with a **grille** to prevent individuals from entering the office to take drugs or to rob the cash drawer.

The increased incidence of robbery and rape makes it extremely important that **snap locks** be used on doors between the office and reception area. Private entry doors to the office should not be left unlocked. Most businesses, especially medical facilities, have security alarm systems which are activated by a computerized code. Usually the last person to leave the facility activates the security system. If the facility has no security system, the doors must be locked and secured before leaving for the day or evening.

You always should be on guard and not let anyone know that you are alone, if ever, so as not to make yourself vulnerable. Your goal should be to provide and maintain a safe environment for all persons related to the facility where you are employed. If you must enter or leave the office after dark, the outside area should be well lighted and security personnel should be available if necessary.

Examination Rooms

The examination table should be cleaned carefully after each patient. Any dropped objects or spills should be cleaned up immediately to prevent slipping or falling. Figure 3–17. Small children will pick up any loose object and put it in their mouth. Extremely ill patients or children should not be left alone on an examination table, where they could fall. All equipment cords should be **concealed** where people will be moving about. No prescription blanks should be left where they can be forged and used illegally for drug **procurement.** Always keep narcotics in a locked cupboard in an area not usually seen by patients.

Anything recognized as a possible office hazard should be remedied. All employees need to follow safety procedures in the proper disposal of drugs. Dated samples should be checked and any that have been kept beyond the expiration date should be properly discarded (flushed down toilet). Potentially dangerous equipment, such as syringes and needles, must be disposed of in biohazard **sharps** containers. Several protective safety adapters are available to reduce the risk of patient-to-staff contamination by accidental needle sticks. Contaminated dressings need to be placed in special disposable biohazard containers.

The medical assistant should take the precaution of washing hands before and after dealing with each patient. When it is necessary to clean up any examination area after any patient, wear latex gloves and use a solution of 20% chlorine and water.

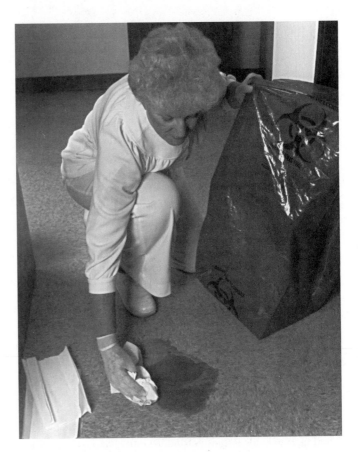

FIGURE 3–17 Always pick up dropped objects or clean up spills immediately to prevent accidents.

Laboratory Area

If chemicals are kept in the office for laboratory work, care must be taken to store them properly. Some chemicals become **volatile** when kept beyond the expiration date, so these dates need to be monitored carefully.

Gloves should always be worn when handling **contaminated** instruments or when processing patient specimens. The Centers for Disease Control in Atlanta has outlined universal precautions to be followed concerning laboratory workers. These precautions are discussed in connection with the clinical procedures in this text.

Every office should have a general safety procedure book that employees must be familiar with through an employee training program. This book should include guidelines for handling of hazardous medical wastes. The U.S. Occupational Safety and Health Administration (OSHA) was established to help the employer provide a safe working environment for the employees. Hazardous medical wastes include blood products, body fluids, tissue cultures, live and **attenuated** vaccines, sharps, table paper with body fluids, gloves, speculums, cotton swabs, and **inoculating loops.**

The laboratory should have an emergency **eyewash** station. Every office laboratory and operating room should be equipped with disposable latex gloves, protective glasses, gowns and masks for the protection of staff and patients.

Every employee should be certified in first aid and cardiopulmonary resuscitation and this certification must be current. The office should have written guidelines outlining the scope of care to be given by medical assistants and the location in the office where this care should be given. A list of all the necessary telephone numbers for police, fire, ambulance, hospitals, and poison control centers should be near each telephone.

The easiest way to be prepared for an emergency is to purchase a prepared emergency kit, which is available through most medical supply houses, Figure 3–18. If your physician feels this is not necessary, you must assemble your own. You should have a supply of sterile dressings, bandage material, and adhesive tape; easily **activated** hot and cold packs; disposable syringe and needle units with adrenaline, narcotics, and **antihistamines.** Adrenaline (epinephrine) is available in cartridge units ready for use. Other supplies include ipecac, an effective **emetic;** tubes of glucose for use in **diabetic** patients suffering from a severe **hypoglycemic** reaction; and an oxygen tank with a mask. Other items your physician might include would be alcohol wipes, aromatic spirits of ammonia, blood pressure cuff, stethoscope, bandage scissors, airways of different sizes, penlight, paper and pencil, and a small bag for **hyperventilation.**

Every office should have guidelines in the office procedure manual regarding methods to handle each type of emergency that might occur in the office. All office personnel should understand their individual roles in handling emergencies in the office.

FIGURE 3–18 Prepared emergency kit.(Courtesy of Banyan International Corporation)

The patient could be involved in an accident in or out of the office. The patient could be suffering from diabetic coma, **anaphylactic shock,** heart attack, or reaction to an **illicit** drug.

Emergencies that might require cardiopulmonary resuscitation are airway obstructions, smoke inhalation, brain injury, chest wall injury, drug or medication reaction, electrocution, drowning, cardiac arrest, trauma, respiratory arrest, **hypothermia,** allergies, electric shock, **asphyxiation,** stroke, and **epilepsy.**

A decision must be made as to who is responsible for recording detailed information in the patient's medical record. The information necessary to be recorded should include:

- date and time of accident or emergency
- full name of injured party
- notation as to whether this individual is a patient, visitor, or office staff member
- address of injured party with telephone number
- location in office where incident occurred
- detailed description of incident
- names of staff involved in any way
- names, addresses, and telephone numbers of witnesses other than staff
- action taken; medications given; physician examined; patient referred to hospital, other medical office, or home
- signature of person preparing report with time and date

The above information should be on a printed form approved by the physician and liability insurance company, Figure 3–19.

When the report of an accident or illness is completed, the office needs to have established guidelines for **disposition** of the form. It may be advisable to have legal input as to whether to place the form in the patient's medical record or file it in a special incident file.

Complete Chapter 3, Unit 5 in the workbook to help you meet the objectives at the beginning of this unit and therefore achieve competency of this subject matter.

Accident Report

Date_____ Time _____ AM/PM

Name _____

(accident victim)

Address _____

Is victim _____ patient _____ staff _____ visitor

Location _____

Detailed description of accident _____

(by victim) _____

_____

_____

Staff members involved _____

_____

_____

Staff member's description of accident _____

_____

Witness(es) other than self _____

_____

Witness(es)'s description_____

_____

Action taken _____

_____

Time _____ Date _____

_____
(signature of preparer)

FIGURE 3–19 Example accident report form

Mr. Right . . .

is always careful when handling specimens and follows all universal precautions when assisting with invasive procedures. He remembers to wash his hands and glove properly before and after each patient with which he comes in contact. He places all waste in the appropriate receptacles.

Promotion outlook: Excellent

Ms Wrong . . .

is careless about following universal precautions and frequently forgets to wear gloves or other protective coverings when assisting with invasive procedures. Other health care team members are tiring of reminding her about disposing of waste appropriately.

Promotion outlook: Poor

REFERENCES

Cody, John P. Cardiopulmonary Resuscitation. "The ABCs of Basic Life Support." *The Professional Medical Assistant.* July–August, 1990.

Fong, Elizabeth, and Ferris, Elvira. *Microbiology for Health Careers,* 4th ed. Albany: Delmar, 1987.

Garza, Diana, and Becan-McBride. *Phlebotomy Handbook.* 3d ed. East Norwalk, CT: Appleton & Lange, 1993.

Jett, Ernestine. "Enforcement of Safety and Security in the Medical Office" *The Professional Medical Assistant.* November–December, 1986.

Joyce, Marilyn and Wallersteiner, Ulrika. *Ergonomics. Humanizing the Automated Office.* Cincinnati: South Western Publishing, 1989.

Keir, A. Lucille. "Safety in the Medical Office." *The Professional Medical Assistant.* September–October, 1986.

Miller, Benjamin F., and Keane, Claire Brackman. *Encyclopedia and Dictionary of Medicine and Allied Health,* 3d ed. Philadelphia: W. B. Saunders Co., 1983.

Mosby's Medical & Nursing Dictionary, 3d ed. St. Louis: C. V. Mosby, 1990.

Nurse's Ready Reference Diagnostic Tests. Springhouse, PA: Springhouse, 1991.

Raphael, Stanley S. Lynch's Medical Laboratory Technology, 3d ed. Windsor, Ontario: W. B. Saunders Co., 1976.

Taber, Clarence W. *Taber's Cyclopedic Medical Dictionary,* 14th ed. Philadelphia: F. A. Davis, 1983.

Ware, Barbara E. *CLIA '88 Physician's Office Laboratory, Are You Ready?* June 1991.

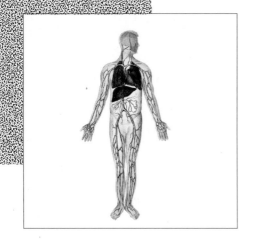

C H A P T E R 4

Anatomy and Physiology of the Human Body

UNIT 1
Anatomical Descriptors and
Fundamental Body Structure

UNIT 2
The Nervous System

UNIT 3
The Senses

UNIT 4
The Integumentary System

UNIT 5
The Skeletal System

UNIT 6
The Muscular System

UNIT 7
The Respiratory System

UNIT 8
The Circulatory System

UNIT 9
The Immune System

UNIT 10
The Digestive System

UNIT 11
The Urinary System

UNIT 12
The Endocrine System

UNIT 13
The Reproductive System

The human body is a fantastic combination of parts that function in an organized manner, far more efficiently and effectively than any machine ever developed. This chapter describes the body's fundamental structure, the body systems, and discusses how the parts work together.

The diseases and disorders affecting the human body are a result of impairment, deterioration, or malfunction of one or more of its component parts. Within this chapter, the anatomy of each body system will be presented as well as how that system functions physiologically within itself and with the other body systems. Following the presentation of each system will be a discussion of characteristic pathophysiological conditions and disorders, many of which result from the body's inability to adapt or defend itself. A basic discussion of the critical role of the immune system in maintaining a healthy state will help you to correlate your knowledge of the body's complex interrelationships. With this understanding you will be able to see how the patient's concerns and complaints, the physician's examination, and the clinical findings fit together to indicate the diagnosis and the plan of treatment the physician prescribes.

U N I T 1

Anatomical Descriptors and Fundamental Body Structure

OBJECTIVES ·······································

Upon completion of this unit, you will meet the following terminal performance objectives by verifying knowledge of the facts and principles presented through oral and written communication at a level deemed competent by the instructor or employer.

1. Describe the anatomical position.
2. Apply the appropriate terminology to points of reference on the human body.

3. Locate the four body cavities.
4. Name the major organ(s) located within each body cavity.
5. Identify the regions of the abdomen.
6. Describe the basic characteristics of the cell.
7. Describe the six ways molecules pass through cell membranes.
8. Describe the four main types of body tissues.
9. Name the 10 systems of the body.
10. Spell and define, using the glossary at the back of the text, all the words to know in this unit.

WORDS TO KNOW ···

abdominal	Golgi apparatus
abdominopelvic	gross anatomy
anatomical	histology
anatomy	histotechnologist
anterior	homeostasis
biochemistry	horizontal
buccal	hypertonic
cardiac	hypochondriac
caudal	hypogastric
cavities	hypotonic
cell membrane	iliac
centrioles	inferior
chromosomes	inguinal
connective	involuntary
coronal	isotonic
cranial	keloid
cytology	lateral
cytoplasm	lumbar
cytotechnologist	lysosomes
dehydration	medial
diaphragm	membrane
diffusion	microscopic anatomy
distal	midline
dorsal	mitochondria
edema	mitosis
elements	muscle
endocytosis	myelin
endoplasmic reticulum	nasal
epigastric	nerve
epithelial	neurilemma
exocytosis	neuron
extremities	normal saline
filtration	nucleolus
frontal	nucleus
gene	orbital
organ	ribosome
organelles	sagittal
osmosis	skeletal
osseous	smooth
pathophysiology	spinal
pelvic	striated
phagocytosis	superior
physiology	system
pinocytosis	thoracic
posterior	tissue
proximal	transverse
pubic	umbilical
quadrant	ventral
retroperitoneal	voluntary

Anatomy and Physiology Defined ··············

Two terms are used in discussing the study of the human body: **anatomy,** which is the study of the physical structure of the body and its organs; and **physiology,** which is the science of the function of cells, tissues, and organs of the body. In other words, anatomy describes the framework and physical characteristics, and physiology explains how everything works together to support life.

Anatomy can be subdivided into various areas of study. For instance, the term **gross anatomy** refers to the study of those features that can be observed with the naked eye by inspection and dissection. As an example, the pathologist, when examining a tissue specimen, will describe its gross **anatomical** surface appearance and then proceed with the dissection and its description.

An area of study known as **microscopic anatomy** deals with features that can be observed only with the use of a microscope. Referring again to the pathologist, a fragment of a specimen can be prepared on a slide and observed with a microscope to complete the description of the specimen's characteristics and formulate an opinion as to its identity or state of condition.

There are two related areas of microscopic anatomy: **cytology,** the study of cell life and formation, and **histology,** the study of the microscopic structure of tissue. Pathologists are assisted by laboratory specialists known as **cytotechnologists** and **histotechnologists** who precisely prepare materials for microscopic examination and diagnosis.

Physiology is the study of the interrelationships of all the functioning structures of the body. When everything is in harmony and all biological indicators are within acceptable limits, the individual is referred to as being in a "steady state," or "normal." When the normal physiology is disrupted to the point of instability and begins to deteriorate, pathophysiological mechanisms are likely to occur and may result in the development of a disease condition. **Pathophysiology** is the study of mechanisms by which disease occurs, the responses of the body to the disease process, and the effects of both on normal function.

Pathophysiology attempts to bring together the clinical signs and symptoms present with the knowledge of the effects of the disease processes on the body, from the cellular level to the total human being. Often close observation of the clinical signs of a disease state has led to the discovery of physiological functions previously unknown. This is currently apparent in the great effort to understand the immune system to find a way to effectively control and eventually eliminate AIDS and cancer.

Fortunately, the healthy body has an enormous capacity to protect itself by compensating, defending, and adapting to the pathophysiological effects of disease. When this fails, however, appropriate medical intervention can often correct or at least control the disease process.

Language of Medicine ....

The members of the health care team must be able to accurately communicate information, findings, and instructions among themselves. Much of the language of medicine is precise and is specific to the field of health care. For instance, it is necessary not only to know about the human body but also to be able to physically as well as verbally locate body structures or describe the site of a patient's complaint or injury. The following fundamental descriptive terminology will be essential to the understanding of body references.

Anatomical Directional Terms ....

Certain directional terms are universally used in describing anatomical structures. A body is said to be in anatomical position when standing erect, with arms down at the sides, and the palms of the hands facing forward, Figure 4–1. This means that when the person is facing you, his or her right side is on your left, as if you were looking in a mirror. When reference is made to a body structure or a specific area, it is in relationship to this anatomical position. The same is true when you are studying illustrations in this textbook or labeling a drawing in the workbook.

Dividing the body vertically down the front will result in a right and left half. This imaginary line is known as the median, or **sagittal,** plane. The right and left designations always refer to right and left in anatomical position. Anything located toward the **midline** is said to be **medial,** whereas anything away from the midline is said to be **lateral.**

Two other terms are used to describe the relationship of the **extremities,** or ends of the body, such as the arms and legs, to the trunk of the body. **Proximal** indicates nearness to the point of attachment, and **distal** indicates distance away from the point of attachment. These terms are also applicable when describing parts of the arms, legs, fingers, or toes. For example, the thumb and great toe have proximal and distal sections, whereas the other fingers and toes have proximal, middle, and distal sections.

If you draw a line vertically through the side of the body, from the top of the head, to the feet, you will make a front and back section, Figure 4–2. This line is known as the **frontal,** or **coronal,** plane. The front is known as the **anterior,** or **ventral** section; the back is called the **posterior,** or **dorsal,** section.

FIGURE 4–1   Anatomical position with directional references

FIGURE 4–2   Anatomical directional references

Finally, drawing an imaginary line **horizontally** (across) the body creates a **transverse** plane. The portion of the body above the line is known as **superior,** or **cranial.** The portion below the line is called **inferior,** or **caudal.** It is not necessary that the body be divided into equal parts. The terms superior and inferior refer to any relationship of structures above or below a "line" and depends on where it is drawn. For example, with a transverse line at the waist, the chest is superior to the abdomen but if at the neck, the chest is inferior to the head. All anatomical directional terms are appropriate only when describing the relationship of one structure to another.

These planes or sections can also be applied to internal structures as well as to the body as a whole. *Incisions* (cuts) made on the body surface or into organs are often made along a plane. The surgeon's description of the operation will identify the location of the incisions made using referencing planes. A tissue specimen cut along the transverse plane is known as a *cross section.*

Body Cavities and Organs

The body is divided into two main **cavities,** an anterior (or ventral) cavity and a posterior (or dorsal) cavity, Figure 4–3. A dome-shaped **muscle** known as the **diaphragm** divides the anterior cavity into an upper, **thoracic** cavity and a lower **abdominopelvic** cavity. The thoracic cavity (chest) has a wall of ribs that protects its vital organs—the heart, lungs, and the great blood vessels, Figure 4–4.

The diaphragm alternately contracts and relaxes to move the lungs, causing breathing to occur.

The abdominopelvic cavity has two parts, an upper, **abdominal** portion and a lower, **pelvic** portion. The abdominal portion extends from the diaphragm to the top edge of the pelvic girdle (bones). The organs found in the abdomen are the stomach, small intestines, most of the large intestine, the liver, spleen, pancreas, and gallbladder. The kidneys are located in the dorsal abdominal area but are behind the peritoneal **membrane** that lines the cavity and so are technically outside the abdominal cavity. This space is referred to as **retroperitoneal,** behind the peritoneum. The pelvic cavity is surrounded by the pelvic girdle, which provides protection for the urinary bladder, the last portion of the large intestine, and the internal reproductive organs.

The cranial cavity is totally encased by the bones of the skull, which provides protection for the brain. The cranial cavity is joined at its base by the **spinal** cavity, which extends through the center of the column of vertebrae (bones). This bony structure contains the spinal cord and protects it from injury.

There are three other small cavities, the **orbital** for the eyes, the **nasal** for the structures of the nose, and the **buccal** or mouth.

Abdominal Regions   The abdomen is such a large area of the body that it is necessary to divide it into regions for purposes of identification or reference. There are two recognized methods of division. One creates **quadrants** known as the right and

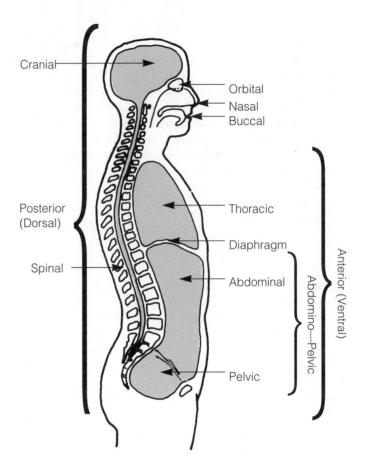

FIGURE 4–3   Body cavities (Copyright by Richardson. Adapted from Caldwell & Hegner, *Nursing Assistant,* 6th ed. Copyright 1992, Delmar Publishers Inc. Used with permission.)

left upper quadrants (RUQ and LUQ) and the right and left lower quadrants (RLQ and LLQ), Figure 4–5.

A more exacting division results in nine regions identifiable by location and an anatomical reference point. The three central areas are called **epigastric** (over the stomach), **umbilical** (around the umbilicus), and **hypogastric** (below the stomach; also called **pubic**). The six side areas are called the right and left **hypochondriac** (below the cartilage, referring to the ribs), the right and left **lumbar** (loin or side region; also called lateral); and the right and left **iliac** (referring to the ileum portion of the pelvic bone; also known as the **inguinal,** meaning groin, region), Figure 4–6, page 75.

The Cell

To understand the structure of the body, you must first learn about its basic building block, the cell. This fascinating wonder is a living, working, microscopic image of the body. It requires food and oxygen to survive, performs specific functions, produces heat and energy, gives off waste products, and can reproduce itself.

Cells vary greatly in size and shape due to their various activities. The body contains about 75 trillion cells. Whenever cells of a particular type are destroyed, the remaining cells of that type divide until they have replaced the missing cells.

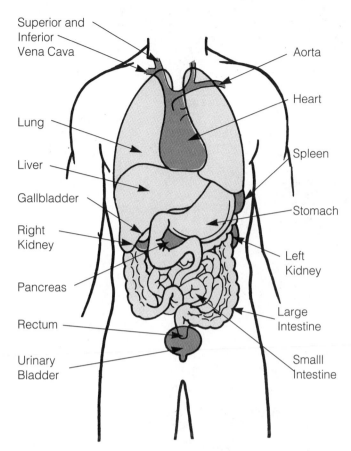

FIGURE 4–4 Thoracic and abdominal organs

Superior and Inferior Vena Cava
Lung
Liver
Gallbladder
Right Kidney
Pancreas
Rectum
Urinary Bladder
Aorta
Heart
Spleen
Stomach
Left Kidney
Large Intestine
Smalll Intestine

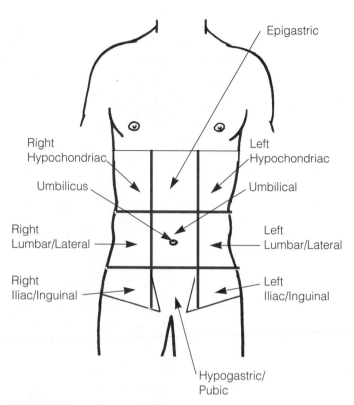

Epigastric
Right Hypochondriac
Umbilicus
Right Lumbar/Lateral
Right Iliac/Inguinal
Left Hypochondriac
Umbilical
Left Lumbar/Lateral
Left Iliac/Inguinal
Hypogastric/ Pubic

FIGURE 4–6 Nine regions of the abdomen (Adapted from Caldwell & Hegner, *Nursing Assistant,* 6th ed. Copyright 1992, Delmar Publishers Inc.)

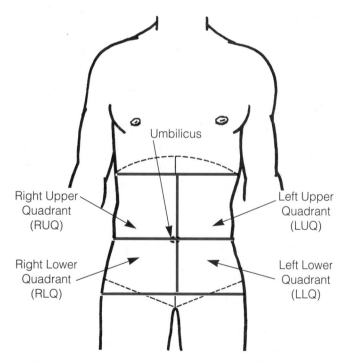

Umbilicus
Right Upper Quadrant (RUQ)
Right Lower Quadrant (RLQ)
Left Upper Quadrant (LUQ)
Left Lower Quadrant (LLQ)

FIGURE 4–5 The four abdominal quadrants (Adapted from Caldwell & Hegner, *Nursing Assistant,* 6th ed. Copyright 1992, Delmar Publishers Inc.)

Cells come in different varieties to perform specific duties. Some secrete materials, some receive and transmit impulses, or some enable us to move. Still others carry nutrients and oxygen, clot blood, or destroy bacteria. Even though they are microscopic in size, their proper function is absolutely essential to life. No manufactured apparatus can match the cell for the number of chemical reactions that occur in such a small space.

A conventional cell is composed of a fluid called **cytoplasm** and is surrounded by a cell membrane, Figure 4–7. The **cell membrane** separates the cell from the surrounding environment. It consists of protein and fat molecules. The membrane controls what enters and leaves the cell; therefore, it plays an important role in the health and welfare of the cell, which will be seen later. Enclosed within the membrane is the sticky semifluid material known as cytoplasm. It is a combination of protein, lipids (fat), carbohydrates, minerals, salts, and water (over 70%). Chemical reactions, such as respiration and protein synthesis, occur in the cytoplasm.

Within the cytoplasm of the cell are many minute bodies called **organelles** that perform amazing tasks. The organelles are the **nucleus, mitochondria, ribosomes, centriole, endoplasmic reticulum, Golgi apparatus,** and **lysosomes.** Scientists still do not understand how some functions are carried out so when describing them they may use the word "magical." They do know that some organelles physically separate the chemical reactions occurring in the cytoplasm because many reactions are not compatible. Organelles also control the time

FIGURE 4–7 Fine structure of a typical animal cell (From Fong, *Body Structures and Functions,* 8th ed. Copyright 1993, Delmar Publishers Inc.)

Within the figure, the following labels appear:

SMOOTH ENDOPLASMIC RETICULUM

MITOCHONDRION

NUCLEOLUS

NUCLEUS

LYSOSOMES

RIBOSOMES

CYTOPLASM

CELL MEMBRANE

CENTRIOLES

PINOCYTIC VESSEL

VACUOLE

© Richardson 1983

ROUGH ENDOPLASMIC RETICULUM

CHROMATIN

GOLGI APPARATUS

when reactions take place, such as producing or processing a molecule in one organelle then later using the molecule in another reaction.

The *nucleus* is a dense mass within the cytoplasm. It is surrounded by its own nuclear membrane. Materials pass in and out of the nucleus from the cytoplasm through pores in the membrane. The membrane is continuous with the endoplasmic reticulum, which often has ribosomes attached. The nucleus is the control center of the cell. It regulates the chemical reactions and controls the process of **mitosis** (cell division) for reproduction. Within the nucleus are the structures called **chromosomes.** Each member of a species has a specific number of chromosomes. Human beings have 46 individual or 23 pairs of chromosomes that store the hereditary material passed on from one generation to another. Twenty-two pairs of chromosomes are autosomes (same in number and kind), and one pair are sex chromosomes—either both X if female, or an X and a Y, if male. Chromosomes have molecules known as deoxyribonucleic acid (DNA), which contain the genes and carry the genetic coding necessary for the exact duplication of the cell.

The DNA structure varies from one cell to another in that

the sequence of the base pairs of the DNA molecule are arranged differently. The sequence is what determines heredity factors. A gene is the specific sequence of about 1000 base pairs. Approximately 100,000 genes compose the DNA molecule of one chromosome. Since humans have 46 chromosomes, we therefore have about 4½ million genes in each cell. This helps explain why there is so much variety in the human race.

The nucleus itself will have at least one **nucleolus.** In a nucleolus, portions of ribonucleic acid (RNA) are assembled with proteins to make subunits of the ribosomes, which then pass through the nuclear pores of the nuclear membrane into the cytoplasm, to become a complete two-part ribosome to synthesize protein. Ribosomes are found circulating in the cytoplasm or attached to the endoplasmic reticulum.

Centrioles are the two cylinder-shaped organelles near the nucleus. During mitosis, the centrioles separate and form spindle fibers that attach to the chromosomes to ensure their equal distribution to the two new daughter cells.

Endoplasmic reticulum crisscrosses the cytoplasm in a network fashion. When attached to the nuclear membrane, it serves as a passageway for the transportation of materials in and out of the nucleus. If grouped together, they can store large amounts of protein. The difference between rough and smooth endoplasmic reticulum is the presence of *ribosomes* on the membrane. Ribosomes give the membrane a coarse and rough appearance.

Mitochondria are round or rod-shaped organelles that supply the cell's energy. There may be from one to more than a thousand in each cell depending on how much energy that type of cell requires. Mitochondria have a double-membraned structure with the inner membrane folding into ridges. Chemicals known as enzymes are located in the ridges. The cell is capable of respiration because the enzymes break down nutrient molecules to provide carbon dioxide and water.

The *Golgi apparatus* is a stack of membrane layers, which are believed to synthesize carbohydrates and combine them with molecules of proteins. The organelle appears to store and prepare secretions to excrete from the cell. Therefore, the cells of the gastric, salivary, and pancreatic glands have large numbers of Golgi apparatus.

Lysosomes are round or oval structures. They have a strong digestive enzyme that consumes protein molecules, such as those found in old worn cells, bacteria, or foreign matter. This is a very important function of the body's natural immune system.

Pinocytic vesicles are pocket-like formations in the cell's membrane. These structures permit large molecules like protein and fat, which cannot pass through the pores of the cell membrane, to enter with the extracellular fluid into the vesicle. Then the "pocket" closes forming a vacuole (bubble) in the cytoplasm. This process is called **endocytosis.** When liquid droplets, instead of protein or fat molecules, are enclosed, the process is known as **pinocytosis,** which means "cell drinking." A related term, **exocytosis,** refers to a similar process whereby substances are moved from the cell to the outside. On entering the cytoplasm, most vesicles fuse with lysosomes and their contents are digested. Special white blood cells known as phagocytes rely on endocytosis to destroy harmful bacteria in

the body. As you learn more about your body, you will begin to appreciate what a magnificent piece of "equipment" it is and how important it is that you care for it properly. You have the physical and mental power to have a great effect on your health and even your very life.

Table 4–1 summarizes the organelles and their role in the function of the cell.

Passing Molecules Through Cell Membranes ....

As stated before, the cell membrane controls materials entering and leaving the cell. This is necessary for the cell to

TABLE 4–1
Summary Table of Cell Organelles

Organelle	Function
Cell membrane	Regulates transport of substances into and out of the cell.
Cytoplasm	Provides an organized watery environment in which life functions take place by the activities of the organelles contained in the cytoplasm.
Nucleus	Serves as the "brain" for the control of the cell's metabolic activities and cell division.
Nuclear membrane	Regulates transport of substances into and out of the nucleus.
Nucleoplasm	A clear, semifluid medium that fills the spaces around the chromatin and the nucleoli.
Nucleolus	Functions as a reservoir for RNA.
Ribosomes	Serve as sites for protein synthesis.
Endoplasmic reticulum	Provides passages through which transport of substances occurs in cytoplasm.
Mitochondria	Serve as sites of cellular respiration and energy production.
Golgi apparatus	Manufactures carbohydrates and packages secretions for discharge from the cell.
Lysosomes	Serve as centers of cellular digestion.
Pinocytic vesicles	Transport of large particles into a cell.
Centrosome and centrioles	Contains two centrioles that are functional during animal cell division.

(From Fong, *Body Structures and Functions,* 8th ed. Copyright 1993, Delmar Publishers Inc.)

acquire substances from its environment to be processed for its use, or for secretion, or for excretion of the waste materials. There are six processes by which materials pass through a cell membrane: **diffusion, osmosis, filtration,** active transport, **phagocytosis** and pinocytosis.

Diffusion is a process whereby gas, liquid, or solid molecules distribute themselves evenly through a medium. When the medium is a fluid and the molecules are solid, they are called solutes, Figure 4–8. When solutes and water pass across a membrane to distribute themselves, they will move from an area of higher concentration to an area of lesser concentration. Diffusion plays a vital role in the body. For example, higher concentrations of oxygen in the alveolus (air sac) of the lung cross the membrane into the lesser concentrated area of the red blood cell in the capillary, Figure 4–8. The blood cell, now with a high concentration of oxygen, circulates in the blood to a body cell with lower oxygen concentration and exchanges its oxygen for the cell's higher concentration of waste products. And so the body's cells "breathe" in a process called *internal respiration.*

Osmosis is a process of diffusion of water or another solvent through a selected permeable membrane, one through which some solutes can pass but others cannot, Figure 4–9. In the illustration, the membrane will only allow the salt and water to pass through; therefore, the salt leaves the greater concentrated area within the membrane to go to the lesser concentrated water. At the same time, the water leaves its higher concentrated area to enter the lesser concentrated area within the membrane. When the water molecules are equal on both sides, the diffusion will stop. The pressure of the water molecules inside the membrane, a state known as the *osmotic pressure,* is then said to be at **equilibrium.**

The osmotic characteristics of solutions are classified by their effect on red blood cells, Figure 4–10, page 79 . If the solution is of the same osmotic pressure as blood serum it is known as an **isotonic** solution. A 0.9% salt (NaCl) solution has the same salt concentration as that of the red blood cell and is called **normal saline.** If the osmolality is lower, the solution is **hypotonic** and the blood cell will swell with water and burst. In a **hypertonic** solution, the cell will release its water and shrink.

Filtration is the movement of solutes and water across a semipermeable membrane as a result of a force, such as gravity or blood pressure. The particles move from a higher to a lower area of pressure. The size of the pores of some membranes allow only small molecules to leave. This process occurs in the kidneys where small molecules of water and waste products are filtered from the blood in the capillaries, but the large protein molecules and red blood cells are retained, Figure 4–11.

Active transport refers to molecules moving across a membrane from an area of low concentration to an area of higher concentration due to the presence of ATP (adenosine triphosphate), a high-energy compound from the cell membrane. It appears as a "carrier" molecule, temporarily binding with another molecule on the outer edge of the membrane. The carrier crosses the membrane and releases its "passenger" into the cytoplasm. The carrier then receives more energy from the membrane and returns to the outer surface to transport another molecule. The carrier can also reverse the process and carry molecules from the inside to the outside.

Phagocytosis is known as "cell eating." White blood cells become phagocytes and engulf bacteria, cell fragments, or damaged cells, Figure 4–12. The white cell forms a vacuole by enfolding its membrane and enclosing the particle. When it is completely enclosed, digestive enzymes enter from the cytoplasm and destroy the trapped material. This process is extremely important to the body's ability to maintain a healthy state.

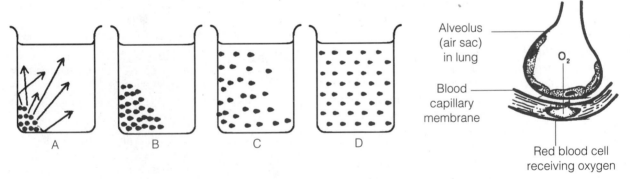

Diffusion:
(A) A small lump of sugar is placed into a beaker of water, its molecules dissolve and begin to diffuse outward. (B&C) The sugar molecules continue to diffuse through the water from an area of greater concentration to an area of lesser concentration. (D) Over a long period of time, the sugar molecules are evenly distributed throughout the water, reaching a state of equilibrium.

Example of diffusion in the human body: Oxygen diffuses from an alveolus in a lung where it is in greater concentration, across the blood capillary membrane, into a red blood cell where it is in lesser concentration.

FIGURE 4–8   The process of diffusion (From Fong, *Body Structures and Functions,* 8th ed. Copyright 1993, Delmar Publishers Inc.)

initial stage

distilled water →

• gelatin • salt • sucrose

(a) Initially, the sausage casing contains a solution of gelatin, salt and sucrose. The casing is permeable to water and salt molecules only. Since the concentration of water molecules is greater outside the casing, water molecules will diffuse into the casing. The opposite situation exists for the salt.

10–12 hours later

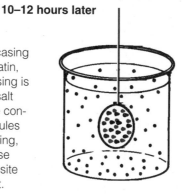

(b) The sausage casing swells due to the net movement of water molecules inward. However, the volume of distilled water in the beaker remains constant.

FIGURE 4–9 Osmosis: the diffusion of water through a selective permeable membrane is illustrated. (A sausage casing is an example of a selective permeable membrane.) (From Fong, *Body Structures and Functions,* 8th ed. Copyright 1993, Delmar Publishers Inc.)

Hypertonic solution

Hypotonic solution

Isotonic solution

Hypertonic solution (seawater)
a red blood cell will shrink and wrinkle up because water molecules are moving out of the cell.

• water molecules

Hypotonic solution (freshwater)
a red blood cell will swell and burst because water molecules are moving into the cell.

Isotonic solution (human blood serum)
a red blood cell remains unchanged, because the movement of water molecules into and out of the cell are the same.

FIGURE 4–10 Movement of water molecules in solutions of different osmolalities. (From Fong, *Body Structures and Functions,* 8th ed. Copyright 1993, Delmar Publishers Inc.)

semi permeable membrane

Filtration: Small molecules are filtered through the semi-permeable membrane, while the large molecules remain in the funnel.

Example of filtration in the human body: Glomerulus of kidney, large particles like red blood cells and proteins remain in the blood, and small molecules like urea and water are excreted as a metabolic excretory product—urine.

FIGURE 4–11 Filtration: a passive transport process (From Fong, *Body Structures and Functions,* 8th ed. Copyright 1993, Delmar Publishers Inc.)

Pinocytosis, as discussed earlier, is called "cell drinking" and involves the engulfing of large molecules of liquid material. Once inside the cytoplasm, the fluid is digested by the cell.

Another area of great importance to the welfare of the human body is its chemistry. The study of chemical reactions within the body is referred to as **biochemistry.** The basic building blocks of all matter are called **elements,** substances in their simplest form. There are 92 natural and at least 13 manufactured elements. Of these elements, about 20 are in all living things. Four of these 20 elements make up 97% of all living matter. They are carbon, oxygen, hydrogen, and nitrogen. The remaining 16 elements are sodium, chloride, magnesium, phosphorus, sulfur, calcium, potassium, iron, copper, manganese, zinc, boron, tin, vanadium, cobalt, and molybdenum. Because the last four occur in the body in such minute amounts, they are known as *trace elements.*

Many elements combine together in specific amounts to form new substances known as *compounds.* Some common compounds are water (hydrogen and oxygen), carbon dioxide (carbon and oxygen), salt (sodium and chloride), hydrochloric acid (hydrogen and chlorine), and sodium bicarbonate (sodium, hydrogen, carbon, and oxygen). Compounds can be classified in one of three groups: acids, bases, or salts. An acid compound will have positively charged ions of hydrogen and negatively charged ions of some other element. They have a sour taste, such as found in some citrus fruits (limes and lemons). An unknown substance, however, should never be tasted to determine its acidity, but rather tested by the special dyes contained in litmus paper. If acid is present, blue litmus paper will turn red.

A base compound is also called an alkali. A base substance will have negatively charged hydroxide ions and positively charged ions of a metal. Bases have a bitter taste and will turn red litmus paper blue. Table 4–2 lists some common acids and bases and identifies where they are found.

When an acid and a base are combined, they form a salt and water. A common example is sodium chloride (table salt), which is the result of combining hydrochloric acid with sodium hydroxide. When the water evaporates, the salt remains.

Frequently the determination of acidity or alkalinity of a body fluid or solution is desired. This measurement is referred to as the pH. A pH value of 7.0 on the pH scale indicates the solution has the same amount of hydrogen ions as hydroxide ions and therefore is neutral. An example of a neutral solution is water. A pH value between 0 and 6.9 indicates an acidic solution. The lower the number the stronger the acid or hydrogen ion concentration. A pH value of 7.1 to 14.0 indicates the solution is basic or alkaline. The higher the number is above 7.0 the stronger the base or hydroxide ion concentration. The pH values of some common acids, bases, and human body fluids and their effect on a pH testing strip are shown in Figure 4–13, page 82.

Cellular Division

The division of cells is known as mitosis and is controlled by the nucleus of the cell, Figure 4–14(a), page 82. When a cell is preparing to divide, the two pairs of centrioles, just outside the nucleus, move to opposite sides of the cell (b). Threadlike substances trail behind them, forming a spindle. The nucleus then duplicates exactly its chromatine material (c). As division begins, the nuclear membrane breaks up, and the pairs of chromosomes attach to the spindles (d) and are pulled to the center of the cell (e). As the spindles enlarge, the centrioles are pushed farther apart (f) until the chromosomes break in half (g). The spindles then dissolve, and a nuclear membrane develops around each new set of chromosomes (h). For unknown reasons, the cell then pinches itself in two, thereby making two new cells (i) called daughter cells. Mitosis results in the formation of two daughter nuclei with the exact same genes as the mother cell nucleus. The purpose of cell division is to provide exact duplication of cells for growth and repair of the body. In the unit on immunity, you will discover what happens when an antigen (foreign matter) interferes with this process.

All cells do not reproduce at the same rate. The blood-forming cells of the bone marrow, the cells of the skin, and the cells of the intestinal lining reproduce continuously. Muscle cells only reproduce every few years; however, muscle tissue formed of voluntary muscle cells may be enlarged with exercise. This is apparent from the great increase in muscle size produced by body builders who use weight and repetitions of

FIGURE 4–12 Phagocytosis of bacteria by a white blood cell. Phagocytosis can occur in the blood stream or white cells may squeeze through capillary walls and destroy bacteria in the tissues.

TABLE 4–2

Names, Location, or Use of Some Common Acids and Bases

Name of Acid	Where Found or Used
Acetic acid	Found in vinegar
Boric acid	Weak eyewash
Carbonic acid	Found in carbonated beverages
Hydrochloric acid	Found in stomach
Nitric acid	Industrial oxidizing acid
Sulfuric acid	Found in batteries and industrial mineral acid

Name of Base	Where Found or Used
Ammonium hydroxide	Household liquid cleaners
Magnesium hydroxide	Milk of magnesia
Potassium hydroxide	Caustic potash
Sodium hydroxide	Lye

(Adapted from Fong, *Body Structure and Functions,* 8th ed. Copyright 1993, Delmar Publishers, Inc.)

routines to achieve muscle definition and enlargement. Cells of the **nerve** tissue, or **neurons,** do not increase in number after birth, and some cannot be regenerated if damaged or destroyed.

There are many kinds of cells with different shapes and sizes. The characteristics shown in Figure 4–7 are common to most cells. Cells like those in the blood (red, white, and platelets) and the nerve cells, however, are very different and perform specialized functions. With this specialization, some of the other cell functions may be lost, such as the ability of some nerve cells to reproduce. Specialization also results in an interdependence among cells to enable them to carry out their activities. One type of cell that is very different is the sex cell (gamete), which is responsible for reproduction. During a process known as meiosis, the ovum from the female and the spermatozoon from the male each reduce their respective 46 chromosomes to 23, one half the normal amount. When fertilization occurs, the two cells combine to form a single cell called a zygote, which will then have the full set of 46 chromosomes, 23 from each parent. The zygote will subsequently, by mitosis, divide again and again until the new being is fully developed. This cellular activity will be more fully discussed in the section on the reproductive system.

Homeostasis

The body has many control systems, some of which operate within the cell. It is important that the fluid within the cell (*intracellular fluid*) maintains the proper chemical balance for the cell to maintain life. The fluid surrounding the cells (*extra-*

cellular fluid) mixes with the fluid of the blood to supply the cell with food and other substances. When the internal environment is functioning properly and all the organs and tissues of the body are performing their appropriate tasks, a condition of **homeostasis** exists. This is a stable condition of the internal environment. This condition continues until one or more of the control systems loses the ability to maintain it. When this occurs, all cells of the body suffer. A moderate dysfunction causes illness; a severe dysfunction leads to death.

Genetic Cellular Change

Several disorders result from improper sex cell division at the time of fertilization or from the inheritance of an altered **gene** or genes. These are collectively called genetic disorders. Some result in structural defects, such as cleft lip, cleft palate, club foot, spinal bifida, and congenital heart disease.

A condition resulting from the absence or alteration of a protein enzyme is known as phenylketonuria (PKU). Before birth the mother's blood supplies the missing chemical compounds, but at birth the baby is unable to handle some metabolic products, thereby impairing brain development, causing profound retardation, seizures, and stunted growth. Checking newborns with a heel-stick blood test permits early diagnosis and dietary treatment to prevent the consequences of the disorder from developing.

A genetic disorder known as galactosemia occurs when a byproduct of lactose (milk sugar) cannot be metabolized. It is caused by the mutation of a single gene. About 1 in 100,000 newborns has this condition. Early symptoms include malnutrition, diarrhea, and severe vomiting. Often the eyes, liver, and brain become damaged. Children who are not treated will die. If the abnormality is detected early enough, infants can be fed a diet including milk substitutes and grow up to be symptom-free as long as they avoid galactose.

Some disorders are known as sex-linked because they are carried by the X or Y chromosome, which differentiates males and females. Probably the best known is hemophilia, a bleeding disorder caused by a lack of protein. The disorder is carried by the female but occurs only in males. This condition is now treatable by administration of factor VIII, a human blood-clotting factor.

Another sex chromosome abnormality is called Turner's syndrome. About 1 in 5000 newborn females will have the disorder. Affected individuals have only 45 chromosomes; because of a failure of the sex cells to divide correctly in meiosis, only one sex chromosome is present in their cells. Turner's syndrome causes a short stature, webbing of the neck, a wide chest with broadly spaced nipples, and poor breast development. The ovaries and secondary sexual characteristics fail to develop, making the female sterile. Often it is not recognized until lack of menses and developing genitalia become apparent. Treatment with estrogen (female hormone) after age 13 to 15, to prevent growth from stopping, will produce a menstrual cycle but will not reverse the sterility.

A similar condition affecting males is called Klinefelter's

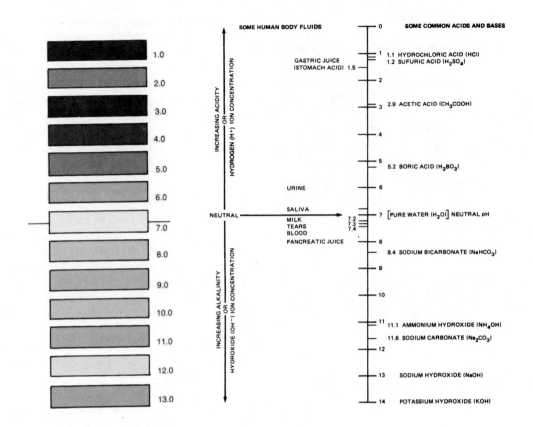

FIGURE 4–13 pH Values of some common acids, bases, and human body fluids and the color changes that can occur to a pH strip when tested. (From Fong, *Body Structures and Functions,* 8th ed. Copyright 1993, Delmar Publishers Inc.)

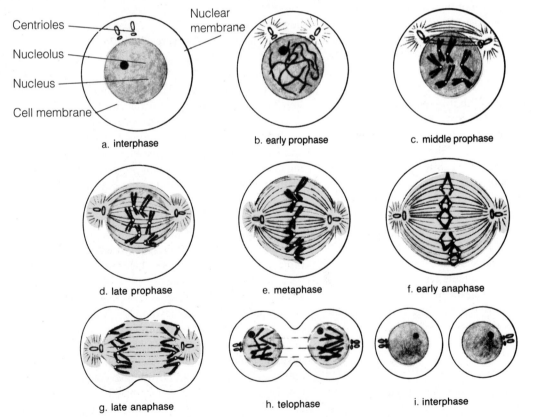

FIGURE 4–14 Stages of mitosis in animal cells (Adapted from Schraer & Stolze, *Biology: The Study of Life,* 2d ed. Copyright 1987, Allyn and Bacon, Inc.)

syndrome and affects, in varying degrees, approximately 1 in 600. It is the result of one or more extra X chromosomes. It usually becomes apparent at puberty when the penis and testicles fail to mature fully, often leading to sterility. The severity depends on the number of extra chromosomes. Other symptoms are breast enlargement, mental retardation, sparse body hair, abnormal body build (long legs with short obese trunk), tallness, a tendency toward alcoholism, and often personality disorders. Treatment with testosterone, the male hormone, if begun early may help reverse the feminine characteristics, but will not reverse the sterility or mental retardation. Psychotherapy is indicated when sexual dysfunction causes emotional maladjustment.

A well-known chromosomal abnormality resulting from improper cell division is Down syndrome. In this disorder, the number 21 chromosome is in triplicate rather than a pair, so that the individual has 47 instead of 46 chromosomes per cell. The *syndrome* (group of features) causes structural defects consisting of slanting eyes, a fold at the inner eye, large tongue, pug nose, and microcephaly (small head). Mental retardation occurs in all cases as well as some degree of growth restriction. About 1 in every 1000 live births in North America develops the disorder.

Amniocentesis, a diagnostic test, is indicated when prenatal interviews indicate the possibility of a genetic problem. A small amount of amniotic fluid, which surrounds the fetus, is removed from the pregnant uterus. Skin cells from the fetus are in the fluid and can be grown in a culture for examination. The test can relieve anxiety or permit early pregnancy termination if findings indicate a cause for concern.

Tissues

As previously stated, not all cells are alike. They may be transparent, as in the eye, or transmit electrical impulses or nutrients. Some have long thin fibers, and others produce secretions. When cells of the same type group together for a common purpose, they form a **tissue.** Tissues are from 60% to 99% water. The essential substances needed by the body are either dissolved or suspended in the tissue fluids. Therefore, water is indispensable to cell life, and lack of it causes death more rapidly than lack of any other substance, except oxygen.

Two common medical terms describe the opposites of tissue fluid balance. When there is too little fluid, the condition is known as **dehydration.** An abnormal accumulation of excess fluid, causing puffiness of the affected tissues, is known as **edema.**

Tissue Classifications
Tissues can be classified into four main types: **epithelial, connective,** nerve, and muscle.

Epithelial. Epithelial tissues form the body's glands, cover the surface of the body, and line the cavities. Epithelium is the main tissue of the skin, which serves as a protective covering for the body. Epithelium also covers all the organs and lines the intestinal, respiratory, and urinary tract, the blood vessels, and the uterus. Some epithelial tissues secrete fluids, such as

mucus and digestive juices. Others selectively absorb nutrients, chemical elements, and water. The epithelium of the urinary bladder is uniquely arranged in folds to allow for expansion as the bladder fills.

Epithelial tissues in glands specialize to provide specific secretions for the body. Glands that secrete directly into the blood in the capillaries are known as *endocrine,* or ductless, glands.

Glands that produce secretions through ducts within the body are classified as *exocrine,* Figure 4–15. Two glands, the liver and pancreas, produce both endocrine and exocrine secretions.

Connective. Connective tissue forms the supporting structure of the body, connecting other tissues together to form the organs and body parts. There are several categories of connective tissue but they can also be simply divided into soft or hard tissues. A soft type is adipose or fat tissue, which stores the body's reserve of food, fills in between tissue fibers, insulates against heat and cold, and pads the body structures, Figure 4–16. Another form of soft connective tissue is stretchable and forms the subcutaneous layer of the skin. A soft but dense connective tissue in the form of tendons, ligaments, and organ capsules serves to support and protect organs and lend elasticity to the walls of arteries, Figure 4–17.

Blood and lymphatic vessels, lymph, the blood, and blood cells are all considered to be connective tissues. Cells in the blood carry nutrients and oxygen to the cells and pick up metabolic wastes for elimination. Lymph fluid consists of water, glucose, fats, and salt and is present in the spaces between the cells of the tissues as well as within the lymph vessels. Soft connective tissue plays a major role in the repair of damaged body tissue. The repair process involves new blood vessel formation and the growth of new connective tissue known as scar tissue. Excessive blood vessel development in the early stages

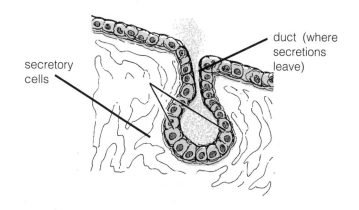

exocrine (duct) gland cell
e.g. sweat and mammary glands

FIGURE 4–15 Epithelial cell tissue of an exocrine gland. (From Fong, *Body Structures and Functions,* 8th ed. Copyright 1993, Delmar Publishers Inc.)

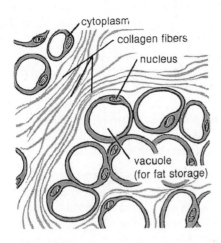

FIGURE 4–16 Adipose tissue throughout the body (From Fong, *Body Structures and Functions,* 8th ed. Copyright 1993, Delmar Publishers Inc.)

FIGURE 4–17 Dense fibrous connective tissue in ligaments and tendons (From Fong, *Body Structures and Functions,* 8th ed. Copyright 1993, Delmar Publishers Inc.)

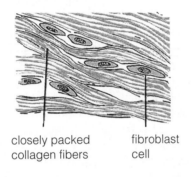

closely packed collagen fibers   fibroblast cell

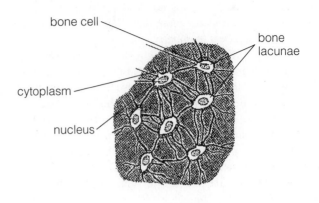

FIGURE 4–18 Hard connective tissue found in bone (From Fong, *Body Structures and Functions,* 8th ed. Copyright 1993, Delmar Publishers Inc.)

results in a condition called "proud flesh." In instances of surgery or suturing (sewing) of a clean wound, the need for tissue regrowth and therefore the resulting scar is reduced because the cut edges are brought together closely by the surgical process. An excessive growth of scar tissue is called a **Keloid.**

Hard connective tissue can be found in the cartilage and bones of the body. Cartilage is located between the bones of the spine (where it acts as a shock absorber and allows for flexibility) and in the ear, nose and voice box (to provide shaping). Bone tissue is actually cartilage with the addition of calcium salts. This addition takes place gradually from birth until the tissue becomes hardened, Figure 4–18.

Bone tissue, which is also called **osseous** tissue, is not a lifeless material. Within most bone is a medullary cavity filled with yellow marrow, which is composed of fat, connective tissue, and blood vessels. Some long bones contain cavities filled with red marrow, which manufactures red blood cells. Because bone is a living tissue with a blood supply and nerves, it can easily repair itself when it is damaged.

Nerve.   Nerve tissue is found throughout the body. It serves as the body's communication network. The basic structural unit of the tissue is the neuron, which consists of a nerve cell body and fibers that resemble tree branches, Figure 4–19, page 85. The dendrites bring impulses to the cell body; the axon

conducts impulses away. Neurons range from a fraction of an inch up to 3 feet in length.

There are three types of nerve cells or neurons. A *sensory neuron* in the skin or sense organs picks up a stimulus and sends it toward the spinal cord and brain. An *interneuron,* or *connecting neuron,* carries the impulse to another neuron. A *motor neuron* receives an impulse and sends a message, which causes a reaction.

Clusters of neurons form the nerve tissue. Nerves throughout the body join together to form the spinal cord, which in turn transmits electrical impulses to and from the brain. Nerves outside the brain and spinal cord are called *peripheral nerves.* The fibers of these nerves are covered with a fatty insulating material called **myelin** sheath, which is then covered with a thin membrane called **neurilemma.** If a sheathed nerve fiber is damaged or cut, it can be surgically repaired and a new fiber may form within the sheath, but nerve tissue recovers very slowly, if at all. Unfortunately, fibers of the brain, spinal cord, optic (eye), and auditory (ear) nerves lack sheaths and cannot be repaired by surgery when damaged or cut.

Muscle.   Muscle tissue is designed to contract on stimulation. Tissue that can be controlled at will with impulses from the brain is called **voluntary** muscle tissue. This type is found connected to the bones of the body, and is called **skeletal** or **striated** muscle, Figure 4–20(a). It gives us the ability to move our bodies.

Involuntary muscle action occurs without control or conscious awareness. There are two types of involuntary muscle tissue. One type, called **smooth** muscle tissue, is found within the walls of all the organs of the body except the heart. This type of tissue moves food and waste material through the digestive tract and changes the size of the iris of the eye and the diameter of arteries, Figure 4–20(b). The other type of involuntary muscle tissue, called **cardiac** muscle tissue, is found only in the heart. Cardiac muscle fibers are joined in a continuous network and must contract together in a forceful, rhythmic action to pump blood throughout the body, Figure 4–20(c).

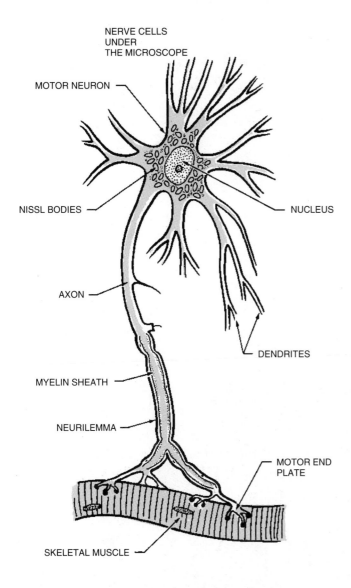

NERVE CELLS
UNDER
THE MICROSCOPE

MOTOR NEURON

NISSL BODIES

NUCLEUS

AXON

DENDRITES

MYELIN SHEATH

NEURILEMMA

MOTOR END
PLATE

SKELETAL MUSCLE

FIGURE 4–19 A motor neuron (From *The Wonderful Human Machine,* Copyright 1979, American Medical Association)

Organs

The **organs** of the body are made of two or more types of tissue that work together to perform a specific body function. For example, the stomach is constructed with walls of smooth muscle tissue to "churn" the food; it is lined with one type of epithelial tissue, which secretes gastric juices, and covered with another type, which protects the organ; connective tissue fills the spaces between the other tissue fibers; nerve tissue controls the rate at which material is emptied from the stomach. (The roles of the organs will be discussed in more detail in the remaining units of this chapter.)

Systems

Organs of the body that perform similar functions are organized into a body **system.** Using the stomach again as an example, it joins with the mouth, throat, esophagus, and small and large intestines to make up the alimentary tract of the

digestive system. The alimentary tract combines with the teeth, tongue, salivary glands, liver, pancreas, and gallbladder to form the total digestive system. The other systems of the body, which will be discussed individually, are the integumentary, skeletal, muscular, respiratory, circulatory, urinary, nervous, endocrine, and reproductive systems.

One additional "system" will also be discussed later in this chapter. The immune system is not normally considered, at least at the present time, as being a "system." The body's health and well-being, however, so directly depend on an intact and effective immune response, that it requires you have a basic knowledge of its role in disease response. As scientists begin to understand better how it functions and what can be done to correct a malfunction, perhaps we can solve the mysteries of cancer and AIDS, as well as many other immunologically based disorders. The basics of the complex subject of immunology are discussed in Unit 9.

Even a body system cannot function alone. All systems must combine their individual contributions for the health and well-being of the total human body. Figure 4–21, page 86 illustrates the body systems.

Note: Figure 4–21 includes the lymphatic system. This system is usually considered as part of the circulatory system.

Complete Chapter 4, Unit 1 in the workbook to help you meet the objectives at the beginning of this unit and therefore achieve competency of this subject matter.

U N I T 2
The Nervous System

OBJECTIVES

Upon completion of this unit, you will meet the following terminal performance objectives by verifying knowledge of the facts and principles presented through oral and written communication at a level deemed competent by the instructor or employer.

1. Name the two main divisions of the nervous system.
2. Identify the two types of peripheral nerves and explain the function of the spinal nerves.
3. Describe simple and complex reflex actions.
4. Describe a synapse and the effects of various substances on its action.
5. Describe the purpose of the automatic nervous system and explain the action of its two divisions.
6. Identify the main parts of the brain and their functions.
7. Name the coverings of the brain and spinal cord and describe their purpose.
8. Describe the function of cerebrospinal fluid.
9. Name common diagnostic tests used to identify neurological disorders and possible reasons for their use.
10. List the functions of the hypothalamus.
11. Describe 21 diseases or disorders of the nervous system.
12. Spell and define, using the glossary at the back of the text, all the words to know in this unit.

centrally located
nucleus

striations

branching of cell

intercalated disc

spindle-shaped cell

nucleus

cells separated
from each other

nucleus   myofibrils

A

B

C

exocrine (duct) gland cell
e.g. sweat and mammmary glands

FIGURE 4–20 (A) Skeletal muscle tissue (straited voluntary) attaches to bone. (B) Smooth muscle tissue in walls of organs and blood vessels. (C) Cardiac muscle tissue of the heart. (From Fong, *Body Structures and Functions,* 8th ed. Copyright 1993, Delmar Publishers Inc.)

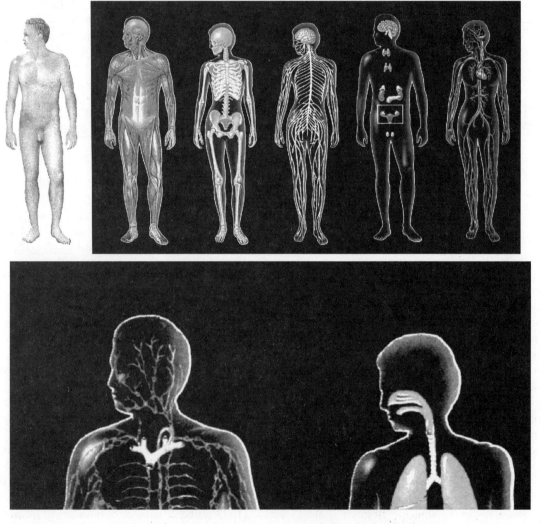

FIGURE 4–21 The body systems (From Starr & Taggart, *Biology, The Unity and Diversity of Life,* 5th ed. Copyright 1989, Wadsworth Publishing Co.)

action potential
angiography
arachnoid
arteriography
auditory
autonomic
axon
brain scan
central
cerebellum
cerebrospinal fluid
cerebrum
computerized axial
  tomography (CAT)
cranium
dendrite
dura mater
electroencephalography
  (EEG)
electromyography
frontal
ganglion
hypothalamus
interneurons
longitudinal fissure
lumbar puncture
magnetic resonance imaging
  (MRI)

medulla oblongata
meninges
midbrain
migraine
motor
myelography
occipital
olfactory
optic
parasympathetic
parietal
peripheral
pia mater
plexuses
pneumoencephalograph
pons
sciatica
sensory
spina bifida
subarachnoid
subdural
sympathetic
synapse
syndrome
temporal
thalamus
thorax
ventricle

The nervous system is the communication network that organizes and coordinates all the body's functions. It is a complex and somewhat difficult system to understand, and in most texts is not usually discussed early in the study of the body systems. In this text, however, it is being presented first. It is believed that this will help you to understand more easily the involvement of the nervous system's regulatory action in the functioning of the other body systems, as they are discussed.

You might think of the system as being something like your telephone system. You can make local, in-state, national, and international calls. You can easily call next door, but the further away you call the more number messages and the more "routing" of signals one needed to complete your call. The phone picks up your voice (stimulus), converts it to impulses, and sends it along a charged line to a bundle of lines and on to phone company switching equipment. Every so often, the impulse is "boosted" to maintain your "voice." It may even be given a special treatment and sent through space and bounced off a satellite, but the message is forwarded to its destination. Your nervous system operates in a similar but much more complicated manner. The system has two main divisions: the **central** nervous system (CNS), which consists of the brain and the spinal cord, and the **peripheral** nervous system, which includes all the nerves that connect the CNS to every organ and area of the body. The **autonomic** nervous system is a specialized part of the peripheral system and controls internal organs and other self-regulating body functions.

Like in all systems, the basic functioning unit is the cell; in this system the unit is a nerve cell, or neuron. As described in Unit 1, there are three types of neurons in nerve tissue: **sensory,** connecting, and **motor.** They receive stimuli or impulses, transmit impulses to other neurons, and deliver response actions to the muscles and glands. Connecting neurons are also called *associative,* or *internuncial, neurons.* Figure 4–22 illustrates the three types of neurons.

All nerve cells have a nucleus, cytoplasm, and a cell membrane. Scattered throughout the cytoplasm are little microscopic granular "dots" called Nissl bodies, see Figure 4–19. They may represent a store of nervous energy. The cell body has processes that are extensions of cytoplasm called **dendrites** and **axons.** A neuron may have many dendrites but only one axon. These extensions are also called *fibers.* Around the long thin axons of peripheral nerves are the Schwann cells. They form a tight protective covering called the myelin sheath and also play a part in the transmission of messages. The myelin is then surrounded by the neurilemma, an elastic sheath covering.

A nerve is composed of bundles of nerve fibers bound together by connective tissue. If a nerve is composed of fibers going from the sense organs to the spinal cord or brain, it is a *sensory,* or *afferent, nerve.* If it is carrying impulses from the brain or spinal cord to a muscle, organ, or gland it is known as a *motor,* or *efferent, nerve.* Some nerves have both kinds of fibers and are known as *mixed nerves.*

Membrane Excitability ....

Nerves carry impulses by creating electrical charges in a process known as membrane excitability. Neurons have a membrane that separates the cytoplasm inside from the extracellular fluids outside the cell, thereby creating two chemically different areas. Each area has differing amounts of potassium and sodium ions and some other charged substances, with the inside being the more negatively charged. When a neuron is stimulated, ions move across the membrane creating a current, which if large enough, will briefly change the inside of the neuron to be more positive than the outside area. This state is known as **action potential.** Neurons and other cells that produce action potentials are said to have membrane excitability.

To understand how impulses are carried along nerves or throughout a muscle when it contracts, we need to learn a little more about membrane excitability. Ions cross a membrane through channels, some of which are open and allow ions to "leak" (diffuse) continuously. Other channels are called "gated" and open only during action potential. Another membrane opening is called a sodium–potassium pump which, by active transport, maintains the flow of ions from higher to lower concentrations levels across the membrane and restores the cytoplasm and extracellular fluid to their original value, after an action potential occurs. This action is in response to the fact there is an imbalance between the cytoplasm and the extracellular fluid. When diffusion takes place, particles move from an area of greater concentration to an area of lesser concentration.

The following simplified description explains how this whole process works.

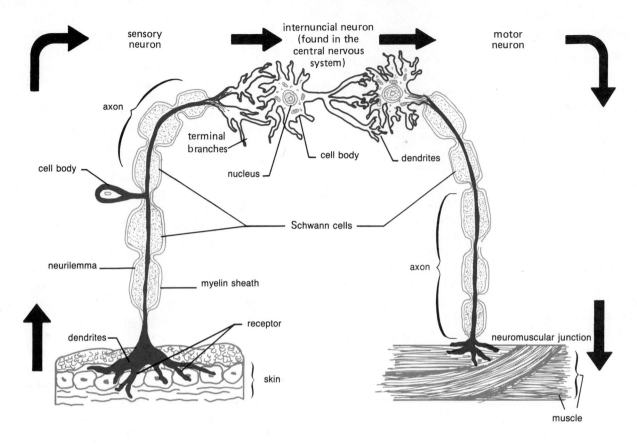

FIGURE 4–22 Classifications of neurons according to function. (From Fong, *Body Structures and Functions,* 8th ed. Copyright 1993, Delmar Publishers Inc.)

1. A neuron membrane is "at rest." There are large amounts of potassium (K$_+$) ions inside the cells but not very many sodium (NA$_+$) ions. The reverse is true outside the cell in the extracellular fluid. Most of the open channels are for potassium to pass through, so it leaks out of the cell.

2. As the K$_+$ ions leave, the inside becomes relatively more negative until some K$_+$ ions are attracted back in and the electrical force balances the diffusion force and movement stops. The inside is still more negative, and the amount of energy between the two differently charged areas is ready to work (carry an impulse). This state is called *resting membrane potential,* Figure 4–23(a). The membrane is now polarized. The sodium ions are not able to move "in" since their channels are closed during the resting state; however, if a few leak in, the membrane pump sends an equal number out.

3. Now suppose a sensory neuron receptor is stimulated by something, a sound for instance. This will cause a change in the membrane potential. The stimulus energy is converted to an electrical signal, and if it is strong enough, it will depolarize a portion of the membrane and allow the gated sodium ion channels to open initiating an action potential, Figure 4–23(b).

4. The sodium ions move through the gated channels into the cytoplasm, and the inside becomes more positive until the membrane potential is reversed and the gates close to sodium ions.

5. Next the potassium gates open, and large amounts of potassium leave the cytoplasm, resulting in the repolarization of the membrane, Figure 4–23(c). After repolarization, the sodium–potassium pump restores the initial concentrations of sodium and potassium ions inside and outside the neuron.

This whole process occurs in a few milliseconds. When this action occurs in one part of the cell membrane, it spreads to adjacent membrane regions, continuing away from the original site of stimulation, sending "messages" over the nerve. This cycle is completed millions of times a minute throughout the body, day after day, year after year.

But what happens when the impulse reaches the end of the neuron? You will recall that impulses travel across a neuron from the dendrites to the cell body and then to the axon. Here there is a minute space between the dendrites of the next neuron called a **synapse,** which the impulse must "jump" chemically. This space is technically called a *synaptic cleft.* Impulses from the sending cell release "transmitter substances" into the cleft, Figure 4–24. These substances are signaling molecules that can cause a rapid change in the membrane potential of the receiving cell. These chemicals can either speed up or slow down the transmission. Normally nerve impulses travel about 200 miles per hour. The intake of alcohol, for instance, seems to aid the chemical that causes impulses to be blocked, and our reactions are therefore slowed down. Other chemicals, such as stimulant drugs and wartime nerve gases, cause the release of a chemical that allows the transmission of impulses to speed up, even to the point of causing a flood of impulses to the brain resulting in the possible breakdown of the body's ability to function.

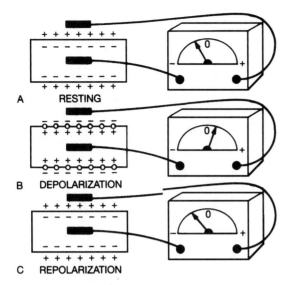

FIGURE 4–23 Sequence of events in membrane potential and relative positive and negative states.
(a). Normal resisting potential—(negative inside/positive outside)
(b). Depolarization—(positive inside/negative outside)
(c). Repolarization—(negative inside/positive outside)

A disease condition called tetanus results from the effects of the bacteria, *Clostridium tetani,* on the nervous and muscular systems. Bacteria invade the body through a puncture wound from a contaminated object or an animal bite. The tissues deep in the puncture do not receive oxygen, so they die off, and the bacteria multiply. A substance is released by the bacteria, which is toxic to the motor neurons that innervate the muscles. A neuron normally stimulates muscle tissue through balanced chemical messages, which alternately contract and relax the muscle tissue. This balance is essential to our ability to maintain erect stature and movement. With the release of the neurotoxin from the bacteria, however, excitation is unbalanced, and the inhibitory synapses of the motor neurons of the brain and spinal cord are affected, thereby allowing excessive contraction of the muscles. (Without the control of the "inhibitor," the message goes on full permission to contract.) The muscles cannot relax and there is a prolonged, spastic paralysis of the muscles, which can result in death.

With this one example, it is apparent how the function of the nervous system affects the total welfare of the body. It is now important to learn how the nerves are organized in the communication network.

Peripheral Nervous System and Spinal Cord

The peripheral nervous system includes 12 pairs of cranial nerves that connect the brain directly to the sense organs (eye, ear, tongue, nose, and skin), the heart, lungs, and other internal organs. Some cranial nerves, like the optic nerve from the eye, have only sensory fibers, whereas others, like those to the heart

and lungs, are mixed nerves containing both sensory and motor fibers. The peripheral system also includes 31 pairs of spinal nerves. The spinal nerves are both motor (to provide a function or movement) and sensory (to perceive stimuli); therefore they are also mixed nerves.

All spinal nerves enter and leave the spinal cord, which is located within the canal created by an opening in each of the bones (vertebrae) of the spinal column. A cross section of the cord would reveal a rounded white mass of myelinated nerve fibers with a notched area on the anterior surface, Figure 4–25. The white matter is mainly axons of **interneurons.** Some axons are grouped together into major sensory nerves going to a specific section of the brain. Others are grouped into major motor nerves going to their muscle or organ destination. Still others connect with each other up, down, and within the gray matter to provide control over activities that occur within the cord itself. In the center of the white area is a gray area in the shape of an H, which is the nerve cell bodies and their fibers without the myelin covering. The gray matter is involved mainly with reflex connections in the spinal cord that deal with the reflexes involved in such things as walking or blinking.

A spinal nerve splits into two roots as it enters the cord. The rear root carrying sensory fibers to the cord enters at the rear horn of the H. The bulge on the rear root contains the sensory nerve cell bodies and is called a **ganglion.** The front root of the nerve leaves at the anterior horn of the H, carrying motor nerve fibers which have their cell bodies inside the gray matter of the cord. Neurons within the cord itself connect sensory to motor nerves.

Sensory neurons transmit messages from millions of special receptor cells to the spinal cord and on to the brain for interpretation and decisions. If a reaction is needed, impulses from the CNS are transmitted to the appropriate muscle or organ over the motor neurons. Connecting interneurons route impulses throughout the body, permitting any nerve to communicate with any other nerve.

In very simple reflex actions in which no interpretation or decision is required, the nerve impulse travels only to the spinal cord and back. The knee jerk test often used by physicians illustrates such a simple reflex and provides an evaluation of the nervous system. When the knee is hanging completely relaxed, the leg should kick up sharply when the tendon below the kneecap is lightly tapped, Figure 4–26. If there is no response, a nervous system disease or disorder can be suspected.

In more complicated reflex actions, such as a hand coming into contact with something hot, the sensory impulse is relayed through nerve cells to the spinal cord and up to the brain, Figure 4–27. There the impulse is interpreted, and the motor neurons carry the message back down the spinal cord and out the appropriate nerves. The eyes see the object, the hand will jerk away, and the voice may speak out.

Autonomic Nervous System The autonomic nervous system is part of the peripheral nervous system. These nerves are involuntary and unconsciously regulate functions, such as breathing, heartbeat, and digestion. The system consists of

FIGURE 4–24 Transmission of a nerve impulse across a synaps is chemical. Acetylcholine and cholinesterase are often the chemical mediators. (From Burke, *Human Anatomy and Physiology in Health and Disease,* 3d ed. Copyright 1992, Delmar Publishers Inc.)

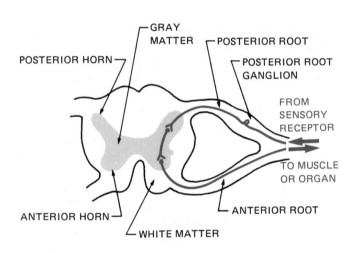

FIGURE 4–25 Cross section of the spinal cord

nerves, ganglia, and **plexuses** (networks of nerves). There are two divisions of the autonomic system. The **sympathetic** division accelerates activity in the smooth, involuntary muscles of the body's organs, and the **parasympathetic** division reverses the action and slows down activity. For example, the sympathetic nerves constrict blood vessels and speed up the heartbeat; the parasympathetic nerves dilate the blood vessels and slow down the heartbeat. These activities continuously balance each other to maintain homeostasis in the body. This on–off mechanism does not apply to all organs, however, because some do not have a dual nerve supply. Also, nerves in both divisions can have excitatory or inhibitory effects. At any given time, the actual effect depends on the net outcome of the two opposing signals.

The *sympathetic nervous system* begins at the base of the brain and runs down both sides of the spinal column in two tracts. These consist of nerve fibers and ganglia. The sympathetic nerves extend to all the vital internal organs, the blood vessels, the iris of the eye, and even to the sweat glands, Figure 4–28, page 93.

The *parasympathetic system* has two important nerves: the vagus and the pelvic nerve. The vagus extends from the medulla oblongata of the brain and branches to the neck, chest, and upper abdominal organs. The pelvic nerve exits the spinal cord around the hip area and branches into the lower abdominal and pelvic organs. Both systems are strongly affected by emotions such as fear, anger, and stress.

The action of the autonomic system is extremely important to our ability to react in an emergency. It is frequently called our "flight–fright mechanism," because it accelerates our body functions to permit escaping or otherwise dealing with danger.

Central Nervous System..........................

The Brain The brain is a large mass of nerve tissue with about 100 billion neurons. It is protected and supported by surrounding membranes known as **meninges,** Figure 4–29, page 94. It is

FIGURE 4–26 The reflex arc. In this example, tapping the knee (patellar tendon) results in extension of the leg, producing the knee jerk reflex. (From Fong, *Body Structures and Functions,* 8th ed. Copyright 1993, Delmar Publishers Inc.)

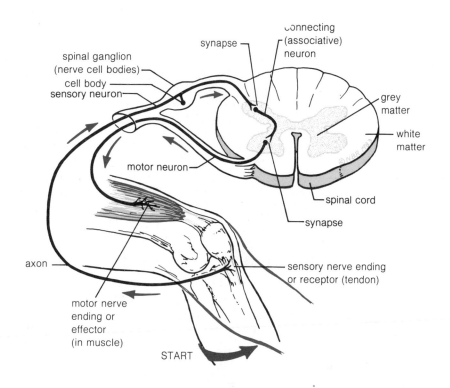

further protected by the **cranium** (skull). The brain surface has extensive deep furrows and folds and is divided into two hemispheres by a **longitudinal fissure.** The hemispheres are connected internally with nerve fibers and share information. The cerebral surface is covered with ridges and furrows known as *fissures,* if they are deep, or *sulci* if they are shallow. The elevated ridges between the sulci are called *convolutions.*

The brain is divided into five parts. The largest is the **cerebrum,** which controls sensory and motor activities. The cerebrum is further divided into lobes, Figure 4–30, page 94. The **frontal** lobe behind the forehead seems to be related to emotions, personality, moral traits, and intellectual functions. The frontal lobe is also the motor area for active voluntary muscle movements as well as two areas that control speech. The **occipital** lobe is the far back portion of the cerebrum. This area is associated with vision. The impulses of color and light received by the eyes are transmitted by the **optic** nerve fibers to the occipital lobe for interpretation. Between the frontal and occipital lobes is the **parietal** lobe. The motor area governing speech lies at its junction with the frontal lobe. It is the parietal lobe that receives impulses from receptors in the hands, feet, and tongue, among others, and sends impulses that cause movement in all these parts in response. This area also receives nerve impulses from sensory receptors for pain, touch, heat, and cold. A small **temporal** lobe lies on the side of the cerebrum. The **auditory** nerve association area is here, which provides us with the sense of hearing. The **olfactory** area, which provides our sense of smell, is within a small projection under the temporal lobe. It is connected by nerve fibers to receptors in the nasal cavity.

Beneath the cerebrum lies the part of the brain known as the

cerebellum. This section is responsible for smooth muscle movement, muscle tone, and coordination of sensory impulses with muscular activity, particularly for equilibrium, walking, and dancing. If the cerebellum is damaged, many activities requiring coordination of muscles cannot be performed.

The **medulla oblongata** is the part of the brain that adjoins the spinal cord. The medulla influences, through the autonomic nervous system, the function of the heart and lungs, stomach secretions, and the size of the openings in blood vessels.

Just above the medulla is the **pons.** This part of the brain also helps to regulate breathing. It is the reflex center for chewing, tasting, and secreting saliva. A small part called the **midbrain** is superior to the pons. This area is the control center for some of the reflex movements of the eyes, such as blinking and changing the size of the pupil. It also conducts impulses between the brain parts above and below it.

In an area between the cerebrum and the midbrain are two major structures, the **thalamus** and the **hypothalamus.** The thalamus acts as a relay station for impulses going to and from the brain as well as those from the cerebellum and other parts of the brain. The hypothalamus lies below the thalamus and is connected to the pituitary gland, midbrain, and thalamus by a bundle of nerve fibers. The hypothalamus performs many vital functions such as:

1. Autonomic nervous control
2. Controling blood pressure by regulating the heart beat and blood vessel constriction and dilation
3. Maintaining body temperature
4. Stimulating the production of an antidiuretic hormone to conserve water in the body and to cause thirst to maintain normal water balance

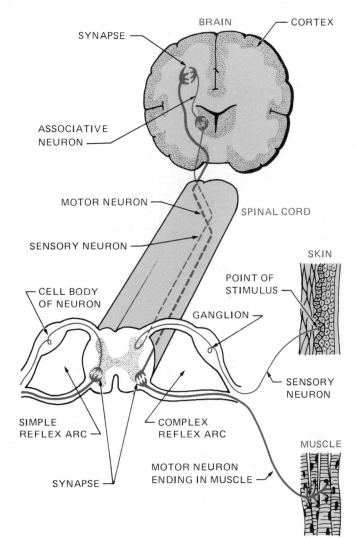

BRAIN — CORTEX

SYNAPSE

ASSOCIATIVE NEURON

MOTOR NEURON

SPINAL CORD

SENSORY NEURON

SKIN

POINT OF STIMULUS

CELL BODY OF NEURON

GANGLION

SENSORY NEURON

SIMPLE REFLEX ARC

COMPLEX REFLEX ARC

MUSCLE

SYNAPSE

MOTOR NEURON ENDING IN MUSCLE

FIGURE 4–27 Complex reflex action (From *The Wonderful Human Machine,* Copyright 1979, American Medical Association)

5. Assisting in the regulation of appetite
6. Increasing secretions and motility in the intestinal tract
7. Playing a role in emotions, such as fear and pleasure
8. Helping maintain wakefulness when it is necessary

The midbrain, pons, and the medulla make up the brain stem. Doctors learned long ago that nerve fibers from the right side of the body cross over in the brain stem to the left side of the brain. The body's left side is likewise controlled by the right side of the brain. Therefore, when a person is paralyzed on the right side, it may be that there is damage to the left side of the brain.

Meninges Because of their common origin, the brain and the spinal cord are covered with the same meninges (membranes), Figure 4–31. Three membrane layers make up the meninges. The innermost layer is called the **pia mater,** a delicate, tight-fitting covering containing blood vessels to nourish the nerve tissue. The middle layer, the **arachnoid,** is a delicate, lacelike

membrane. The outer layer, called **dura mater,** is a tough, fibrous tissue which protects the CNS from being damaged from contact with the bony surfaces of the skull and spine. The space between the dura mater and the arachnoid is called the **subdural** space. The **subarachnoid** space is between the arachnoid and the pia mater.

Cavities of the Brain and Spinal Cord Within the brain are several hollow areas called **ventricles.** They extend into the lobes of the cerebrum and into contact with the other sections of the brain by means of small passageways. The central canal of the spinal cord is directly associated with the most inferior ventricle. There are also connections from the ventricles into the subarachnoid space of the meninges.

Cerebrospinal Fluid The hollow cavities within the brain and spinal cord are filled with a liquid called **cerebrospinal fluid (CSF).** This fluid acts as a watery cushion or shock absorber to provide additional protection for the delicate tissues of the CNS. The fluid transports nutrients, primarily proteins, and carbohydrates to the brain and spinal cord. CSF is formed continuously within the ventricles of the brain at the rate of 450 mL (15 ounces) per day. Only 150 mL are present at any one time in a normal adult. The fluid circulates within the cavities of the brain and spinal cord and the subarachnoid space, being reabsorbed into the blood vessels in special structures called *arachnoidal villi.*

Diagnostic Tests ....

Diagnosis of neurological disorders and diseases may require the use of specific tests. Some of the more common tests and a few possible findings are as follows:

■ **Arteriography**—(cerebral angiography)—A catheter (small tube) is inserted into an artery and threaded up to the carotid artery in the neck. A dye is injected through the catheter to show the cerebral blood vessels when X rays are taken. This test can detect an aneurysm, hemorrhage, evidence of a cerebrovascular accident, and arteriosclerosis.

■ **Brain scan**—Radioisotopes are injected into the blood and then measured by a special scanner to detect abnormal masses or blood vessel lesions within the brain. This test is used less frequently due to development of magnetic resonance imaging.

■ **Computerized axial tomography (CAT)** scan—A series of X rays of layers of the brain to construct a three-dimensional picture. Useful for identifying tumors, bleeding, a blood clot, decrease in brain size, and brain edema.

■ **Electroencephalography (EEG)**—A brain wave test to detect abnormal electrical impulses which could be caused by a tumor, epilepsy, retardation, or psychological disorder. New technology has developed an ambulatory EEG monitor that helps diagnose neurological conditions, including fainting "spells" and seizures, by permitting continuous monitoring.

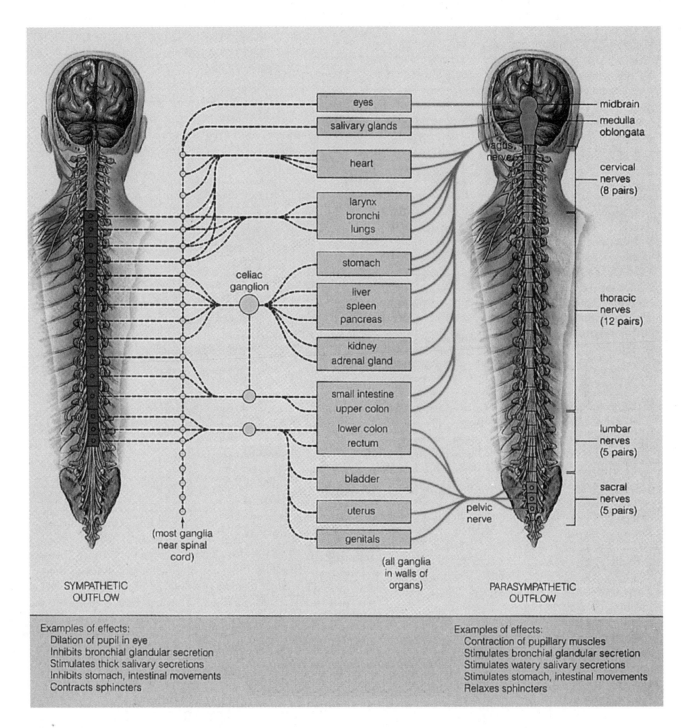

FIGURE 4–28 Autonomic nervous system. Shown here are the main sympathetic and parasympathetic pathways leading out from the central nervous system to some major organs. As the lists of examples suggest, in some cases the sympathetic and parasympathetic nerves operate antagonistically in their effects on the organ. Keep in mind that both systems have paired nerves leading out from the brain and spinal cord. (From Starr & Taggart, *Biology, The Unity and Diversity of Life,* 5th ed. Copyright 1989, Wadsworth Publishing Co.)

- **Electromyography**—Needles are inserted into selected skeletal muscles. When the patient contracts the muscles, the nerve impulses are recorded and the conduction time is measured to detect neuromuscular disorders or nerve damage.
- **Lumbar puncture**—A spinal needle is inserted into the subarachnoid space between the vertebrae of the lower back, and CSF is removed for examination, Figure 4–32.

The procedure is indicated when infection is suspected, when there is hemorrhage from injury, or when the fluid pressure must be measured. When measurement is desired, a calibrated glass tube is attached to the needle and the level of the fluid is observed and recorded.

- **Magnetic resonance imaging (MRI)**—Uses magnetic waves to give results similar to a CAT scan but has much

FIGURE 4–29   Cross section of brain (Adapted from Smith, *Medical Terminology, A Programmed Text,* 6th ed. Copyright 1991, Delmar Publishers Inc.)

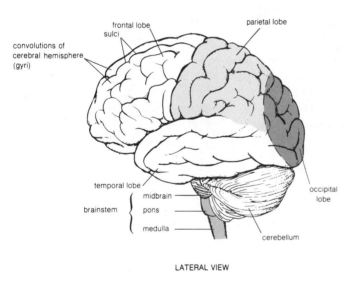

LATERAL VIEW

FIGURE 4–30   The parts of the brain (From Fong, *Body Structures and Functions,* 8th ed. Copyright 1993, Delmar Publishers Inc.)

better quality. It is very useful for detecting problems with the spine and the brain.

■ **Myelography**—A lumbar puncture is performed, removing CSF and instilling a dye to outline the structures on X ray. This will show irregularities or compression of the spinal cord. If air is instilled following removal of CSF to visualize cerebral cavities, the procedure is called a **pneumoencephalograph.** Used less frequently due to new technology.

■ **Skull X ray**—To identify fractures and dense areas which indicate a tumor or increased pressure within the skull.

Diseases and Disorders ....

Amyotrophic Lateral Sclerosis (ALS; Lou Gehrig's disease). ALS is a common motor neuron disease causing degeneration of the upper motor nerves in the medulla oblongata and the lower nerves in the spinal cord. It results in atrophy (wasting away) of the muscles. The onset occurs between the ages of 40 and 70 and is usually fatal within 3 to 10 years due to aspiration pneumonia or respiratory failure. The rate of incidence is 2 to 7 people for every 100,000. It affects men four times as frequently as women. About 10% of the cases are from an inherited autosomal trait. Other causes are from vitamin E deficiency, which damages cell membranes; metabolic interference in the production of nucleic acid by the nerves; an

FIGURE 4–31   A diagrammatic representation of the meninges and the circulation of cerebral spinal fluid from its formation in the choroid plexus until its return to the blood in the cranial venous sinus. (Adapted from Burke, *Human Anatomy and Physiology in Health and Disease,* 3d ed. Copyright 1992, Delmar Publishers Inc.)

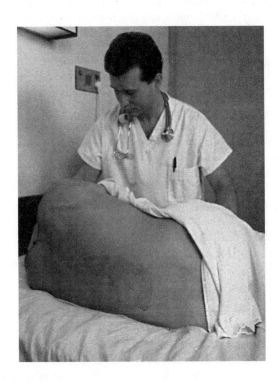

FIGURE 4–32(A)   Positioning of patient

autoimmune disorder; and the effects of a nutritional deficiency of the motor neurons.

Factors that often precipitate the development of ALS are trauma, acute viral infections, and physical exhaustion. The symptoms are muscular atrophy and weakness, especially of the hands and forearms, plus problems with speech, chewing, and swallowing. If the brain stem is involved, respirations will be affected, as well as occasional choking and excessive drooling. Mental deterioration does not usually occur; therefore, the patient is acutely aware of the progressive physical deterioration, so depression due to the consequences of the disease, may happen. No effective treatment is available, only methods to control symptoms and provide emotional and physical support.

Bell's Palsy.   This disease of unknown origin of the seventh cranial nerve causes weakness or *paralysis* on one side of the face. It occurs suddenly and within 1 to 8 weeks will usually spontaneously subside. The symptoms are drooping mouth (on the affected side) with drooling of saliva, a distorted sense of taste, and an inability to close the affected eye. Occasionally pain in the area of the jaw's angle may be present.

Treatment with steroids aids in reducing the associated edema. Moist heat applied to the face and jaw helps relieve any pain, but care must be taken to avoid burning the skin. It may be

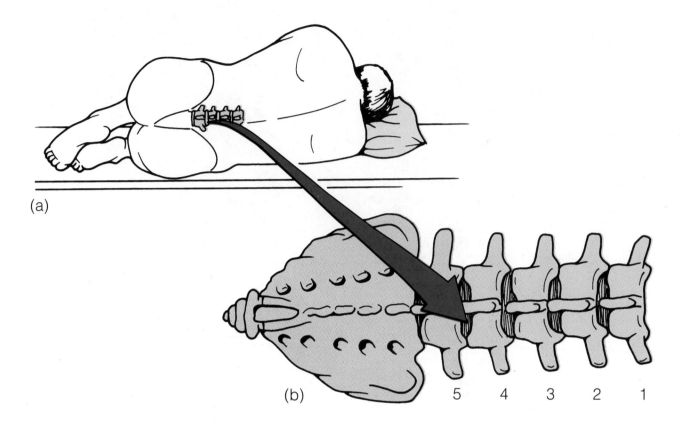

(a)

(b)   5   4   3   2   1

FIGURE 4–32(B)   Site of lumbar puncture

advisable to protect the eye with an eye patch while outdoors or if exposed to dust or pollutants.

Cerebral Palsy.   This disorder is associated with birth and involves both nerves and muscles. It is the most common crippler of children. Cerebral palsy appears in about 15,000 live births per year, 25% of which are either small or premature, weighing less than 5½ pounds. There are three forms of cerebral palsy: spastic, athetoid, and ataxic. About 70% of those affected have the spastic type. Characteristics of this form are hyperactive tendon reflexes, rapid alteration between muscular contraction and relaxation, contracture tendency (permanent muscle shortening), and underdevelopment of the affected extremities. Approximately 40% of the children affected are also mentally retarded, 25% have seizures, and 80% have speech impairment.

Cerebral palsy is probably caused by conditions that resulted in a lack of oxygen to the brain, hemorrhage, or brain damage. Prenatal conditions include rubella (German measles), toxemia, maternal diabetes, and malnutrition. At the time of birth such difficulties as forceps delivery, breech presentation, premature placental separation, premature birth, and either a too rapid or too prolonged labor are considered causative factors.

There is no cure for cerebral palsy, only supportive treatment, including physical, occupational, and speech therapy; psychological assistance; braces or splints; perhaps orthopedic surgery for severe contractures; muscle relaxors; and, when indicated, barbiturates and anticonvulsants to control seizures.

Encephalitis.   This severe brain inflammation, usually caused by a virus-bearing mosquito or tick, can also be contracted from the viruses that cause polio, herpes, or mumps or following measles, rubella, or a vaccination. The fluids from the lymphatic system infiltrate the brain tissue, causing edema and nerve cell destruction.

The disease onset is sudden and acute. Symptoms include fever, headache, and vomiting and progress to a stiff neck and back, drowsiness, and eventual coma. The disease is treatable with supportive drug therapy to control restlessness and convulsions, reduce edema, and relieve headache. Antiviral agents are ineffective except against herpes virus encephalitis.

Epilepsy.   This seizure disorder affects 1% to 2% of the population. It is associated with abnormal electrical impulses from the neurons of the brain. It is believed to be caused by either abnormal brain chemistry or several other possibilities, including birth trauma, anoxia (lack of oxygen), meningitis, encephalitis, ingestion of toxins (mercury, lead, carbon monoxide), brain tumor, PKU, and head injury.

The disorder is characterized by either petit or grand mal seizures. Petit mal seizures are of short duration and mild.

Grand mal seizures may last up to 5 minutes, with convulsions, loss of control of bodily functions, and unconsciousness.

Diagnosis is made upon evidence of seizure characteristics, a positive EEG, and various X-ray procedures. Treatment consists of drug therapy to control the seizures, and psychological support.

Headache. Headaches are commonly classified as vascular, muscle contraction (tension), or traction–inflammatory. Both muscle contraction and traction–inflammatory types cause dull, persistent aching and a feeling of a tight band around the head, with tender spots on the head or neck. Most chronic headaches result from tension that may be caused by emotional stress, fatigue, or environmental conditions. Other causes include inflammation of the sinuses, diseased teeth, and muscle spasms of the neck and shoulder.

Vasodilators, such as nitrates, alcohol, and histamine, expand arteries causing pressure against the brain's nerve endings and are often the causative factors. Many people are affected by anything aged or fermented, such as cured or processed meats and wine, especially red wine. Other foods or additives cause headaches by the vasoconstricting action of amines in such things as MSG, chocolate, and aspartame. A condition known as hypoglycemia (low blood sugar) can result in vasodilation and headaches but can be easily avoided by eating three meals a day, preferably five smaller ones.

A **migraine** headache is characterized by prodromal (beginning) symptoms, which may include fatigue, visual disturbances, such as zig-zag lines and bright lights; sensory symptoms, such as tingling of the face and lips; and sometimes motor symptoms, such as staggering. Migraines frequently occur in people with compulsive personalities and within families. They usually happen on weekends and holidays. A migraine headache is a severe throbbing pain caused by initial constriction then dilation of the blood vessels in the brain. Frequently, it is accompanied by sensitivity to light, nausea, and vomiting. The headache can occur suddenly and last from a few hours to a few days. It cannot be prevented, but medication can reduce frequency and intensity. Ergotamine, especially with caffeine, seems to be fairly effective, if taken early; it is available in suppository form if vomiting prevents oral administration. There is no cure for migraine headaches, only control. Drugs known as beta blockers and tricyclic antidepressants appear to be very effective in controlling symptoms.

It seems to be best to lie quietly in bed in a darkened room until the symptoms subside. Limited relief may be obtained from regular analgesics, and some people feel an ice bag to the head and a wet cloth over the eyes and forehead are beneficial. Usually, it is just a matter of waiting out the episode.

When headaches are frequent, unusual (such as causing awakening in the middle of the night), or persistent or become increasingly more intense, medical attention should be sought. It may be important to rule out the presence of pathology, such as an aneurysm, abscess, intercranial bleeding, or tumor.

Herpes Zoster (shingles). This is an acute inflammation of the dorsal root ganglion by the herpes virus that also causes chickenpox. It is characterized by fluid-filled vesicle lesions on the skin and severe pain from the affected nerves. The onset is characterized by fever and discomfort followed by severe deep pain, itching, and abnormal skin sensations. The vesicles erupt in about 2 weeks, spreading around the **thorax** or vertically on the extremities. The episode may last from 1 to 4 weeks.

Treatment consists of medication, sometimes even narcotics, to relieve the pain and itching, plus a systemic antibiotic if infection develops.

Hydrocephalus. This excessive accumulation of CSF within the ventricles of the brain, occurring most frequently in newborns, may result from overproduction of CSF, obstruction of the flow of CSF, or a lack of absorption. The increased fluid compresses the brain tissue resulting in brain damage. Hydrocephalus is characterized by an abnormally enlarged head; distended scalp veins; fragile, shiny scalp skin; a high-pitched, shrill cry; irritability; and vomiting.

Surgery is the only treatment for hydrocephalus. A shunt (passageway) is inserted into a ventricle in the brain to drain off excess fluid into either the peritoneal cavity or the atrium (upper chamber) of the heart for absorption by the body.

Meningitis. This inflammation of the meninges of the brain and spinal cord is due usually to a bacterial infection from the ears, sinuses, or lungs (pneumonia), or a brain abscess. Mortality is 70% to 100% if left untreated.

Meningitis is characterized by a high fever, chills, headache, vomiting, and specifically by positive Brudzinski's and Kernig's signs, Figure 4–33, page 98. Brudzinski's sign is demonstrated by the flexing of the hips and knees when the head and neck of a dorsal recumbent person are raised and pulled forward. Kernig's sign is demonstrated by pain and resistance when the knee is straightened after flexing at the thigh and knee.

Diagnosis of meningitis is confirmed by a lumbar puncture that shows elevated pressure, cloudiness from the excess white cells, and identification of the causative organism after culturing. Treatment consists of antibiotics, medication to reduce cerebral edema, pain relievers for headache, and an anticonvulsant. Isolation may be indicated in certain instances.

Multiple Sclerosis (MS). This disease, causing the demyelination of the white matter of the brain and spinal cord, results in double or blurred vision and sensations of tingling and numbness. Onset occurs between the ages of 20 and 40. MS is usually characterized by a series of attacks and periods of remission. Its symptoms are tremor, muscular weakness, paralysis, urinary frequency, incontinence, and emotional swings. Symptoms and extent of remission depend on the body's ability to remyelinate and restore synaptic function.

The cause of MS is unknown. Theories suggest the cause could be a slow-acting virus, an allergic reaction to an infectious agent, trauma, lack of oxygen, or nutritional deficits, in addition to others. Treatment consists of ACTH (adrenocorticotropic hormone) and steroids to relieve symptoms and hasten remission. Drugs for the emotional swings, urinary prob-

FIGURE 4-33 Two telltale signs of meningitis: (a) Brudzinski's sign (b) Kernigs signs

lems, and muscular spasticity are used as required. Bed rest to prevent fatigue is important during acute phases.

Neuralgia. Severe cutting pain along the course of a nerve may be due to inflammation, pressure on the nerve, toxins, or a change in the root ganglia. The term is used to describe general nerve pain.

Neuron and Spinal Cord Damage. This results in a loss of sensation and voluntary motion due to destruction of the neurons.

Hemiplegia is paralysis on one side of the body because of damage to the opposite side of the brain. Trauma, a tumor, or cerebrovascular accident (CVA) are the usual causative factors. Hemiplegia is characterized by unilateral paralysis of the tongue, face, arm, and leg, causing muscular contractures. Often the patient has difficulty comprehending written or verbal communication and is unable to perceive sensory stimuli on the affected side.

Paraplegia is a motor or sensory loss in the lower extremities due to spinal cord injury from trauma, most frequently from automobile, motorcycle, or sports–related accidents. Incomplete spinal cord injury is evident when ability to flex toes, control bodily functions, and feel perianal sensations is present. With complete spinal cord injury, there is a total lack of sensation and muscular control for at least 24 hours, and return of functions is unlikely. Accurate assessment of the extent of paralysis cannot be made until a year after the injury.

Quadriplegia is paralysis of the arms, legs, and body below the level of the injury to the spinal cord. It usually occurs from

injury sustained in an automobile or a sporting accident and is often in the area of the fifth to seventh cervical vertebrae. Spinal cord injuries above the fifth vertebrae dramatically affect body systems, such as the respiratory and the circulatory, in addition to body paralysis. A complete physical and neurological examination is necessary to assess remaining motor function and determine if the cord injury is complete or partial. The condition occurs most frequently among young men. Athletic activities, such as diving, gymnastics, and trampoline usage, are often the cause of spinal cord injury.

Parkinson's Disease. This condition is characterized by severe muscle rigidity, a peculiar gait, drooling, and a progressive tremor. The body becomes bent forward, with head bowed. The steps become faster and faster with increasing forward body inclination, which often results in falling.

There is no known cure for the disease, although a drug called levodopa relieves most of the symptoms until the necessarily increased dosage begins to cause serious side effects. In selected patients a surgical procedure can either freeze, electrically coagulate, or radioactively destroy a small area of the brain to prevent the involuntary motions.

Reye's Syndrome. This acute childhood illness causes fatty infiltration of the liver and increased intracranial pressure (ICP). Further damage from fat infiltration occurs in the kidneys and possibly the muscle of the heart. The **syndrome** (group of symptoms) affects children from infancy to adolescence, occurring equally in males and females, but affects whites more than blacks. There also appears to be a positive correlation between Reye's syndrome and aspirin ingestion. Reye's syndrome almost always follows within 1 to 3 days of an acute viral infection, such as influenza, upper respiratory infection, or chickenpox.

The syndrome prognosis depends on the degree of CNS depression from ICP. At one time, mortality was 90%; now with early treatment and ICP monitoring, the rate has been reduced to 20%. Death usually results from cerebral swelling, respiratory arrest, or coma.

The symptoms occur in stages of severity beginning with vomiting, lethargy, and liver dysfunction, then progression to hyperventilation, delirium, hyperactive reflexes, and coma. The condition worsens as symptoms of rigidity, deepening coma, large fixed pupils, seizures, and eventual respiratory arrest occurs.

Sciatica. Inflammation and severe pain of the **sciatic** nerve causes sharp, piercing pain in the back of the thigh extending down the inside of the leg. Primary causes may be exposure to wet and cold, impingement on the nerve by the spinous processes (bony projections of the vertebrae), or uneven length of the legs, causing improper vertebral alignment. Treatment consists of bed rest, heat, medication for pain, and sometimes the use of traction.

Spinal Cord Defects (Spina bifida, meningocele, myelomeningocele). These spinal cord defects result from failure of tissues to properly close during the first 3 months of pregnancy. They occur most frequently in the lumbosacral area.

Spina bifida occulta is the most common, characterized by the incomplete closure of one or more vertebrae, but without protrusion of the spinal cord or meninges, Figure 4–34. There is usually a depression, a tuft of hair, a port wine nevi, or a combination of these signs over the defect. In spina bifida with meningocele, the sac contains meninges and CSF. Spina bifida with myelomeningocele contains meninges, CSF, and a portion of the spinal cord or nerve roots.

The incidence is approximately 5% of live births, or about 100,000 infants per year, and is highest among persons of Welsh or Irish descent. Treatment and prognosis depend on the extent of the defect. Neurological symptoms range from minimal weakness of the feet and some bladder and bowel problems to permanent neurological dysfunction such as paralysis, inability to control the bladder and bowels, hydrocephalus, clubfoot, and sometimes mental retardation. If CSF and meninges are involved, surgical closure is required to prevent further injury. Unfortunately, the neurological conditions cannot be reversed. With hydrocephalus present, a shunt will be implanted to relieve the fluid pressure.

Subarachnoid Hemorrhage.

This is a collection of blood in the subarachnoid space, usually due to the spontaneous rupture of a weakened blood vessel. The patient may complain of a sudden, severe headache and experience nausea and projectile vomiting. This may be accompanied by motor disturbances, seizures, and deviations in sensory perception, particularly in vision. Precipitating factors include hypertension, oral contraceptives, malformations of cranial blood vessels, and family history.

Subdural Hematoma.

A collection of blood within the subdural space, usually resulting from injury due to a fall or accident, is a slow process in which the gradually accumulating blood causes progressive symptoms such as motor disturbances, facial weakness on the side opposite the hematoma, generalized seizures, and a decreasing level of consciousness. Surgical intervention is indicated to remove the pressure on the brain tissues caused by the hematoma when symptoms and intracranial pressure reach a significant state.

Transient Ischemic Attack (TIA).

This temporary condition lasting 12 to 24 hours is characterized by symptoms such as double vision, slurred speech, dizziness, staggering gait, and falling. TIA is a warning sign of impending thrombotic CVA (stroke from a blood clot). It results from microscopic clots temporarily closing off tiny arteries in the brain and impairing blood flow. Treatment includes the use of aspirin and an anticoagulant to reduce blood clot formation to minimize the risk of thrombosis and the resulting CVA.

Trigeminal Neuralgia (tic douloureux).

This disorder of the fifth cranial nerve, on one side of the face, produces episodes of excruciating facial pain on stimulation of a trigger zone. It frequently follows exposure to heat or cold, a draft from air, smiling, or drinking hot or cold liquids. The episodes may last from 1 to 15 minutes, recurring from several times daily to a few times a year. Persons with the disorder live in fear of the next attack.

Treatment consists of oral medication, injection of alcohol or phenol into the nerve branch, or both oral medication and injection. With frequent, severe attacks, a surgical procedure is indicated that severs the nerve, thereby relieving the pain, but also results in loss of sensation to the innervated area. Care must be taken afterward to protect the affected eye, avoid burns from hot food, guard against dental decay, and avoid biting the inner cheek and lip.

Complete Chapter 4, Unit 2 in the workbook to help you meet the objectives at the beginning of this unit and therefore achieve competency of this subject matter.

a. Spina Bifida Occulta

b. Meningocele

c. Myelomeningocele

FIGURE 4–34   Spinal cord defects: (a) Spina bifida occulta (b) Meningocele (c) Myelomeningocele

UNIT 3
The Senses

presbyopia
pupil
receptor
retina
retinopathy
sclera
semicircular canals

sensorineural
stapes
strabismus
tinnitus
tympanic membrane
vitreous humor

OBJECTIVES

Upon completion of this unit, you will meet the following terminal performance objectives by verifying knowledge of the facts and principles presented through oral and written communication at a level deemed competent by the instructor or employer.

1. Name the senses of the human body identifying the corresponding organ(s) responsible for perception.
2. Identify on an anatomical illustration the structures of the eye, ear, nose, tongue, and skin.
3. Trace the path of a visual image from the cornea to the visual center of the brain.
4. Explain the effects of the lens and cornea upon the focusing of images.
5. Trace the path of sound from the entrance of the ear to the auditory center of the brain.
6. Explain the balance function of the inner ear.
7. Describe the anatomy of the olfactory organ and explain how an odor is perceived.
8. Name the taste sensations and identify the corresponding areas on the surface of the tongue.
9. Name the types of contact receptors found in the skin.
10. Describe 14 diseases or disorders of the eye, 8 of the ear, 3 of the nose, and 2 of the mouth and tongue.
11. Spell and define, using the glossary at the back of the text, all the words to know in this unit.

WORDS TO KNOW

accommodation
amblyopia
aqueous humor
astigmatism
auditory
cataract
cerumen
choroid
cochlea
conjunctiva
cornea
enucleation
epistaxis
eustachian tube
fovea centralis
glaucoma

hyperopia
incus
insidious
iris
lacrimal
lens
malleus
Ménière's disease
myopia
optic disc
organ of Corti
otitis
otosclerosis
papillae
polyps
presbycusis

The human being is able to communicate with the surrounding environment because of a miraculous network of nerves coordinated with the organs of the five special senses, which allow us to see, hear, taste, smell, and touch. Knowledge of the environment requires the cooperation of three factors: the sense organs to perceive, intact cranial nerves to transmit, and a functioning area of the brain to interpret the received stimuli.

A stimulus is anything the body is able to detect by means of its **receptors.** Receptors are the peripheral nerve endings of sensory nerves that respond to stimuli. They are not all alike and do not respond to the same kinds of stimuli. Some respond to environmental chemical energy from ions or molecules that are dissolved in body fluids. These are chemoreceptors and are associated with the sense of taste and smell. Changes in position or pressure or the effects of acceleration create mechanical energy, which is detected by mechanoreceptors. These are associated with touch, hearing, and equilibrium. The detection of energy from light is possible due to the photoreceptors in the eyes. Thermoreceptors detect radiant energy from heat and are in the skin or connective tissues.

The stimulus, regardless of its form, is converted into energy. If the stimulus is sufficient enough to cause an action potential in the neuron, the message will travel along the sensory nerve to the brain. The reason messages are interpreted differently, such as being hot, a color, or an odor, is that certain nerves always end up in the same specific part of the brain. In other words, the sensation of heat or pain and the "seeing" of a color actually occurs in the brain, not at the point of stimulus. The ability to distinguish between hot, cold, red, or blue, for example, is the outcome of messages being received in an appropriate section of the brain, undergoing routing, being compared with stored past experiences and producing the interpretation of the stimulus.

The primary organs of the senses are familiar: the eye and the sense of sight; the ear and the sense of hearing; the tongue and the sense of taste; the nose and the sense of smell; and the skin and the sense of touch. These organs cannot perform their functions, however, without the cooperation of the corresponding nerves and section of the brain.

The Eye and the Sense of Sight

The structure of the eyeball is frequently compared to that of a camera. The outside of the camera is made of a strong plastic or metal to protect its interior structures. To protect the eye, it is located within the bony orbital cavity of the skull. For additional protection, the outside of the eye is covered with tough, white fibrous tissue called the **sclera,** Figure 4–35. The sclera helps maintain the shape of the eyeball. Six extraocular, or extrinsic (outside), muscles are attached to the sclera and anchored in the skull; these contract or relax as pairs to move the eyeball within its cavity. This permits rolling of the eyes in up–down, in–out, and combinations of these directions, to permit a large field of vision without moving the head, Figure 4–36, page 102. Under the sclera is another covering called the **choroid,** which contains the blood vessels that serve the tissues of the eye. This layer has a nonreflective pigment that makes it dark and opaque and prevents light from reflecting within the eye.

Focusing the Image

Both the eye and the camera have a lens to focus an image onto a surface for "recording." In the camera this surface is the film. In the eye it is the **retina.** In the camera, the distance between the film and the camera lens is adjusted to bring the picture into focus before it is recorded on the film. In the eye, the shape of the elastic **lens** is automatically altered by ciliary muscles of the ciliary body to focus objects onto the retina. When the ciliary body contracts, the lens becomes rounder, in a process known as **accommodation** for permitting near vision. With relaxation, the lens thins out to accommodate focusing on distant objects. The shape of the lens is convex on both the anterior and posterior surfaces. The shape is quite rounded in childhood, becoming more convex with age until it is nearly flat in the elderly, causing difficulty with accommodating near vision.

Controlling Light

The aperture of the camera is similar to the **iris** of the eye; the size of their openings is adjusted to allow varying amounts of light to enter. The iris is the colored circular muscle which surrounds the central opening called the **pupil.** The amount of melanin (color) and its location in the iris determines the color of the eye. When melanin is present only in the posterior area, the iris appears blue, if it is scattered throughout, it will go from green to brown to black, depending on the amount of pigment. In the eye, the two intrinsic (inside) muscle structures of the iris regulate the amount of light that enters the eye. When the light is bright, the circular muscle fibers of the iris contract, reducing the size of the pupil, thereby permitting less light to enter. If it is dark or dimly lit, the pupil will dilate (enlarge) as the radial muscle fibers of the iris contract to pull it outward, permitting more light to enter.

The Cornea

The **cornea** is a transparent extension of the sclera that lies in front of the pupil. This covering has no blood vessels to interfere with vision so the tissue is nourished by lymph fluid circulating through the cellular spaces. It has both pain and touch receptors, which cause it to be extremely sensitive to any foreign body that touches its surface. If an injury to the cornea results in scarring, vision will be impaired.

The curvature of the cornea "corrects" some of the unclear image that the edge of the lens projects. If the cornea develops an abnormal shape, vision becomes blurred, and the result may be a disorder known as **astigmatism.**

Surface Membranes

A mucous membrane called the **conjunctiva** lines the inner surfaces of the eyelids and covers the anterior sclera surface of the eye. At the margin of the cornea, the conjunctiva merges with the transparent epithelium covering that protects the cornea. The conjunctiva and cornea are lubricated by tiny glands that secrete an oily substance. Further protection for the eye is provided by **lacrimal** glands, which secrete tears to moisten and cleanse the surface of the membrane.

conjunctiva (conjunctiv/o)
cornea (corne/o) (kerat/o)
iris (irid/o)
pupil (core/o)
path of light
lens (phac/o)
anterior chamber (aqueous humor)
posterior chamber (vitreous humor)
suspensory ligament
cyliary body and muscle (cycl/o)

retina (retin/o)
fovea centralis (fone/o)
retinal arteries and veins
optic nerve
choroid coat
sclera (scler/o)

FIGURE 4–35 Internal view of the eye (From Fong, *Body Structures and Functions,* 8th ed. Copyright 1993, Delmar Publishers Inc.)

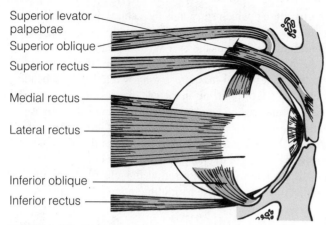

Superior levator
palpebrae
Superior oblique
Superior rectus
Medial rectus
Lateral rectus
Inferior oblique
Inferior rectus

FIGURE 4–36 Extraocular (extrinsic) muscles of the eye

Cavities and Humors   The eyeball is divided into two main areas separated by the lens and its supporting ciliary body structures. The more anterior area is subdivided into the anterior chamber, which is between the cornea and the iris, and the posterior chamber, which lies between the iris and the lens. A salty, clear fluid known as the **aqueous humor** fills and circulates between the chambers. It maintains the curvature of the cornea and assists in the refraction process. The eyeball behind the lens, sometimes called a vitreous chamber, or vitreous body, is filled with a thick, jellylike substance called the **vitreous humor.** This material not only aids in refraction but also maintains the shape of the eyeball. Injury with the loss of an appreciable amount of the humor may cause damage to the eyeball, which could necessitate surgical removal of the eye by a procedure called **enucleation.**

The Retina   The inside layer of the eyeball is the retina, a multilayered nervous tissue. Specialized nerve cells called rods and cones transmit the stimuli focused on the retinal surface through the optic nerve to the visual center in the brain where the image is "seen." The cones, about 7 million in number, are sensitive to colors and function only in well-lighted environments. Most of them are located in a depression on the posterior surface of the retina called the **fovea centralis,** the area of sharpest vision. There are about 100 million rods in the more peripheral areas of the retina. The rods are very sensitive to light and permit us to see, without color, in dimly lit or nearly dark surroundings.

Optic Disc.   Two other types of nerve cells in the retina relay impulses from the rods and cones. The axons of one type form the fibers of the optic nerve. Where the optic nerves exits the retina, there are neither rods or cones so it is referred to as the **optic disc** or blind spot.

The Path of Light   The process of sight begins with the passage of light rays through the cornea, on through the aqueous humor, the pupil, and the lens into the vitreous humor, to focus at the back of the eyeball on the retina. Here the image is picked up by the rods and cones, transformed into nerve impulses, and transmitted over the optic nerve to the

thalamus. Here some of the fibers cross over to the nerve tract of the other eye. From the thalamus, other neurons relay the impulses to the visual center in the occipital lobe of the cerebrum, where the impulses are "developed" into pictures and "seen."

Refraction Error   Each part of the eyeball refracts (deflects) the light to cause the image to focus on the retina, Figure 4–37(a). This does not always occur correctly, however. When the image is improperly refracted and focuses in front of the retina (b), the person is said to be nearsighted, or to have **myopia.** When the image focuses behind the retina (c), the person is said to be farsighted, or to have **hyperopia.** These conditions may result from abnormal curvature of the lens or cornea, or from an abnormally shaped eyeball. Note that images are inverted when they pass through the lens due to the curvature deflecting the image. Eyeglasses provide a means of refracting light to correct abnormal deflection of the image. They perform artificially what the eye's structures fail to do.

Diseases and Disorders of the Eye ....

Amblyopia (lazy eye).   A condition known as **amblyopia** usually results from one eye turning inward, causing blurring of vision. The brain therefore suppresses the visual impulses from the inward-turning eye. The condition is treated by covering the "good eye," thereby stimulating development of the "lazy eye." Amblyopia is most prevalent in children under age 5. For a good prognosis, therapy should begin before the age of 8; otherwise, eventual blindness of the affected eye may result.

Blepharitis.   This inflammation is caused by the sebaceous glands producing excess secretions, which lead to greasy scales and sticky, crusted eyelids. The condition is usually associated with seborrhea of the scalp (dandruff). The itching and burning sensations cause an unconscious rubbing of the eyes resulting in red-rimmed eyelid margins. Treatment consists of frequent shampoos of the hair and daily cleansing of the eyelids with a mild shampoo to remove the scales.

Cataract.   This gradually developing opacity (cloudiness) of the lens occurs most frequently in persons over 70 years of age, as part of the aging process. The probable cause of **cataracts** is a change in the composition of the proteins of the lens. The condition causes a painless, gradual blurring and loss of vision. The pupil turns from black to a milky white as the lens becomes visible. People with cataracts frequently complain of seeing halos around lights or being blinded at night by oncoming automobile headlights.

Cataracts are treated by surgical removal of the lens and postoperative substitution of cataract eyeglasses. Other options are possible for some patients. Contact lenses can be fitted and provide much better correction than glasses. Frequently an intraocular lens (IOL) is implanted directly behind the cornea when the cataract surgery is performed. A new "taco" style

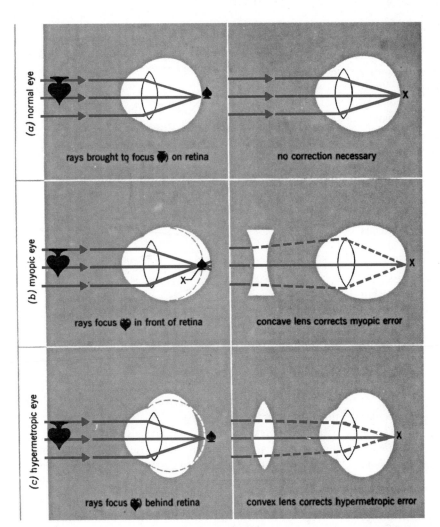

(a) normal eye

rays brought to focus on retina

no correction necessary

(b) myopic eye

rays focus in front of retina

concave lens corrects myopic error

(c) hypermetropic eye

rays focus behind retina

convex lens corrects hypermetropic error

FIGURE 4–37
The refraction of an image (a) Normal vision (b) Nearsightedness (c) Farsightedness and the type of lens required to correct the vision. (From Burke, *Human Anatomy and Physiology in Health and Disease,* 3d ed. Copyright 1992 Delmar Publishers Inc.)

lens is inserted in a folded-over state through a very tiny incision popping open after it is implanted. Cataract surgery is now being done on an outpatient basis, with the patient detained only a few hours.

Sometime after surgery the capsule that held the lens in place, and is now behind and supporting the IOL, may become clouded, once again obstructing the path of light into the eye. This problem can be easily solved without invasive surgery, using a laser beam to make a tiny opening in the capsule, which lets in light and restores vision.

Conjunctivitis (Pinkeye). This condition results in redness, pain, swelling, and occasionally a discharge, due to inflammation of the **conjunctiva.** It is usually caused by an infectious organism, such as bacteria (*Streptococcus* or *Staphylococcus*) or a virus (herpes simplex). Allergic reactions and environmental irritants can also cause the condition.

It usually begins in one eye, spreading rapidly to the other from contamination by a wash cloth or by the hands. Since it is highly contagious, other family members should not share towels, wash cloths, pillows, and other such belongings with the infected person. The causative organism is identified by stained smears of the drainage and indicates the method of treatment. Bacterial conjunctivitis responds to antibiotics and sulfa drug therapy; the herpes viral type does not.

Corneal Abrasion. A scratch or trauma to the cornea, usually from a foreign body in the eye, is most often caused by dirt that becomes imbedded under the eyelid, small pieces of wood, metal, or paper, or an injury from a fingernail. Even if the eye waters profusely to cleanse the surface, the scratch (abrasion) remains, causing redness, tearing, and irritation. Abrasions may also occur when people fall asleep wearing hard contact lenses. Vision may be affected if the location and extent of injury are significant. Foreign bodies embedded in the cornea require removal following application of a topical anesthetic. Treatment consists of antibiotic eyedrops or ointment and application of a pressure eye patch to prevent blinking. Corneal epithelium heals rapidly within 24 to 48 hours.

Corneal Ulcers. These result from bacterial, viral, or fungal infections. The first signs are pain, aggravated by blinking, and excessive tearing. Blurred vision results from the ulcerations, the corneal surface appears irregular, and exudate (pus) may be present. Instillation of an ophthalmic dye will permit confirmation of the diagnosis. A culture of the drainage to determine the causative organism will indicate appropriate medication. Broad-spectrum antibiotics are used initially to prevent corneal scarring and the resulting impairment of vision. Certain bacterially caused ulcers progress so rapidly that, without proper treatment, the cornea will perforate (be pierced with holes), and vision in the eye will be lost within 48 hours.

Diabetic Retinopathy. This form of vascular **retinopathy** results from juvenile or adult diabetes. Approximately 75% of patients with juvenile diabetes develop diabetic retinopathy within 20 years after the onset of diabetes. Incidence in adults with diabetes increases with the length of time a person is diabetic. About 80% of patients with diabetes of 20 to 30 years' duration develop retinopathy. The condition is a result of an interference with the blood supply to the eyes. It is the leading cause of acquired blindness in adults.

Symptoms result from an edematous retina, which causes light to scatter. Tiny capillary walls thicken and show evidence of dilation, twisting, and hemorrhage. This causes glare, blurred vision, and reduced visual acuity. If diagnosed and treated early, prognosis is good for simple forms; in extensive forms, prognosis is poor, with 50% becoming blind within 5 years. Treatment consists of sealing holes that have developed in the retina and coagulating the leaking vessels with a laser beam. If new abnormal vessels have grown onto the retina and into the vitreous body, it is possible for the retina to detach from the choroid layer, resulting in vitreous hemorrhage and blindness. With this advanced condition, open surgery will be required.

Glaucoma (Chronic). This condition of excessive intraocular pressure results in atrophy (wasting away) of the optic nerve. **Glaucoma** causes severe visual impairment and eventually blindness. It occurs in 20% of adults over age 40 and accounts for 15% of all blindness in the United States. It is the most easily prevented cause of blindness.

The condition results from either an overproduction of the aqueous humor produced by the epithelium of the ciliary body or the obstruction of its outflow circulating mechanisms to Schlemm's canal for absorption into venous circulation, Figure 4–38. With chronic open-angle glaucoma, fluid cannot drain because of a blockage of the trabecular meshwork. Symptoms are **insidious** (gradual) and are often not recognized until late in the disease. They include mild aching, a loss of peripheral (side) vision, seeing halos around lights, and difficulty seeing at night.

In acute closed-angle glaucoma, fluid cannot drain because the iris presses against the cornea, closing off the canal of Schlemm. There is a rapid onset of symptoms, and it is considered an emergency. There is pain and redness of the affected eye with a feeling of pressure. The pupil is moderately dilated and nonreactive to light. There is blurred and decreased visual acuity as well as sensitivity to light. Unless the pressure is relieved quickly, blindness will occur within 3 to 5 days. Usual treatment consists of aggressive drug therapy and a peripheral iridectomy (removal of a piece of the iris) to permit outflow of the aqueous humor.

Glaucoma is diagnosed with evidence of increased intraocular pressure as measured by a tonometer and confirmed by viewing, through an ophthalmoscope, characteristic changes in the optic disk. Initial treatment usually consists of systemic drugs to reduce the production of aqueous humor and eye drops to aid in the outflow. With inadequate response, a surgi-

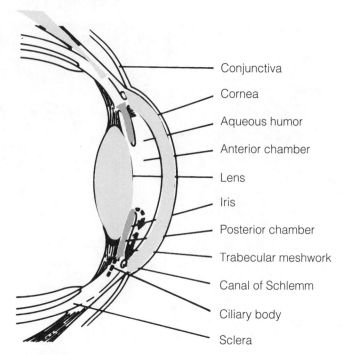

FIGURE 4–38 Normal flow of aqueous humor

cal procedure is required to create an opening for the circulation of the fluid.

Laser surgery is a quick, less expensive, and relatively painless solution to both open- and closed-angle glaucoma. In open-angle, if medication is ineffective, a laser beam is directed to open the trabecular meshwork. In closed-angle, the laser makes a tiny opening in the iris to allow the fluid to drain. A second treatment may be necessary in closed-angle glaucoma. Laser eye surgery is more effective in the early stages of the disease.

Hordeolum (Stye). This localized infection of a gland of the eyelid produces an abscess around an eyelash. The eye is red, painful, and swollen. Treatment consists of applying warm, wet compresses to relieve pain and promote drainage, and the use of eye drops or ointment to take care of the infection.

Iritis. An inflammation of the iris is often caused by an improperly healed corneal abrasion, especially if damage is from a sharp object. Iritis produces moderate to severe eye pain, photophobia, and a small nonreactive pupil due to the spasm of the iris. Prompt treatment is required to prevent complications. The pupil is dilated with mydriatics to allow the eye to rest to prevent the formation of posterior synechiae (adhesions of the iris to the lens). Corticosteroid drops are used to reduce the inflammation.

Presbyopia. This condition is characterized by inability of the lens to accommodate for near vision because of loss of elasticity. **Presbyopia** occurs as part of the normal aging process. The condition can be corrected by the fitting of contact lenses or eyeglasses.

Ptosis. Drooping of the upper eyelid may be a congenital condition (a condition one is born with), the result of aging, the presence of an excess fatty fold, or a neurological factor. Treatment may be required if vision is restricted or the appearance is cosmetically undesirable. A surgical procedure on the eyelid muscles will correct the disorder, or a device can be attached to the eyeglass frame to elevate the eyelid.

Retinal Detachment. This disorder is characterized by the separation of the retina from the choroid layer of the eyeball. The separation may occur with aging, which causes the normal vitreous support to shrink away. This results in a small hole or tear that permits the humor to seep between the layers and cause separation. Other causative factors include severe high blood pressure, diabetes, trauma, and other systemic diseases.

Diagnosis can be made from the patient's complaints of seeing floating spots, flashes of light, and a gradual vision loss. Confirmation is possible after pupil dilation and ophthalmoscopy reveal a gray and opaque retina with indefinite margins in the affected areas. Folds, tears, and a ballooning inward of the retina may be seen. Treatment consists of limiting eye movements with a patch, bed rest, sedation, and appropriate positioning of the head. Spontaneous reattachment is rare. A coagulation laser beam can repair simple tears in the retina by "spot welding" the area with several rows of "welds," but once separation has occurred, other treatment will be necessary. Both heat and cold therapies are used to create a sterile inflammatory reaction, which causes the retina to readhere. A tight band is placed around the eyeball, inside the sclera layer, which makes the choroid "indent" against the retina to maintain its closeness. Various surgical procedures to reattach the retina to the choroid can be performed.

Strabismus. In this condition, one eye deviates, with the gaze being abnormally inward (cross-eyed), outward (walleyed), higher, or lower than that of the other eye. This condition may result from muscle imbalance or attempts to compensate for farsightedness. **Strabismus** is frequently associated with Down syndrome, cerebral palsy, and mental retardation. Diagnosis is made on observation of the obvious visual symptoms and the complaint of blurred or double vision. Conservative initial treatment consists of a patch on the normal eye, corrective glasses, and specific eye exercises. Surgery to adjust the muscles that control eye placement and movement may be indicated. If strabismus develops before age 5, the deviated eye may be suppressed, resulting in amblyopia that could cause loss of vision if not treated.

The Ear and the Sense of Hearing...............

The ear is capable of receiving vibrations in the air and translating them into the sounds we recognize: the more vibrations per second, the higher the frequency, or pitch, of the sound, the stronger the vibration, the louder the sound.

The Outer Ear   Vibrations are picked up by the pinna (auricle) of the outer ear and directed down the external **auditory** canal to the **tympanic membrane** (eardrum), Figure 4–39.

The Middle Ear   The sound waves vibrate the membrane and the **malleus** (hammer) attached to its inner surface. The malleus in turn "strikes" the **incus** (anvil), which moves the **stapes** (stirrup). These three small bones and the space around them are called the middle ear. The middle ear communicates the vibrations to the inner ear by the stapes pushing against the fluid in the vestibule of the inner ear through the oval window.

The middle ear is connected by means of the **eustachian tube** to the throat. The tube is responsible for equalizing air

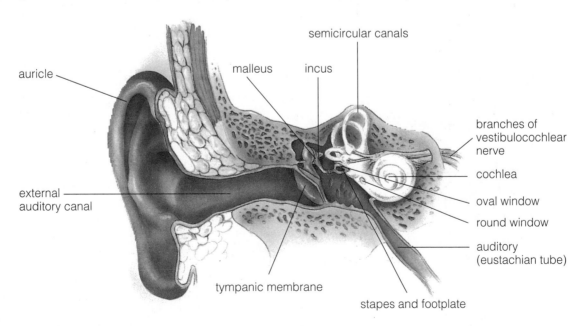

FIGURE 4–39   The ear (From Smith, *Medical Terminology, A Programmed Text*, 6th ed. Copyright 1991, Delmar Publishers Inc.)

pressure in the middle ear with the outside atmospheric pressure. Unfortunately, infections from the throat often pass through the tube into the middle ear. Rapid changes in altitude, harsh blowing of the nose, or a forceful sneeze may cause temporary air pressure inequities.

The Inner Ear   The vibrations from the middle ear continue through the coiled **cochlea,** which contains the **organ of Corti,** a collection of specialized nerve cells, Figure 4–40. These cells transmit the impulses to the auditory nerve, which passes them on to the auditory center of the temporal lobe of the cerebrum for interpretation.

The inner ear also contains three **semicircular canals.** These structures are responsible for maintaining equilibrium (balance). Inside the canals, hairlike nerve cell receptors are embedded in a gelatin-like material. When the head moves, the material pushes against the receptors, which transmit to the brain the change in position.

Another nerve receptor network in the semicircular canals is similarly constructed inside two small sacs. The gelatin surface here is covered with a layer of tiny limestone grains. When the head moves, the grains shift causing the hair cells to send out impulses.

DETAIL OF SENSORY ENDING (CRISTA) IN SEMICIRCULAR CANAL

GELATINOUS SUBSTANCE

NERVE FIBERS

SUPERIOR SEMICIRCULAR CANAL

HAIR CELLS

POSTERIOR SEMICIRCULAR CANAL

VESTIBULAR NERVE
COCHLEAR NERVE

LATERAL SEMICIRCULAR CANAL

VESTIBULE

OVAL WINDOW

COCHLEA

FIGURE 4–40   Enlarged view of the inner ear (From *The Wonderful Human Machine*, Copyright 1979, American Medical Association)

Diseases and Disorders of the Ear ....

Auditory Canal Obstruction.   The auditory canal can be obstructed by impacted **cerumen** (ear wax) or a foreign body, such as a bean, pea, pebble, bead, or insect. Children often put objects into their ears. Some obstructions may cause discomfort and a degree of hearing loss. Treatment consists of a removal technique appropriate to the obstruction. Cerumen can be removed by gentle scraping with a cerumen spoon or irrigation by syringe or an aerated water jet (see Chapter 6). Irrigation should be stopped immediately if it causes pain. Removal of insects can be accomplished easily after killing with an instillation of 70% alcohol. Similar objects can also be removed after irrigation with alcohol if they cannot be reached with forceps. Water must be avoided if it may cause swelling of the object, such as a bean or pea.

Hearing Loss.   This condition of reduced ability to perceive sound at normal levels can be either a conductive loss due to the inability to carry sound waves through the structures of the ear or a nerve loss **sensorineural,** due to transmission failure of the nerves within the inner ear or the auditory nerve. Loss can also be caused by a combination of lack of conduction and impulse transmission.

Conductive loss may be caused by an obstruction from a buildup of cerumen (wax), a foreign body, swelling within the auditory canal, middle ear infection, or otosclerosis.

Sudden loss of hearing without prior impairment is considered a medical emergency because prompt treatment may restore hearing. Common causes are acute infection, head trauma, brain tumor, toxic drugs, or metabolic and vascular disorders.

Hearing loss can also be noise-induced and can be temporary or, over time, permanent. It follows prolonged exposure to noise in excess of 85 to 90 db (see Chapter 6). It is common among people who work in constant industrial noise, military personnel, and rock musicians. This loss is preventable with the enforcement of the use of protective devices, such as ear plugs, as mandated by law in occupational exposure.

Bone- and air-conduction hearing loss is assessed by the Rinne and Weber tests. An audiometer can be used to give a pure-tone audiometry examination to measure the threshold and degree of loudness at which sound can be perceived (see Chapter 6). A gradual loss of hearing occurs normally as part of the aging process and is known as **presbycusis.**

Ménière's Disease.   The condition known as **Ménière's disease** is characterized by severe vertigo (dizziness), **tinnitus** (ringing in the ears), and nerve loss, apparently from degeneration of the hair cells in the cochlea and vestibule of the inner ear. Violent attacks may last from 10 minutes to hours and cause severe nausea, vomiting, and perspiration. Often the vertigo causes loss of balance and results in the person falling. Treatment consists of drugs to reduce fluid, antihistamines, and mild sedation. If frequent severe attacks occur, surgical destruction of the cochlea may be indicated at the cost of permanent hearing loss.

Motion Sickness. This is characterized by loss of equilibrium, perspiration, headache, nausea, and vomiting brought on by irregular motion. The disorder probably results from excessive stimulation of the inner ear receptors or confusion in the brain between the visual stimulus and movement perception. Treatment consists of avoiding the causative motions, lying down, and closing the eyes. When avoidance is not possible, the head should be kept still and vision focused on distant and stationary objects. Medications to prevent vomiting are usually beneficial.

Otitis: Externa. This infection of the external auditory canal is usually caused by bacteria. **Otitis** causes pain and hearing loss. Otitis externa can result from contaminated swimming water (swimmer's ears); cleaning the canal with bobby pins or introducing an organism on a cotton swab; regular use of earphones or plugs which can trap moisture, creating optimal growing conditions; and scratching the ear canal with a fingernail. It is best treated with heat, pain medication, and antibiotic ear drops, following thorough cleaning.

Otitis: Media. An infection of the middle ear often associated with respiratory infections, otitis media can also result from obstruction of the eustachian tube, which causes a negative pressure to develop and "pull" serous fluid from the blood vessels into the middle ear. Otitis media is characterized by a severe, deep, and throbbing pain; fever; hearing loss; nausea and vomiting; and dizziness. The tympanic membrane may be reddened and bulge into the external canal. Excessive pressure may cause it to rupture, resulting in drainage into the canal. Recurring episodes may scar and thicken the membrane, causing a conduction hearing loss. Holes and tears from a rupture will also cause a loss of hearing.

Treatment requires antibiotics, such as penicillin or erythromycin (with a sulfa drug if allergic to penicillin), in addition to pain medication. A myringotomy (incision of the tympanic membrane) is indicated if bulging and severe pain are present. Young children and infants are prone to ear infections. Anatomically, their eustachian tubes slant horizontally, which allows fluid to collect more easily and become a medium for bacterial growth. Infants who are allowed to take a bottle while lying down, especially on their backs, may get fluid into their eustachian tubes if they cough or cry. With chronic fluid collection due to obstruction, it may be necessary to insert a tiny polyethylene tube through the membrane temporarily to equalize the pressure.

Otosclerosis. The most common cause of conductive deafness is **otosclerosis.** The loss is slow and progressive and may be accompanied by tinnitus. It is characterized by the formation of spongy bone, which immobilizes the stapes in the oval window of the vestibule, disrupting the conduction of vibrations from the tympanic membrane to the cochlea. It appears to result from a genetic factor and often occurs among family members. Incidence in Caucasians is at least 10%, affecting twice as many females as males, usually between 15 and 30 years of age. Treatment for otosclerosis consists of surgically removing the stapes (stapedectomy) and inserting an artificial substitute, which results in partial or complete return of hearing. An appropriate type of hearing aid may be of some assistance, if a stapedectomy is not possible.

Presbycusis (Senile Deafness). This hearing loss is an effect of aging and results from deterioration of the auditory system and a loss of the hair cells in the organ of Corti. It is sensorineural in nature, normally manifesting itself through the loss of high-frequency sounds. It is usually accompanied by an annoying tinnitus. The patient has difficulty understanding the spoken word and may become depressed due to inability to communicate. Presbycusis is irreversible but can be somewhat overcome with an effective and properly-fitted hearing aid.

The Nose and the Sense of Smell ....

The sense of smell is due to the olfactory organ in the top of the nasal cavity, Figure 4–41. The nerve fibers in the organ are chemoreceptors that respond to stimuli from ions or molecules dissolved in the moisture from the mucous membranes. The organ is connected by nerve fibers, which run through tiny holes in the skull bone above the nasal cavity, to the olfactory center in the brain. The nerve fibers connect with hair cells in the mucous membrane of the nose. These odor detectors can "smell" something only after it is dissolved in the mucus secretions.

Diseases and Disorders of the Nose ....

Epistaxis (Nosebleed). This usually occurs after injury, either external or internal, such as a blow to the nose, nosepicking, or foreign body insertion. Less frequent causes

FIGURE 4–41 The sense of smell (From *The Wonderful Human Machine*, Copyright 1979, American Medical Association)

of **epistaxis** are chronic conditions, such as nasal or sinus infection, that result in capillary congestion and bleeding, or the inhalation of irritating substances. Predisposing systemic factors include high blood pressure, anticoagulation drugs, chronic aspirin use, and blood diseases, such as anemia, hemophilia, and leukemia.

Treatment varies depending on the cause, location, and severity. Even moderate bleeding is considered severe if it persists longer than 10 minutes after pressure is applied. Symptoms may include lightheadedness, a drop in blood pressure, rapid pulse, dyspnea, pallor, and other indications of shock. Initial first aid treatment may consist of: elevating the head; compression of nostrils against the septum continuously for 5 to 10 minutes; application of ice or cold compresses to nose and back of neck; preventing the swallowing of blood (to determine the amount lost); avoiding talking or blowing the nose; and observing for amount of blood loss and signs of shock.

Advanced treatment includes: for anterior bleeding, applying epinephrine-saturated cotton ball or gauze to the bleeding site and the use of external pressure, followed by cauterization by electric cautery or silver nitrate; for posterior bleeding, the insertion of a nasal pack for 48 to 72 hours may be required. Small catheters are passed through each side of the nose into the mouth. Rolled gauze packs are attached to the catheters and drawn back through the mouth and up into the posterior nasal cavity where they become lodged, making pressure against the leaking blood vessels. If necessary, anterior bleeding can be treated by packing for 24 to 48 hours. Other treatment may include supplemental vitamin K, blood transfusions, and surgical ligation (tying) of the bleeding artery.

Nasal Polyps. These benign growths, usually multiple and in both sides of the nose, often occur in large enough numbers and size to distend the nose and obstruct the airway. They are caused by prolonged mucous membrane edema associated with allergies, chronic sinusitis, rhinitis, and recurrent nasal infections. Diagnosis is made by visual observation through a nasal speculum or X rays of posterior nasal passages and the sinuses. Treatment with antihistamines, cortisone, and antibiotics if infected, will temporarily reduce the size of the **polyps.** Surgical removal is the treatment of choice, however, and is usually necessary.

Rhinitis (Allergic). This reaction to airborne allergens causes sneezing, profuse watery discharge, itching of the eyes and nose, conjunctivitis, and tearing. Many symptoms are the result of the body's attempt to dilute or remove irritants coming into contact with its mucous membranes. Treatment consists of eliminating environmental antigens when possible, the use of antibiotics, and systemic corticosteroids. Long-term management includes injections of the offending allergens to cause desensitization, the use of air conditioning, and, if severe and persistent, relocation to a safe environment.

The Tongue and the Sense of Taste ....

The ability to taste flavors is located in the receptors of the taste buds on the tongue. They are located at the tip, sides, and back, grouped by the taste that can be perceived, Figure 4–42. The sweet area is at the tip, the salty areas are next along the sides, followed by the sour areas and another area of salty perception. The large **papillae** (raised areas) at the back transmit the bitter sensations. Like the sense of smell, taste is possible because of the chemoreceptors that receive stimuli from ions or molecules and initiate the impulses. As with smell, taste is not possible unless the substance is moistened. This moisture is supplied by the salivary glands, in sufficient quantities to affect taste.

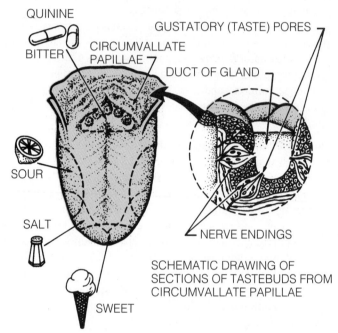

FIGURE 4–42 The sense of taste (From *The Wonderful Human Machine,* Copyright 1979, American Medical Association)

Diseases and Disorders of the Mouth and Tongue ....

Glossitis. Inflammation of the tongue caused by an organism, irritation, injury, or nutritional deficiencies is known as glossitis. Such agents as tobacco, alcohol, spicy foods, and jagged teeth may cause glossitis. The condition results in a red, swollen tongue, pain on chewing, difficult speech, and occasionally an obstructed airway. Treatment includes topical anesthetic mouthwash, systemic pain medication, good oral hygiene, and the avoidance of alcohol and hot, cold, or spicy foods.

Oral Cancer. In recent years, a significant increase in the incidence of oral cancer has been noted. There seems to be evidence that people have switched from cigarettes to smokeless forms of tobacco in an effort to avoid the development of lung cancer. In exchange, the use of products, such as chewing tobacco and snuff, has caused extensive disease of the gums tongue, and other oral structures and often results in the development of cancer within the oral cavity.

The Skin and the Sense of Touch ....

The sense of touch requires direct contact with the body through contact receptors, Figure 4–43. The sense of touch involves mechanical energy, such as pressure or traction, which activates mechanoreceptors and radiant energy, such as heat or cold, which activates thermoreceptors. The design of the receptor varies with its location on the body. Touch receptors are most concentrated in the fingertips. Pain receptors are simply bare nerve endings in the skin and other organs. Separate skin receptors perceive heat and cold. Each of the contact receptors in the skin has its own perceptive function enabling us to feel the many different sensations of pain, touch, pressure, heat, cold, traction, and tickle. This sense aids us in protecting ourselves, identifying injury, feeling pleasure, and maintaining contact with our environment. The skin is the subject of the next unit.

Complete Chapter 4, Unit 3 in the workbook to help you meet the objectives at the beginning of this unit and therefore achieve competency of this subject matter.

PAIN TOUCH HEAT PRESSURE TRACTION COLD TICKLE

FIGURE 4–43 The sense of touch (From *The Wonderful Human Machine,* Copyright 1979, American Medical Association)

U N I T   4

The Integumentary System

OBJECTIVES ....

Upon completion of this unit, you will meet the following terminal performance objectives by verifying knowledge of the facts and principles presented through oral and written communication at a level deemed competent by the instructor or employer.

1. List the five functions of the skin.
2. Explain how the skin regulates body temperature.
3. Describe how the body cools its surface.
4. Name the three layers of skin tissue and the characteristic structures of each layer.
5. Describe the process that causes wrinkles.
6. Explain what causes a suntan to develop.
7. Identify the ABCD rules and other warning signs of melanoma and the factors that contribute to its development.
8. Explain what causes blushing, birthmarks, moles, and albinism.
9. Identify 20 diseases or disorders of the skin.
10. Spell and define, using the glossary at the back of the text, all the words to know in this unit.

WORDS TO KNOW ....

albino	macule
alopecia	melanin
carbunculosis	melanocytes
constrict	pediculosis
dermatitis	perception
dermis	pigment
dilate	psoriasis
eczema	pustule
epidermis	receptors
erythema	sebaceous
follicle	sebum
folliculitis	slough
furuncle	subcutaneous
herpes simplex	transdermal
herpes zoster	urticaria
integumentary	verrucae
inunction	vesicle
keloid	wheals
Lyme disease	whorl

The word **integumentary** refers to an external covering, or skin. You may never have thought of the skin as a "body system," but according to the definition of a system in Unit 1, the skin with all its structures qualifies: it is many tissues (nerve, connective, muscle, epithelial), forming organs (sweat and oil glands), to perform a function. The skin is not usually listed as one of the body's systems, however. Most anatomists classify the skin as an organ. When listed in this category, it becomes the largest organ of the body. An average adult has about 3000 square inches of skin surface. The skin makes up about 15% of the total body weight, which would be approximately 20 pounds of a 145 pound person. The skin varies in thickness from very thin over the eyelids to quite thick on the soles of the feet.

The skin is so important to survival that the loss of even a small percentage of its vital function is a cause for concern. If about one-third of the skin of a healthy young adult is lost, death may result. Skin covers all the body's surface, preventing the tissue fluids from escaping and foreign materials in the environment from entering. At the openings to the body, such as the nose, mouth, or anus, it joins with the mucous membranes that line the openings into the respiratory and digestive systems to make a continuous internal and external covering.

Functions

The skin performs five important functions for the body: protection, perception, temperature control, absorption, and excretion. The skin protects against the invasion of bacteria by serving as a barrier. It is effective, however, only as long as it remains intact. A cut or scrape of the surface allows bacteria to enter. It also protects the delicate underlying tissues from injury by the damaging rays of the sun. Equally important, it protects the body's tissues from loss of fluid. This is of great concern when large areas of skin are lost as a result of burns, for example, which allows fluids to escape and bacteria to enter.

The skin serves as an organ of **perception** in cooperation with the nervous system and the sense of touch. A square inch of skin contains about 72 feet of nerves and hundreds of **receptors** registering pain, heat, cold, and pressure.

In that same square inch are about 15 feet of blood vessels, which provide food and oxygen, and also regulate the body's temperature. This function is of such importance to the body that the skin receives approximately one-third of the blood circulating throughout the body. When the body's temperature control center in the brain senses the body is becoming too warm, the nervous system sends messages to the surface vessels to **dilate,** which allows heat from the blood to escape through the skin and therefore cool the body. If heat must be retained, the vessels are ordered to **constrict** to reduce the loss of heat so that body temperature can be maintained at an adequate level. This important function is discussed in greater detail in Chapter 5, Unit 4, Vital Signs.

The skin also contains sweat glands, which are likewise controlled by the heat regulator in the brain. When the air temperature rises, the body produces sweat, which evaporates from its surface to provide a cooling effect and thereby reduce the amount of heat within the underlying blood vessels.

The skin is capable of absorbing some materials from its surface through the hair **follicles** and the glands. This function can be of use to the physician in treating certain conditions. Perhaps the two most common applications are antimotion sickness medication, which is placed on the skin's surface behind the ear, and a medicated paste strip, which is placed on the chest to treat certain heart conditions. A trend seems to be developing toward a greater amount of medications being administered through the skin. Primarily the advantages are "timed release," which spreads medication evenly over a long period of time, thereby not only eliminating repeated dosage, but also the digestive system side effects from certain oral drugs. This form of drug administration is called **inunction,** or **transdermal.**

Several substances known as lipid-soluble (e.g., vitamins A, D, and K, the sex hormones, etc.) and almost all gases (e.g., oxygen, hydrogen, and nitrogen, etc.) can pass through the skin. It is interesting to note that carbon monoxide cannot pass.

The skin's function of excretion consists primarily of eliminating water and salt plus a minute amount of other waste products. Excessive fluid loss as a result of strenuous activity or highly elevated temperature can be a matter of concern. Fluid must be replaced to maintain a proper fluid balance. The skin also combines the ultraviolet rays from sunlight with compounds normally present in the skin to produce vitamin D while screening out any harmful ultraviolet rays.

A great number of microscopic skin structures are located within an area of only one square centimeter. This is illustrated in Figure 4–44, as a small circle on the back of the hand. That this large group of anatomical structures could be located in such a small area seems inconceivable. These microscopic wonders perform an invaluable service for the body.

Structure of the Skin

The skin is composed of three layers: the **epidermis** on the top, the **dermis** in the middle, and the **subcutaneous** layer on the bottom, Figure 4–45, page 111. The subcutaneous layer is filled with fat globules, blood vessels, and nerves. The dermis contains blood vessels, nerves, hair follicles, and sweat and oil glands. This layer is usually referred to as the "true skin." The top of the dermis is covered with cone-shaped papillae, which create an uneven surface. The epidermis is full of ridges that fit snugly over the papillae on top of the dermis. These ridges form the **whorls** and patterns on the fingertips that we call fingerprints. Since no two people have exactly the same pattern of

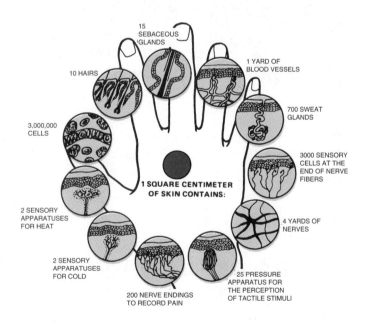

FIGURE 4–44 Structures of the skin (From *The Wonderful Human Machine,* Copyright 1979, American Medical Association)

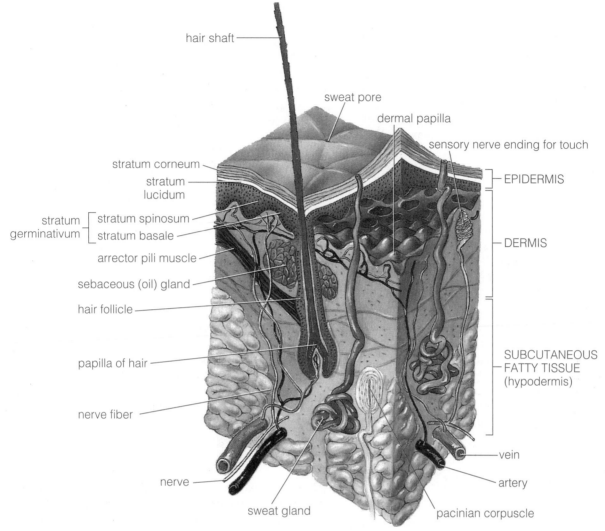

FIGURE 4–45 Cross section of skin (From Smith, *Medical Terminology, A Programmed Text,* 6th ed. Copyright 1991, Delmar Publishers Inc.)

ridges, they will not have the same fingerprints, making this characteristic a suitable means of identification. Similar patterns of ridges appear on the soles of the feet and are used for identification of newborns. New cells are formed deep in the epidermis. Here rapid cell division pushes cells toward the surface of the skin to replace those that wear away, die, and flake off. The process from division to flaking off takes about 30 to 45 days. Because of the skin's ability to reproduce cells rapidly, it can repair itself quickly following cuts and abrasions.

The skin is strong, soft, flexible, and elastic in young people because of the presence of keratin in the epidermis and collagenous fibers in the dermis. Also, some dermis cells store fat. The action of the keratin and cell membranes allows skin to act as a barrier to prevent dehydration. With age, the fatty underlying tissue is absorbed and the elastic fibers decrease, leaving an excess in the outer layer which develops folds or wrinkles.

The skin has four appendages: the sweat and oil glands, hair, and the nails. The dermis contains the sweat and **sebaceous** (oil) glands. Sweat glands are tiny coiled tubes deep in the dermis

with corkscrew tubules leading to the surface. Oil glands are located in or near hair follicles over the entire skin surface except for the palms of the hands and the soles of the feet.

A sebaceous gland contains an oily substance which helps prevent the hair and skin from becoming dry and brittle. Unfortunately, oil glands often become plugged by cell overgrowth. The gland continues to produce oil, which fills the duct and results in development of a blackhead or pimple.

Every hair has a root, which is inside a follicle (shaft) that extends deep into the dermal layer. With long hair, the root extends into the subcutaneous layer. Attached to each follicle is a small involuntary muscle. With certain emotions or sensations of coldness, the muscle contracts, causing the hair to stand erect and producing what we call "goose flesh." An inner layer of cells in the shaft of hair contains a **pigment** which gives the hair its color. Hair that is white has cells that contain air in place of pigment.

The hair and nails are composed of hard keratin (soft keratin is found in the epidermis). They are similar, but the hard keratin is more permanent and does not **slough** (drop) off, which means they must be cut occasionally.

Skin Color

A brown-black pigment called **melanin** is produced by cells called **melanocytes**, which are present in the epidermis to protect the underlying tissues from damage by the sun. The amount of melanin affects the color of the skin as does another pigment, carotene, which is yellow. The presence of blood vessels in the dermis also contributes to the coloration of the skin. When the skin is exposed to the sun, it may become reddened due to dilation of the superficial blood vessels. The condition is known medically as **erythema,** but it is commonly known as sunburn. If it is not severe, the skin will acquire a brown coloration or suntan, which is produced by the melanin pigment increasing and moving to the surface to protect the underlying tissues. New melanin will replace the old in the lower cell layer. Freckles are actually small areas of melanin pigment.

Skin coloration is affected by many factors. The rich supply of blood vessels causes reddening of the skin, due to dilation, when we blush. Birthmarks may be due to coloration from a concentration of blood vessels or from patches of skin pigment. Moles are also pigmented patches. A person whose skin has little or no pigment to give it color is said to be an **albino.** An albino's hair also lacks pigment and will be white. Because pigment is also lacking in the coloration of the eyes, the sun and artificial light cannot be filtered out. Therefore the eyes of a person with albinism are very sensitive to light. People with this disorder must wear sunglasses or tinted lenses for comfort and to prevent eye damage.

The Skin as a Diagnostic Testing Site

The skin is often used to test and diagnose disorders and diseases of the body, specifically in the area of allergies. Because of its natural capacity to defend the body from foreign substances, it makes an excellent medium for testing the reaction to minute amounts of allergens. Following injection of common substances, usually on the back or inner surface of the forearm, the skin will form variously-sized areas around the injection sites, reacting to those materials that initiate an allergic response. Physicians can then identify causative substances and recommend measures to reduce the problems associated with the allergic disorder. (See Chapter 8, Diagnostic Tests, X rays, and Procedures.)

Diseases and Disorders

Acne Vulgaris.   This inflammatory disease of the follicles of the sebaceous glands mainly affects adolescents. The true cause is unknown. Research has determined that dietary habits appear to be less of a factor than originally thought. Present findings seem to suggest that hormonal dysfunction and an oversupply of **sebum,** oil from the sebaceous glands, are the probable underlying causes. It collects at the openings to the glands, hardens, and closes off the natural flow of oily secretion, causing blackheads or cysts to develop. Sometimes the area will become filled with leukocytes that cause pus to accumulate and pimples to develop.

Usual treatment for severe acne includes a topical antibacterial product either alone or in combination with a topical vitamin A product. Often antibiotics applied to the skin are helpful. Antibiotics are systematically used to decrease bacterial growth. Occasionally with females who have severe disease, estrogens may be used to control the androgen (male hormone) activity, which stimulates the growth of sebaceous glands and the production of sebum.

Alopecia.   This is loss of hair, usually occurring on the scalp. There are two types of **alopecia.** A scarring type causes irreversible hair loss and is usually the result of physical or chemical trauma or chronic tension on the hair shaft from such things as braiding or tightly rolling the hair. Certain diseases, such as lupus erythematosus, bacterial or viral infections, and skin tumors, may also cause scarring alopecia.

The most common form of nonscarring alopecia is male-pattern baldness. It seems to be primarily due to aging and androgen levels. There is a tendency for genetic influence and it will often be displayed among male family members. Women may also exhibit the male pattern but at a lesser degree.

Other forms of nonscarring alopecia are: physiologic, which is usually temporary and occurs suddenly in infants or the mother's diffuse loss after childbirth; areata, which is of unknown cause but is self-limiting and occurs among both sexes from young to middle age; and trichotillomania, which is the pulling out of one's own hair and is most common among children. These people may also pull out other hair, such as the eyebrows.

There is no known "cure" for male-pattern baldness; however, recent specific drug usage seems to prevent further loss and encourage some regrowth in many men. Surgical grafting of hair follicles from other parts of the scalp have proved successful. Areata alopecia usually reverses itself within 4 to 6 weeks. Trichotillomania alopecia can be controlled by a behavioral change or if necessary, psychiatric counseling.

Hair loss as a result of chemotherapy is common. Certain chemical agents destroy the cells of the hair, which result in the massive loss of hair over a 2- or 3-day period soon after the initiation of the drug. Normally, some fine hair will remain, but is very sparse. Fortunately, about 3 months after treatments end, hair will begin regrowth, sometimes a different color or texture.

Cancer.   The skin may be the site of different forms of cancerous lesions, such as basal cell carcinomas, squamous cell carcinomas, and malignant melanomas. Nevi (moles) are considered to be potentially malignant and require careful observation. Bleeding, itching, or a change in color, size, shape, or texture of a mole suggests a possible conversion to a malignant state.

Basal cell carcinoma is caused primarily by prolonged exposure to the sun and occurs where there are abundant sebaceous follicles, especially on the face. It is more prevalent in persons over 40, especially blond, fair-skinned males. It is the most common malignant tumor affecting Caucasians.

There are basically three types of basal cell carcinoma lesions, each with its own distinctive characteristics and usual location. They are diagnosed by appearance and surgical biopsy.

Nodulo-ulcerative lesions occur most often on the face and are small, smooth, pinkish and translucent papules. As they enlarge, the centers become depressed and the borders elevated and firm. *Superficial* basal cell carcinoma are often multiple and commonly occur on the chest and back. They are oval or irregularly shaped with sharply defined, threadlike borders that are slightly elevated. *Sclerosing* basal cell lesions occur on the head and neck. They appear yellow to white, are waxy, and do not have distinct borders.

Squamous cell carcinoma is predisposed by sunlight, presence of premalignant lesions, X-ray therapy, environmental carcinogens, and chronic skin irritation. Its incidence is highest in fair-skinned Caucasian males over the age of 60. Living in sunny climates and working in outdoor employment greatly increase the risk of development.

This form of carcinoma is commonly found on the face, ears, and back of the hands as well as other sun-damaged areas. The lesions have a tendency to metastasize. Those located on unexposed skin have the greatest incidence. Lesions of the lower lip and ears are exceptionally metastatic.

Malignant melanoma develops from pigment-producing cells and occurs in three forms: superficial spreading, modular malignant, and lentigo maligna melanomas. It spreads through the lymphatic and circulatory systems, metastasizing to the lymph nodes, liver, lungs, and CNS. Prognosis varies with the characteristic of the lesion. Superficial tumors are curable, whereas deeper lesions tend to metastasize. The American Cancer Society recently released facts about the incidence of malignant melanoma. For the year 1993, about 32,000 people were diagnosed; about 6500 died. This incidence translates into 1 in every 105 United States residents as compared with only 1 in every 1500 in 1935. If the trend continues, the incidence is projected to be 1 in 75 by the year 2000.

The major cause of malignant melanoma is exposure to the sun. The sun produces ultraviolet rays, mainly UVA and UVB. UVBs cause sunburn, premature aging of the skin, and skin cancers. Most sunscreens provide a degree of protection against this ray. Recent evidence, however, seems to suggest that the UVA rays may also be damaging the skin, perhaps aiding the cancer-forming ability of UVB.

The Cancer Society cited the primary reasons for the increase to be weekend leisure time, which results in intense bursts of exposure to UVB, the loss of the ozone layer protection, UVA rays not being blocked by sunscreens, and the tendency of people to purposely lie flat in the sun for hours at a time, which allows deeper penetration of the rays. People most at risk are those who have had severe blistering sunburns during their teens or twenties.

Other contributing factors are blond or red hair, fair skin, blue eyes, and a tendency to sunburn. Persons who work or spend many hours outdoors or who live in places with intense year-round sunshine are also at risk. Arizona has the highest incidence reported. The peak of incidence occurs between 50 to 70 years of age. Incidence is slightly higher among women than men.

Dermatologists recommend avoiding sun altogether from 10:00 A.M. to 3:00 P.M. (perhaps from 8:00 A.M. to 6:00 P.M. if the ozone condition worsens), and using a sunscreen of at least 15 SPF that will block both UVA and UVB during exposure. Sunlamps, tanning pills, and tanning salons should be avoided. The information and photos in Figure 4–46, page 114, show the ABCD rules and appearance signs of melanoma.

Dermatitis. The term means inflammation of the skin and can refer to any form of skin condition such as: seborrhea, eczema, contact **dermatitis** (from irritants), exfoliative dermatitis (large pieces of peeling skin), or stasis (from lack of blood supply). Dermatitis is often caused by allergens, such as wool; detergent; cosmetics; pollen; or foods, such as eggs, milk, seafood, or wheat products. Common symptoms are dry skin, redness, itching, edema, formation of lesions, and scaling. It is treated by avoiding known allergens, applying anti-inflammatory products to the skin, systemic steroids, antihistamines, and other measures specific to the type of dermatitis.

Eczema. This noncontagious skin disease is characterized by dry, red, itchy, and scaly skin. It can be acute or chronic and sometimes produces a watery discharge. Several things may initiate **eczema,** such as diet, cosmetics, clothing, medications, soaps, occupational or environmental substances, and emotional stress.

Treatment consists primarily of removal of the causative agent when possible and the local application of ointments to alleviate the symptoms. Oral steroids are indicated to reduce inflammation, and antibiotics are used if secondary infection is present.

Follicular Infections. A staphylococcal infection of the hair follicle that results in the formation of a pustule is known as **folliculitis.** It can be of a superficial form, involving only the surface area around a single follicle, or deep, involving the total hair follicle. Treatment consists of thorough cleansing of the area and the application of wet heat to promote drainage from the lesion as well as the use of topical antibiotics. If recurrent, systemic antibiotics may be indicated.

Folliculitis may lead to the development of **furuncles** (boils), which are hard, painful nodules that enlarge over several days until they rupture, releasing pus and dead cells through one draining point. The area remains red and swollen for a short time, but the pain lessens. Furuncles may be caused by irritation, pressure, or friction of the follicular site. Treatment consists of the measures used for folliculitis with wet heat to relieve pain and encourage "ripening" of the lesion. Often incision and drainage are required to allow complete expulsion of the material. Patients must be cautioned not to squeeze a boil because it may rupture into the surrounding tissues.

Carbunculosis follows persistent staphylococcal infection and furunculosis and is characterized by deep follicular abscesses of several follicles with multiple draining points. It is extremely painful and usually associated with fever and general malaise. Carbunculosis requires treatment with systemic antibiotics in addition to the localized heat applications and drainage. Wash cloths and towels, bed sheets, and clothing used by the infected person must not be shared with other

What is the Difference Between a Melanoma and an Ordinary Mole?

A normal mole is an evenly colored brown, tan, or black spot in the skin. It is either flat or raised. Its shape is round or oval and it has sharply defined borders. Moles are generally less than 6 mm in diameter (about the size of a pencil eraser). A mole may be present at birth or it may appear spontaneously, usually in the first few decades of life. Sometimes several moles appear at the same time, especially on sun-exposed areas of the skin. Once a mole has fully developed, it normally remains the same size, shape, and color for many years. Most moles eventually fade away in older persons.

Almost everyone has moles, on the average of about 25. The vast majority of moles are perfectly harmless. A sudden or continuous change in a mole's appearance is a sign that you should see your physician. However, a melanoma is more complicated than a mole.

Here's the simple **ABCD** rule to help you remember the important signs of melanoma:

A. **Asymmetry.** One half does not match the other half, Figure 4–46(a).

B. **Border irregularity.** The edges are ragged, notched or blurred, Figure 4–46(b).

C. **Color.** The pigmentation is not uniform. Shades of tan, brown, and black are present. Red, white, and blue may add to the mottled appearance, Figure 4–46(c).

D. **Diameter greater than 6 mm.** Any sudden or continuing increase in size should be of special concern, Figure 4–46(d).

Other Warning Signs of Melanoma

Change in the surface of a mole—scaliness, oozing, bleeding, or the appearance of a bump or nodule; spread of pigment from the border into surrounding skin; redness or a new swelling beyond the border; change in sensation—itchiness, tenderness or pain.

(The above information reprinted, with permission, from a brochure titled *Why You Should Know About Melanoma,* distributed by the American Cancer Society and developed in cooperation with the American Academy of Dermatology.)

(a) Asymmetry

(b) Border irregularity

(c) Color

(d) Diameter

FIGURE 4–46   The signs of melanoma (Courtesy of the American Academy of Dermatology) family members to prevent spreading the bacteria. A patient with recurring furuncles should see a physician to rule out any underlying cause, such as diabetes.

Herpes Simplex. This viral infection results in cold sores or blisters on the mouth or face. It is equally prevalent among males and females and occurs throughout the world. Diagnosis is made from the typical lesions that appear as vesicles with a red base that eventually ruptures making a painful ulcer. **Herpes simplex** has a 2- to 12-day incubation period during which tingling and itching signal the oncoming vesicle. A yellow crust develops following vesicle rupture, and healing is complete after approximately 3 weeks.

Treatment consists of topical applications of tincture of benzoin at initial indication followed by various ointments to the lesion to alleviate cracking and discomfort. Some people feel that an ice cube to the lesion when it appears produces quicker healing.

Herpes Zoster. This is an acute infectious process by the virus that also causes chickenpox. In **herpes zoster infection,** also known as shingles, the dorsal root ganglia are inflamed, causing severe neuralgic pain along the area of the involved nerves. It is characterized by fever, malaise, and the eruption of vesicles in the painful area, which spread unilaterally around the back, chest, back of neck, or vertically on the extremities. (See Unit 2.)

Hirsutism. This disorder usually appears in women and children; excessive body hair develops in an adult male pattern of growth. There may be a family history of the disorder, or it could be related to an endrocrine problem resulting from either pituitary dysfunction, ovarian lesions, or adrenal gland enlargement.

The most common symptom is growth of facial hair but other masculinization signs, such as deepening voice, increased muscle mass, menstrual irregularity, and breast size reduction may be exhibited. Treatment consists of hair removal by shaving, depilatory creams, or waxing as well as bleaching to minimize the appearance of hair. Electrolysis will permanently destroy the hair follicles but is slow and expensive. If hormonal causes are evident, treatment may involve counteracting or controlling endocrine secretions in specific situations.

Impetigo. This contagious, superficial skin infection is usually seen in young children. Predisposing factors include anemia, malnutrition, and poor hygiene, but these are not essential to the development of the disease. The causative organism is either streptococcal or staphylococcal. If strep, a small red **macule** (flat area with definite edge) turns into a **vesicle** (raised lesion containing serous fluid), then to a **pustule** (lesion with purulent material), within a relatively short period of time. (The terms *macule*, *vesicle*, and *pustule* refer to any skin lesion that demonstrates these descriptive characteristics, not to impetigo alone.) When the lesions break, a characteristic yellow crust develops from the exudate (drainage). Other sites develop from contact with the lesions or the drainage. The staph lesion is characterized by a thin-walled vesicle, which forms a thin, clear crust from the exudate. Both forms characteristically have a clear central area and definite outer rims. The lesions appear primarily on the face, neck, and other exposed areas of the body. Contamination of others is prevented by avoiding contact through wash cloths, towels, and bed linens. Scratching of the lesions must be prohibited. Therapy includes washing the areas two to three times daily to remove the exudate, and a systemic antibiotic to prevent secondary infection.

Keloid. A scar that developes excess dense tissue as it progresses through the healing process is known as **keloid.**

Lyme Disease. This disease is caused by a spirochete (corkscrew bacteria) carried by the deer tick. **Lyme disease** was named after Old Lyme, Connecticut, where it was first identified. The deer tick is known as a three-host tick and has a 2-year life cycle. In spring, eggs are deposited and six-legged larval ticks hatch, attaching themselves to small mammals or birds to obtain their first meal of blood. The tick larvae over winter, molting to a larger eight-legged nymphal stage, which attaches to dogs, squirrels, and deer. Next they molt to the adult stage in the summer and attach to a larger mammal, primarily a deer. After gorging on blood and mating, they later drop off to lay eggs. The tick can transmit the disease during any stage. Bites seem to occur most often during summer or late autumn. The ticks apparently go from these hosts to woods and field underbrush where they are picked up by people and pets.

The disease was first recognized and reported in the United States in the mid 1970s with the incidence almost doubling from 4882 cases in 1988 to 8551 cases in 1989. There were 22,570 cases reported between 1982 and 1989, with over one-third being in 1989 alone. About 80% of the cases are reported in California, Connecticut, New Jersey, New York, Pennsylvania, Rhode Island, and Wisconsin. Symptoms begin with a distinctive bullseye rash, but it is not always apparent on everyone. Usually there is a small red bump and rash at the bite site. This site can expand to an oval or round area 2 to 3 inches in diameter. The rash will fade after a few weeks, with or without treatment. Early symptoms include profound fatigue, stiff neck, flulike headache, chills, muscle aches, and fever. Later stages may produce heart and nervous system involvement with subsequent chronic arthritis beginning up to a year later.

Fortunately, treatment with antibiotics for 2 to 3 weeks is effective, especially if begun early in the disease process. The best line of treatment is defense. When hiking or camping in a wooded or brushy area, use repellents with a high concentration of Deet, applied sparingly to adult skin, but not to a child's. Use only as directed. Wear long sleeves and trousers tucked into either socks or boots to prevent tick contact with the skin. Light-colored clothing also makes it easier to spot the ticks. The most common sites are underarms, groin, or behind the knees, and on the heads of children. Pets should also be checked. The deer tick is very small, about the size of a pinhead, orange-brown with a black spot near the head. It resembles a crab. If detected on a human, it should be removed, alive if possible, and shown to a doctor or sent to proper health authorities for positive identification. When removing, grasp with forceps or tweezers at the mouth parts where attached and pull straight out. If you have to use your fingers, cover them with a tissue. Cleanse the site with antiseptic and wash clothing because ticks hide in seams and creases.

Ticks can be tested for spirochete infection. About 30% to 60% of Northeastern ticks are positive. Even if positive, you may not develop Lyme disease. If the tick is removed within 24 hours, your risk is minimal. The longer attached, the greater the chance of infection. Ticks require 18 to 48 hours to transmit the bacterium into a victim. Lyme disease is an increasingly serious public health problem, now ranked as the second most prevalent infectious disease in the United States, surpassed only by AIDS.

Pediculosis. There are three types of **pediculosis** caused by three varieties of parasitic lice: capitis from head lice; corporis from body lice; and pubis from pubic lice, commonly called crabs. The lice feed on human blood and lay eggs known as nits on body hairs or fibers of clothing. The nits hatch and will die in 24 hours unless they feed on a host. Nits mature in 2 to 3 weeks.

Capitis is the most common form and is found primarily among children, especially girls. It is caused by poor hygiene and overcrowding. It spreads through shared combs, brushes, clothing, and hats. It is identifiable as an oval grayish, dandruff-like fleck that cannot be shaken off. Its symptoms are itching and scalp abrasions with matted, foul-smelling hair in severe cases. Nits are easily treated with gamma benzene hydrochloride (GBH) cream rubbed into the scalp at night followed by GBH shampoo the next morning. A follow-up treatment is required the next night. Nits can then be removed with a fine-tooth comb.

Pediculosis corporis lives in clothing seams except when feeding on the host. Initially small red papules appear, which itch. The resulting scratching causes rashes and wheals to develop. The usual cause is prolonged wearing of the same clothes, overcrowding, and poor hygiene. It is spread through shared clothing and linens. Treatment consists of bathing with soap and water and the use of GBH if infestation is severe. All clothing and linens must be washed or dry-cleaned.

Pediculosis pubis is found attached primarily to pubic hair and is transmitted through sexual intercourse or contact with infected clothes, bedding, or towels. The lice cause itching, which results in skin irritation from scratching. Treatment consists of local applications of GBH ointment, lotion, or cream, which must remain for 24 hours or shampooing with GBH. Treatment must be repeated in a week. All clothing and linens must be washed. Sexual contacts must also be treated, or reinfection will occur.

Psoriasis. This chronic disease is characterized by itching and red papules (solid, elevated masses) covered with silvery scales. **Psoriasis** is recurrent, with alternating periods of remission or increased severity. Contributing factors are environmental (cold weather causes flare-ups), endocrine changes, pregnancy, and emotional stress.

Psoriasis cannot be cured. Scales can be softened with applications of ointments and then removed in an oatmeal bath. Ultraviolet light, either artificial or from the sun, retards cell production. Normal cells require about 2 weeks to move from their place of production to the skin surface and after another couple of weeks of wear and tear, are sloughed off. Psoriatic cells require only 4 days, which does not permit the cell to mature and results in marked proliferation of the epidermis. Steroid creams, tar preparations, and sometimes the use of coverings, such as plastic gloves or plastic wrap worn overnight, may help to control the disease.

A recent accidental discovery may hold promise of treatment. An experimental drug, FK 506, used to block organ transplant rejection, rapidly cleared psoriasis according to researchers at the University of Pittsburgh Medical Center. The drug suppresses a T cell in the immune system. Since psoriasis is somewhat genetically determined, and researchers have identified the presence of certain antigens, it is believed it could be caused by an autoimmune deficiency.

Ringworm. This fungus may affect the scalp (tinea capitis), the body (tinea corporis), or other areas, such as the groin, beard, or feet (tinea pedia, or athlete's foot). On the body, it is characterized by flat lesions, which are dry and scaly or moist and crusty. When they enlarge, clear central areas develop leaving an outer ring from which it gets its name. On the scalp, small papules occur causing scaly patches of baldness.

Treatment consists of systemic medication and topical applications of antifungals. Since the disease is contagious, care must be taken to prevent its spread by refraining from sharing bed linens, combs, and towels.

Scabies. This skin infection is caused by the itch mite. The female mite burrows into the skin, laying eggs that later hatch into larvae. The larvae emerge, mate, and then reenter the skin. The condition causes an itching which becomes intense at night. The lesions are characteristically threadlike red nodules, approximately $\frac{3}{8}$ inch long. They occur between fingers, at the inner wrist area, the elbows, in axillary folds (armpit), about the waist, on genitalia (external sex organs) of males, and on the nipples of females. The infection is spread by skin contact or sexual activity.

Treatment consists of bathing with soap and water followed by an application of pediculicide, such as Kwell. It must remain on the skin for 24 hours and be repeated in 1 week to destroy the developing mites. An antipruritic (against itching) or steroid may be applied topically to help reduce the itching.

Urticaria (hives). This is a self-limiting reaction to allergens, such as drugs, food, insect stings, and airborne agents. **Urticaria** often occurs during especially stressful or emotional times. The reaction produces distinct, raised **wheals** surrounded by a reddened area. They may be few in number or cover the entire body. Often they are accompanied with itching.

Urticaria is treated by eliminating or limiting the causative allergen or, when that is not possible, by gradual desensitization through interdermal injection of the allergen. Antihistamine is used to reduce itching and swelling. A barbituate may be required when the causative factor is emotional stress.

Verrucae (warts). This is a benign (noncancerous) viral infection of the skin, probably transmitted by direct or self-contact. Common **verrucae** are characterized by a rough, elevated, rounded surface, usually on the extremities, especially the hands and fingers. Plantar warts occur primarily at pressure points on the soles of the feet. Condyloma accuminatum (venereal warts) are moist, soft, pink to red warts occurring singly, but most often in large clusters, on the penis, vulva, or anus. This type of wart is transmitted by sexual contact.

Treatment of warts varies with the type, size, and location. Common types often disappear spontaneously. When removal is necessary, they can be destroyed by methods using electricity, acid, liquid nitrogen, or solid carbon dioxide. Venereal warts are treated with applications of podophyllum and tincture of benzoin.

Table 4–3 summarizes different types of skin lesions and their characteristics, which may help you to identify some common conditions.

Complete Chapter 4, Unit 4 in the workbook to help you meet the objectives at the beginning of this unit and therefore achieve competency of this subject matter.

U N I T   5
The Skeletal System

OBJECTIVES ....

Upon completion of this unit, you will meet the following terminal performance objectives by verifying knowledge of the facts and principles presented through oral and written communication at a level deemed competent by the instructor or employer.

1. Name the two divisions of the skeletal system and the bone groups in each division.
2. Describe the structure of the long bones.
3. Explain how long bones grow.
4. Identify the elements which make up bone tissue.
5. Identify the major bones of the body.
6. List the six functions of the skeletal system.
7. Name the divisions of the spinal column and the number of vertebrae in each division.
8. Describe fontanels and explain why they are essential.
9. Describe the structure of the rib cage and its primary function.
10. Identify three kinds of synovial joints and give examples of each.
11. List the parts of a synovial joint and identify the purpose of each part.
12. Name the seven types of fractures and the characteristics of each.
13. Outline the treatment of a fracture.
14. Describe the healing process of a fracture.
15. Define the term *fatty embolus,* explaining its origin and what might occur with one.
16. List situations predisposing to amputation.
17. Define the phantom limb sensation.
18. Discuss two diagnostic examinations.
19. Explain why the symptoms of carpal tunnel syndrome occur.
20. Name the three types of spinal curvatures, describing their physical characteristics.

TABLE 4–3
Different Types of Skin Lesions, Their Characteristics, Size, and Examples

Type of Skin Lesion	Characteristics	Size	Example(s)
Bulla (blister)	Fluid-filled area	Greater than 5 mm across	A large blister
Macule	A round, flat area usually distinguished from its surrounding skin by its change in color	Smaller than 1 cm	Freckle Petechia (small hemorrhage spot)
Nodule	Elevated solid area, deeper and firmer than a papule	Greater than 5 mm across	Wart
Papule	Elevated solid area	5 mm or less across	Elevated nevus (mole)
Pustule	Discrete, pus-filled raised area	Varying size	Acne
Ulcer	A deep loss of skin surface that may extend into the dermis that can bleed periodically and scar	Varies in sizes	Venous stasis ulcer
Tumor tumor	Solid abnormal mass of cells that may extend deep through cutaneous tissue	Larger than 1–2 cm	Benign (harmless) epidermal Basal cell carcinoma (rarely metastasizing)
Vesicle	Fluid-filled raised area	5 mm or less across	Chickenpox Herpes simplex
Wheal	Itchy, temporarily elevated area with an irregular	Varies in size	Hives

(Adapted from Fong, *Body Structures and Functions,* 8th ed. Copyright 1993, Delmar Publishers Inc.)

21. Identify 17 diseases and disorders of the skeletal system.
22. Spell and define, using the glossary at the back of the text, all the words to know in this unit.

WORDS TO KNOW ....

alignment	laminectomy
amputate	ligament
appendicular	lordosis
arthritis	marrow
articulation	metacarpal
axial	metatarsal
bunion	osteoporosis
bursa	patella
callus	periosteum
carpal	phalanges
cartilage	phalanx
cervical	phantom limb
clavicle	prosthesis
coccyx	radius
comminuted	reduce
compound	sacrum
cranium	scapula
depressed	scoliosis
diarthrosis	simple
dislocation	skeletal
embolus	spinal fusion
epiphyses	spiral
femur	sprain
fibula	sternum
fracture	symphysis pubis
greenstick	synovial
humerus	tarsal
ilium	tibia
impacted	traction
intervertebral	ulna
ischium	vertebrae
kyphosis	xiphoid

The **skeletal** system consists of organs called bones. It may be difficult to think of bones as living, functioning organs, but they use food and oxygen and perform functions just as other organs do.

The skeleton is divided into two sections. The spinal column, skull, and rib cage make up the **axial** skeleton. The bones of the arms, hands, legs, feet, shoulders, and pelvis make up the **appendicular** skeleton, Figure 4–47.

The primary purpose of the skeletal system is to support the body. This support must be strong yet not heavy. Bone is said to be as strong as cast iron, yet it is much lighter and more flexible. The skeleton must be flexible enough to endure pressure, stress, and shock without shattering.

Bone Structure ....

Over 20% of the weight of bone is water. Two-thirds of the remainder are minerals and one-third, organic matter. The main minerals are calcium, phosphorus, and magnesium. The organic matter is primarily collagen, a type of protein fiber that forms the matrix (intercellular substance) of the bone.

The ends of long bones have articulating (connecting) surfaces that fit together with other bones to form joints, Figure 4–48, page 120. These ends are separated by cartilage to facilitate movement. The ends and parts of the shaft are filled with a meshlike network of spongy bone. The openings in the spongy bone are filled with red **marrow.** The inside of the shaft of the bone is filled with a fat or yellow marrow.

A tough membrane called **periosteum** covers the surface of the bone. Blood vessels and nerves pass through the periosteum and into the bone through a network of openings called Haversian canals. Some larger vessels pass directly into both the yellow and red marrow.

Number of Bones ....

At birth, a baby has 270 bones. As the child grows, some of the bones fuse together so that at adulthood there are only 206. For example, at the lower end of the spinal column five **vertebrae** have fused to form the **sacrum** and the last four have fused into the **coccyx** (tailbone), Figure 4–49, page 121. The smallest bones in the body are the malleus, incus, and stapes of the middle ear.

Functions of the Skeleton ....

The skeleton serves at least six functions for the body. One, as previously indicated, is to support the body. The bones provide a framework for the distribution of the body's fat, muscles, and skin.

Two, the bones also serve to protect the body's vital organs. The brain and spinal cord are both located within bony cavities. The cranium also provides protection for the inner ear and parts of the eye. The heart and lungs are positioned within the rib cage. The internal reproductive organs and the urinary bladder lie within the bony pelvis.

Third, the bones are the points of attachment for skeletal muscles. When the muscles contract, they allow the joints of the skeleton to rotate, bend, or straighten, thereby providing for movement and flexibility. Fourth, the bones, along with the muscles, give shape to the body.

A fifth and vital function of bone is the formation of red blood cells. The red marrow in the spongy areas of the long bones, the ribs, and the vertebrae produces millions of red blood cells a minute. This rate is necessary to replace the cells, which live only a few weeks. When the body needs

FIGURE 4–47 Bones of the skeleton (Axial in gray, appendicular in red) (From Fong, *Body Structures and Functions,* 8th ed. Copyright 1993, Delmar Publishers Inc.)

more red cells than the red marrow can produce, some of the yellow marrow is converted to red.

Finally, bones store most of the body's supply of calcium. Calcium is needed by the heart to beat, by the muscles to contract, and by the blood to clot. When the calcium in the body is inadequate for all its needs, the blood takes calcium from its storage in the bone. The bone minerals are constantly being borrowed and replaced through the blood flow within the body.

Spinal Column

The spinal column is a stack of vertebrae that supports the head and keeps the trunk erect. As noted earlier, it provides protection for the spinal cord, which descends from the brain through its canal. The bones of the column are separated by

intervertebral cartilage disks between their rounded front portions, Figure 4–50. The disks permit the column to bend or twist and also absorb much of the shock received from walking, running, or jumping. The vertebrae in the column are named for the area of the body in which they are located: **cervical** (neck), thoracic (chest), lumbar (back), sacral (posterior pelvic girdle), and coccygeal (tailbone), Figure 4–51, page 122.

The spinal nerves enter and leave the spinal cord through foramen (openings) between the vertebrae. The disks maintain adequate spacing between vertebrae to prevent damage to the spinal nerves from bone-to-bone contact.

Typical vertebrae as shown in Figure 4–50 have descriptive parts, mainly the large solid part called the *body,* the winglike side projections called the *transverse processes,* a posterior projection called a *spinous process* (the part you can feel if

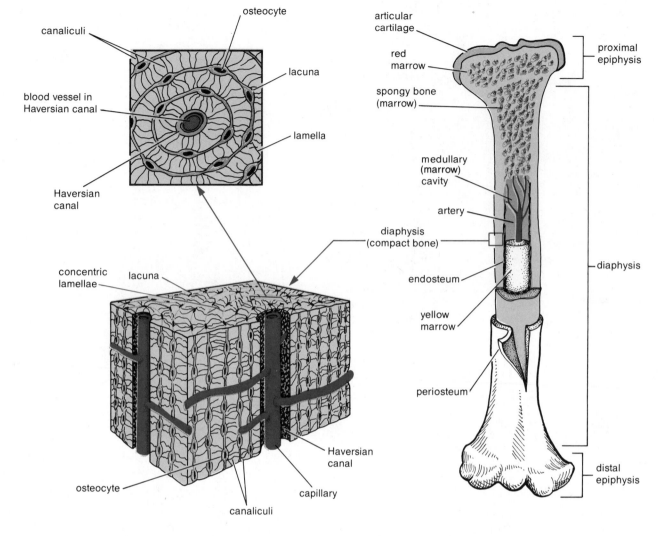

FIGURE 4–48 A typical long bone (From Fong, *Body Structures and Functions*, 8th ed. Copyright 1993, Delmar Publishers, Inc.)

you arch your back) and the *foramen* through which the spinal cord passes. Other processes called *articular* are where parts of two vertebrae touch.

The Skull

The skull is the bony structure of the head. It consists of a cranial and a facial portion. The **cranium** is actually a fusion of eight cranial bones, with the vital function of protecting the brain from injury, Figure 4–52, page 123. The main bones of the cranium are: the frontal (the forehead and upper eye sockets), two parietal bones, two temporal, and the occipital (back of the skull). The facial bones are: the mandible (lower jaw), the maxillae (upper jaw), the zygomatic (cheek bones), and the several small bones about the eyes, nose, and palate.

The cranium is not solid bone at birth. Spaces between the bones are soft incomplete bone to allow for the molding of the skull during the birth process and for enlargement of the skull as growth occurs. A large diamond-shaped anterior area where the frontal and parietal bones meet and a triangular space posteriorly where the occipital bone meets the parietals are known

as *fontanels* or "soft spots," and can easily be felt. Other smaller fontanels are located along the sides of the skull. Without these areas for growth, the brain could not increase in size during late pregnancy and early infancy. The fontanels gradually close, turning the membrane and cartilage into solid bone after about 2 years. The irregular lines marking the former growth areas are called *sutures.*

The skull does not grow remarkably when compared with the rest of the body. It makes up about one-fourth of the total length of the infant's body but only one-eighth of the adult's total length.

The Rib Cage

Thoracic vertebrae serve as the posterior attachment points for 12 pairs of ribs, Figure 4–53, page 123. The top 10 pairs are also attached by cartilage strips to the **sternum** (breast bone) anteriorly. The flexibility of the cartilage attachment allows the rib cage to move when the lungs are inflated to breathe. The bottom two pairs of ribs are called floating ribs because they are attached only to the spinal column and not the sternum.

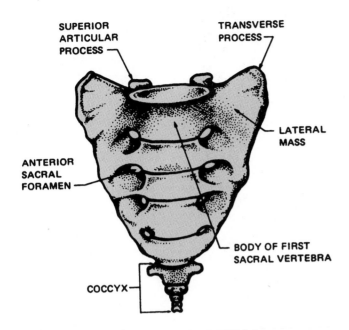

FIGURE 4–49 The sacrum and coccyx (From *The Wonderful Human Machine,* Copyright 1979, American Medical Association.)

Labels in figure: SUPERIOR ARTICULAR PROCESS, TRANSVERSE PROCESS, LATERAL MASS, ANTERIOR SACRAL FORAMEN, BODY OF FIRST SACRAL VERTEBRA, COCCYX

Long Bones

The long bones of the body are found in the extremities. To a great extent, the long bones of the lower extremities determine our height. Long bones are shaped generally like hollow cylinders to be strong with the least amount of weight. A typical long bone has a main shaft, or diaphysis, and ends called **epiphyses.** Early in life the epiphysis is mainly **cartilage.** Later the cartilage becomes a strip or "growth plate" which permits new tissue growth and bone length. At maturity, growth stops and the cartilage is replaced by bone.

The **femur** (thigh bone) is the longest bone in any species, extending from the hip joint to the knee. (Refer to Figure 4–47, page 119.) The thickness of the femur wall depends on the size and needs of the species. For example, large animals, such as the bear, have a thick, heavy femur to support their weight and accommodate slow movements, whereas the deer has a very thin and light femur to permit speed. The **tibia** (shin bone) and **fibula** complete the long bones of the leg. The small bone at the knee is known as the **patella.**

The long bones of the upper extremities are the **humerus** of the arm and the **radius** and **ulna** of the forearm. The radius extends from the thumb side of the wrist to the elbow, and the ulna extends from the little finger side to the elbow joint.

The rib cage is sometimes described in terms of true and false ribs. When this division is made, the first seven pairs of ribs are considered "true" ribs because of their posterior and direct anterior attachment. The last five pairs are "false" ribs because they attach anteriorly to the cartilage of the rib above or have no anterior attachment.

Three other bones of the thoracic area should be mentioned. They are the **clavicle** (collar bone) anteriorly and the **scapula** (shoulder blade) posteriorly. A small bony process called the **xiphoid** is attached to the inferior edge of the sternum.

Bones of the Hands and Feet

The bones of the hands and feet are similar in structure, Figure 4–54, page 124. The wrist has eight bones, known as **carpals** and the ankle has seven, called **tarsals.** In the palm area of the hand there are five **metacarpals** that correspond to the five **metatarsals** of the instep of the foot. The **phalanges** (fingers and toes) are further subdivided into individual sections called a **phalanx.** There are three phalanx sections in each finger and toe except the thumb and great toe, which have only two. The sec-

A typical vertebra

Labels in figure: articular process, vertebral arch, spinous process, body, transverse process, lamina, intervertebral disc, foramen, lamina, transverse process, pedicle, foramen (space for spinal cord), spinous process, pedicle, body, articular process, spinal cord in vertebral canal

FIGURE 4–50 Vertebrae structure (From Fong, *Body Structures and Functions,* 8th ed. Copyright 1993, Delmar Publishers Inc.)

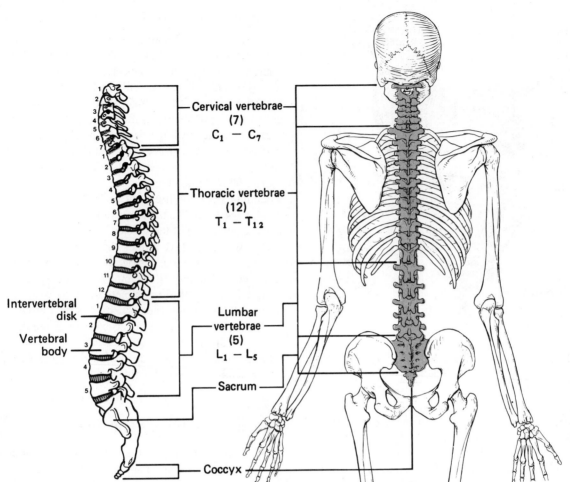

FIGURE 4–51 The spinal column (From Kinn, *Medical Terminology, Building Blocks for Health Careers,*.Copyright 1990, Delmar Publishers Inc.)

tion of a phalanx is identified as distal, medial, or proximal by its relationship to the metacarpals or metatarsals.

The Pelvic Girdle

The pelvic girdle provides the structure for the hip area. Two large bones called *os coxae* (hip bones) are joined posteriorly with the sacrum. The top blade-shaped portion is called the **ilium,** Figure 4–55, page125. The anterior lower portion is called the pubis, with the point of attachment (right and left pubis) called the **symphysis pubis.** The posterior lower portion of the bone is called the **ischium.** The hip bone provides the recessed area where the head of the femur fits. The anatomical name for the socket is *acetabulum.*

Joints

The place where two or more bony parts join together is known as an **articulation** or joint. Strong, flexible bands of connective tissue called **ligaments** hold long bones together at joints. Ligaments can stretch and often become torn as a result of injury.

There are three main types of joints, classified primarily by their degree of movement. A movable joint such as the knee or elbow, is called **diarthrosis,** or **synovial** joint. A partially movable joint such as where ribs attach to the spine or between the vertebrae, is known as *amphiarthrosis,* or *cartilaginous.* An immovable joint such as a cranial suture, is called *synarthrosis,* or *fibrous.*

Most of the body's joints are diarthrotic. They may have three distinct parts, articular cartilage, a **bursa** (saclike capsule), and a synovial cavity. The articulating joint surfaces of bones are covered with the articular cartilage, which provides a slippery, smooth surface and enables the joint to absorb shock. An articular capsule of tough, fibrous tissue encloses the articulating surfaces and is lined with a synovial membrane, which secretes synovial fluid into the cavity, lubricating the joint and reducing friction.

The joint is surrounded with ligaments, tendons, and muscles that hold the joint together but still allow for movement. Some synovial joints have cushionlike sacs called bursa, which form from the synovial membrane and are filled with synovial fluid. These are generally located between tendons and bones. In addition, synovial membranes may also form sheaths that wrap around the tendons. Bursa and tendon sheaths cushion and lubricate tendons and help reduce friction between the tendons and the bone.

The synovial joints of the body have been copied by human engineering to develop many useful devices, Figure 4–56,

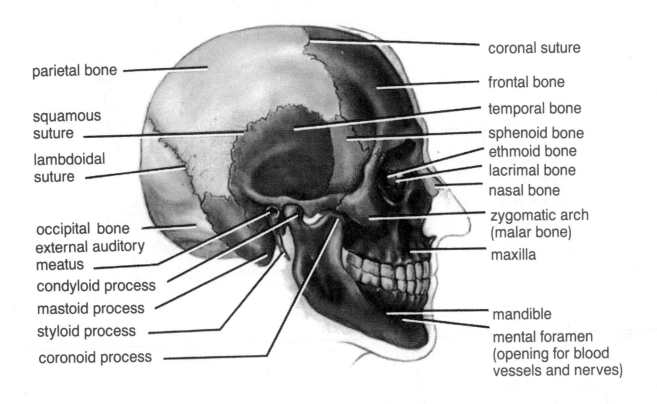

parietal bone

squamous suture

lambdoidal suture

occipital bone
external auditory meatus

condyloid process

mastoid process

styloid process

coronoid process

coronal suture

frontal bone

temporal bone

sphenoid bone

ethmoid bone

lacrimal bone

nasal bone

zygomatic arch (malar bone)

maxilla

mandible

mental foramen (opening for blood vessels and nerves)

FIGURE 4–52 The skull (From Smith, *Medical Terminology, A Programmed Text*, 6th ed. Copyright 1991, Delmar Publishers.)

VERTEBRAE IN THE BACK

CLAVICLE (COLLAR BONE)

MANUBRIUM

RIBS (COSTALS)

TRUE RIBS

STERNUM (BREAST BONE)

COSTAL CARTILAGE

XIPHOID PROCESS

FLOATING RIBS

FALSE RIBS

SPINAL COLUMN

© *Richardson 1983*

FIGURE 4–53 The rib cage (Copyright by Richardson. From Fong, *Body Structures and Functions*, 8th ed. Copyright 1993, Delmar Publishers Inc. Used with permission.)

FIGURE 4–54 Bones of the hand and foot (Copyright by Johnson. From Fong, Ferris, & Skelley, *Body Structures and Functions*, 8th ed. Copyright 1993, Delmar Publishers Inc. Used with permission.)

page 126. The ball and socket type of joint found in the hip or shoulder can be seen in the movement of a desk pen set. The action of the fingers, knees, and elbows is like that of a hinge. An unusual pivot type of joint appears at the wrists and elbows. When the palm of the hand is up, the radius and ulna are side by side. As the palm is turned down, the radius crosses over the ulna in a pivoting action. This type of motion is independent of the elbow's hinge action. Joints found in the wrists and ankle are formed by bones with curved surfaces, which allow for various angular movements.

Fractures

The bones of children contain a high percentage of cartilage and are much more flexible than those of an adult. Frequently the bone will crack under pressure but will not break all the way through. This type of fracture is called a **greenstick**, Figure 4–57(a).

A complete bone break in which there is no involvement with the skin surface is known as a **simple** fracture, Figure 4–57(b). When broken bone protrudes through the skin's surface, it is known as a **compound** fracture, Figure 4–57(c). This causes additional concerns because of the possibility of infection to the area. A more involved type of fracture is called **impacted,** Figure 4–57(d), which indicates that the broken ends are jammed into each other. A **comminuted,** Figure 4–57(e) fracture is one with more than one fracture line and several bone fragments. A **spiral,** Figure 4–57(f) fracture may occur with a severe twisting action as in a skiing accident, causing the break to wind around the bone. A **depressed,** Figure 4–57(g) fracture may occur with severe head injuries in which a broken piece of skull is driven inward. The Colles fracture, Figure 4–57(h), involves the distal end of the radius and results in its dislocation, causing a characteristic bulge at the wrist. Often the ulna is also fractured, resulting in a greater wrist deformity. It is a common fracture of children from falls while skating, riding bikes, and climbing. It is generally caused by falling on an outstretched hand.

In treating fractures, immobilization of the affected part and prevention of shock are the main concerns. The extremity is splinted, extending above and below the area of fracture. Elevation of the part and application of a cold pack or ice helps prevent swelling. When there is also damage to the surrounding tissues, especially to the exterior, control of bleeding may be indicated. This may require direct pressure over the wound.

When long bones are broken, they are usually pulled by the muscles attached to their surfaces into abnormal positions, often causing overlapping of their broken parts. Before the bone can be set, **traction** (pulling) either manually or by a system of ropes and pulleys, must be used to stretch the muscles and pull the bone pieces back into **alignment.** This procedure is known as **reducing** the fracture. Once the ends fit together properly, a splint or cast can be used to maintain the position until the bone has healed.

With involved fractures, such as compound or comminuted, an additional surgical procedure is often necessary either to repair the skin and surrounding tissues or to place all the small bone fragments in position. This procedure is called an *open reduction* because it involves an opening into the fractured bone through the skin and overlying tissues, to achieve alignment of the bone. Sometimes the use of pins or wire is required to hold the fragments together.

Bone Healing Process　When a fracture occurs, healing begins with a sticky material, which is secreted by the blood. This material forms a bulgy deposit called a **callus** around the break, which holds the ends together, Figure 4–58, page 128.

ACETABULUM
SYMPHYSIS PUBIS
OBTURATOR FORAMEN
ISCHIUM

NARROWER ANGLE
IN MALE

WIDER ANGLE
IN FEMALE

ILIUM
SACRUM
COCCYX
SYMPHYSIS PUBIS

FALSE PELVIS

FALSE PELVIS

INLET OF TRUE PELVIS

MALE

FEMALE

FIGURE 4–55   The pelvic girdle (Copyright by Johnson. From Fong, Ferris, & Skelley, *Body Structures and Functions*, 8th ed. Copyright 1993, Delmar Publishers Inc. Used with permission.)

As time passes, the callus turns first to cartilage and then to bone. Certain bone cells build the new bone tissue while others remove the cartilage and then slowly smooth the repaired section back to approximately its original size.

A complication which may occur after a fracture of long bones is a fat **embolus.** An embolus is a mass of foreign material circulating within the blood vessels. This potentially fatal complication may follow the release of fat droplets from the marrow of the long bones. The trauma of the event can also cause the body to release catecholamines, which in turn activate fatty acids. The fatty acids can develop into a fatty embolus and circulate in the blood, becoming lodged in the lungs or even the brain. If the embolus causes an *infarction* (blocked blood vessel) of a large enough vessel, death can occur.

Usual symptoms and signs include apprehension, sweating, fever, rapid heart rate, pallor, difficulty breathing, bluish discoloration of the skin, convulsions, and coma. If the complication occurs, it is usually within 24 to 48 hours, but may occur as late as 3 days after the fracture.

Amputation

Severe trauma, a malignant tumor, lack of circulation, or complications of other conditions, such as diabetes, may result in the need to **amputate** an extremity. The change in the patient's body image and function causes emotional as well as physical difficulties in coping with daily activities. Following

amputation a condition often occurs known as the **phantom limb** sensation: the feeling that the missing extremity is still present. It is often described as an itching or tingling sensation. This may last for quite some time but will usually subside eventually. It is considered normal to experience the sensation.

When the amputated stump has healed sufficiently, a **prosthesis** (artificial part) may be fitted. Lower limbs are either attached directly to the remaining extremity, fastened by means of straps or belt to the waist, or hung from the shoulder. The method depends to a great extent on the amount of the remaining extremity. Upper limbs may be replaced by a "hook" device that can be opened and closed to grasp objects. A prosthesis that closely resembles a real arm and hand is often desired, even though it lacks the flexibility of the "hook."

Diagnostic Examinations

- Arthroscopy—This endoscopic procedure permits direct visual inspection of a joint, most often the knee. It is frequently used to evaluate injuries suffered by athletes. Arthroscopy is useful in detecting **arthritis,** torn meniscus, cysts, or loose pieces of tissue. Some surgical procedures can be performed through the scope to repair damaged joint structures, thereby eliminating open surgery.
- X ray—A frequently used test that evaluates the condition of bones in such cases as dislocations, sprains, and fractures. X

FIGURE 4–56 Types of joints (Adapted from *The Wonderful Human Machine*. Copyright 1979, American Medical Association.)

ray can also be used to determine bone structure changes like those occurring in some metabolic conditions, such as acromegaly (giantism), **osteoporosis,** or with Paget's disease.

Diseases and Disorders ....

Arthritis, Osteoarthritis. This common form of arthritis causes progressive deterioration of joint cartilage, most often at the hips and knees. It is accompanied by joint pain, stiffness, aching (particularly with weather changes), "grating" during joint motion, and fluid around the joint.

Osteoarthritis is best treated with aspirin, nonsteroidal anti-inflammatories, intraarticular joint injections of steroids, and reducing pressure on joints through the use of a cane, crutches, a cervical collar, and so forth. Occasionally, disability and uncontrollable pain will require surgical intervention. This can range from scraping deteriorated bone fragments from the joint to replacing joint bone parts with prosthetic appliances (artificial joints).

Arthritis, Rheumatoid. A chronic inflammatory disease attacking joints and surrounding tissues, this is an intermittent disease with periods of remission. It is three times more common in females than males, most often striking between the ages of 35 and 45. The cause of the condition is not thoroughly understood. The disease attacks the joint synovial membrane, causing edema and congestion. Tissue layers become granulated and thicken, eventually involving the cartilage and destroying the joint capsule and bone. Scar tissue formation, bone atrophy, and malalignment cause visible deformities, pain, and often immobility.

Bursitis. This is a painful inflammation of the bursa. A bursa is a sac located around a joint and containing lubricating fluids that allow muscles and tendons to move freely over bony surfaces. Bursitis occurs most frequently at the hip, shoulder, or knee. It is usually associated with middle age and results from recurring trauma or stresses on a joint or from inflammatory arthritis.

Treatment consists of joint rest, often immobilization, a pain medication, and joint injection with a steroid combined with an anesthetic. It may be necessary to remove joint fluid by aspiration (withdrawal through a needle) and institute a program of physical therapy to preserve joint motion.

Carpal Tunnel Syndrome. This condition results from the compression of the median nerve at the wrist. The carpal tunnel is a passageway for nerves, blood vessels, and flexor tendons to the fingers and thumb. It is formed by the carpal bones and the transverse ligament. The tendon sheaths become inflamed, causing swelling, which presses the median nerve against the transverse ligament, resulting in pain, tingling, numbness, and weakness of the hand. It involves only the thumb and index and middle finger. The patient will be unable to make a fist.

The condition occurs most frequently among women between the ages of 30 and 60 and is usually occupationally related. Persons most likely to develop the syndrome are those who use their hands strenuously in grasping, twisting, or turning actions, such as assembly line workers and packers. Other systemic conditions that cause the carpal tunnel to swell are diabetes mellitus, pregnancy, menopause, hypothyroidism, benign tumors, and others.

Diagnosis can be made on examination that reveals decreased sensitivity of the first two fingers and the thumb on pricking with a pin, X rays showing bony abnormalities, and an electromyogram showing delayed motor nerve conduction. Patients may also have an *atrophy* (shrinking) of the muscle on the palm side of the thumb due to decreased innervation.

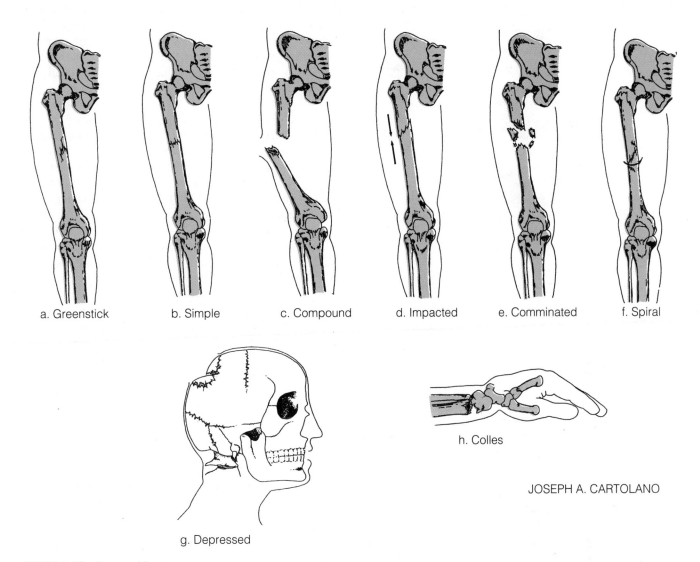

a. Greenstick   b. Simple   c. Compound   d. Impacted   e. Comminated   f. Spiral

g. Depressed

h. Colles

JOSEPH A. CARTOLANO

FIGURE 4–57 Types of fractures

If the syndrome is of short duration, treatment will consist of immobilizing the hand and forearm in a splint, local injections of corticosteroids, and systemic anti-inflammatory medication. It may be necessary to seek new employment if a work-related connection is determined. If conservative treatment does not correct the problem, a surgical procedure may be indicated to section the transverse ligament and "freeup" the nerve. Usually conservative treatment is not successful and only surgery will relieve the symptoms.

Congenital Hip Dysplagia.   This abnormality of the hip joint is present at birth. It is the most common hip disorder of children, affecting one or both joints. It is present in three forms: unstable, with the hip in place but easily dislocated by manipulation; incomplete dislocation, with the head of the femur on the edge of the acetabulum; and complete dislocation, with the head totally outside the hip socket. Signs of hip dysplagia include the appearance of one leg being shorter than the other or one hip being more prominent. If both hips are involved the child has a characteristic "duck waddle" or, if one hip only, a

limp. Early treatment is essential to normal development. In infants, a splint device is used for 3 to 4 months to maintain proper positioning. Older babies may be placed in traction, or the hips may be reduced and a cast applied for a period of 4 to 6 months.

Dislocation.   Displacement of bones at a joint so that the regular meeting surfaces are no longer in contact is a **dislocation.** This occurs most frequently at joints of the fingers, shoulder, knee, and hip. Prompt reduction (relocation) is essential to limit damage to surrounding tissues. It is extremely painful and is often accompanied by joint surface fractures. Following reduction, a splint, cast, or traction (depending on the joint involved) to immobilize the area is indicated. From 2 to 8 weeks will be needed to allow surrounding ligaments to heal completely.

Epicondylitis (Tennis Elbow).   This is an inflammation of the forearm extensor tendon at its attachment to the humerus. It probably begins as a tear and is common among people who grasp things forcefully or twist the forearm. Pain occurs at the

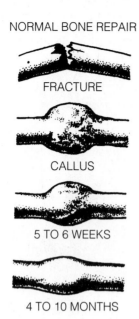

NORMAL BONE REPAIR

FRACTURE

CALLUS

5 TO 6 WEEKS

4 TO 10 MONTHS

FIGURE 4–58 Normal bone repair (From *The Wonderful Human Machine*. Copyright 1979, American Medical Association.

elbow and becomes intense. There is tenderness over the area where the radius articulates with the humerus.

The condition is best treated with an injection of a steroid and a local anesthetic, aspirin, an immobilizing splint, heat, and physical therapy. If the disorder is not treated, it may result in a disability.

Gout (Gouty Arthritis).   This metabolic disease results in severe joint pain, especially at night. It most often affects the great toe but can involve other joints. The pain results from deposits of urates (uric acid salts), which are overproduced or retained by the body. Often gout is associated with another disease, such as leukemia, due to cell destruction by chemotherapy. Gout may also follow drug therapy that interferes with urate excretion. Gout can be a progressive disease, initially causing severe pain and a hot, tender, inflamed joint. This attack will be followed by a symptom-free period of approximately 6 months to 2 years, when a second episode will occur. Additional attacks usually involve other joints of the feet and legs. Eventually the condition becomes chronic (ongoing), involving many joints that are persistently painful and become degenerated, deformed, and disabling.

Gout is best treated with medication to suppress uric acid formation and promote excretion of the urates. Dietary restrictions must be followed, such as avoiding alcohol, primarily beer and wine, and purine-rich foods such as liver, sardines, kidneys, and lentils.

Hallux Valgus.   This is a lateral deviation of the great toe with enlargement of the first metatarsal head and a **bunion** formation. A bunion is a bursa with a callus formation. The bursa becomes inflamed, filled with fluid, and tender. The overlying skin will be red. It is common in women, most often caused by prolonged pressure on the foot from narrow, high-heeled shoes. The condition can also result from degenerative arthritis. Hallux valgus will cause bone deformity, and the change will alter the person's weight-bearing pattern. Early treatment with proper shoes, and the use of padding and straightening devices as well as exercises, may correct the situation. A severe deformity and disabling pain will require surgical removal of the bunion.

Herniated Disk (Ruptured Disk).   In this situation, the soft gellike material within an intervertebral disk has been forced through its outer surface. The extruded material may cause pressure on a spinal nerve exiting the spinal cord or may impinge on the spinal cord itself. A herniated disk may result from severe trauma or strain, but it is frequently related to degeneration of the intervertebral joints. It occurs most often in the lumbar or lumbosacral regions. Herniated disks usually occur in adults, mainly men, under age 45. In elderly people with disk degeneration, herniation can occur from a minor trauma. The classic symptom is severe lower back pain, frequently radiating deep into the buttocks and down the back of the leg. It is usually unilateral (one sided). Sensory loss results from nerve compression, and the patient experiences numbness, muscle spasm, motor difficulty, and eventually weakness and atrophy of the leg muscles.

Conservative treatment consists of prolonged bed rest, often with pelvic traction, heat applications, and specific exercises. A **laminectomy** is indicated if there is neurological involvement that does not improve with conservative therapy. This procedure involves removing a portion of the lamina (flattened portion of the vertebral arch) to remove the protruding disk material. A new type of treatment, chemonucleolysis, which involves injecting an enzyme into the disk to dissolve the tissue, is being tried as an alternative to laminectomy surgery.

If pain still persists, a surgical procedure, **spinal fusion,** is performed to stabilize the adjoining vertebrae. This is accomplished by vertically "notching" the spinous process of the two or three involved vertebrae and placing a long sliver of bone taken from the ilium into the notches. When the bone heals, the joined vertebrae can no longer move independently to impinge on the nerve or spinal cord.

Kyphosis (Roundback, Humpback).   This is a bowing of the back, usually at the thoracic level, due to improper vertebral alignment, Figure 4–59(a). In children and adolescents **kyphosis** is caused by growth retardation or a disturbance in epiphysis development during rapid growth periods. It occurs often in youths engaged in excessive sports activities. Adult kyphosis may result from aging and the degeneration of intervertebral disks or the collapse of vertebrae due to osteoporosis.

Kyphosis as a result of poor posture during childhood can be treated by therapeutic exercise, a firm mattress, and a Milwaukee brace to straighten the spine until spinal growth is complete. If neurological damage or disabling pain occurs in adolescents and adults (which happens rarely) a surgical procedure may be indicated, which involves posterior spinal fusion, bone grafting, and casting to straighten the severe curvature. With full skeletal maturity and debilitating curvature, a posterior spinal fusion can be accomplished with the use of a stainless steel Harrington rod mechanism to align the vertebrae.

Lordosis. This abnormal anterior convex curvature of the lumbar spine is commonly referred to as swayback, Figure 4–59(b). The body's spine normally curves in at this point; however, an exaggerated curvature is considered to be **lordosis.** This condition can be improved, or at least prevented from progressing, by appropriate exercises, improving posture and having proper footwear.

Lumbar Myositis. This inflammation of the lumbar region muscles of the back causes low back pain. It is common and is due primarily to a straining of the back muscles. The condition is best treated with rest, mild analgesics, and muscle relaxers. When improved, a program of stretching exercises is prescribed to condition and strengthen the muscles.

Osteoporosis. **Osteoporosis** is a metabolic bone disorder, characterized by acceleration of the rate of bone resorption while the rate of bone formation slows down, which causes a loss of bone mass. The loss of calcium and phosphate from the bone allows it to become porous, brittle, and prone to fracture. The cause of primary osteoporosis may be a combination of prolonged inadequate dietary intake of calcium, faulty metabolism due to estrogen deficiency, or a sedentary life style. This type is also known as senile, or postmenopausal, osteoporosis because it affects primarily elderly, postmenopausal women. Recent statistics show the condition may affect 25 million older Americans. Secondary osteoporosis can occur following

prolonged steroid therapy, bone immobilization or lack of use (with paralysis), malnutrition, alcoholism, scurvy, and hyperthyroidism. It is usually discovered following injury from bending to lift something. The individual hears a snapping sound and then feels instant pain in the lower back. The sound and pain are from the collapse of a vertebra. Other common signs are slowly developing kyphosis, loss of height, fractures of the forearm or hip from minor falls, and spontaneous vertebral fractures. The condition is treatable to prevent additional fracturing by increasing exercise, giving an estrogen supplement, and taking calcium and vitamin D to support normal bone metabolism.

Recently, scientists in Philadelphia, using new biotechnology equipment, believe they have discovered the cause of postmenopausal osteoporosis. They have linked the condition to a defect on chromosome 7, leading them to think that it may be possible to develop a test that will predict who will develop osteoporosis so that preventive measures may be taken long before the symptoms would become evident.

Scoliosis. A lateral curvature of the spine (usually in the thoracic region), known as **scoliosis,** results from rotation of the spinal column. It may also be lumbar or involve both, Figure 4–59(c). The thorax usually curves to the right while the lumbar curves left. Because the body has to maintain balance, the cervical spine will also curve left, which gives the spine an "S" curve appearance.

There are two forms of scoliosis: functional, caused by poor posture or uneven leg lengths, and structural, resulting from vertebral body deformities. Structural scoliosis can be caused

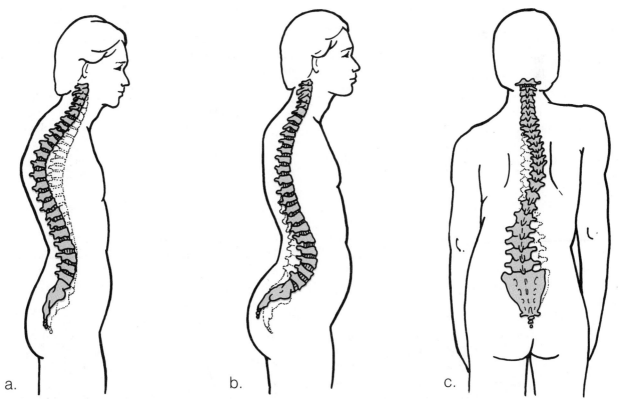

FIGURE 4–59 Abnormal curvatures of the spine. (a) Kyphosis (b) Lordosis (c) Scoliosis (Adapted from Fong, *Body Structures and Functions*, 8th ed. Copyright 1993, Delmar Publishers Inc.)

by congenital defects of the vertebrae, muscular dystrophy or paralysis, or a transmitted trait that develops during the growth process. An infantile type of transmitted scoliosis occurs primarily in boys from birth to age 3 and causes left thorax and right lumbar curves. Another type known as juvenile scoliosis affects both sexes between the ages of 4 and 10. The third type, called adolescent, affects primarily girls between 10 and maturity of the skeleton, and results in varying types of curvatures. Adolescent scoliosis can be easily diagnosed. Classic symptoms are apparently uneven hemlines or unequal pants legs, one hip appearing to be higher than the other, and one shoulder appearing higher and perhaps the scapula more pronounced.

Treatment includes observation, exercises, and a brace. With curvature beyond 60 degrees, an immobilizing cast or preoperative traction system is followed by surgical correction using posterior spinal fusion and a Harrington rod for stabilization. Note the following parent teaching aid for detecting scoliosis.

How to Detect Scoliosis

Parents:
To check your child for scoliosis (abnormal curvature of the spine) perform this simple test. First, have your child remove his or her shirt and stand up straight. As you look at the child's back, answer these questions:

- Is one shoulder higher than the other, or is one shoulder blade more prominent?

- When the child's arms hang loosely at his or her sides, does one arm swing away from the body more than the other?

- Is one hip higher or more prominent than the other?

- Does the child seem to tilt to one side?

Ask your child to bend forward, with arms hanging down and palms together at knee level. Can you see a hump on the back at the ribs or near the waist?

If your answer to any of these questions is "yes," your child needs careful evaluation for scoliosis. Notify your doctor.

Sprain.   This complete or incomplete tear in the supporting ligaments of a joint follows a severe twisting action. **Sprains** are characterized by pain, swelling, and a black-and-blue discoloration. The ankle is the most common site. Care of sprains should follow the easy to remember R.I.C.E. method—Rest, Ice, Compression, and Elevation. Treatment consists of (1) controlling pain and swelling by elevating the joint and applying ice intermittently for the first 12 to 24 hours, (2) immobilization using an elastic wrap or, if very severe, a soft cast, and (3) the use of crutches to eliminate stress on the joint. If healing does not occur normally in 3 to 4 weeks, the torn ligaments may require surgical repair, especially if sprains reoccur.

Subluxation.   This partial or incomplete dislocation of the articulating surfaces of joint bones usually results from injury or a disease process. If it results from injury, it can be painful and involve the surrounding nerves, blood vessels, ligaments, and soft tissues. Symptoms include joint deformity, impaired motion, pain, and change in length if an extremity is involved. Common sites are shoulders, elbows, wrists, knees, fingers and toes, hips, and ankles. Diagnostic X ray is usually indicated to rule out or confirm accompanying joint fracture.

Treatment consists of reduction as soon as possible to minimize swelling and muscle spasms, which make reduction difficult. Depending on the joint involved, medication is used to control muscle spasm and pain and possibly a splint or cast is used to immobilize and support the joint while ligaments heal.

Complete Chapter 4, Unit 5 in the workbook to help you meet the objectives at the beginning of this unit and therefore achieve competency of this subject matter.

U N I T   6
The Muscular System

OBJECTIVES ···

Upon completion of this unit, you will meet the following terminal performance objectives by verifying knowledge of the facts and principles presented through oral and written communication at a level deemed competent by the instructor or employer.

1. Explain how muscular activity increases body heat.
2. List six functions of skeletal muscles.
3. Name and describe the three types of muscular tissue and the purpose of each.
4. Describe the purpose of a muscle team and give an example.
5. Explain what muscle tone means.
6. Describe the structure and function of a tendon and identify the body's strongest tendon.
7. Explain the terms origin and insertion.
8. Describe a muscle sheath and a bursa and the purpose of each.
9. Identify the muscles of respiration and describe how their function results in breathing.
10. Name the major skeletal muscles of the body.
11. Describe the smooth muscle action of peristalsis.
12. Explain the structure and function of a sphincter.
13. Describe four disorders or diseases of the muscular system.
14. Spell and define, using the glossary at the back of the text, all the words to know in this unit.

abduction

Achilles tendon

adduction

anchor

aponeurosis

atrophy

biceps

contracture

cramp

deltoid

dystrophy

extensor

fascia

flexor

gastrocnemius

gluteus maximus

hamstring

insertion

intercostal

latissimus dorsi

muscle team

muscle tone

musculoskeletal

origin

pectoralis major

peristalsis

quadriceps femoris

sartorius

sheath

spasm

sphincter

sternocleidomastoid

strain

tendon

tendonitis

tibialis anterior

torticollis

trapezius

triceps

There are approximately 600 muscle organs in the human body. Muscles are composed of muscular tissue, which is constructed of bundles of muscle fibers about the size of a human hair. The larger the muscle, the greater the number of fibers. Muscles perform their duties by alternately contracting and relaxing. All muscle activity is directed by the nervous system. Motor neuron axons innervate several muscle cells within a muscle. Signals from the brain go through the axons and cause all the cells under their control to contract at the same time. That group of cells and its motor neuron are called a *motor unit.* When only one stimulus acts on the unit causing a contraction, it is called a *twitch.* This quick, simple contraction naturally occurs occasionally as a spontaneous event in a muscle. Scientists can study these units by using an electrical stimulus, which will also activate the motor unit. A muscle contraction is a quick progression of events following a stimulus—a very brief interval before the contraction begins, then it intensifies to a peak, and decreases to relaxation. If a second stimulus is received before the first is completed, the contraction will strengthen. When repeated stimulation occurs without a relaxation time, the muscle is maintained in a state of contraction called *tetanus* (not to be confused with the disease of the same name). This occurs when we experience muscle **cramps** and **spasms.**

At all times, motor units are alternately either contracted or relaxed; there is no other state in which they exist. The units that make up the muscles are contracted in sufficient number to meet whatever need is necessary. During sleep, for instance, only a few would be contracted at a given time, yet during strenuous activity, a great number would be called on to contract, a process known as *muscle recruitment.*

Some muscles work in partnership with the bones and can be controlled voluntarily by the motor nerves of the peripheral nervous system. Other muscles function continuously without the slightest conscious concern. The autonomic nervous system directs their activities to provide the body with essential services. It is the action of these muscles that causes us to breathe and our blood to circulate.

Muscle Fuel ....

All body tissues must have food and oxygen to survive. The muscles receive an ample supply of both because of their importance to the body's safety and well-being. The body stores carbohydrates in its muscles in the form of a starch called *glycogen.* When muscles function, they use the stored glycogen, changing it to glucose, as their source of energy. Heat is released as this fuel is used, thereby warming the body. Strenuous exercise burns a great deal of stored glycogen and therefore often results in overheating the body.

Functions of Muscle ....

In addition to providing heat and the ability to move, muscles support the structures of the body and hold the body upright. The muscles along the back, shoulders, and neck hold the trunk and head erect while permitting great flexibility in movement.

The structure of the skeletal muscles protects the blood vessels and nerves that lie throughout the body. The contraction of lower leg muscles aids in the return flow of blood to the heart by squeezing the veins of the legs. Muscles also provide protective padding to shield delicate internal organs and structures from injury.

Visually, the muscles add greatly to our appearance by giving shape to the body. Body-building enthusiasts spend years developing the degree of muscle enlargement and definition they feel is desirable. Muscle fiber, and therefore the muscle, hypertrophies (grows larger) with exercise; the number of fibers does not increase, however.

Muscle Growth ....

Muscle tissue changes slightly with age. During infancy, muscles have little connective tissue, often being attached to the bone directly. With maturity, the connective tissue increases as do the elastic fibers. Muscles grow in relation to the structures to which they are attached. Muscles of the eye, for example, grow very little, but the large muscles of the lower extremities grow considerably.

Types of Muscle Tissue ....

There are three types of muscle tissue, Figure 4–60. First, there is the *skeletal* type. Skeletal muscles are attached to

HEART

NERVE

SKELETAL MUSCLE

SMOOTH MUSCLE

STOMACH

FIGURE 4–60 Types of muscle tissue (From *The Wonderful Human Machine*. Copyright 1979, American Medical Association.)

bones and therefore permit movement. Since we have some control over movements, this type of muscle tissue is also called voluntary. Skeletal muscle cells are long and strong, some reaching lengths up to 12 inches. These cells are held together by connective tissue to form a muscle bundle. The bundles in turn are enclosed in a tougher connective tissue **sheath** to form the muscle organs, such as the **biceps** of the arm. The larger the muscle organ, the greater the number of fibers.

The second type of muscle tissue is *smooth*. Smooth muscle tissue is made of small, delicate muscle cells and is found throughout the internal organs of the body, except for the heart. Smooth muscle activity occurs continuously in such actions as breathing, moving food through the intestinal tract, changing the size of the pupil of the eye, and dilating or constricting blood vessels. These muscles function without conscious direct control, so they are also called involuntary.

The third type is *cardiac* muscle tissue. As the name implies, this type is found in the heart. These cells are joined in a continuous network without sheath separation. The membranes of adjacent cells are fused at places called *intercalated disks*. A communication system at the fused areas will not permit independent cell contraction. When one cell receives a signal to contract, all neighboring cells are stimulated and they contract together to produce the action of a heart beat. This type of muscle tissue is also involuntary, which is fortunate. It would be a full-time job to consciously contract the heart muscle 70 times a minute, 100,800 times a day.

Skeletal Muscle Action ....

When muscles contract they become shorter and thicker. A good example is the skeletal muscle of the upper arm, the biceps. When the biceps contract to bend the elbow, the shorter, and thicker muscle causes a bulge in the upper arm, Figure 4–61.

The skeletal muscle that bends a joint is called a **flexor,** whereas the action of straightening the joint is done by the **extensor** muscle. The extensor muscle that straightens the elbow is the **triceps.** The flexor and its partner, the extensor muscle, form what is known as a **muscle team** to bend and straighten joints, Figure 4–62, page 134. Muscles also contract to move extremities away from the body's center line, which is known as **abduction,** or toward the center line, which is known as **adduction,** Figure 4–63, page 134.

Muscle Tone ....

Most skeletal muscles are partially contracted at all times to maintain the body's erect position. It is believed that some fibers contract while others rest and that they then exchange places. This constant state of contraction is known as **muscle tone.** Physicians frequently refer to muscle tone when examining patients. Evaluation of muscle tone aids in determining the status of the CNS and the motor function of the peripheral nerves.

DELTOID

PECTORALIS
MAJOR

BICEPS
(EXTENDED)

TRICEPS

BICIPITAL
FASCIA

FLEXORS OF
HAND AND
WRIST

FLEXORS OF
HAND AND
WRIST

BICEPS
(CONTRACTED)

BRACHIALIS

TRICEPS

FIGURE 4–61 Action of the biceps/triceps muscle team (From *The Wonderful Human Machine*. Copyright 1979, American Medical Association.)

Loss of muscle tone can occur when muscles are not used, as with severe illness, old age, paralysis, or temporarily when an extremity has been immobilized in a cast. With prolonged lack of use muscles will **atrophy,** which is a progressive wasting away of the muscle tissue. Atrophy renders a muscle useless. Another muscular condition that develops from lack of use is called **contracture.** Here flexor muscles become shorter and permanently bend the joints. This is a common condition with paralyzed or unconscious patients. The most common sites are the fingers, elbows, knees, and hip joints.

Muscle Attachment ·····························

Skeletal muscles are attached to bone in various ways. In some instances the connective tissue within the muscle is attached directly to the bone periosteum. Some muscular connective tissue sheaths extend to form a strong fibrous structure known as a **tendon,** which is attached to rough surfaces on a bone. Tendons are extremely strong and do not stretch. A tendon 1 inch thick reportedly will support 9 tons of weight. Because of this characteristic, a bone will sometimes fracture before the tendon attached to it will separate. The thickest and strongest tendon in the human body is the **Achilles tendon,** which attaches the **gastrocnemius** muscle in the calf of the leg to the heel bone.

A similar type of connective tissue is called a ligament, but it does not perform the same function. A ligament is a flexible, fibrous tissue which supports organs and connects bone to bone at joints. Ligaments, unlike tendons, do stretch.

Another form of muscular attachment is by **fascia,** a sheet-like, tough membrane that forms sheaths to cover and protect the muscle tissue. The term **aponeurosis** designates either a fascia or a flat tendon type of muscle attachment.

Origin or Insertion   When skeletal muscles join bones that meet at joints, one of the bones becomes the **anchor** on which the muscle has its **origin.** The bone to be moved becomes the **insertion** end for the muscle. For example, the biceps has its origin at the shoulder and its insertion on the radius. When the biceps contracts, being firmly anchored at the shoulder, it pulls upon the insertion location on the forearm, and the arm flexes (bends).

The terms origin and insertion can also apply to muscle attachments other than at joints. Essentially, the end nearest the center of the body is described as the origin, and the distal end is referred to as the insertion. Usually the origin is relatively immobile, and the insertion is into a movable structure.

Sheaths and Bursae ·····························

To protect the moving parts of the muscles, muscle groups are separated from each other by membranes called *sheaths* to reduce the friction from movement. Within muscle groups, individual muscles are also separated by membranes. The tendons that extend from the muscle group are also enclosed in lubricated sheaths to protect them from damage by rubbing against other tendons, bone, or cartilage.

FIGURE 4–62 Flexor–extensor muscle team action

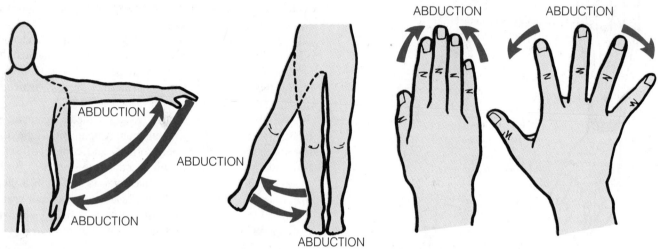

FIGURE 4–63 Abduction–adduction muscle team action

A sheath which is shaped like a sac and has a slippery fluid lining is known as a bursa. A bursa functions as a water cushion to minimize pressure and friction over bony prominences and under tendons. The most common bursae are located at the elbow, knee, and shoulder.

Major Skeletal Muscles

The muscle most important in breathing divides the chest cavity from the abdominal cavity. This muscle is called the *diaphragm,* Figure 4–64. It is a dome-shaped muscle with tendons that attach it in the back to the spinal column, in the front to the tip of the sternum, and along the sides to the cartilage edge of the ribs. When the muscle contracts, it becomes shorter and therefore flatter, creating a vacuum which causes the lungs to draw in air. When the muscle relaxes, it returns to its dome shape and forces air out of the lungs. The diaphragm also plays a role in coughing, sneezing, or laughing. Spasmodic contractions of the diaphragm, followed by spasmodic closure of the space between the vocal cords cause the common hiccough.

The orbicularis oculi and orbicularis oris are circular muscles around the eye and mouth, Figure 4–65, page 136. Their contrac-

tion enables us to squint or wink and to whistle or pucker the mouth. The **sternocleidomastoid** and the **trapezius** are the major muscles of the neck and upper back, which hold the head erect and assist with its movement, Figure 4–66, page 137. The trapezius not only supports the head but extends down the back and shoulders, giving us the ability to raise and throw back the shoulders.

The **pectoralis major** is the main upper chest muscle. It extends from the sternum to the head of the humerus, enabling us to flex the arm across the chest. The **intercostal** muscles lie beneath the pectoralis major, between the ribs. These serve as accessory muscles to the diaphragm by enlarging the thoracic cavity during inspiration.

The abdomen is covered by three main muscle layers that run in different directions to make a strong wall to protect the abdominal organs. The external oblique is first, with the internal oblique beneath, and the transversus abdominis the innermost layer. A long, narrow muscle, the rectus abdominis, extends from the pubis to the bottom of the rib cage in the center of the abdomen. It overlies and is surrounded by connective tissue layers from the other three muscles.

The back is covered by a large muscle called the **latissimus dorsi.** Its main function is to extend and adduct the arm, as

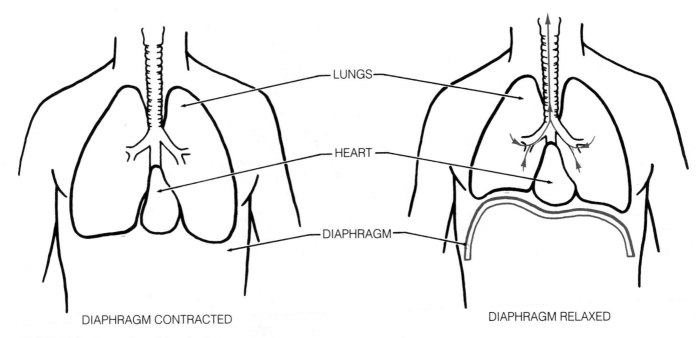

LUNGS

HEART

DIAPHRAGM

DIAPHRAGM CONTRACTED

DIAPHRAGM RELAXED

FIGURE 4–64   The action of the diaphragm muscle

when swimming. Thick vertical groups of four different muscles overlap and extend from the sacrum and lower vertebrae to the occipital bone and upper cervical vertebrae to support and move the spinal column.

The shoulders are protected by a triangle of muscle called the **deltoid,** which abducts the arm. The deltoid, if of adequate size, may be used for small injections of medication that must be given intramuscularly.

Lower Extremity Muscles
The muscles of the lower extremities involve about one-half of the body's total muscle mass. The buttocks are formed by the large **gluteus maximus** muscles, which support much of the body's weight and enable us to stand erect. The upper outer quadrant of the buttocks is the site of choice for intramuscular injections, especially for large amounts of a slowly absorbing material.

The front of the thigh has the longest muscle of the body, the **sartorius.** It anchors on the iliac spine and crosses diagonally down the front of the thigh to insert on the medial surface of the tibia. The sartorius flexes the hip and knee joints to turn the thigh outward, making it possible to sit cross-legged on the floor. The **quadriceps femoris,** with four separate parts (rectus femoris, vastus lateralis, vastus medialis, and vastus intermedius) makes up the bulk of the anterior thigh musculature. It is a powerful extensor of the knee and is used when we rise from a sitting position, kick a ball, or swim.

The **tibialis anterior** is in the front of the leg. When it is flexed, it is possible to walk on your heels with the rest of the foot off the ground. It also serves to invert the foot, turning it toward the other foot.

The posterior thigh is the site of the **hamstring** group, which includes the biceps femoris, semitendinosus, semi-

membranosus, and a portion of the adductor magnus. Their primary function is to flex the knee by pulling on the insertion at the fibula and tibia. The tendons are easily identified by palpation behind the knee. The gastrocnemius is the main muscle in the calf of the leg. Its tendon, the Achilles, has been mentioned. Contraction of the gastrocnemius permits you to stand to tiptoe since it acts as the flexor of the plantar surface (sole) of the foot.

Muscles of Expression
A number of muscles in the face enable us to show our feelings. The frontalis (forehead) can be raised to express surprise or lowered to show a stern glance. Raising one side of the obicularis oris about the upper lip will result in a sneer. The obicularis oris also allows us to whistle, kiss, smile, grin, grimace with pain, or pout.

The obicularis oculi around the eyes help complete the frown as well as enabling us to squint or wink. The large muscle of the lower jaw, the masseter, in cooperation with other smaller muscles, opens and closes the mouth to express emotions of surprise and disbelief but also is powerful and is responsible for our ability to chew and grind the food we eat.

Muscle Strain and Cramps ....

Occasionally, too much stress is applied to skeletal muscles while exercising or participating in athletic activities. This may result in a **strain,** but the muscles will recover with a period of rest. Athletes frequently "pull" their hamstring group during strenuous competition. Another frequent occurrence is a muscle cramp or spasm, caused by a muscle that has contracted but cannot relax. It can usually be treated by working the extremity or rubbing the muscle.

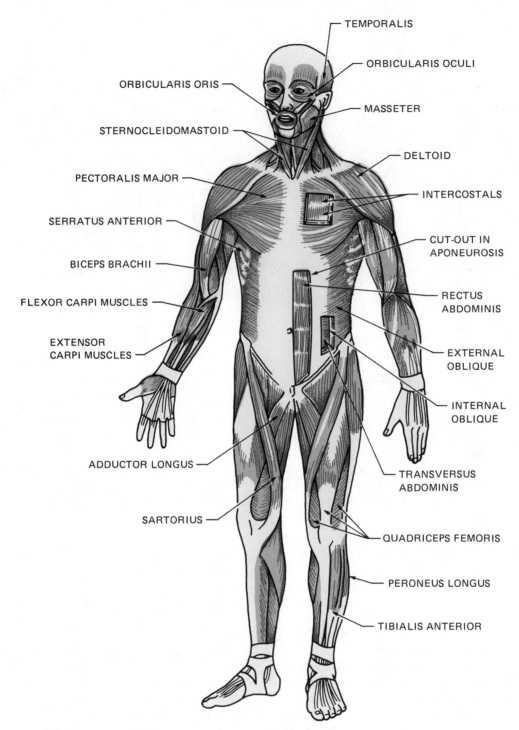

TEMPORALIS

ORBICULARIS OCULI

ORBICULARIS ORIS

MASSETER

STERNOCLEIDOMASTOID

DELTOID

PECTORALIS MAJOR

INTERCOSTALS

SERRATUS ANTERIOR

CUT-OUT IN APONEUROSIS

BICEPS BRACHII

RECTUS ABDOMINIS

FLEXOR CARPI MUSCLES

EXTENSOR CARPI MUSCLES

EXTERNAL OBLIQUE

INTERNAL OBLIQUE

ADDUCTOR LONGUS

TRANSVERSUS ABDOMINIS

SARTORIUS

QUADRICEPS FEMORIS

PERONEUS LONGUS

TIBIALIS ANTERIOR

FIGURE 4–65 Principal muscles (anterior view) (Copyright by Johnson. From Fong, Ferris, & Skelley, *Body Structures and Functions*, 8th ed. Copyright 1993, Delmar Publishers Inc. Used with permission.)

Muscle Fatigue   Prolonged strenuous exercise can result in muscle fatigue. Muscles require large amounts of oxygen to sustain the conversion of glycogen stored in the muscle into energy (adenosine triphosphate, or ATP), a function of the many mitochondria within muscle cells. Vigorous exercise is believed to cause an oxygen deficit within the muscle because the body cannot take in and circulate oxygen fast enough to keep up with the demand. When this occurs, lactic acid begins to accumulate, the glycogen is depleted, and the muscle's supply of ATP runs low. The muscle loses its ability to contract effectively and finally becomes incapable of reacting at all to the stimulus to contract. This occurs primarily in marathon runners who sometimes even collapse from muscle fatigue. Most of us simply stop our activities long before this happens.

Oxygen debt is "paid back" by the rapid and deep breathing that follows exercise. When the accumulated lactic acid is removed and the amount of oxygen restored to once again pro-

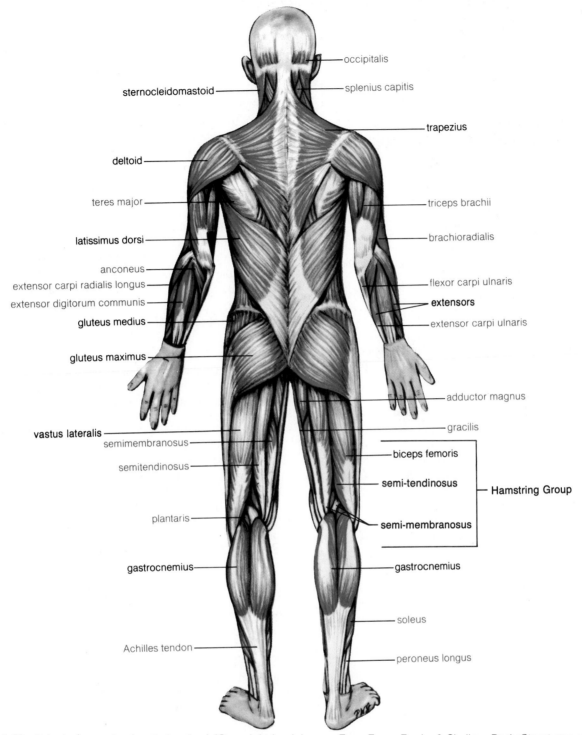

occipitalis

splenius capitis

sternocleidomastoid

trapezius

deltoid

triceps brachii

teres major

brachioradialis

latissimus dorsi

anconeus

flexor carpi ulnaris

extensor carpi radialis longus

extensors

extensor digitorum communis

extensor carpi ulnaris

gluteus medius

gluteus maximus

adductor magnus

gracilis

vastus lateralis

semimembranosus

biceps femoris

semitendinosus

semi-tendinosus ⎤

plantaris

Hamstring Group

semi-membranosus ⎦

gastrocnemius

gastrocnemius

soleus

Achilles tendon

peroneus longus

FIGURE 4–66   Principal muscles (posterior view) (Copyright by Johnson. From Fong, Ferris, & Skelley, *Body Structures and Functions*, 8th ed. Copyright 1993, Delmar Publishers Inc. Used with permission.)

duce ATP, the muscle can again respond to a stimulus and contract.

Smooth Muscle Action ....

Smooth, involuntary muscles can be found throughout the internal organs and structures of the body. They are controlled automatically by signals from the autonomic nervous system.

In the esophagus (the structure that connects the mouth with the stomach), the muscle tissue changes from voluntary mus-

cles at the top that assist in swallowing, to smooth, involuntary muscles that move the food to the stomach. A two-layer muscle structure in the lower esophagus continues into the stomach and intestines. One layer of smooth muscle is circular and contracts to narrow the tube. Another layer is longitudinal and contracts to shorten the tube. The alternating action of both layers, contracting and relaxing, works the food through the body in a wavelike action called **peristalsis,** Figure 4–67. The stomach has a third layer in the muscle wall because of its need to break up and churn the food that is swallowed, which must be in a

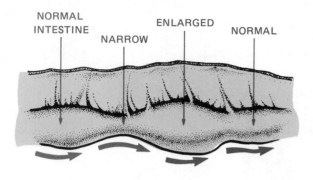

NORMAL INTESTINE   NARROW   ENLARGED   NORMAL

PERISTALTIC WAVE

FIGURE 4–67 Peristaltic action (From *The Wonderful Human Machine.* Copyright 1979, American Medical Association.)

near-liquid state before it can be passed on to the small intestine.

Sphincters Throughout the digestive system and inside the blood vessels of the body are smooth, doughnut-shaped muscle structures called **sphincters.** These pinch shut intermittently to control the flow of food, liquid, or blood. Sphincters in the digestive system are capable of remaining contracted for hours if necessary. Both ends of the stomach have sphincter muscles to hold the contents securely inside while muscular action and chemical processes digest food. When the food is in the proper state, the lower sphincter opens slightly to allow small amounts of the liquid to escape into the small intestine.

An example of smooth muscle sphincter action that can be easily observed is the pupil of the eye. When available light is decreased, the radial muscles of the iris contract to enlarge the pupil, permitting more light to enter, thereby increasing the ability to see. When light is focused on the eye, the circular sphincter muscles of the iris that surround the pupil contract, making the pupil smaller, thereby limiting the amount of light striking the retina. The physician will usually check light reflex action of the eyes in assessing the condition of the brain and autonomic nervous system.

Disorders and Diseases ....

Bursitis/Tendonitis (See Unit 5). **Tendonitis** is a painful inflammation of the tendon and tendon–muscle attachments to bone, usually at the shoulder, hip, heel, or hamstrings. Bursitis is an inflammation of the bursa that covers and lubricates the muscles and tendons, and occurs most often at the shoulder, elbow, or knee. Both conditions are painful and result in limited movement of the extremities.

Tendonitis normally follows a sports-related activity that damages the muscle–tendon structure. It can also result from misaligned posture and other **musculoskeletal** disorders. With injury, apply ice initially for the first 12 to 24 hours. Later, applications of heat will usually aid in relief of the joint pain. If calcium deposits have formed within the tendon it becomes

weak, and the condition will be aggravated by heat. The calcium deposits are visible on X ray to confirm the diagnosis. Application of ice packs will help relieve discomfort from calcified tendonitis.

Both conditions may be treated by resting the joint, oral does of pain medication, and intraarticular injections of a mixture of a corticosteroid and a local anesthetic. If fluid has accumulated within the area, it may require aspiration prior to the injection treatment. When pain has subsided, a physical therapy regime may be indicated to maintain joint function and prevent muscular atrophy.

Epicondylitis (Tennis Elbow) (See Unit 5). This is inflammation of a forearm tendon at the attachment on the humerus at the elbow. The initial elbow pain gradually worsens and often involves the forearm and the back of the hand when an object is grasped or the elbow is twisted. There is tenderness over the head of the radius and the projection of the humerus at the elbow joint. Epicondylitis probably begins as a partial tear of the tendon from its attachment.

Injection of the area, as with tendonitis, is effective. Immobilization, heat therapy, and manipulation of the tendon attachment are used before resorting to surgical excision of the tendon for recurring and continual inflammation.

Fibromyositis. This is inflammation of the soft tissue, which results in painful muscles. Often the cause is unknown. It is believed to be stress- and tension-related. Headaches usually occur as well. The main diagnostic finding is the presence of a "trigger point" which causes pain when pressed. Treatment consists of nonsteroidal antiinflammatory drugs, muscle relaxants, exercise, and physical therapy.

Muscular Dystrophy. This group of congenital disorders results in progressive wasting away of skeletal muscles. There are several types of muscular **dystrophy.** Duchenne's, which represents 50% of the cases, is an X-linked chromosomal disorder affecting only males. The onset is usually in early childhood, ages 3 to 5, with death occurring after 10 to 15 years. Initially the leg and pelvic muscles are affected, making all activities involving the lower extremities difficult. Children are usually confined to a wheelchair by ages 9 to 12. The disease progresses from skeletal to smooth muscles, affecting the heart and diaphragm and eventually resulting in cardiac or respiratory failure.

Erb's, or juvenile, muscular dystrophy and a similar type do not reduce life expectancy. These forms progress much more slowly and occur later in childhood or adolescence. Weakness of the facial muscles and inability to raise the arms are among the main symptoms.

The fourth is a mixed type of dystrophy occurring generally between ages 30 and 50, affecting all voluntary muscles and resulting in rapid, progressive deterioration. Death usually results in about 5 years from onset.

A positive diagnosis of dystrophy can be made from a typical medical history and evaluation of voluntary muscle movements. Confirmation is possible by a biopsy of the muscle tissue, which shows characteristic deposits of fat and connective tissue. There is no treatment to stop the progression of the disease.

Torticollis (Wryneck). This neck deformity is caused by shortening or spasm of the sternocleidomastoid neck muscle, which bends the head to the affected side and rotates the chin toward the opposite side. It can be congenital or acquired. The congenital form usually follows a difficult (eg. breech) birth and occurs mostly in firstborn females. It is thought to develop from malposition before birth, prenatal injury, or the rupture of muscle fibers with resulting scar tissue development. Acquired **torticollis** results from muscle damage by disease, a cervical spine injury, or muscle spasms due to a CNS disorder. Acquired torticollis can also develop as a result of hysteria.

Treatment of the congenital type consists of stretching the shortened muscle through passive exercises and positional arrangement of the head during sleeping. Surgical correction of the muscle can be accomplished if conservative methods are not effective. Acquired torticollis is treated by correcting the underlying cause whenever possible. Application of heat, cervical traction, a neck brace, exercise, psychotherapy (if hysteria-related), and massage are indicated.

Complete Chapter 4, Unit 6 in the workbook to help you meet the objectives at the beginning of this unit and therefore achieve competency of this subject matter.

U N I T   7
The Respiratory System

OBJECTIVES

Upon completion of this unit, you will meet the following terminal performance objectives by verifying knowledge of the facts and principles presented through oral and written communication at a level deemed competent by the instructor or employer.

1. Describe the source and importance of oxygen.
2. Trace the path of oxygen to the internal cell.
3. Describe the structure and function of the nose, pharynx, epiglottis, larynx, trachea, bronchus, bronchiole, and alveolus.
4. Explain how voice sounds are produced.
5. Differentiate between external and internal respiration.
6. Describe the structure and function of the pleural coverings of the lungs and chest cavity.
7. Describe the relationship of the diaphragm and brain to breathing.
8. Discuss five normal occurrences that alter breathing patterns and explain why they occur.
9. Identify ten diagnostic examinations for respiratory assessment.
10. Explain the role of surfactant in the lungs.
11. Differentiate between perfusion and ventilation scans.
12. Describe 26 diseases or disorders of the respiratory tract.
13. Spell and define, using the glossary at the back of the text, all the words to know in this unit.

WORDS TO KNOW

allergic rhinitis	larynx
alveoli	Legionnaires' disease
angiography	liter
apnea	lung
arteriography	orthopnea
asthma	oxygen
atelectasis	perfusion
bronchi	pharynx
bronchiole	pleura
bronchitis	pleurisy
carbon dioxide	pneumoconiosis
chronic obstructive pulmonary disease (COPD)	pneumonia
	pneumothorax
cilia	pulmonary
cyanosis	pulmonary edema
dyspnea	pulmonary emoboli
emphysema	respiratory
empyema	rhinitis
epiglottis	septum
epistaxis	sinusitis
expectoration	spirometer
expiration	spontaneous
hemothorax	sputum
hiccoughs	sudden infant death syndrome (SIDS)
hiccup	
histoplasmosis	surfactant
hyaline membrane disease (HMO)	trachea
	tracheotomy
hypoxia	tuberculosis
influenza	upper respiratory infection (URI)
inspiration	
intubation	ventilation
laryngectomy	vital capacity

Oxygen (O_2) is provided continuously by plants on land and in the sea. Plants use sun, water, and **carbon dioxide** (CO_2) to make oxygen, which they release into the air. Humans breathe O_2 and exhale CO_2 and water. This cycle provides the means for supporting life.

Oxygen in the air is essential to the survival of living cells. An adult human being carries 2 quarts of O_2 in the blood, lungs, and tissues. This supply is adequate for about 4 minutes. The respiratory system is responsible for taking in air, removing the oxygen content, and sending it in the blood to the cells of the body. The oxygen content of inhaled air is about 24%.

The respiratory system must also take from the blood the waste product CO_2 and exhaust it from the lungs. Exhaled air still contains about 16% oxygen. When the level of CO_2 in the blood rises to a certain point, the respiratory center in the brain is triggered and a breath is taken. This function is so vital to life that its interruption for just a few minutes will result in death.

The Pathway of Oxygen ....

The Nose Air enters the body through the nose, Figure 4–68. Here the air is filtered, warmed, and moistened by the structures within the nasal cavity. The nose is divided by a wall of cartilage called the **septum.** Near the middle of the

nasal cavity, on each side, are a series of three scroll-like bones called conchae, or turbinates. The conchae are covered with mucus-producing epithelium, which adds moisture to the air, and are supplied with abundant blood vessels, which warm the air. Just inside the nostrils are hairs called **cilia,** which trap particles in the air so they do not enter the lungs.

The mucus from the lining also helps trap dust and bacteria. When irritating substances come in contact with the lining, extra mucus is produced to dilute the irritant. This is why sneezing occurs and the nose "runs." Both actions are methods of removing irritants.

Ciliated mucosa in the posterior portion of the nose and in the pharynx (throat) help propel inhaled particles into the back of the pharynx to be swallowed. Particles in the trachea and bronchi must first be propelled upward past the epiglottis, in an action called *mucus streaming.* The particles can then be

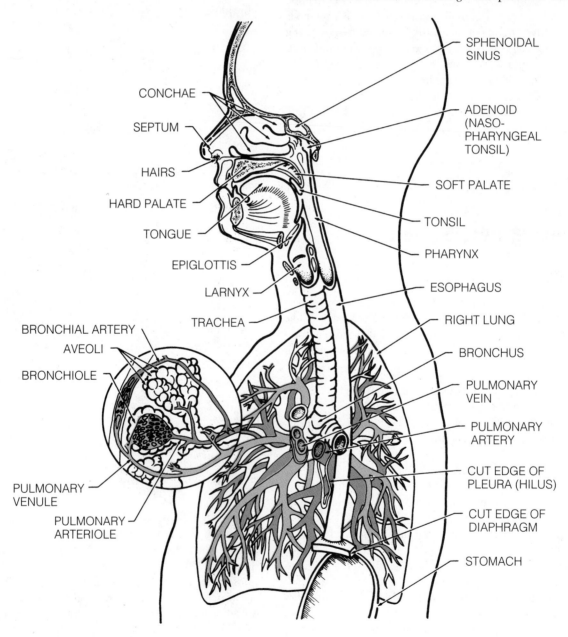

FIGURE 4–68   The respiratory system (From *The Wonderful Human Machine.* Copyright 1979, American Medical Association.)

directed toward the esophagus and swallowed. The constant beating action of the cilia and the flow of the mucus-secretions cleanse the air passages. This beneficial function is temporarily halted by the effect of smoking, which paralyzes the cilia and mucus-streaming action, thereby allowing foreign particles to enter the lungs. The paralysis lasts for several minutes.

The sinuses of the head are lined with the continuation of the nasal membranes, Figure 4–69, page 141. This explains why sinusitis occurs frequently with nasal infections, usually the result of spreading the organism by blowing the nose too forcefully.

The Pharynx, Larynx, and Epiglottis

After the air is filtered, warmed, and moistened in the nose, it enters the **pharynx.** The pharynx serves as a passageway for both air and food. Except for an occasional mistake, it is not possible to swallow food and breathe at the same time. When this does occur, the result is choking, which can be very serious.

Normally, when food is swallowed, a cartilage "lid" called the **epiglottis** is pushed by the base of the tongue to cover the opening into the **larynx.** At the same time, the larynx moves up to help close the opening. With the opening to the larynx covered by the epiglottis, food is directed down the esophagus into the stomach.

When air passes under the open epiglottis, it enters the larynx, commonly called the voice box. The larynx is a tube with a series of nine separate cartilages to maintain its opening, Figure 4–70, page 142. The thyroid cartilage is the largest and is located anteriorly. Its prominent projection is known as the Adam's apple, and its action can be observed when a person swallows. The larynx is lined with mucous membrane, which

also forms two folds called the vocal cords. The cords are attached to the front of the larynx wall by cartilage. Muscles attach to the cartilage, and when they contract or relax the vocal cords move either toward or away from the center of the larynx, Figure 4–71.

During breathing, the vocal cords are near to the wall of the larynx so that air can pass freely in and out. When speaking, the vocal cords move across the larynx and are held tense by the contracting muscles. The degree of tension and the length of the cords determine the pitch of the voice. The tighter and longer the cords, the higher the pitch. The pressure on the air being expelled from the lungs determines the volume or loudness of the voice as it vibrates the vocal cords. Note that speech is most easily accomplished during the exhaling of air. Inhaling does not create sufficient air pressure, nor can it be sustained long enough to produce speech.

Part of the mucous membrane lining of the larynx is loosely attached and of a different type of epithelium. It may become swollen, actually preventing respirations. In this emergency situation, an airway may be achieved by **intubation** (passing a tube through the mouth into the larynx) or by making an external opening into the **trachea,** called a **tracheotomy,** and inserting a tube to permit air to enter.

The Trachea, Bronchi, and Bronchioles

The next passageway for air is the trachea, Figure 4–72. It is commonly called the windpipe and extends from the neck into the chest, directly in front of the esophagus. The trachea is held open by a series of C-shaped cartilage rings. The wall between the rings is elastic, enabling the trachea to adjust to different body positions.

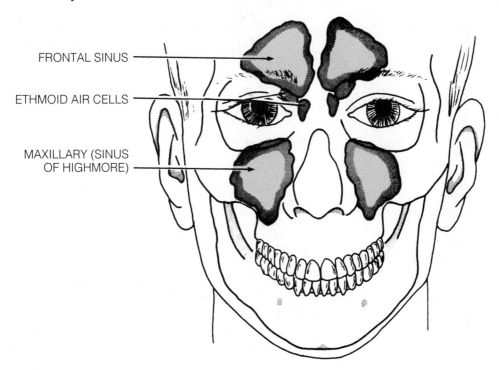

FRONTAL SINUS

ETHMOID AIR CELLS

MAXILLARY (SINUS OF HIGHMORE)

FIGURE 4–69 Paranasal sinuses (frontal view) (From Anderson & Burkard, *The Dental Assistant.* Copyright 1978, Delmar Publishers, Inc.)

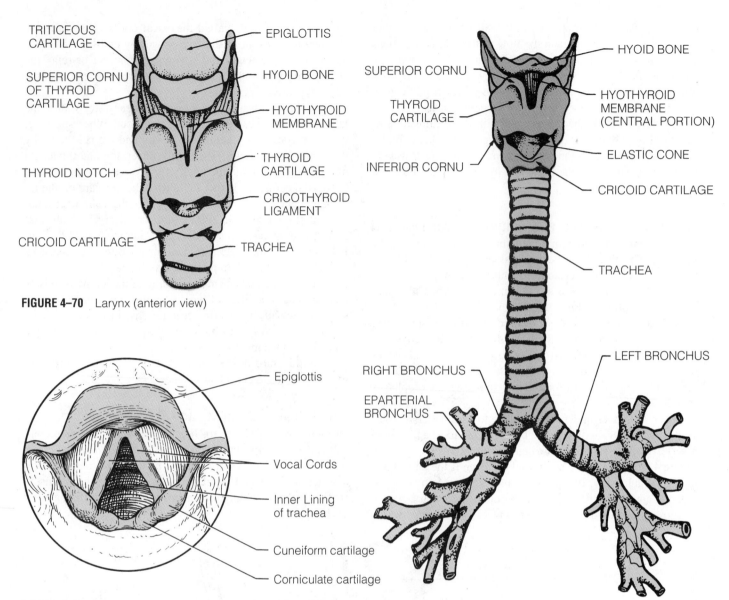

FIGURE 4–70 Larynx (anterior view)

FIGURE 4–71 The vocal cords in the larynx (From Kinn, *Medical Terminology, Building Blocks for Health Careers,* Copyright 1990, Delmar Publishers Inc.)

FIGURE 4–72 The larynx, trachea and bronchi

About the middle of the sternum, the trachea divides into two sections called the right and left **bronchi.** The structure of the two main bronchi is similar to that of the trachea, with incomplete cartilage rings to maintain the air passageway. Each bronchus divides and subdivides into many increasingly smaller bronchi, each with the cartilage-ringed structure, until they are barely visible without a microscope. These tiny air passageways have walls of muscle cells and are called **bronchioles.**

The Alveoli   Each bronchiole ends in a grapelike cluster of microscopic air sacs called **alveoli.** It is estimated that the body contains about 500 million alveoli, approximately three times the amount necessary to sustain life. The membrane walls of the alveoli are only one cell thick and are surrounded by a network of microscopic blood vessels called capillaries, Figure 4–73, page 143.

Respiration ....

The structure of the **respiratory** apparatus has been compared to an upside-down tree, with the trunk, branches, twigs, and leaves corresponding to the trachea, bronchi, bronchioles, and alveoli.

On **inspiration,** air enters the body, eventually arriving in an alveolus. Here O_2 passes through the wall of the alveolus into the surrounding capillary as CO_2 leaves the capillary and enters the alveolus. When **expiration** occurs, CO_2 exits from the bronchial tree and is exhaled from the body. The process of getting O_2 from the nose to the alveolus and into the capillary and the return of CO_2 to the nose is known as *external respiration,* Figure 4–74(a), page 144.

At the same time, oxygen from the alveolus is circulating through the body to every cell. First the oxygen enters the capillary surrounding the alveolus, then it circulates through a

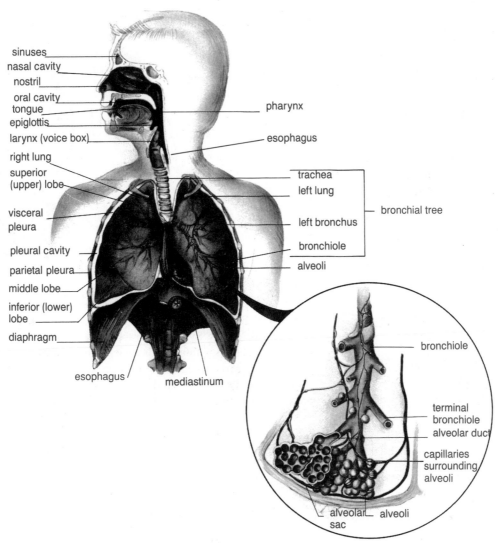

FIGURE 4–73 Aveoli (Adapted from Smith, *Medical Terminology, A Programmed Text*, 6th ed. Copyright 1991, Delmar Publishers, Inc.)

venule, a vein, back to the heart, out an artery, to an arteriole, and into a capillary next to a body cell. Here the O_2 in the blood is given to the cell while CO_2 from the cell is picked up by the capillary. The exchange of O_2 and CO_2 at the cell is known as *internal respiration*, Figure 4–74(b), page 144.

Oxygen and carbon dioxide in the alveolus and the cell exchange by the process of *diffusion*. It should be remembered that materials move across a membrane from an area of higher concentration to an area of lower concentration. In the alveoli of the lung, O_2 concentration is greater than in the surrounding capillary, so it diffuses into the blood. At the same time, CO_2 is in higher concentration in the blood than in the alveolus so it leaves the blood and enters the alveolus and is exhaled during the next respiration. At the cell the O_2 content in the capillary is greater than that within the cell, so the O_2 leaves the blood and enters the cell. On the other hand, CO_2 level within the cell is greater than in the capillary, so CO_2 diffuses out of the cell into the blood. This process of external and internal respiration is continuous throughout the life span of a person.

The Lung and the Pleura

The structures of the bronchial tree are contained in an organ known as the **lung.** The tissue of the lung is so filled with the alveoli that it is spongy and extremely light. It will float if placed in water. Prior to birth and breathing, the lung is solid and will sink in water. At birth, the lungs begin to fill with air, inflating the alveoli. The degree of inflation depends on the presence of **surfactant,** a fatty molecule on the respiratory membrane. The surfactant maintains the inflated alveolus so it does not collapse between breaths. About 2 weeks are required to completely inflate the lungs. Surfactant is not present in sufficient amounts to cause adequate inflation in premature infants and sometimes also in those born with other conditions. This results in *respiratory distress syndrome* (RDS), which is characterized by labored breathing with resulting exhaustion from the expenditure of energy required to reinflate alveoli after each breath. Many infants die each year even though current technology can supply continuous positive pressure to maintain open alveoli and therefore accomplish O_2

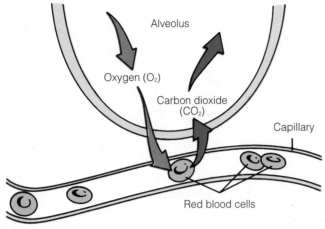

Alveolus

Oxygen (O_2)

Carbon dioxide
(CO_2)

Capillary

Red blood cells

a. External respiration in the lungs

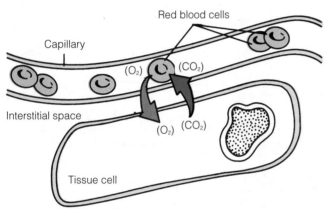

Red blood cells

Capillary

(O_2)   (CO_2)

Interstitial space

(O_2)   (CO_2)

Tissue cell

b. Internal respiration at the cell

FIGURE 4–74   Simplified external and internal respiration

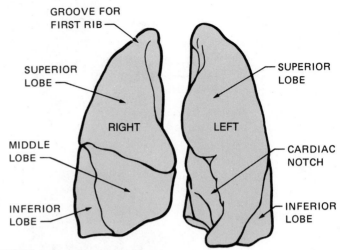

GROOVE FOR
FIRST RIB

SUPERIOR
LOBE

SUPERIOR
LOBE

RIGHT   LEFT

MIDDLE
LOBE

CARDIAC
NOTCH

INFERIOR
LOBE

INFERIOR
LOBE

FIGURE 4–75   Anterior lung surface

and CO_2 exchange. The lungs continue to mature throughout childhood, with additional alveolar formation. It has been determined that smoking at an early age retards the maturing of the lungs, and the additional alveoli never develop.

The lung is divided into a right and left lung, Figure 4–75. The right lung has three lobes: superior, middle, and inferior. The left lung has two: superior and inferior. The heart lies on the medial surface of the left lung in a space called the *cardiac notch*. Each lung with its blood vessels and nerves is enclosed in a membrane called the visceral **pleura.** A membrane also lines the thoracic cavity, and is called the parietal pleura. The airtight space between the pleural membranes is known as the pleural space or cavity. It contains a lubricating fluid to prevent friction as the membranes rub together during respiration. The "space" is virtually nonexistent in healthy lungs because the lungs fill the thoracic cavity within the rib cage, pressing the visceral against the parietal pleura. As will be discussed later, however, certain conditions and diseases cause an abnormal presence of fluid or air within the pleural space.

The Muscles of Breathing ....

The action of the diaphragm and the muscles of the rib cage

were discussed in Unit 6. It is important to remember that the lung itself is not capable of any breathing action. It is acted on primarily by the contraction of the diaphragm producing a vacuum within the thoracic cavity to draw in air. At this time there is a negative pressure within the lungs; the pressure inside is less than the atmospheric pressure outside. When the inside pressure exceeds outside atmospheric pressure, it becomes positive and causes expiration to again equalize inside–outside pressure. When the diaphragm returns to its relaxed state, air is forced out of the lungs, Figure 4–76.

Breathing action is controlled by the respiratory center in the brain. An increase of CO_2 or a lack of O_2 in the blood will trigger the center. Since we can somewhat voluntarily control breathing, it is possible to force rapid respirations and deplete the CO_2 in the blood, temporarily interrupting breathing and possibly losing consciousness. Children will occasionally hold their breath to frighten their parents and receive concessions. Usually, there is no need to be overly concerned because sooner or later a breath has to be taken. If consciousness is lost, the automatic system resumes control and breathing returns to normal.

Other situations can alter a breathing pattern for perfectly normal reasons, such as.

- Coughing—When a deep breath is taken followed by a forceful exhalation from the mouth to clear something from the lower respiratory structures.
- **Hiccoughs** (also spelled **hiccups**)—Caused by a spasm of the diaphragm and a spasmodic closure of the glottis (space between the vocal cords). It is believed to be the result of an irritation to the diaphragm or the phrenic nerve, which innervates its muscle.
- Sneezing—Occurs like a cough except air is forced through the nose to clear the upper respiratory structures. Usually results from mucous membrane contact with an irritant.
- Yawning—A deep prolonged breath that fills the lungs, believe to be caused by the need to increase oxygen within the blood.
- Crying (or laughing)—Alters the breathing pattern in response to emotions.

(a) Inspiration   (b) Expiration

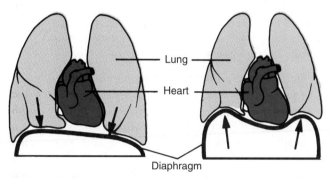

FIGURE 4–76 Position of diaphragm and ribs during inspiration (a) and expiration (b)

Diagnostic Examinations

- Arterial blood gases—Blood taken directly from an artery to evaluate the exchange of O_2 and CO_2 in the lungs. The test measures the partial pressures of both gases and determines the pH of the blood. The PO_2 (partial pressure of oxygen) indicates how much oxygen the lungs are delivering to the blood. The PCO_2 (partial pressure of carbon dioxide) indicates how efficiently the lungs eliminate carbon dioxide. The pH determines the acid–base level, which indicates the hydrogen (H^+) ion content. If acid, there is excess hydrogen ion; alkalinity indicates a deficit. Results aid in the diagnosis and treatment of many disorders and conditions, such as CNS depression from drugs or injury, hypoventilation, hyperventilation, anxiety, certain kidney diseases, and many others.
- Bronchoscopy—The insertion of an instrument, the bronchoscope, into the trachea and bronchial tree to view the tissues, obtain a secretion or tissue sample, or remove a foreign body.
- Chest X ray—A radiological examination to determine the general health of lung and surrounding tissues or to identify a disease process.
- Lung **perfusion** scan—An examination of the lung following intravenous (IV) injection of a radioactive contrast medium to provide a visual image of pulmonary blood flow. It is useful in diagnosing blood vessel obstruction, such as pulmonary emboli (foreign substance in an artery).
- Lung **ventilation** scan—An examination following the inhalation of a mixture of air and radioactive gas from a mask and bag. The test indicates the areas of the lung that are ventilated during respiration. It determines the distribution pattern of the gas and illustrates obstructed airways or areas of consolidation, such as occur with pneumonia.
- Pulmonary **angiography/arteriography**—A radiological examination of the pulmonary circulation following the injection of a radiopaque iodine material through a catheter that is placed in the pulmonary artery or one of its branches. The catheter is inserted into a vein at the inner surface of the elbow or in the groin, and passed through the veins and through the first half of the heart into the pulmonary artery. The test aids in diagnosing pulmonary emboli, especially when the lung scan was not conclusive. It is also used to evaluate pulmonary circulation in certain heart conditions before surgery.
- **Pulmonary** function tests—To measure lung volume in a normal breath, lung capacity when forcing air into and out of the lungs, and other variables during a specified period of time. Many tests can be performed in a specialized hospital pulmonary laboratory; however, the most common test and one that is appropriate to the physician's office, is the **spirometer** to measure ventilation function. The spirograph reveals the patient's normal breathing capacity volume, the extra forced expiration volume possible, the extra forced inspiration volume possible, and the total extra forced inspiration and expiration volume possible. The total volume exchange achieved is called the **vital capacity** of the lung. (See Chapter 8 for additional information.)
- Pulse oximeter—The pulse oximeter is a small electronic device that fits over the end of the index finger and is connected by a wire to a machine. The device determines the amount of oxygen in the blood and displays it digitally in the window of the machine. Frequently, postoperative patients are monitored for oxygen content as are patients with cardiac and respiratory conditions. If the pulse oximeter indicates the oxygen level is too low, oxygen will be administered at a proper amount to supplement that being circulated by the body.
- **Sputum** analysis—A laboratory examination of material coughed up from the bronchial tree or trachea. If properly prepared it can aid in the diagnosis of infectious organisms or cancer cells.
- Thoracentesis—Withdrawing of fluid from the pleural space by needle aspiration following local anesthetic, Figure 4–77. Fluid may be present as a result of excessive production or inadequate reabsorption of the pleural fluid that may be associated with cancer, tuberculosis, or a blood or lymphatic disorder. A specimen is often withdrawn for analysis to determine the presence of organisms, malignant cells, blood, or lymph fluid properties.

Disorders and Diseases

Allergic Rhinitis. A reaction to airborne allergens, causes sneezing, profuse watery nasal discharge, itching of the eyes

FIGURE 4–77 Thoracentesis. Fluid is being removed from the pleural cavity (From Burke, *Human Anatomy and Physiology in Health and Disease*, 3d ed. Copyright 1992, Delmar Publishers Inc.)

and nose, red and swollen eyelids, and nasal congestion. **Allergic rhinitis** may be seasonal, as with hay fever, or perennial, caused by house dust, mold, cigarette smoke, and the like.

Treatment consists primarily of administering antihistamines and avoiding the allergens. The use of air conditioning filters allergens, keeps down dust, and removes excess moisture from the air. The use of steroid nasal sprays may also be helpful. Desensitizing injections of the allergens before or during the season is indicated for long-term management. In severe or persistent cases, it may be necessary to relocate to a relatively pollen-free environment.

Asthma. This chronic allergic disorder results from sensitivity to allergens, such as pollen, dust, animal dander, certain foods, and a number of other substances. It can also develop from an infectious process or from unknown causes. **Asthma** is characterized by bronchospasms, which narrow the bronchioles, increased mucus secretions that block passageways of air, and edema of the mucosal lining. These reactions decrease the lung's capacity to exchange air. Symptoms usually occur as a sudden onset of wheezing, **dyspnea**, and tightness of the chest. They are often accompanied by coughing and **expectoration** of thick sputum. The patient may become frightened and experience feelings of suffocation to the point that speech is nearly impossible. The symptoms of airway obstruction may be present to some extent between acute attacks.

Determination of the offending allergens is usually accomplished with a series of skin tests. Minute amounts of the most common causative agents are introduced just below the skin by a needle prick or applied as patches to the skin surface. The presence of a reddened area about a site after a specified amount of time is evidence of sensitivity.

The treatment of choice for asthma is prevention by eliminating allergens. This is not always possible, however. Desensitization to specific allergens through injections may be helpful. During attacks, limited inhalation of specific bronchodilating drugs and administration of epinephrine, followed by corticosteroids, should alleviate symptoms. With severe attacks, O_2 administered at approximately 2 **liters** per minute helps to ease breathing and increase O_2 within the arteries.

Atelectasis. The lack of air in the lungs due to the collapse of the microscopic structures of the lung; **atelectasis** may occur following abdominal or thoracic surgery or with pressure from pleural effusion (fluid, air, pus, blood, or lymph) in the pleural cavity. It can be chronic, caused by mucous plugs in the bronchial tree in patients with cystic fibrosis and obstructive pulmonary disease and in heavy smokers. Bronchial occlusion can also result from cancer or inflamed tissues. Acute (sudden) atelectasis may occur with any condition that causes pain on deep breathing, such as rib fractures, traumatic injury, surgical procedures, or **pleurisy.**

Chronic Obstructive Pulmonary Disease (COPD). A condition characterized by chronic obstruction of the airways resulting from emphysema, chronic bronchitis, asthma, or any combination of these disorders. Usually, there is more than one condition, most often a combination of bronchitis and emphysema.

Bronchitis is an inflammation of the bronchial walls with distortion and narrowing of the airways. The presence of mucus results in a productive cough and dyspnea on exertion. Bronchitis can be an acute disease, caused by an infection, or a chronic disease, caused by damaged cilia, enlarged mucous glands, and chronic inflammation. The severity of chronic bronchitis is related to the amount and duration of smoking. Wheezing and prolonged expiration time may be observed.

Acute bronchitis is managed with antibiotics to treat the infection, expectorants to help remove excessive mucus, and avoiding smoking. Chronic bronchitis also requires bronchodilators, respiratory therapy to loosen mucous secretions, and corticosteroids in some cases. Adequate fluid intake is important.

Emphysema is an irreversible enlargement of the air spaces in the lungs due to destruction of the alveoli wall. Emphysema results in the inability to exchange O_2 and CO_2 in the affected areas and to exhale stale air from the lungs. Symptoms include a chronic cough, weight loss, barrel chest, the use of accessory muscles to breathe, prolonged expiration, rapid pursed-lip breathing, cyanosis, and, eventually, respiratory failure and death. Treatment and control are the same as those for COPD.

The incidence of COPD is increasing. Until recently, it occurred most often in men, primarily due to their heavier smoking habits. With increased use of tobacco by women, the difference is decreasing. Other causes of **chronic obstructive pulmonary disease** are chronic respiratory infections and allergies. Smoking is the most important factor, however, because it impairs ciliary action, causes inflammation in airways, destroys alveolar walls, and results in peribronchiolar fibrosis (formation of scar tissue around the bronchioles).

COPD is a progressive disease; symptoms occur gradually and become worse with age. Initially there is a productive cough and a decline in the ability to exercise. As the disease progresses, the individual becomes dyspnic with minimal exertion, has frequent respiratory infections, develops thoracic deformities (usually barrel chest from muscular changes caused by attempting to breathe), suffers severe respiratory failure and hypoxemia (insufficient O_2 in the blood), and eventually dies.

Treatment consists of methods to halt the progression of the disease and control its present state. Damaged structures cannot be restored. Prime emphasis is placed on avoiding smoking and other respiratory irritants. In addition, the use of bronchodilators, prompt treatment of respiratory infections, effective breathing and coughing instructions, proper diet, and the use of O_2 are indicated. The most important factor in prevention is *not* smoking.

Epistaxis (Nosebleed).

(See Unit 3.) Nosebleeds usually follow injury, either external or internal, such as a blow to the nose, nosepicking, or foreign body insertion. Less frequent causes of **epistaxis** are chronic conditions, such as nasal or sinus infection that results in capillary congestion and bleeding, or the inhalation of irritating substances. Predisposing systemic factors include high blood pressure, anticoagulation drugs, chronic aspirin use, and blood diseases, such as anemia, hemophilia, and leukemia.

Treatment varies depending on the cause, location, and severity. Even moderate bleeding is considered severe if it persists longer than 10 minutes after pressure is applied. Symptoms may include lightheadedness, a drop in blood pressure, rapid pulse, dyspnea, pallor, and other indications of shock. Initial first aid treatment may consist of elevating the head, compression of nostrils against the septum continuously for 5 to 10 minutes, application of ice or cold compresses to nose and back of neck, preventing the swallowing of blood (to determine the amount lost), avoiding talking or blowing the nose, and observing for amount of blood loss and signs of shock.

Advanced treatment includes: for anterior bleeding, applying epinephrine-saturated cotton ball or gauze to the bleeding site and the use of external pressure, followed by cauterization by electric cautery or silver nitrate; for posterior bleeding, the insertion of a nasal pack for 48 to 72 hours may be required. Small catheters are passed through each side of the nose into the mouth. Rolled gauze packs are attached to the catheters and drawn back through the mouth and up into the posterior nasal cavity where they become lodged, making pressure against the leaking blood vessels. If necessary, anterior bleeding can be treated by packing for 24 to 48 hours. Other treatment may include supplemental vitamin K, blood transfusions, and surgical ligation (tying) of the bleeding artery.

Histoplasmosis.

A fungal infection, occurring worldwide, **histoplasmosis** is caused by an organism found in droppings from birds or bats, or in soil near their roosts, as in barns, caves, chicken coops, around buildings, and under bridges. It has also been determined to come from cat feces due to ingested birds.

In the United States, histoplasmosis occurs in three forms: primary acute, progressive disseminated, and chronic pulmonary. Symptoms vary with the form contracted. The primary acute resembles a severe cold. The progressive involves the liver, spleen, and lymph glands, and may cause inflammation of the heart muscle and the pericardium (covering membrane), as well as the meninges of the brain and spinal cord. The chronic form resembles tuberculosis, causing a productive cough, dyspnea, weakness, and cyanosis.

Hyaline Membrane Disease (HMD).

This condition results from immature alveolar and bronchiolar development and a weak intercostal musculature in premature infants (before week 37 of gestation). If untreated, 14% of infants weighing less than 5.5 pounds will die within 72 hours. Incidence in the United States alone is 40,000 newborn deaths per year. **Hyaline membrane disease (HMD)** occurs more frequently in infants born to diabetic or smoking mothers and those delivered by cesarean section or whose birth is precipitated by hemorrhage.

HMD causes respiratory distress due to the collapse of the alveoli and the immature capillary system resulting in an inadequate oxygen supply. Frequently the infant breathes normally at first, but as the collapse progresses, respirations become rapid and shallow. The intercostal muscles and the sternum retract, and the nostrils flare, providing evidence of increased breathing difficulty. A characteristic "grunting" on expiration can be heard. With progression the heart rate decreases and respirations stop. Low body temperature, due to inadequate body fat, and an immature nervous system add to the difficulties.

Aggressive treatment is required, preferably in a neonatal intensive care unit. Heat is supplemented by an isolette, and O_2 is supplied as needed. Fluids are given intravenously or directly by catheter into the stomach, when the infant is too weak to eat. A few of the infants who survive will still have abnormally developed bronchopulmonary tissue.

Influenza (flu).

This acute, highly contagious respiratory infection usually occurs in colder months and in infrequent epidemics (widespread incidence, not of local origin). It is more prevalent in school children aged 6 to 14 and adults over age 40. **Influenza** can be fatal to the elderly or people with chronic heart, lung, or kidney disease. The disease is directly transmitted by droplets inhaled from an infected person's sneezing or coughing, or by indirect contact with contaminated objects, such as a drinking glass. Influenza viruses have the ability to alter their influence on the population. As people develop immunity to a virus after having contact with it, the virus alters its composition and a new strain results to which people have little or no resistance. Hence an epidemic or pandemic (present in many areas of the world at the same time) develops.

Influenza viruses are classified into three types:

1. Type A—the most lethal, occurring every 2 to 3 years with a major new strain developing every 10 to 15 years.

2. Type B—occurring every 4 to 6 years resulting in epidemics.

3. Type C—endemic (of local origin) and causing infrequent cases.

Symptoms of flu are the sudden onset of chills and a fever of

101° to 104°F (38°–40°C), headaches, muscle aches, a nonproductive cough, and **rhinitis.** Pneumonia is the most common complication, developing 3 to 5 days after infection begins.

Treatment consists of bed rest, adequate fluid intake, and aspirin or similar medication to relieve the pain and fever. Antibiotics have no effect on the virus and should not be used except for secondary bacterial infection. Flu immunizations, which provide protection for 3 to 6 months, are recommended for the high-risk population. The vaccine is only 75% effective, however, because the serum is determined by the previous year's strain.

Laryngectomy.   This is surgical removal of the larynx, usually the result of cancer caused by smoking. The earliest symptom of internal disease of the larynx is persistent hoarseness. With involvement externally, it is a lump in the throat or pain, or burning when drinking hot liquids or citrus juices.

Diagnosis can often be made by viewing with a laryngoscope. This examination is often followed with radiological studies to confirm. With positive diagnosis, the larynx may be partially or totally removed. With total removal, a permanent opening called a stoma is made in the neck through which air can be taken in and exhaled, Figure 4–78. Coughing results in material being expelled through the stoma.

A great deal of patient support is necessary to assist in developing alternative methods of communication prior to surgery. The patient may need psychiatric assistance to cope with the loss of speech, sense of smell, ability to blow the nose, and related problems. Much support can be obtained from organizations established to aid in rehabilitation of **laryngectomy** patients. Local chapters of the "Lost Chord Club," made up of persons who have lost their larynx, volunteer their services to speak with new patients and help them learn techniques of producing speech. The American Cancer Society and the International Association of Laryngectomies also provide assistance with speech methods which use esophageal air that is swallowed and released slowly, the artificial larynx, and other mechanical devices.

The individual in Figure 4–78 has a voice prosthesis inserted into the stoma. By placing his finger over the opening in the prosthesis, he is able to produce a good quality of speech. A "patch" of thin foam is placed over the opening to prevent inhaling foreign materials. The foam is porous and permits easy exchange of air.

Laryngitis.   This inflammation of the vocal cords occurs in both acute and chronic forms. Acute laryngitis usually results from an infectious process, excessive use of the voice, inhalation of smoke or fumes, or accidental aspiration of chemicals. Chronic laryngitis develops from other preexistent chronic conditions, such as sinusitis, bronchitis, and allergies or from smoking, abuse of alcohol, and continual exposure to irritants.

Laryngitis is treated by resting the voice, using medication for underlying infection, if present, and eliminating coexistent causes (in the case of chronic laryngitis).

Legionnaires' Disease.   This acute bronchopneumonia derived its name from a highly publicized incident in which 182 people

A

B

FIGURE 4–78   Laryngeal stoma (a) with voice prosthesis and (b) inserter, following laryngectomy

developed the disease at an American Legion Convention in Philadelphia in 1976. **Legionnaires' disease** usually occurs in late summer or early fall.

The bacillus that causes the disease is probably transmitted through the air. In past epidemics, it was spread through air conditioning systems and cooling towers. It does not spread person to person. Symptoms include nonspecific signs, such as diarrhea, lack of appetite, headache, chills, weakness, and an unremitting fever that develops within 12 to 48 hours. Temperature may reach 105°F (40.5°C). A cough then develops, which becomes productive, with grayish sputum. Other symptoms are nausea, vomiting, confusion, dyspnea, chest pain, and, in 50% of the patients, a slow pulse rate. Severe symptoms are evidence of complications and include low blood pressure, irregular heart beat, respiratory failure, kidney failure, and shock (which is usually fatal). Smokers are three to four times more likely to develop Legionnaires' disease than nonsmokers.

Treatment consists of antibiotics, medication to reduce the fever, maintaining fluid balance, and measures to support adequate respiration, such as oxygen and mechanical ventilation by inhalation therapy.

Lung Cancer. This is the leading cause of cancer deaths among men and increasingly prevalent in women, despite the fact that it is largely preventable. It is attributed to inhalation of carcinogens in tobacco and the environment. The inhalation of carcinogens causes a progressive destruction of the cells in the lungs. There is a correlation between the risk of cancer and the number of cigarettes smoked daily, the depth of inhalation, the age at which smoking began, and the nicotine content of the tobacco. An individual over 40 who began smoking as a teenager and has averaged a pack a day for at least 20 years is most susceptible. Lung cancer can take 20 to 30 years to develop. An estimated 85% of lung cancer in men and 75% in women is caused by cigarette smoking. Less than 10% of lung cancers occur among nonsmokers.

Other inhalants that increase *susceptibility* are industrial air pollutants, such as asbestos, arsenic, iron oxides, chromium, radioactive dust, vinyl chloride, and coal dust. There also is an indication that there is a familial tendency link to lung cancer. The combination of industrial pollutants and cigarettes is very risky. For example, asbestos workers who also smoke increase their risk of developing lung cancer by 60 times.

Involuntary smoking, that which the nonsmoker gets "second hand" from a spouse or others, though less concentrated, still contains the same harmful substances. For example, wives exposed to husbands who smoke 20 or more cigarettes a day at home, have double the risk of lung cancer when compared with wives of nonsmokers. Children of smoking parents are also affected. They are more prone to respiratory infections and more likely to develop lung diseases later in life.

The prognosis for lung cancer patients is very poor, because by the time a diagnosis is made, two-thirds of the patients have passed the stage where it might be curable. Only 13% of all lung cancer patients (all races and all stages) live 5 or more years after diagnosis. This is primarily due to delayed diagnosis because of lack of symptoms. The first indication of squamous or oat cell carcinoma is a smoker's cough, wheezing, dyspnea, and hemoptysis (spitting of blood). If the carcinoma is anaplastic or adenocarcinoma, the symptoms are fever, weakness, weight loss, and anorexia. The disease metastasizes to many other sites within the thoracic cavity and throughout the entire body.

Treatment consists primarily of surgical excision when appropriate, radiation, and chemotherapy. Usually since the disease is advanced before treatment begins, little more than temporary reduction in symptoms and discomfort is expected. The best treatment is obviously prevention. Quitting smoking or never starting is the best defense against lung cancer.

Figure 4–79 is a reprint of a brochure distributed by the American Cancer Society that illustrates the effects of emphysema and cancer on the tissues of the lung.

Pleurisy. An inflammation of the visceral and parietal pleura in the thoracic cavity, **pleurisy** develops as a complication of pneumonia, tuberculosis, chest injury, and other factors. Sharp, stabbing pain is experienced on respiration due to irri-

NORMAL LUNG

The lung is our breathing machine. It draws in air, filters it, separates out life-giving oxygen for the body's use and expels what is left over—mostly carbon dioxide. The normal adult lung is about the size of a football.

When we inhale, air enters the lung through tubes, or passageways, called bronchi. These bronchi are lined with vibrating hairlike structures called cilia, which whip back and forth some 900 times a miunute, to help keep solid pollutants in the air from entering the lung. The air is carried down through smaller and smal-ler bronchi until it reaches tiny air sacs which are uniform in size. This is where the oxygen/carbon dioxide exchange takes place.

Unfortunately, damage to the lung often takes place before there are any symptoms.

CANCER

Cancer ravages the lungs with an army of wildly multiplying cells. It begins most often with the constant irritation of the lining of the bronchi by cigarette smoke.

Under the onslaught of this irritation, the hairlike cilia which filter the air we breathe disappear from the lining of the bronchi. Although extra mucus is secreted to substitute for the cilia and trap pollutants, this mucus itself becomes a problem. It remains trapped until finally forced out of the lung by a "smoker's cough."

If a smoker quits before cancerous lesions are present, the bronchial lining will return to normal. If not, the abnormal cell growth spreads, blocking the bronchi and then invading the lung tissue itself.

In the latter stages of lung cancer, abnormal cells break away from the lung and are carried by the lymphatic system to other vital organs, where new cancers begin.

Because lung cancer is difficult to detect early, it is very difficult to treat successfully. It is often fatal. Yet if no one smoked cigarettes, 83% of lung cancers would eventually disappear.

Research now shows that even involuntary smoking exposures result in enough inhaling of smoke to increase the risk of developing lung cancer as well as other respiratory illnesses and risk to the fetus during pregnancy. A new study found that women exposed to husbands who smoked 20 or more cigarettes a day at home had double the risk of lung cancer compared to women married to nonsmokers.

It has been said that if the effects of cigarette smoking appeared on our skin instead of in our lungs—where it can't be seen—no one would smoke. Now you have seen the ugly inside story.

Call your local Unit of the American Cancer Society for information on how to quit smoking.

EMPHYSEMA

Emphysema is a disease which destroys the lung's elasticity, and therefore its ability to inhale and exhale properly.

Tissue affected by emphysema can never be repaired or replaced and the disease, progressing slowly but steadily, turns its victims into respiratory cripples. Patients spend years gasping for breath, and when death comes, it frequently is due to an overworked heart.

Emphysema changes the lung's normal appearance. Some of the air sacs burst and collapse, creating tiny craters in the lung, while others balloon in the body's desperate struggle to obtain oxygen and expel carbon dioxide.

Emphysema used to be a relatively rare disease, but today it is becoming increasingly common. It has been stongly associated with the cigarette habit because of the intense air pollution caused by cigarette smoke in the lungs.

AMERICAN CANCER SOCIETY®

FIGURE 4–79 Normal and diseased lung tissue (Courtesy of the American Cancer Society) tation of the pleural nerve endings as the lungs move, rubbing against the inner chest wall. As a result, lung movement on the affected side may be limited, and dyspnea occurs.

Treatment is generally symptomatic, with bed rest and medications to reduce the inflammation and relieve the pain. Some physicians may partially immobilize the chest with a restrictive support to lessen movement of the chest wall and reduce friction. If fluid collects within the pleural space, a thoracentesis is indicated to prohibit lung compression by the fluid or to determine, by laboratory examination, a causative agent (see Figure 4–77).

Paroxysmal Nocturnal Dyspnea (PND).   This symptom, associated with chronic lung disease or left ventricular failure (heart disease), occurs at night. Individuals awaken from sleep with a feeling of suffocation. They often run to open a window and gasp for air. Just sitting upright will help some people because of the effect of gravity on fluid in the lungs. The episode will resolve itself usually within a few minutes.

Pleural Effusion.   This presence of excess fluid in the pleural space can result from overproduction or inadequate reabsorption of the pleural fluid. Some effusions result from chronic diseases, such as congestive heart failure, liver disease, tuberculosis, malignancy, lupus erythematosus, and rheumatoid arthritis. When the effusion becomes symptomatic, depressing lung tissue and reducing the lungs' ability to exchange O_2 for CO_2, resulting in **hypoxia** (lack of O_2), oxygen will be administered to increase concentration to the remainder of the lung. If the fluid is a result of an infectious process, exudate (pus) and dead tissue will be present, and the effusion is known as **empyema.** Drainage of the material by thoracentesis and insertion of chest tubes may be necessary. Antibiotics are required to destroy the causative organism. Effusion that contains blood is called a **hemothorax** and will require drainage to prevent fibrothorax (scar tissue) formation.

Pneumoconiosis.   These are lung diseases developed after years of contact with environmental or occupational causative agents. Basically, there are three types of **pneumoconiosis.** One form, *silicosis,* occurs from exposure to silica sand dust in occupations, such as sand blaster and foundry worker, in manufacturing of ceramic and sandstone products and construction materials, and in mining of gold, lead, zinc, and iron. Nodules develop where specific disease-fighting cells have ingested the silica particles but then been unable to dispose of the ingested material. The cells die, causing the release of an enzyme that attracts more cells to assist in destroying the invading material. A fibrous (scar) tissue results, and the process continues until large areas of the lung tissue are destroyed.

Another form, *asbestosis,* can develop 15 to 20 years after regular exposure to asbestos has ended. Asbestosis is most prevalent in the construction, fireproofing, and textile industries, and in brake and automotive occupations dealing with clutch linings. The general public may also develop the condition from exposure to fibrous dust or the waste piles of asbestos factories. Asbestosis is the result of inhaling minute asbestos fibers, which enter the bronchioles and penetrate the

alveolar walls. The fibers become encased, and fibrosis of the lung tissue develops, obliterating the air passages. Fibers also cause fibrotic changes in the parietal pleura.

A third type, coal worker's, or *black lung disease,* is a progressive nodular form resulting from exposure to coal dust. It is found in two forms: simple, which produces small lung lesions, or complicated, which produces masses of fibrous tissue. The development usually occurs after 15 years or more of exposure and depends to some extent on the amount of dust, the type of coal mined, the silica content, and the location of the mine.

Initially, the body's fighting cells ingest the dust and become filled, forming macules in the terminal bronchioles, which are surrounded by dilated alveoli. The supporting tissue atrophies (wastes away), resulting in permanent dilation of the small airways. When the disease changes from a simple to a complicated form, one or both lungs can become involved. The fibrous tissue masses enlarge, causing destruction of the alveoli and airways.

Treatment of all types is essentially the same: avoiding respiratory infections, use of bronchodilators to aid in respiration, chest vibration, oxygen supplement, and other respiratory therapy to improve removal of bronchial secretions.

Pneumonia.   This is an acute infection of the principal tissues of the lungs, which may impair the exchange of O_2 and CO_2. Chances for recovery from **pneumonia** are good for persons with normal lungs, but pneumonia is the fifth leading cause of death in debilitated (weakened) patients.

Pneumonia is classified in several ways: by microbiological origin (bacterium, virus, fungus, protozoan, etc.); by location (bronchus, lobar, or lobular); or by type (primary, caused by inhaled pathogens, or secondary, following lung damage by an inhaled chemical or by an infection spread from another area of the body).

Pneumonia often occurs with chronic weakening illnesses, such as cancer, or after surgery. It is also associated with malnutrition, smoking, COPD, age, and with a decreased level of consciousness. Symptoms range from coughing, sputum production, and pleural chest pain to chills and fever. Treatment consists of bed rest, an appropriate antibiotic, adequate fluid intake, respiratory support measures, such as oxygen or mechanical breathing therapy, and medication for pain.

Pneumothorax.   In this condition air or gas has accumulated between the parietal and visceral pleurae, causing some degree of collapse of the lung tissue. If it is **spontaneous,** air has leaked from the lung tissue as the result of a disease process or a ruptured blisterlike lesion. A traumatic **pneumothorax** results from a penetrating chest wound, as by a knife or gunshot, from thoracic surgery, or from the insertion of tubing into the blood vessels of the chest. Fractured ribs can penetrate the thorax causing collapse of the lung. Since the atmospheric pressure outside is greater than that within the pleural cavity, it compresses the lung tissue as it enters. Frequently blood is also present with an injury and, if located between the pleura, it is referred to as a hemothorax.

In tension pneumothorax, air enters the pleural space as the result of trauma but is unable to leave by the same route.

Each inspiration results in additional trapped air being sucked in. Eventually, pressure is exerted against the large chest veins, interfering with blood flow returning to the heart. If severe, the great vessels of the chest and the heart may be pushed toward the uninjured side of the chest.

The primary symptoms of pneumothorax are sudden, sharp pain made worse by breathing or coughing, unequal chest wall movement, shortness of breath, and **cyanosis.** As the degree of collapse increases, respirations become more stressful, the pulse becomes rapid and weak, and the patient becomes pale. Death may result without prompt treatment.

Treatment varies with the degree of collapse. If it is spontaneous, with 30% or less involvement and no dyspnea or apparent sign of increasing difficulty, it may be treated with bed rest, careful monitoring of vital signs, and perhaps needle aspiration of the air mass. With greater than 30% collapse, the lung is slowly reexpanded by low suction through a tube inserted into the chest. If there is evidence of trauma, the tissue must be repaired, the chest closed, and the wound drained by means of chest tubes.

Pulmonary Edema.   Accumulation within the tissues of the lungs of fluid that has escaped from the blood vessels due to increased pressure, **pulmonary edema** is common with heart disorders causing left ventricular failure. Symptoms include dyspnea on exertion, coughing, **orthopnea** (ability to breathe only in an upright position), and rapid pulse and respiration. With progression, respirations become more labored, noisy, and rapid. A cough that produces frothy, bloody sputum may develop. As the condition worsens, the patient becomes cold, clammy, and cyanotic. Confusion and a depressed level of consciousness occur in cases of severe heart failure.

Treatment consists of procedures to decrease the accumulated fluids and improve the exchange of O_2 and CO_2. Diuretics (water pills) bronchodilators, and high concentrations of oxygen may be indicated.

Pulmonary Embolism.   Obstruction of a pulmonary artery or arteriole by a circulating thrombus (blood clot) or another substance such as air, purulent matter, or fatty material is called a **pulmonary embolism.** The obstruction causes dyspnea, chest pain, rapid heart rate, a productive cough, and a low-grade fever. The symptoms vary with the extent of obstruction. In massive embolism, with over 50% obstruction of arterial circulation, death occurs rapidly.

Predisposing factors include long-term immobility, which permits slow-moving blood to clot within the vessels, varicose veins, surgery, pregnancy, vascular injury, obesity, fractures, and many chronic pulmonary and circulatory diseases.

Treatment consists of measures to maintain adequate heart and lung function while the obstruction is being resolved, usually within 10 to 14 days. Medication is given to inhibit the blood from forming additional clots, as well as break up the present occlusion. Supportive oxygen therapy is used as needed. If the embolus is caused by purulent material from an infectious process, then aggressive antibiotic therapy is indicated.

Sinusitis.   Inflammation of the paranasal sinus cavities, **sinusitis** usually results from the common cold organism or chronically from persistent bacterial infection. Symptoms include nasal congestion, low-grade fever, headache pain over cheeks and upper teeth, pain over eyes or eyebrows, and a nonproductive cough. Treatment consists of analgesics for pain, medication to decrease secretions, steam inhalations to encourage drainage, and application of heat to relieve pain and congestion. Surgical drainage of the affected sinus cavity may be necessary in persistent, severe conditions.

Sudden Infant Death Syndrome (SIDS).   This is a mysterious condition that kills apparently healthy infants between the ages of 4 weeks and 7 months. It is unexplainable even after autopsy. **Sudden infant death syndrome** kills 6000 to 7000 infants annually in the United States. It occurs more frequently in winter, in poorer families, to mothers under 20, and among underweight babies. Study of the syndrome suggests that the infant may have had undetected respiratory dysfunctions which caused prolonged periods of **apnea** (absence of breathing), resulting in extreme hypoxemia (lack of oxygen in the blood), and serious irregular heartbeat.

Diagnosis of SIDS requires an autopsy to rule out other causes of death. Several characteristics of the syndrome confirm the diagnosis. Parents need a great deal of support to deal with the death, as they often feel they were somehow to blame. There is a National Sudden Infant Death Foundation with local chapters of parents whose babies have died of the syndrome. Many local health organizations provide counseling and information services. These resources can be of great assistance.

Tuberculosis (TB).   An acute or chronic infection causing nodular lesions and patchy infiltration of the lung tissue is known as **tuberculosis.** The body reacts to the invading causative organism by converting the destroyed tissue into a cheeselike material. This material may localize and become fibrotic, or it may develop into cavities within the lung tissue. The cavities are filled with the multiplying bacilli, and the infected debris spreads throughout the tracheobronchial tree.

On initial contact with the tubercular bacillus, most people's immune defense system kills the organism or walls it off in a nodule. These dormant organisms may become active later causing an acute phase.

Symptoms of primary infection include fatigue, weakness, lack of appetite, weight loss, night sweats, and low-grade fever. On reactivation, symptoms may include a productive cough characterized by purulent mucus, occasionally mixed with blood, and chest pains.

Treatment consists of isolation until the contagious phase has passed. Care must be taken in handling the nasal and expectorated discharges. Bed rest and an adequate diet are very important. Medication specifically for TB must be continued for a year or more to effect a cure. After 2 to 4 weeks, the disease is no longer infectious and the person can resume a normal life.

Upper Respiratory Infection.   This term is used to refer to symptoms associated with the common cold. An **upper respiratory infection (URI)** may be caused by several different viruses and be transmitted by respiratory droplets, contaminated objects, or hands. Children are the main transmitters of the organism. The disease is usually self-limiting after a 1- to 4-day incubation period. It is characterized by sore throat, nasal congestion, headache, burning and watery eyes, fever, and general lethargy. A cough may be present, which is nonproductive and hacking, often at night. Symptoms usually persist for a week before subsiding. Secondary bacterial infections affecting the lower respiratory tract are uncommon.

Complete Chapter 4, Unit 7 in the workbook to help you meet the objectives at the beginning of this unit and therefore achieve competency of this subject matter.

U N I T   8
The Circulatory System

OBJECTIVES ....

Upon completion of this unit, you will meet the following terminal performance objectives by verifying knowledge of the facts and principles presented through oral and written communication at a level deemed competent by the instructor or employer.

1. Name the four main parts of the circulatory system.
2. Describe the anatomy of the heart, identifying the internal and external structures.
3. Differentiate between pulmonary, systemic, and portal circulation.
4. Describe the heart sounds, including the actions producing the sounds and where they can be ausculated.
5. Locate the pacemaker, explain its action, and tell how the heart rate is influenced by the body.
6. Explain how the cardiac conditions of heart block and fibrillation relate to the pacemaker.
7. Explain the purpose of an artificial pacemaker and how it functions.
8. Name the five types of blood vessels and their purpose and structure.
9. Describe the function of a capillary bed.
10. Trace the pathway of blood through the pulmonary and systemic circulation.
11. Explain the function and structure of the lymphatic system.
12. Name the components of whole blood and the role of each.
13. Describe the clotting process.
14. Name the blood types and explain their importance to recipients of transfusions.
15. Explain the importance of the Rh factor in pregnancy and transfusions.
16. Identify eight cardiovascular tests and the reasons for giving them.
17. Describe 25 diseases or disorders of the circulatory system.
18. Spell and define, using the glossary at the back of the text, all the words to know in this unit.

WORDS TO KNOW ....

accelerator	leukemia
adenitis	leukocyte
ambulate	lubb dupp
anemia	lymph
aneurysm	lymphatic system
angina	lymphocyte
angioplasty	metastasize
anticoagulant	mitral
aorta	MUGA scan
arrhythmias	murmur
arterioles	myocardial infarction (MI)
arteriosclerosis	myocardium
artery	nodes
atherosclerosis	pacemaker
atrium	papillary muscles
AV node	pericardium
bicuspid	phlebitis
bradycardia	plasma
capillary	platelet
cardiac	portal
cardiovascular	Rh factor
cerebrovascular accident (CVA)	SA node
compatible	semilunar
congestive heart failure (CHF)	septum
	sickle cell
coronary	spleen
cross-match	stasis ulcer
diastole	systole
electrocardiograph (ECG)	tachycardia
embolism	thrombophlebitis
endocardium	thrombosis
erythrocyte	transfusion
exudate	transient ischemic attack (TIA)
fibrillation	
heart block	tricuspid
hemoglobin	vagus
hemorrhage	valve
Holter monitor	varicose
hypertension	vein
hypotension	vena cava
infarction	ventricle
ischemia	venule

The circulatory system transports oxygen and nutrients to the body's cells and carbon dioxide and other waste products from the cells, to be eliminated from the body. The blood, which flows through a closed circuit of vessels, is the transportation vehicle. A very efficient muscle, the heart, is the force behind the system. A few minutes' interruption of the circulatory system can result in death.

The circulatory system is composed of four main parts: (1) a pump, the heart; (2) the plumbing, the blood vessels; (3) the circulating fluid, the blood; and (4) an auxiliary fluid system, the **lymphatic system.** Each day the heart pumps the equivalent of 4000 gallons of blood, at 40 miles per hour, through an estimated 70,000 miles of blood vessels. To achieve this, the heart must forcefully contract, squeezing out blood, at an average rate of 72 times per minute, or about 100,000 times each day. In a year's time, the heart will contract 40 million times, resting only a fraction of a second between beats. To appreciate this phenomenal organ, alternately open and close your fist a little more often than once a second for just one minute by the clock. You will notice that not only your hand but also your forearm muscles begin to tire. Scientists have estimated that the work of the heart is about equal to the energy needed to lift a 10-pound weight 3 feet off the floor twice a minute for a lifetime. The condition of the blood vessels and the composition of the blood are major factors in the amount of force the heart must exert to circulate the blood.

The Heart ....

The heart is about the size of a clenched fist and is located behind the sternum, between the lungs, with two-thirds of it on the left side of the chest. It is constructed of several layers of muscles arranged in both circular and spiral fashion. When the muscles contract, blood is squeezed out of the heart chambers. During the relaxation phase, the heart fills with blood entering from the great **veins.** There is a considerable difference in the size of the heart during the phases, as shown in Figure 4–80.

The contraction phase is known as **systole** and the relaxation phase is called **diastole.** Systole is the period when the heart exerts the greatest pressure on the blood. This corresponds to the beat phase of the heart and can be heard over the heart with a stethoscope or felt as the pulse in an **artery.** The systolic pressure can be determined by measurement with blood pressure equipment and is represented by the larger, or top, number of the blood pressure reading. Diastole is the period of least pressure and is the time when the heart rests. This phase cannot be felt as a beat, but the diastolic pressure can be heard and determined by measurement. It is represented by the smaller, or bottom, number of the blood pressure reading.

External Heart Structures
The outer wall of the heart is surrounded by a sac called the **pericardium.** Like the

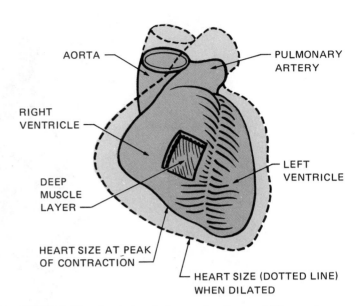

FIGURE 4–80 Heart size during contraction and filling actions (From *The Wonderful Human Machine,* Copyright 1979, American Medical Association)

pleura of the lungs, the pericardium has one layer called the parietal, which lines the sac, and another layer, the visceral, which covers the heart itself. The pericardial fluid between the layers prevents friction when the heart beats. The heart structure does not receive its blood supply from the blood pumped through its interior, but from a number of small blood vessels which cover the surface of the heart, Figure 4–81. These blood vessels, called the **coronary** arteries and veins, carry oxygen, nutrients, and waste products to and from the heart muscle. The right and left coronary arteries enter the top of the heart from the **aorta.** Blood from the coronary veins returns to the right atrium by a small opening called the coronary sinus.

The muscle wall of the heart is called the myocardium. The wall of the left lower chamber is thicker because it must pump blood through the entire general, or systemic, circulation, as discussed later.

Internal Heart Structures
A tissue known as **endocardium** lines the interior surface of the heart, Figure 4–82, page 155. The lining also covers the heart valves and the interior surface of the blood vessels to allow for the smooth flow of blood. Internally, the heart is a double pump, divided into a right and left side by a muscular wall called a **septum.** The septum prevents the blood on the right side from mixing with that on the left. The sides are further divided into upper and lower chambers. The right upper chamber is called the right **atrium,** the lower, the right **ventricle.** The left side is similarly divided into a left atrium and left ventricle.

The chambers are separated by one-way **valves** which keep the blood flowing in the right direction. The **tricuspid** valve is between the right atrium and ventricle, and the **bicuspid,** or

right common carotid artery

right subclavian artery

brachiocephalic artery

superior vena cava

right pulmonary artery

ascending aorta

right auricle

right coronary artery

right coronary vein

right ventricle

pericardium

left common carotid artery

left subclavian artery

aortic arch

left pulmonary artery

left auricle

left coronary artery

left coronary vein

left ventricle

anterior coronary artery

apex

FIGURE 4–81 External heart structures (From Smith, *Medical Terminology, A Programmed Text,* 6th ed. Copyright 1991, Delmar Publishers Inc.)

mitral, valve is between the left atrium and ventricle. **Papillary muscles** are attached by cords to the undersurfaces of the valve cusps or leaflets. When the atria contract, the papillary muscles also contract to pull open the valves, allowing the blood from the atria to enter the empty ventricles. Then the muscles relax, which allows the valves to close as the atria refill. The closed valves prevent the blood from reentering the atria when the ventricles contract.

At the contraction of the ventricles, blood is forced out to the great arteries of the body. The right ventricle sends the blood through a semilunar valve into the pulmonary artery on its way through the pulmonary circulation in the lungs for a supply of oxygen. The left ventricle forces the blood past a semilunar valve into the aorta to be distributed throughout the systemic circulation of the body.

A specific sequence of events occurs within the body as the blood is circulated. Blood flow occurs in two distinct patterns, *pulmonary circulation* between the heart and the lungs and *systemic circulation,* between the heart and the rest of the body. Figure 4–83, page 155, and the following material describe the flow of blood through the pulmonary system.

Pulmonary Circulation

1. Deoxygenated (without O_2) blood carried in the superior vena cava from the arms, neck, and head and carried in the inferior vena cava from the lower extremities and internal organs (except the heart itself) enters the right atrium. Circulation from the heart also empties into the atrium by way of the coronary sinus.

2. The right atrium contracts, squeezing blood through the tricuspid valve, which is opened by the papillary muscles, into the right ventricle. Then the valve closes.

3. The right ventricle contracts, sending blood out through the semilunar valve into the pulmonary artery. (Remember, this artery carries deoxygenated blood but is still an artery because it is leaving the heart.)

4. The pulmonary artery divides into a right and left branch, one going to each lung. The division continues into smaller arteries, arterioles, and then to the capillaries in the alveolar sacs. Here the deoxygenated blood gives up its CO_2 and picks up O_2.

5. With a fresh supply of O_2, the capillaries join the venules, then become veins and reenter the heart as four pulmonary veins, two from each lung, emptying into the left atrium. (This is the only time veins carry oxygenated blood, but they are still veins because they are returning to the heart.)

6. The left atrium contracts, forcing blood through the mitral, or bicuspid, valve into the left ventricle, and the valve immediately closes.

7. The left ventricle contracts forcefully, sending blood racing out of the heart past the semilunar valve into the aorta.

The action of the chambers of the heart just described occurs simultaneously in both sides of the heart. In other

FIGURE 4–82 The heart and it's valves (Adapted from Fong, *Body Structures and Functions,* 8th ed. Copyright 1993, Delmar Publishers Inc.)

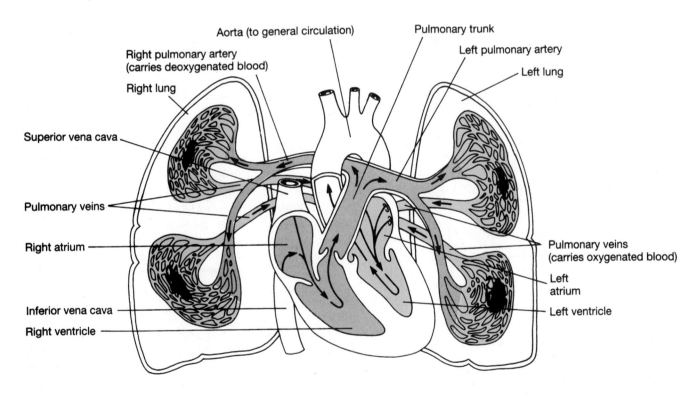

FIGURE 4–83 Pulmonary circulation (Copyright by Johnson. From Fong, Ferris, & Skelley, *Body Structures and Functions,* 8th ed. Copyright 1993, Delmar Publishers Inc.)

words, both atria contract at the same time, as do the ventricles. The chambers must work in unison or blood being pushed forward would have no place to go (this situation does occur in certain cardiovascular disorders and will be discussed later). The total action just described occurs each time the heart beats.

Heart Sounds

The physician listens at specific locations on the chest wall to hear specific functions of the heart. Figure 4–84 illustrates the anatomical location of the valves and the corresponding auscultatory areas. When a stethoscope is used to listen to the heartbeat, two distinct sounds can be heard. They are referred to as the **lubb dupp** sounds. The lubb sound which is heard first, is caused by the valves slamming shut between the atria and the ventricles. The physician refers to this sound as the S_1. It is heard loudest at the apex of the heart.

The dupp, heard second, is shorter and higher pitched. It is caused by the semilunar valves closing in the aorta and the pulmonary arteries. This sound is known as the S_2. It is loudest at the second intercostal space on each side of the sternum. With a little practice, the valves' condition and level of function can be evaluated from their sounds.

Certain conditions cause changes in the action of the heart valves. Normally the right heart valves close a fraction of a second before the left, due to the lower pressure in the right side of the heart. When the ventricles are distended, an audible vibration may occur, which is referred to as an S_3, or a ventricular gallop. Occasionally, just before S_1, at the end of diastole, the atria may contract, forcing blood into an already filled

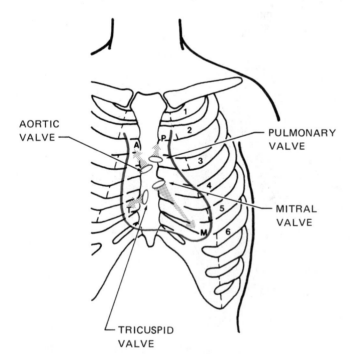

AORTIC VALVE

PULMONARY VALVE

MITRAL VALVE

TRICUSPID VALVE

FIGURE 4–84 Anatomical location of the heart valves and the accompanying auscultatory location. Valves are shown as oval structures and the auscultatory location by the letters A, T, M, and P. The rib levels are numbered.

ventricle. This causes a rise in the ventricular pressure and vibrations known as atrial gallop, or S_4.

The Pacemaker

The normal heart beats rhythmically as long as the cells receive the correct balance of sodium, calcium, and potassium and an adequate supply of oxygen and nutrients. Another essential element is the "spark" from the group of nerve cells in the right atrium called the sinoatrial or **SA node,** also called the **pacemaker,** Figure 4–85, page 157. The node generates the electrical impulse that starts each wave of muscle contraction in the heart. The impulse in the right atrium spreads over the muscles of both atria, causing them to contract simultaneously, sending blood into the ventricles. The impulse apparently triggers the atrioventricular, or **AV, node,** located between the atria and the ventricles, even though there is no direct connection between the nodes. The AV node has nerve fibers which extend through the septum and are called the *bundle of His.* The bundle divides into a right and left branch, infiltrating the muscles of each ventricle with a system of Purkinje fibers. The AV node causes the contraction of the ventricles.

Rhythm Disorders

The self-generating impulse of the heart is one of the body's miracles. Even if the heart were removed from the body it would continue to beat as long as it was supplied with the necessary nutrients. In a **cardiac** condition known as **heart block,** there is an interruption in the message from the SA node to the AV node. The interruption can occur in varying degrees. The abnormal rhythm patterns can be viewed on an **electrocardiograph** (heart action recording, or **ECG**). *First-degree block* is characterized by a momentary delay at the AV node before the impulse is transmitted to the ventricles. *Second-degree block* can be of two forms. One occurs in cycles of delayed impulses until the SA node fails to conduct to the AV node, then returns to near normal. A second form is characterized by a pattern of only every second, third, or fourth impulse being conducted to the ventricles. This causes a marked decrease in heart output and is usually progressive to the third degree. *Third-degree heart block* is known as "complete heart block." There is no impulse carried over from the pacemaker. Because the heart is essential to life, there is a built-in safety factor. The atria continue to beat at 72 times per minute, while the ventricles contract independently at about half the atrial rate, adequate to sustain life but resulting in a severe decrease in cardiac output.

Other rhythm disorders are known as **arrhythmias** (absence of rhythm). Premature contractions cause arrhythmia and occur when an area of the heart, not the SA node, "sparks" and stimulates a contraction of the rest of the myocardium. This area is known as an ectopic (abnormal place) pacemaker. There are three types of premature contractions, each identified by the area of its location; atrial, ventricular, or AV junctional.

FIGURE 4–85 SA and AV nodes and the conduction pathway of the heart's electrical impulse (Adapted from Smith, *Medical Terminology, A Programmed Text,* 6th ed. Copyright 1991, Delmar Publishers Inc.)

Atrial are known as PACs, *premature atrial contractions,* and cause the atria to contract ahead of the anticipated time. *Premature junctional contractions* (PJCs) have the ectopic pacemaker focused at the junction of the AV node and the bundle of His. Usually PACs and PJCs are of no clinical significance and are usually caused by nicotine, caffeine, fatigue, or tension.

Premature ventricular contractions (PVCs) are a different matter. They originate in the ventricle and cause contraction ahead of the next anticipated beat. They can be benign or deadly. If frequent, 5 to 6 per minute or in pairs, they may require immediate intervention to decrease the irritability of the cardiac muscle to maintain cardiac output. If the PVCs occur every other beat, it is a *bigeminal rhythm;* if they occur every third beat, it is a *trigeminal rhythm.* PVCs can be caused by electrolyte and acid–base imbalance, drug therapy, myocardial infarction (see diseases), or oxygen deficit.

In another malfunction of the impulse mechanism known as **fibrillation,** the rhythm breaks down and the muscle fibers contract at random without coordination. This results in very ineffective heart action and is a life-threatening condition. An electrical device called a *defibrillator* is used to discharge a strong electrical current into the patient's heart through electrode paddles held against the bare chest wall. The shock should interfere with the uncoordinated action and allow the SA node to resume its control.

Artificial Pacemaker When the natural pacemaker of the heart fails to maintain a normal heart rate and cardiac drug therapy designed to cause effective, regular beats fails to correct the situation, an artificial pacemaker may be indicated.

The device consists of a small battery-powered pulse generator with an electrode catheter, Figure 4–86. The electrode is inserted into a vein and threaded through the vena cava, the right atrium, and into the right ventricle at the apex. The procedure is accomplished while observing the path of the electrode by fluoroscopy. The action of the heart throughout the procedure, and for at least the first 24 hours following, is monitored carefully by frequent electrocardiograph (ECG) tracings. The stimulation threshold of the pacemaker to maintain myocardial contractions is determined by noting the number of milliamperes (mA) which produce the desired QRS complex (ECG tracing of contraction). This milliamperage and the desired rate can be set in the pacemaker.

It should be noted that when the heart is totally dependent on artificial pacing, the heart rate will always be that which is artificially set, regardless of the level of activity. The artificial pacemaker will not increase the rate to meet the needs of increased activity.

A pacemaker can be attached temporarily to the chest wall, upper arm, or waist. It can also be "permanently" inserted surgically into a muscular pocket on the chest wall. Permanent units are self-contained and will operate for about 3 to as many as 20 years. Pacemakers can also be of either the fixed or the demand type. Fixed units fire continuously at a predetermined rate. Demand types sense the person's own rate and fire only when required. An external unit can be programmed to change the mode of firing of some implanted types.

Pacemakers are of benefit to patients with a slow, irregular heart rhythm, complete heart block, or a slow ventricular rate due to congenital or disease conditions.

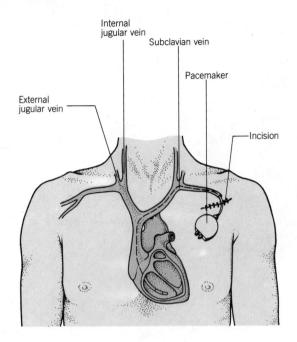

FIGURE 4–86 Artificial pacemaker (From Burke, *Human Anatomy and Physiology in Health and Disease,* 3d ed. Copyright 1992, Delmar Publishers Inc.)

FIGURE 4–87 Nerves influencing the heart rate

Controlling the Rate

Two nerves, the **vagus** and the **accelerator,** have fibers in the muscle of the heart and have some control over the natural rate of the heartbeat, Figure 4–87. The vagus nerve, also called the decelerator, slows down the heart rate while the accelerator nerve increases the rate. The nerves, however, are stimulated by many things. Heart rate can increase as the result of fear, anger, or excitement and can decrease with severe depression. The amount of oxygen, carbon dioxide, and electrolytes (sodium, potassium, magnesium, phosphates, and chlorides) present in the blood affect the rate of the heart. A heart rate which is consistently rapid (over 100 beats per minute) is known as **tachycardia.** When the rate is consistently slow, less than 60 beats per minute, it is referred to as **bradycardia.**

The Blood Vessels ....

Blood vessels are divided into three main types: arteries, veins, and **capillaries,** Figure 4–88, page 159.

Arteries

An artery always carries blood *away* from the heart and usually carries fresh, oxygenated blood. The one exception is the pulmonary artery, which leaves the right ventricle of the heart on its way *to* the lungs to pick up oxygen. Arteries are constructed with layers of elastic fibers that allow the walls to expand and recoil in response to the injection of blood when the ventricles contract. In the systemic circulation, this action causes a wavelike effect within the arteries, which can be felt as the pulse at the pulse points of the body. Figure 4–89, page 160, shows the main arteries of the human body. In areas where arteries lie over firm or bony structure, such as at the wrist, the

side of the neck or inner elbow surface, the pulse can be felt if the artery is pressed against the underlying structure.

As the arteries divide and branch off into smaller and smaller vessels, they become known as **arterioles.** Eventually, the arterioles join the microscopic blood vessels known as capillaries. When the blood enters the vast network of capillaries, called a capillary bed, it is so dispersed that the rate of flow is reduced to a slow trickle, permitting time for O_2 and nutrients to enter the cells in exchange for CO_2 and waste products, Figure 4–90, page 161.

Capillary walls are thin, one-cell structures that allow the passage of molecules into the fluid-filled tissue spaces surrounding the cells. The molecules pass through the fluid to enter either the cell or the capillary. Tiny openings in the capillary walls permit white blood cells to leave the blood and enter the fluid of the tissue spaces to destroy bacteria. **Plasma** also seeps through the capillary walls, adding to the amount of tissue fluid. Excess fluid, certain waste products, and other substances are removed by an adjoining capillary of the lymphatic system, an action that will be discussed later in this unit.

The vast number of capillaries within the body would be more than capable of holding all the body's supply of blood. Therefore, an automatic system permits a group of cells being served by one section of a capillary bed to receive blood for only a short period of time. Then another section is served and the first section must wait for another turn. This control is maintained by a series of capillary sphincters, which open and close the entrances to the capillary beds.

Body cells, in order of importance, have a predetermined priority for receiving the available blood supply. At any given time, only two of the three major body functions can be served. The brain and other central nervous system structures always have first priority. Next come the skeletal muscles that enable us to move and therefore provide a degree of protection to the body with the fight or flight options. Last is the supply to the internal organs of the digestive system. This means that if you have eaten recently and you decide to run, swim, or exercise strenuously, your stomach may complain with cramps because the muscles are not getting enough blood supply to digest its contents.

When the blood leaves the capillary bed, it is carrying CO_2 and waste products from the cells to be circulated to the proper

tunica interna, or intima
endothelium,
areolar, and elastic tissue

tunica media
smooth muscle

tunica externa, or adventitia
connective tissue

elastic
fibers

valve

endothelium

capillary

lumen

artery

a. Types of blood vessels and their general structure

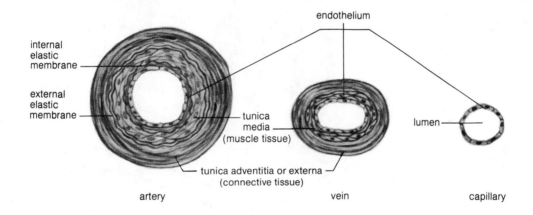

endothelium

internal
elastic
membrane

external
elastic
membrane

tunica
media
(muscle tissue)

tunica adventitia or externa
(connective tissue)

lumen

artery

vein

capillary

b. Cross section of blood vessels

FIGURE 4–88   Comparative structure of blood vessels (From Fong, *Body Structures and Functions,* 8th ed. Copyright 1993, Delmar Publishers Inc.)

organ for disposal. Capillaries join with **venules,** which are tiny branches of the veins. As they return blood toward the heart, venules join together forming veins, which eventually enter the heart, from the lower body by the inferior **vena cava** and from the upper body by the superior vena cava.

Veins
Veins are similar to arteries in construction except that the walls are thinner and they lack the elastic fiber lining that lets arteries alter the size of their openings. The pressure that is present in arteries is absent in veins, and therefore they can collapse when they are not filled. The major veins of the body are shown in Figure 4–91, page 162.

Veins carry deoxygenated blood back to the heart to be sent to the lungs for exhaling of CO_2 and to pick up a new supply of O_2. Every time the heart beats, blood is forced through the arteries and arterioles to the capillaries, where the pressure from the heart is dissipated in the vast capillary network. With each successive beat, additional blood is forced through the capillaries into the venules and veins, which move it back toward the heart. Special valve structures are located throughout the veins to maintain the flow of blood in the proper direction, Figure 4–92, page 163. Veins in the lower extremities especially contain many valves since they are returning blood "uphill" so to speak. During the relaxation phase of the heartbeat, the venous blood could flow back toward the capillaries, but the valves close as relaxation begins, and the blood is trapped in the veins until the following beat forces it to move forward.

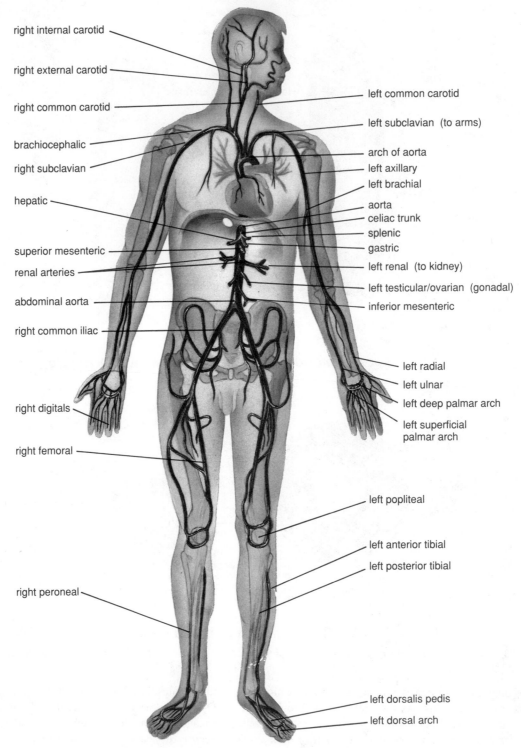

right internal carotid

right external carotid

right common carotid

brachiocephalic

right subclavian

hepatic

superior mesenteric

renal arteries

abdominal aorta

right common iliac

right digitals

right femoral

right peroneal

left common carotid

left subclavian (to arms)

arch of aorta

left axillary

left brachial

aorta

celiac trunk

splenic

gastric

left renal (to kidney)

left testicular/ovarian (gonadal)

inferior mesenteric

left radial

left ulnar

left deep palmar arch

left superficial
palmar arch

left popliteal

left anterior tibial

left posterior tibial

left dorsalis pedis

left dorsal arch

FIGURE 4–89   Major arteries of the body (From Smith, *Medical Terminology, A Programmed Text*, 6th ed. Copyright 1991, Delmar Publishers Inc.)

Another factor helps move blood in veins back to the heart. The veins of the extremities are located in and around the large skeletal muscles. When the muscles contract, they squeeze the veins, thereby aiding in the movement of the blood, Figure 4–93, page 163.

Blood flows to every cell in the body through the systemic circulation. Refer to Figures 4–89 and 4–91, as you read the following description of the flow through the major arteries and veins.

Systemic Circulation

1. As the blood leaves the left ventricle, it enters the huge aorta. Immediately, the right and left coronary arteries to

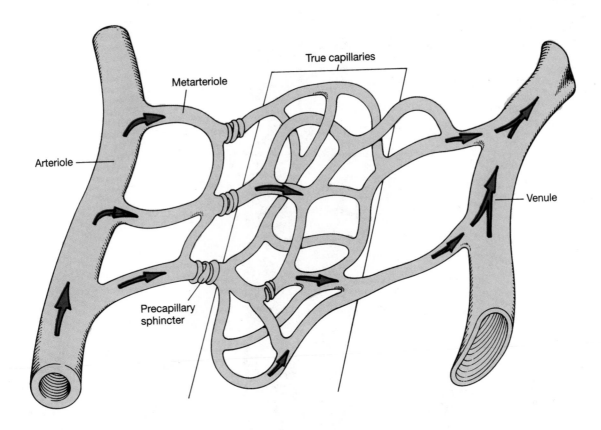

FIGURE 4-90 Capillary bed connecting an arteriole with a venule (Copyright by Richardson. From Fong, *Body Structures and Functions*, 8th ed. Copyright 1993, Delmar Publishers Inc. Used with permission.)

the heart exit from the aorta at its arch. Other great arteries, the common carotid, the subclavian, and the innominate, which becomes the brachial and radial arteries of the arm, also exit from the arch, divide into right and left branches and supply blood to the head, neck, and upper extremities.

2. As the aorta descends through the body, the thoracic and abdominal portions give origin to the large arteries supplying the organs of the thorax and abdomen.

3. When the aorta reaches the level of the fourth lumbar vertebra, it divides into two large common iliac arteries with the external branch descending down the legs and the internal branch leading to the pelvic organs and genitalia (external sex organs).

4. The external branch of the iliac artery becomes the femoral artery in the thigh and continues down the leg as the tibial branch.

5. Eventually all systemic arteries throughout the body subdivide until they become arterioles and then join the capillaries. In this circuit, the capillaries deliver the O_2, water, and nutrients to the body's cells and pick up the cells' CO_2 and wastes.

6. Upon leaving the capillaries, the blood is considered deoxygenated. The capillaries join venules, which eventually become veins.

7. The major lower extremity veins are the anterior and posterior tibial, the small and great saphenous, the popliteal, and the femoral. These join with pelvic veins and enter the inferior vena cava.

8. The major veins of the upper extremities are the basilic, median, and cephalic. These join with the subclavian, internal and external jugular, the innominate, and the sinuses from the head to enter the superior vena cava.

9. The superior vena cava and inferior vena cava empty into the right atrium of the heart and systemic circulation is completed.

Portal Circulation The preceding was a simplified description of the body's general circulation. Another "circuit," however, leaves and reenters the system just described. It is called the **portal** circulation, Figure 4-94, page 164. The details of its function are beyond the scope of this text, but it can be described in general terms.

As the aorta descends through the abdomen, arteries branch off to the internal organs: the stomach, liver, spleen, pancreas, kidneys, and so on. Each organ receives substances on which it reacts. These substances may be sugar, salt, hormones, a toxic chemical, nutrients, waste products from the cells of other organs—everything you eat, drink, inhale, or inject into your body eventually enters the circulatory system.

The blood leaving certain organs (ones without a pair) empties into the special portal circulation and eventually becomes the portal vein. This vein goes to the liver to permit the blood from the large and small intestines, stomach, pancreas, and spleen to come into contact with the liver's specialized cells. Many life-preserving functions are performed by

superior sagittal sinus
inferior sagittal sinus
straight sinus

right external jugular
right internal jugular

brachiocephalic
superior vena cava

right hepatic
inferior vena cava
superior mesenteric
right renal
right ovarian or testicular
right common iliac

right palmar arch

right femoral
right great saphenous

right small saphenous

left subclavian
great cardiac
left cephalic
left axillary
left basilic
left brachial
left hepatic
hepatic portal
splenic
left renal
left ovarian or testicular
inferior mesenteric

left external iliac

left palmar digitals

left femoral
left great saphenous
left popliteal

left posterior tibial
left anterior tibial

left dorsal venous arch

FIGURE 4–91   Major veins of the body (From Smith, *Medical Terminology, A Programmed Text*, 6th ed. Copyright 1991, Delmar Publishers.)

these liver cells. For example, here nutrients that enter the blood from the digestive system are altered, stored, or released into the main circulatory system, as needed. After passing through the liver, the blood is carried by the venous system to the inferior vena cava and is recirculated.

The Lymphatic System

The lymphatic system consists of **lymph,** a straw-colored fluid similar to blood plasma; lymph **nodes;** lymph vessels; and the

spleen. In addition, the lymphatic tissue, which produces **lymphocytes** (a type of blood cell), is often considered to be part of the system. This includes the tonsils, the thymus gland, and the intestinal lymphoid tissue.

Lymph   Lymph is composed of blood plasma that filters out of the capillaries, lymphocytes, hormones, and many other substances, which are the products of cellular activity, such as water, digested nutrients, salts, oxygen, carbon dioxide, and urea. It is a continuous-forming process. Lymph fills the

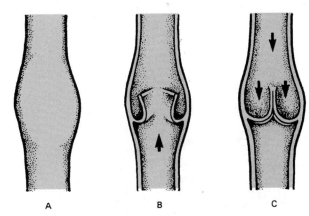

FIGURE 4-92 Vein valves (a) External view shows dilation at site of valve (b) Vein opened and valves opened (c) Valves closed to prevent backflow of blood

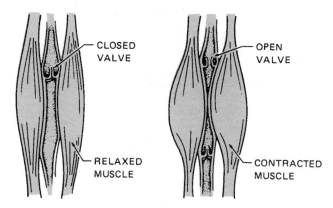

FIGURE 4-93 How muscles help move blood through internal viens

spaces between the cells and is also referred to as intercellular, or *interstitial, fluid.* Lymph acts as the "bridge" between cells and capillaries. Lymph is moved through the body primarily by contraction of the skeletal muscles. There is no pump like the heart to move lymph. Lymph vessels are constructed like veins, however, with valves to prevent the backflow of fluid.

Lymph Vessels
Vessels carrying lymph are located throughout the body, somewhat like veins. Lymphatic capillaries absorb fluid and other substances from the tissues and return it to the circulatory system, Figure 4-95. It is a one-way system only, however, from the cells toward the heart. There are no separate vessels bringing lymph to the cells.

The vast network of lymph capillaries joins to form small lymph vessels that in turn form larger vessels called *lymphatics.* Lymphatics eventually form two main ducts. The right lymphatic duct receives lymph from the right side of the head, the right arm, and the upper right trunk. The thoracic duct receives lymph from the rest of the body, Figure 4-96, page 166.

Lymph Nodes
Lymph nodes are small round or oval structures located usually in clusters along the lymph vessels at various places in the body. Lymph enters the nodes from four afferent lymph vessels, filters

through a mesh of sinuses, and leaves by way of a single efferent vessel. Lymphocytes, a type of white blood cell, are derived from stem cells in the bone marrow. They enter the bloodstream and go to the lymph tissue to "live." Their action is essential to the immune system of the body. When needed, they divide by mitosis, greatly increasing in number. Phagocytes, another type of white blood cell, can also be found in lymph nodes. The structure of the nodes and the cell's function purify the lymph by removing harmful substances, such as bacteria or malignant cells. The nodes increase and decrease in size in relation to the amount of material being filtered. In acute infections, they become swollen and tender due to the collection of cells gathered to destroy the invading substances. This condition is known as **adenitis.** With extensive involvement, the node may break down and an abscess will form.

Physicians palpate for nodes when patients have infectious conditions or when a malignancy is known or suspected. With malignancy, the cancer cells are abnormal and so are identified by the cells in the lymph node to be removed from the circulating fluid. As more cells accumulate, the node becomes enlarged and is therefore palpable. Early detection of lymph node involvement is critical to the prognosis of patients with cancer, for it is through the lymphatic system that a malignancy often **metastasizes** (spreads) to other sites. The extent of lymph node involvement is an important indicator of the ultimate prognosis of the patient.

The Spleen The spleen is an organ composed of lymphatic tissue, lying just beneath the left side of the diaphragm, in back of the upper portion of the stomach. The spleen produces lymphocytes, stores red blood cells, keeps the appropriate balance between cells and plasma in the blood, and removes and destroys worn-out red cells. The organ functions like a large lymph node. It is soft and elastic and varies in size according to the flow of blood through the organ. During an acute infection, it will become enlarged and tender. Patients with leukemia may have an enlarged, firm spleen that is palpable on examination. The spleen is filled with excess immature cells to be destroyed.

The Blood

Blood is the life-giving fluid of the body. It flows through the blood vessels transporting substances essential to the maintenance of life. The average adult has 8 to 10 pints of blood. A loss of 2 pints, or about 20%, is cause for concern. The blood carries oxygen from the lungs to the cells, nutrients from the digestive system to the cells, and cellular wastes from the cells to the appropriate organ for excretion. It picks up hormones excreted from endocrine glands and distributes them throughout the body to the appropriate receiving organ. Blood also delivers the minerals necessary for muscular contraction, heartbeat, stimulation of the respiratory system, and the homeostasis of cells. This vital substance is composed of only two main parts—the plasma and the cells—but each part has many essential components.

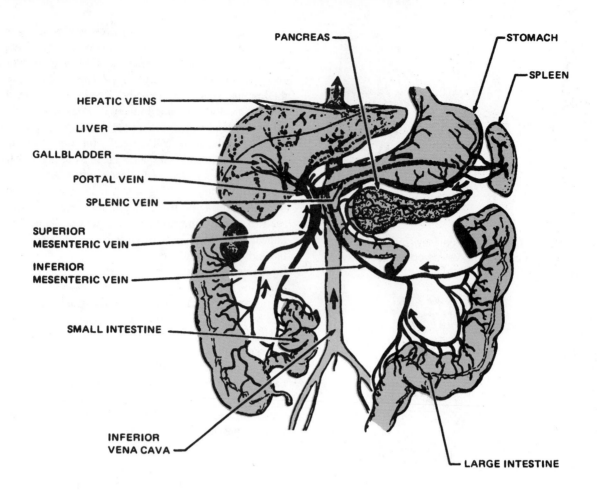

PANCREAS — STOMACH — SPLEEN

HEPATIC VEINS — LIVER — GALLBLADDER — PORTAL VEIN — SPLENIC VEIN — SUPERIOR MESENTERIC VEIN — INFERIOR MESENTERIC VEIN — SMALL INTESTINE — INFERIOR VENA CAVA — LARGE INTESTINE

FIGURE 4–94 Portal circulation

Plasma

Plasma is a straw-colored liquid that makes up a little over half the volume of blood. It is about 90% water, the remainder consisting of minerals, such as calcium, sodium, potassium, phosphorus, and bicarbonates. The minerals are commonly referred to as *electrolytes*. These elements are processed by the body from the foods that are eaten and play a major role in maintaining the acid–base balance of the blood.

Plasma contains other vital substances, such as vitamins, hormones, enzymes, nutrients absorbed from the digestive system (such as glucose, fatty acids, and amino acids). Oxygen, carbon dioxide, and other waste products from the cells are also carried in the plasma.

In addition, three important proteins are found in plasma: fibrinogen, which is necessary to clot blood; serum albumin, which aids in maintaining blood pressure by regulating the exchange of water between the cells and the blood; and serum globulin, which assists in the formation of antibodies. A substance called prothrombin is a type of globulin formed by the liver, with the aid of vitamin K. It plays an important role in the clotting of the blood.

Cells

The cellular portion of the blood can be divided into three types of cells: red, white, and platelets, Figure 4–97.

Red Blood Cells.

Erythrocytes (red blood cells) are biconcave disks with very thin centers to enable them to fold over if necessary to pass through a narrow opening. Red cells number about 25 trillion in the body or about 5 million to a cubic millimeter of blood. It is the red cells which give blood its color. A red blood cell lasts about 4 months. They are produced in the bone marrow at a rate of about a million a second, the same rate at which they wear out.

Erythrocytes obtain their color from **hemoglobin,** which is a combination of a protein and an iron pigment. It is hemoglobin that attracts and carries the oxygen and carbon dioxide in the blood. When hemoglobin is carrying a lot of oxygen it is bright red in color. As the oxygen is given up to the cells and exchanged for carbon dioxide, the color changes to the dark reddish blue that is visible in surface veins.

White Blood Cells.

White blood cells are called **leukocytes.** Leukocytes are present in the blood at approximately 5000 to 9000 per cubic millimeter, or about one white cell for every 600 to 700 red blood cells. White cells are about twice the size of red blood cells. Leukocytes play a vital role in defending the body against invasion, moving through capillary walls into the tissue fluid to chase down bacteria.

Leukocytes are divided into two major groups—granulocytes and agranulocytes—depending upon the presence of granules and certain staining characteristics.

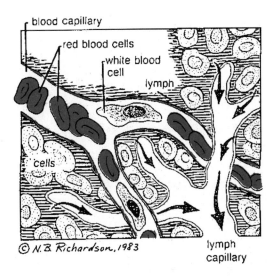

blood capillary

red blood cells

white blood cell

lymph

cells

© N.B. Richardson, 1983

lymph capillary

FIGURE 4–95 Lymph circulation (Copyright by Richardson. From Fong, *Body Structures and Functions*, 8th ed. Copyright 1993, Delmar Publishers Inc.)

Granulocytes are produced in red bone marrow and last for only a few days. There are three types. *Neutrophils* phagocytize (destroy) bacteria by surrounding, swallowing, and digesting them. *Eosinophils* are thought to consume the toxic substances in tissues since they are found in increasing numbers when the body has had a foreign protein injected or an allergic reaction or has been infected by a parasite. The third type, the *basophils,* are also thought to participate in phagocytosis since their numbers increase with chronic inflammation or during healing from an infection.

Agranulocytes are of two types: *lymphocytes,* which are produced by bone marrow and lymphoid tissues, such as the nodes and spleen; and *monocytes,* which are formed in the bone marrow. Lymphocytes primarily specialize in providing immunity for the body by attaching themselves to foreign bodies and destroying them, and by developing antibodies. The monocyte assists with phagocytosis. Some enlarge greatly when they enter tissue and become fixed.

When an inflammation occurs, white cells can divide and proliferate into capsule-like structures around foreign objects that cannot be digested, such as silica dust and carbon particles, or causative organisms of infections, such as tuberculosis. This action effectively walls off involved tissue in an attempt to contain the foreign material or prevent the spread of disease. The evidence of a phagocytic reaction to invading bacteria or a foreign object is the presence of **exudate** (pus). Exudate is composed of lymph, bacteria, and dead white cells.

Platelets. The third kind of cell is the **platelet.** These cells are the smallest of the three and are present in the blood at a rate of 200,000 to 400,000 per cubic millimeter. They are also formed in the bone marrow from cell fragments.

Platelets function in the life-saving process of clotting blood. When a blood vessel is cut or damaged it is believed that the rough surface may catch or attract platelets to the area. This reaction occurs only when there is an incidence of bleed-

ing; otherwise the clotting process would stop circulation within the blood vessels. When there is a cut, platelets pile up at the site to form a small mass. Once attached firmly to the damaged area, they release the chemical, serotonin, which causes the blood vessel to spasm, resulting in a narrowing of the vessel and a decrease in blood loss until the clot can be formed, Figure 4–98. At the same time, platelets and injured tissues release thromboplastin, which triggers the clotting process to begin. The thromboplastin cooperates with calcium ions and other blood-clotting factors in the blood, to convert prothrombin (present in plasma) into thrombin. The thrombin acts on another protein in the plasma called fibrinogen. This reaction results in the formation of fibrin, tiny threads which form a network of fine mesh fibers over the cut. This net begins to catch the red blood cells, other platelets, and plasma, forming the clot. It should be remembered that unless the cut blood vessel is small, a clot may not be able to form. The force of the flow of blood will wash away the body's efforts to form fibrin nets, and therefore will be unable to collect the ingredients of the clot. Clotting can be assisted by applying pressure over the area to stop the blood flow until a clot can form. When major vessels are cut, it may be necessary to surgically close the opening with sutures to control the bleeding. Fortunately, internal bleeding vessels can also undergo the clotting process. Complications can occur from the clotted mass, especially if the clot or its fragments break loose and enter the circulation before the body's natural "housekeeping" function can gradually remove it from the blood vessel.

Bleeding Time The length of time required for blood to clot from an induced puncture wound is useful information when preparing a patient for a surgical procedure or evaluating the effects of certain disorders or medications. The normal range of bleeding time for the template puncture method is from 2 to 8 minutes. The length of time varies with the method used.

Blood Types There are four types of blood: A, B, AB, and O. The type of blood a person has depends on the presence of a protein factor called agglutinogen, or antigen on the surface of the red blood cell. Type A blood has an A agglutinogen, type B has a B agglutinogen, type AB has both agglutinogens, and type O has neither, Figure 4–99.

Similarly, a protein is present in blood plasma known as agglutinin, or antibody. Type A blood has a b agglutinin, type B blood has an a agglutinin, type AB has no agglutinins, and type O has both a and b.

The term *agglutinate* refers to the process of clumping, or sticking together. Blood clumps and forms clots in the blood vessels if agglutinins and agglutinogens of the same type are mixed together. This reaction can be fatal. Therefore, it is extremely important to determine the blood types of both the recipient and the donor when blood **transfusions** are required. A laboratory test known as type and **cross-match** is necessary to make this determination prior to the administration of either whole blood or packed cell transfusions. Not only is the blood typed, but it is also mixed and observed to ensure that aggluti-

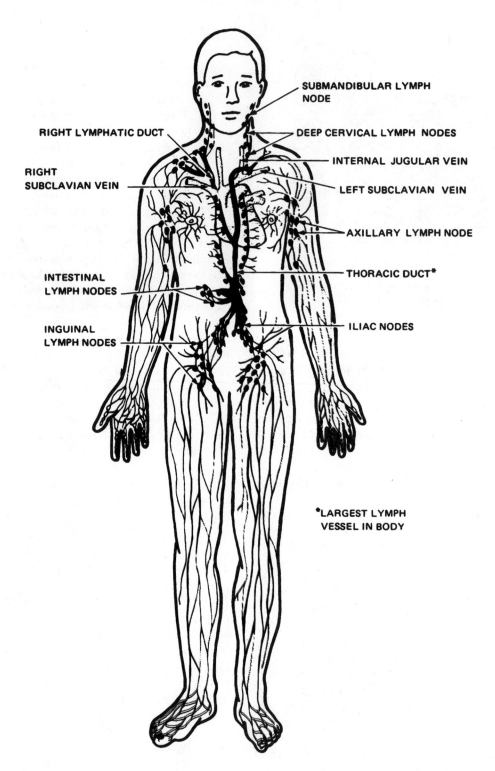

FIGURE 4–96 Lymphatic system

nation does not occur. Cross-matching will also detect the presence of subtypes and an agglutinogen known as H.

Rh Factor
Red blood cells may have another factor known as the **Rh factor.** It is an antigen that was first detected in the blood of a Rhesus monkey, therefore the name Rh. If the red cell has the factor it is said to be Rh positive, or Rh+. If the

factor is absent, then the blood is said to be Rh negative, or Rh−. Blood must also be checked for the presence of this antigen when a transfusion is to be given. If an Rh negative person receives Rh positive blood, the antigen is "foreign" to the recipient's bloodstream. Within 2 weeks, the individual will produce antibodies in response to this invasion of a foreign substance. Usually no problems occur unless, at a later

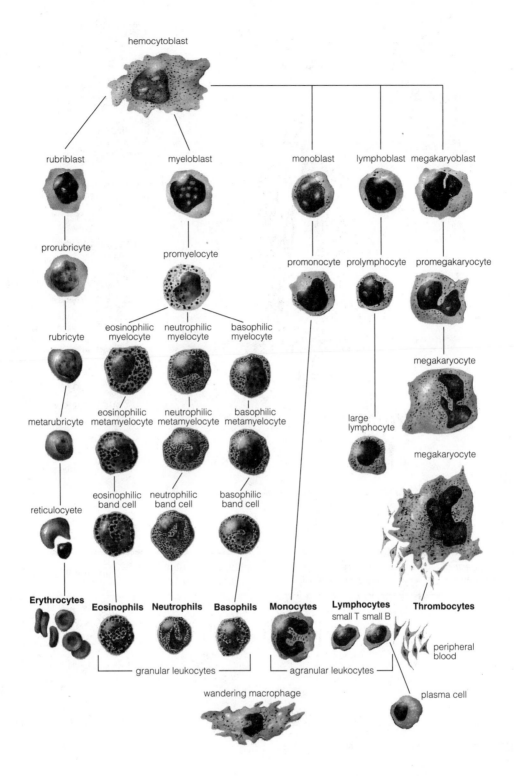

hemocytoblast

rubriblast

prorubricyte

rubricyte

metarubricyte

reticulocyete

Erythrocytes

myeloblast

promyelocyte

eosinophilic neutrophilic basophilic
myelocyte myelocyte myelocyte

eosinophilic neutrophilic basophilic
metamyelocyte metamyelocyte metamyelocyte

eosinophilic neutrophilic basophilic
band cell band cell band cell

Eosinophils **Neutrophils** **Basophils**

— granular leukocytes —

wandering macrophage

monoblast lymphoblast megakaryoblast

promonocyte prolymphocyte promegakaryocyte

megakaryocyte

large
lymphocyte

megakaryocyte

Monocytes **Lymphocytes** **Thrombocytes**
small T small B

— agranular leukocytes —

peripheral
blood

plasma cell

FIGURE 4–97   Types of blood cells (Adapted from Smith, *Medical Terminology, A Programmed Text*, 6th ed. Copyright 1991, Delmar Publishers.)

date, the person receives another Rh positive transfusion. This time the developed antibodies will react to the antigen being received and may cause serious complications.

It should be noted that persons who are Rh positive can receive either Rh positive or Rh negative blood, provided it is properly typed and cross-matched, because they already have the factor, and the Rh negative blood is without the antigen.

When the two blood samples can mix without evidence of any clumping and the Rh factor is appropriate, the blood is said to be **compatible.**

The Rh factor is also of concern with pregnancy. If a female who is Rh negative becomes pregnant with an Rh positive baby, a few positive cells may enter the mother's blood at delivery and cause the production of antibodies. The firstborn

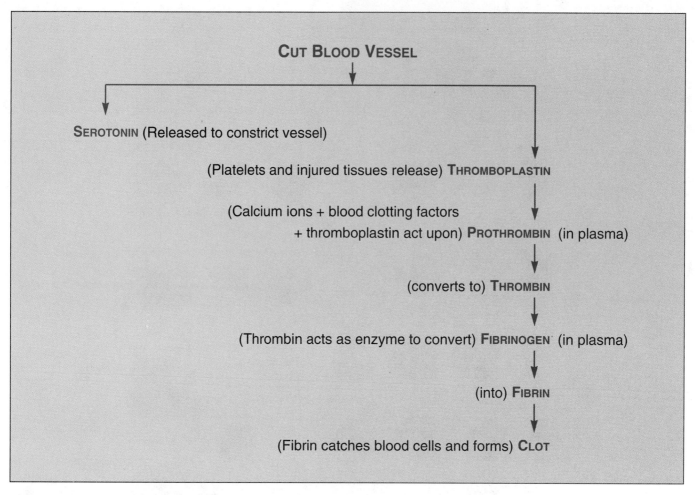

FIGURE 4–98 Process of blood clot formation

Blood Type	Percent of Population	Antigen/Agglutinogen on Red Blood Cells	Antibody/Agglutinin in Plasma	Can Receive	Can Donate To
A	41%	A	Anti-b	A or O only	A or AB only
B	12%	B	Anti-a	B or O only	B or AB only
AB	3%	A and B	none	A, B, AB, O Universal recipient	AB only
O	44%	None	Anti-a and b	O only	A, B, AB, O Universal donor

FIGURE 4–99 Blood types

will not be affected, but later pregnancies, if Rh positive, may be affected by the antibodies which have been developed. These antibodies slowly filter into the fetal circulation and destroy the Rh positive red cells, making the newborn profoundly anemic and jaundiced. The situation must be treated vigorously, with steps taken to alter the infant's blood.

This potentially fatal situation can be avoided by determining the Rh factor of the mother. If she is negative, then the father's factor must be determined before the first child is born. At the time of delivery, if the baby is positive, the Rh negative mother is given an injection of an Rh(D) immune human globulin, which prohibits the production of antibodies against the baby's Rh positive blood. Only when the mother is negative and the fetus positive is there cause for concern. If the father also happens to be negative, there is no need to treat for the antibodies unless the mother could have, at some previous time, received an Rh positive blood transfusion.

In the next unit on the immune system, we will take a

deeper look into the function of leukocytes and how they maintain our immunity. We will also learn more about the antigen–antibody process.

Cardiovascular Tests

Many sophisticated tests can be performed on the circulatory system, but most of them are best studied at a more advanced level. A few of the more frequently encountered **cardiovascular** diagnostic procedures will be discussed briefly here. Common studies done on blood are discussed in Chapter 7.

■ Arteriograph (angiograph)—a radiological examination of an artery or arteries after injecting a contrast medium, usually into the femoral artery. The test is used to indicate the status of blood flow, collateral circulation, malformed vessels, an aneurysm, or the presence of **hemorrhage.**

■ Cardiac catherization—A catheter to the right side of the heart is inserted into a vein at the antecubital space of the right arm. A catheter to the left side of the heart is inserted into the brachial artery at the left antecubital space. The femoral artery or vein may also be used. The catheter is passed through the blood vessels until it reaches the heart. When it is determined, by fluoroscopy, that the catheter is properly positioned, a contrast medium is injected to permit visualization of the heart's activity. The heart's chambers and valves and the coronary arteries or the pulmonary artery may be viewed, depending on the side being catheterized. The procedure can also be used to measure blood pressure within the pulmonary artery and some portions of the heart.

■ Doppler ultrasonography—Sound waves are transmitted through the skin and are reflected by the cells in the blood moving through the blood vessels, Figure 4–100. This diagnostic tool can evaluate the major blood vessels of the body to determine deep vein **thrombosis** (DVT), peripheral arterial **aneurysms,** and occluded carotid arteries.

■ Echocardiograph—A test using ultrahigh-frequency sound waves directed through the chest wall into the heart. The waves reflect from the heart through a mechanical device to produce a record of the structures of the heart and its chambers. The test evaluates cardiac function and structure and can reveal valve irregularities, defects in the interior walls, and the presence of fluid between the layers of the pericardium.

■ Electrocardiograph (ECG)—This test is also called EKG, usually when referred to verbally; it can be written in either form. It is perhaps the most common tool used to evaluate heart performance. The ECG is a graphic recording of the electrical activity of the heart. It identifies rhythm, abnormalities in conduction, and electrolyte imbalance. The graph is useful in documenting diagnosis and provides a method of measuring progression of cardiac disease conditions. The ECG also helps evaluate the effectiveness of an artificial pacemaker and cardiac medications.

The test may be taken while the patient is lying in a comfortable position, or in an exercise mode, such as bicy-

cling or walking a treadmill. The exercise mode measures the effects of controlled physical stress and is referred to as a *stress ECG.* Frequently, abnormalities of cardiac action are more evident upon exertion.

Another type of ECG is called the **Holter monitor,** or **ambulatory** (walking) ECG. The ECG electrodes are attached to the patient's chest wall and a portable cassette recorder (monitor) is placed in a belt about the waist. For a 24-hour period the patient's heart action is recorded, and a diary is kept of daily activities and any associated symptoms. At the end of the test, the recording is analyzed by computer and a report is printed. This type of test is most beneficial for symptoms which occur irregularly or to evaluate the status of recovering cardiac patients. Another version permits the patient to activate the recording device only when experiencing symptoms. This patient-activated monitor can be worn for several days. (See Chapter 8.)

■ **MUGA scan**—MUGA is an acronym for MUltiple Gated Acquisition; it is a test to evaluate the condition of the myocardium of the heart. The test can be done in a resting or exercise mode. Isotopes are injected intravenously and are taken up by the myocardium. The scintillation camera records the motion of the heart. The test permits measurement of ventricular contractions to evaluate the strength of the heart wall. Patients who receive a chemotherapeutic drug that has cardiac toxicity side effects are monitored periodically by MUGA scans due to the drug's tendency to damage the myocardium.

■ Stress thallium ECG—A test to evaluate myocardial blood flow and the condition of the cells. The ECG electrodes are attached to the patient before performing the stress test on either a treadmill or a bicycle. The blood pressure and pulse rate are carefully monitored. When the patient reaches peak

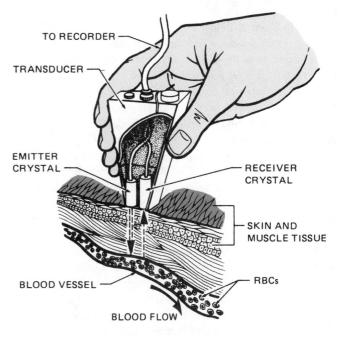

HOW THE DOPPLER PROBE WORKS

TO RECORDER

TRANSDUCER

EMITTER CRYSTAL

RECEIVER CRYSTAL

SKIN AND MUSCLE TISSUE

BLOOD VESSEL

RBCs

BLOOD FLOW

FIGURE 4–100 Doppler ultrasound

stress, the thallium is injected intravenously into the anticubital vein and the exercise continued for an additional minute to ensure circulation of the isotope to the heart. The ECG electrodes are removed, and within 3 to 5 minutes the patient is positioned under the scintillation camera. The scanner records the amount of thallium uptake by the heart over the next several minutes. Areas of the heart with normal blood supply and healthy cells rapidly take up the isotope. Areas of poor blood flow or damaged cells do not take up the material and appear as dark spots on the scan; these are known as cold spots.

The test is indicated for assessing myocardial condition, demonstrating the location and extent of a **myocardial infarction (MI),** diagnosing coronary artery disease, and determining the effectiveness of artery grafts and angioplasty procedures.

■ Venogram—A radiographic examination using a contrast medium to determine the condition of the deep veins of the legs. It is especially useful in determining the presence of deep vein thrombosis (DVT), which may occlude the vein systems and lead to pulmonary embolism, a potentially lethal situation. DVT may result from vein injury, prolonged bed rest, surgery, childbirth, irregularity in the coagulation process, and the use of oral contraceptives.

Diseases and Disorders ....

Anemia.   This term indicates that certain elements are lacking in the blood. There are various types of **anemias.** The most common form of anemia is iron deficiency anemia, or the presence of an inadequate supply of iron to form normal red blood cells. When the body's supply of iron decreases, so does the number of red blood cells and as a result, the hemoglobin. This reduces the body's ability to carry oxygen to the cells and causes symptoms of fatigue, listlessness, pallor, inability to concentrate, and difficulty in breathing on exertion. Iron deficiency anemia develops from an inadequate dietary intake of iron or inability of the body to absorb iron, as the result of diarrhea, partial or total removal of the stomach, or certain diseases. It can also be caused by intestinal bleeding, heavy menstruation, colon cancer, or bleeding ulcers. It is most common among premature infants, children, adolescents (especially girls), and women before menopause. Iron deficiency anemia can be treated with oral iron preparations, once the cause is determined. Another form of anemia is known as aplastic. It is a disease resulting from injury or destruction of the blood cell formation function of the bone marrow. This disease generally produces a fatal bleeding episode or a systemic infection, often as a result of infectious hepatitis.

Anemia is a term that is used to describe conditions of low red blood cell count occurring over extended periods of time. Low red blood cell count can also occur, however, following an acute blood loss and is referred to by some as acute blood loss anemia. In this instance, there is a sudden loss of red blood cells and therefore hemoglobin and iron. The rapid loss of blood volume can be fatal. Acute blood loss can result from

severe trauma, the inability to coagulate the blood, ruptured gastric or intestinal ulcers, postoperative bleeding, postpartum (after birth) hemorrhage, or a ruptured aneurysm. A loss of 20% to 30% of blood volume causes circulatory insufficiency with symptoms of shock; restlessness; low blood pressure; rapid pulse; perspiration; and cool, clammy skin. With a loss greater than 30%, the circulatory system may fail and be followed by shock and then coma. Blood loss beyond 40% is life-threatening, and the patient will die unless blood volume is immediately replaced.

Aneurysm.   The ballooning out of the wall of an artery is due to a weakening of the wall structure. Often an aneurysm is associated with **atherosclerosis** or **arteriosclerosis** and the resulting hypertension. A slight break or weakness in the muscular layer of an artery allows the pressure of the blood to push the walls of the blood vessel out, Figure 4–101. The larger the bulge, the thinner the arterial wall becomes. Eventually, the wall gives way, and a hemorrhage occurs. The extent of the bleeding and its effects on the body depend to a great extent on the location of the aneurysm and the size of the involved blood vessel.

Aneurysms are found primarily in cerebral arteries, the thoracic or abdominal section of the aorta, and the femoral and popliteal arteries of the leg. Some aneurysms are without symptoms and are discovered by accident or an X ray.

A cerebral aneurysm, depending on its location, may rupture and cause bleeding within the subarachnoid space, or an artery within the brain tissue itself may rupture. If the hemorrhage is not too massive, the blood clots. Later the body will slowly reabsorb the blood clots and function will return. Hemorrhage may be fatal, however, due to increased intracranial pressure from the blood, which compresses and damages brain tissue. Remember, the skull is a solid structure that does not stretch; therefore when bleeding occurs the delicate tissues of the brain are displaced and damaged. Cerebral aneurysms are graded from I to V depending on the amount of bleeding. Rebleeding after 7 to 10 days is not uncommon. When the initial blood has clotted, the body resumes its normal function of removing clotted material, which may lead to a renewed and often fatal recurrence.

Aneurysms of the aorta occur due to the great pressure in the artery. Rupture of the aorta is usually fatal. If the thoracic aneurysm begins by "splitting" of the wall, the person may experience a tearing or ripping sensation accompanied by chest pain, pallor, rapid pulse, shortness of breath, loss of pulses below the neck, and other symptoms. Surgery can be accomplished to remove the damaged segment of the aorta and replace it with a Dacron or Teflon blood vessel graft.

An abdominal aneurysm is usually without symptoms but is detectable on palpation as a pulsating mass in an area around the umbilicus (navel). If it ruptures, the patient may experience pain similar to that of kidney spasms. About 20% of such patients die immediately; however, if the bleeding is in the retroperitoneal space (behind the peritoneal lining of the abdomen) the limited space puts pressure on the tear as it fills with blood, closing off the opening. An abdominal aneurysm

(a) Saccular – unilateral pouchlike bulge

(b) Fusiform – a spindle-shaped bulge
of the entire artery wall

FIGURE 4–101 Types of aneurysms

is repaired like an aneurysm of the thoracic aorta. In addition, an external Dacron prosthesis (artificial part) may be applied around the aneurysm and sutured into place to support the weakened wall.

Aneurysms in the lower extremities may interfere with circulation and cause severe **ischemia** (lack of blood) and gangrene (tissue death), which may require amputation of an affected portion or the total extremity.

Angina ....

This heart condition causes severe chest pain that radiates down the inner surface of the left arm, usually associated with emotional stress or physical exertion. The pain is believed to be caused by a spasm of one or more coronary arteries, which results in ischemia to a portion of the heart muscle. The episode may last from a few seconds to several minutes. Symptoms, in addition to the pain, include irregular heart rate, lowered blood pressure, anxiety, and perspiration. The treatment consists of nitroglycerin, in a tablet form, placed under the tongue or applied to the body in a paste form. The nitroglycerin dilates the constricted artery or arteries to permit the flow of blood to the heart tissue. When **angina** pain persists after 10 minutes and the use of three sublingual tablets, the patient should go directly to the nearest hospital emergency room.

The patient must be instructed to have nitroglycerin available at all times. Tablets must be kept in a dark, tightly closed bottle, without cotton, and be protected from heat and sunlight. Tablets over 3 months old should be discarded. Nitroglycerin has recently been produced in a patch form to permit prolonged release of the drug in measurable doses. It is also available as an oral spray.

Arrest (Cardiac). This is complete, sudden cessation of heart action. The condition is rapidly fatal, producing irreversible brain damage after 5 minutes. It is believed to result from a failure in the body's ability to transport calcium, which interferes with its electrical and mechanical functions. It is associated with severe lack of blood to the myocardium. Cardiac arrest can also be caused by heart failure, electrical shock, fibrillation, drowning, anesthetics, respiratory failure, and severe electrolyte imbalances.

Arrest is treated initially by external cardiac massage (CPR, or cardiopulmonary resuscitation technique), then supplemented by defibrillation, IV drug therapy, and ventilation procedures. Death is certain if function cannot be restored quickly.

Arrhythmia. This term is used to identify any abnormal changes in heart rhythm. Arrhythmias vary in severity from mild to life-threatening, as with fibrillation. They are classified according to the origin of the irregularity; for example, PVC or atrial flutter. The more the heart action is affected, the greater the consequences on the cardiac output and the blood pressure, which in turn determines the clinical significance.

Arteriosclerosis. A "hardening" of the arteries and arterioles is caused by changes in their structural walls. The muscular and elastic tissue is gradually replaced by fibrous tissue and calcification. Since the vessels are no longer capable of expanding and recoiling with each heartbeat, the heart must exert more pressure on the blood to pump it through the more rigid vessels. Arteriosclerosis results in high blood pressure and may lead to an aneurysm and cerebral hemorrhage.

Atherosclerosis. This condition is characterized by the deposit of fatty material along the linings of the arteries, Figure 4–102. As the material builds up, the opening of the artery may become partially or totally closed, thereby reducing or eliminating the flow of blood to the area. Atherosclerosis can also result in elevated blood pressure, but the greatest danger results from the atherosclerotic plaque deposits breaking loose and circulating through the bloodstream as emboli.

Athletic Heart Syndrome. This is a series of cardiac changes resulting from strenuous exercise. Primarily the heart enlarges (cardiomegaly), particularly the ventricles, because of its adaptive ability to meet the body's need for increased output. Since the heart is a muscle, it reacts just as the biceps do to physical endurance training. This syndrome is increasing due to the emphasis on physical fitness.

The athletic heart usually produces no symptoms except perhaps pounding or irregularity after strenuous activity. Bradycardia of 40 beats per minute is common and may be considered "normal" due to the heart's increased efficiency upon contraction.

Carditis. Literally, inflammation of the heart, the term is usually used with one of three prefixes that define the portion of the heart that is involved. The inflammation results from an infectious process caused by a viral, fungal, or bacterial invasion. Other causes vary with the form of inflammation, as follows.

■ *Pericarditis*—An inflammation of the pericardium, the fibroserous tissue sac which covers the heart. It may result in a purulent or bloody exudate forming within the sac, or the tissue may become thickened and fibrous, constricting the filling action of the heart. Pericarditis can follow injury to the heart, an infarction, or cardiac surgery.

DEPOSITS OF
LIPIDS AND
FATTY SUBSTANCES

NORMAL
ARTERY

LESS
DISTENSIBLE

BLOCKED
LUMEN

FIGURE 4–102   Atherosclerosis of an artery

Acute pericarditis typically causes sharp, sudden pain that begins at the sternum and radiates across the back to the shoulders and arms. It is similar to pleurisy, becoming more intense on inspiration but decreasing when sitting upright and leaning forward. A very serious condition will occur if the collection of fluid within the pericardium is rapid. Pressure within the sac prevents ventricular filling during diastole, thereby severely decreasing cardiac output and resulting in pallor, hypotension, and eventually cardiovascular collapse and death. Emergency treatment to remove the fluid by needle aspiration or surgical incision will result in a dramatic improvement.

Pericarditis that causes a gradual fluid accumulation allows time for the pericardium to stretch, often to hold 1 to 2 liters (L) of fluid. Chronic pericarditis that results in constriction or recurrent collection of fluid may necessitate partial removal of the pericardium to allow escape of the fluid or, if constriction, a total pericardectomy (removal of the pericardium).

Myocarditis—An inflammation of the myocardium (heart muscle). It can occur in both acute and chronic forms. Symptoms produced are generally nonspecific, such as fatigue, palpitations, fever, and dyspnea. It is usually an uncomplicated disease and is self-limiting in nature. Normally, it is associated with a recent upper respiratory infection (URI) and fever. Myocarditis may produce mild chest soreness and a feeling of pressure but not the anginal type of pain. Occasionally, myocarditis may initiate a degenerative process of the tiny fibrils (small fibers) in the muscular tissue. This may result in heart failure, enlargement, and arrhythmia. Myocarditis is treated with antibiotics, bed rest, and appropriate measures for complications that may develop.

Endocarditis—Infection of the endocardial lining, heart valves, tissue adjoining artificial valves, or the blood vessel linings. The infecting organism in acute endocarditis is usually a streptococcus, staphylococcus, or pneumococcus. The gonococcus is also capable of causing endocarditis. Intra-

venous drug abuse may lead to infections from staph or fungi normally present on the skin surface. A subacute form may affect persons with valve or other cardiac lesions that may be acquired or congenital. In the infectious process, fibrin and platelets collect where the invading circulating organisms have produced wartlike vegetations on the valves and often the surrounding structures. The vegetative growths may cause serious complications if they embolize to the spleen, kidneys, or lungs.

If endocarditis is left untreated it usually results in death. Recovery is improved to 70% with proper treatment. When severe valve damage occurs, resulting complications may include insufficient cardiac action and congestive failure due to improper valve function. Damaged valves can be surgically removed with open heart surgery and replaced with artificial valves. If the infection involves an artificial valve, surgery to replace the prosthesis will be required.

Cerebrovascular Accident (CVA).   A condition commonly known as a stroke, CVA is the sudden impairment of the flow of blood to the brain, thereby diminishing or interrupting the supply of oxygen and causing serious damage or destruction of brain tissue. A **cerebrovascular accident** is the result of high blood pressure, which ruptures an artery; artherosclerosis, which occludes an artery; or thrombosis (a blood clot), which interrupts the flow of blood. When a large enough area is involved, death will result.

CVAs are classified according to their course of progression. **Transient ischemic attacks (TIAs)** are small, temporary interruptions of blood flow. A progressive stroke is one which is in progress, such as with a thrombosis. It begins with some neurological symptoms and worsens within a day or two. A complete stroke is at its maximum when it occurs. Approximately one-half of CVA patients die as a result of the condition.

Symptoms vary with the area of the brain that is involved. CVAs involving posterior cerebral arteries affect the vision and often result in coma. Anterior artery involvement results in confusion, weakness, loss of coordination, personality changes, and numbness, especially in the legs. If the CVA occurs in the right hemisphere of the brain, symptoms are produced on the left side of the body, and if in the left hemisphere, on the right side. A CVA may leave the patient with many varied symptoms, which may include slurred speech, amnesia, dizziness, paralysis (one extremity, one side, or total), inability to speak, coma, double vision, incontinence (inability to control bladder and bowels), and rigidity.

Congestive Heart Failure (CHF).   This group of cardiac dysfunctions results in poor performance of the heart with related congestion of the circulatory system. Usually the myocardium of the left ventricle is affected, often as a result of prolonged high blood pressure. **Congestive heart failure** can also be a complication of coronary artery disease or a result of a mechanical disorder involving the heart's valvular functions.

With left-sided heart failure, cardiac output is decreased due to poor emptying of the ventricle. The left atrium continues to force blood into the ventricle, however, resulting in increased pressure and volume within the ventricle. As this backup continues, the left atrium becomes congested, backing up blood into the pulmonary veins and then the pulmonary capillary beds. The fluid in the capillaries fills the alveolar spaces, resulting in pulmonary edema. There is a lack of oxygen exchange, and a decrease in the emptying capability of the right ventricle. Symptoms of left-sided failure are shortness of breath, inability to breathe while lying down, periods of gasping for air, weak and rapid pulse, cool and clammy skin, and an ashen gray or cyanotic skin coloring. Often a cough produces pink, frothy sputum.

Right-sided heart failure is usually a result of failure on the left side. It can occur however, in isolation as a result of pulmonary disease, a malfunctioning tricuspid valve, or a congenital defect. With right-sided failure, returning blood flow becomes congested in the systemic circulation, eventually causing fluid to enter the interstitial spaces. Initially, the fluid can be viewed as edema in the lower extremities, but as the failure continues edema is present in the upper extremities and in various organs throughout the system. Right-sided failure symptoms include swelling of the extremities, enlarged liver and spleen, and ascites (fluid in the abdominal cavity) due to filtration from portal circulation venous pressure.

Heart failure is extremely serious. Treatment involves the use of drugs to quickly increase cardiac output and remove congested fluids. Arterial vasodilators increase the efficiency of heart action. Bed rest is enforced and antiembolism stockings are used to prevent thromboembolism due to venous stasis. Continued treatment involves the use of cardiac drugs, frequent periods of rest, the use of elastic support stockings, skin care of the lower extremities, and dietary adjustments to reduce sodium intake and ensure proper nutrition.

Coronary Artery Disease. This disease of the arteries that surround the heart, carrying oxygen and nutrients to the myocardium, characteristically results from atherosclerosis, which narrows the vessel openings, thereby reducing the volume of blood flow to that portion of the heart muscle served

by the arterial branch. Consequent lack of oxygen causes the typical symptoms of angina: tightness of the chest and crushing substernal chest pains radiating to the left arm, neck, and shoulder blades. Other symptoms may be nausea, vomiting, fainting, and perspiring. When angina pain persists, it suggests an infarction.

Coronary artery disease may be diagnosed by the ECG during an attack or during a treadmill or exercise bicycle test. An angiograph, also called an arteriograph, allows visualization by X-ray examination of the arteries following injection of a contrast medium into an artery.

Narrowed, clogged arteries can be treated by three methods. First is the use of nitrates to dilate the vessel. Nitroglycerin in tablet form is placed under the tongue or can be applied in an ointment form to the skin surface. Second, an **angioplasty** can be performed during catheterization of the heart. A balloon-like device is inflated to compress the fatty deposits against the arterial walls, thereby opening the constricted vessel, Figure 4–103. A third method is coronary bypass surgery. This entails bypassing clogged arteries by redirecting blood through vein grafts surgically transplanted from the legs to the heart's surface.

Coronary artery disease is best treated by prevention, which includes weight control; a diet low in salt, fats, and cholesterol; regular active exercise; reduction of stress; and refraining from smoking.

Embolism. An embolus is defined as foreign matter that enters and circulates in the bloodstream. Emboli (more than one) can result from various situations. A thrombus that forms within a blood vessel becomes an embolus when it breaks loose and begins to circulate. When the embolus obstructs a blood vessel it is called an **embolism.** An embolus can also result from air introduced into a blood vessel. An infection may produce a circulating clump of exudate, as discussed under endocarditis. Skeletal fractures are known to cause the formation of fat emboli. One theory holds that minute fat globules from the

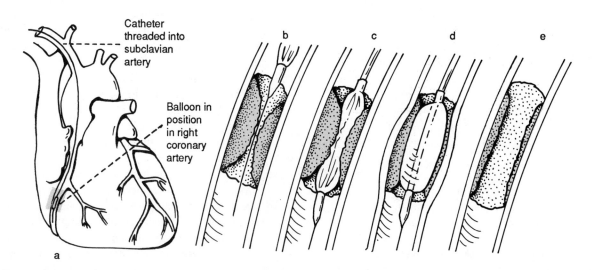

FIGURE 4–103 Balloon angioplasty (From Burke, *Human Anatomy and Physiology in Health and Disease*, 3d ed. Copyright 1992, Delmar Publishers Inc.)

bone marrow enter the damaged blood vessels at the fracture site. The greatest danger of fat emboli is that they may circulate to the capillary beds in the lungs and block the alveolar exchange, resulting in an insufficient supply of oxygen.

An embolus of any type is potentially lethal if the circulating mass is of adequate size to obstruct the blood supply to a significant portion of an organ. The resulting **infarction** (interference with circulation) is especially rapid when it occurs within a major pulmonary artery or in one of the coronary arteries, and it can prove fatal. Infarction of a kidney, the spleen, or the brain will produce symptoms related to the degree of tissue damage. If a nonvital organ is extensively destroyed, surgical removal may be indicated.

Hypertension. In this condition, blood pressure is consistently elevated above 140/90 for persons under age 50 and 150/90 for those over 50. The severity can be gauged by the diastolic pressure, or the least amount of pressure present during the resting phase of the heartbeat. Mild **hypertension** diastole is about 100 mm Hg, moderate is 110, and severe is over 120 mm Hg.

Hypertension may be classified as *essential* (unknown cause) or *secondary* (resulting from another disease or disorder). Essential hypertension is correlated with family history, race (higher among blacks), obesity, stress, a diet high in saturated fats and salt, oral contraceptives, and aging.

Secondary hypertension may be the result of kidney disease; thyroid, pituitary or parathyroid dysfunction; or neurological disorders that interfere with blood pressure regulation. Treatment of the primary cause will reduce the blood pressure.

Hypertension may also be classified as *benign* or *malignant*. In the benign form, the pressure rises moderately over a fairly long period of time. Malignant hypertension is characterized by an accelerated, rapid, and severe increase, which may not respond to treatment.

Hypertension is the foremost contributing factor to CVAs, kidney damage, and various cardiac conditions. It is predictably more severe among individuals who smoke, because the nicotine in tobacco causes constriction of the blood vessels.

Treatment of hypertension is directed at reducing the elevated pressure and maintaining an acceptable level. It is of great importance to prevent complications of the disease. Treatment focuses on diet, the control of sodium (currently being questioned), the use of diuretics to encourage elimination of retained body fluids, and antihypertensive drugs to reduce vasoconstriction or increase kidney filtration or both. It is of the utmost importance that the patient maintain the treatment regimen, since hypertension is not curable, only treatable. Patients must be encouraged to continue with their medication even though they have no symptoms of hypertension. Compliance with dietary and drug therapy is the only means of preventing life-threatening complications.

Hypotension. Defined as blood pressure below the normal range, **hypotension** can result from an acute blood loss, heart failure, shock, kidney failure, thyroid disease, and certain other infectious conditions. Hypotension may become life-

threatening when the circulation of blood becomes impaired and the exchange of gases is inadequate. The treatment of hypotension is determined by the underlying cause. Options include transfusion and intravenous fluid replacement, cardiac stimulants, thyroid medication, and other appropriate drugs.

Leukemia. This is a malignant disease of the bone marrow (myelogenous) or lymphatic tissue (lymphocytic). **Leukemia** can be present in either an acute or chronic form. In the acute phase, a great number of immature white blood cells are produced in the bone marrow or lymph tissue. The excessive amount of white cells cause pressure and discomfort within the bones, swelling and pain in the lymph nodes, and greatly elevated white cell count in the blood. The earliest symptoms of the disease are fever, pallor, fatigue, swelling of lymphoid tissue (spleen, liver), and a tendency toward large bruises.

Even in the presence of great numbers of leukocytes and lymphocytes, the body has little defense against infection due to the immaturity of the cells. The major complication of leukemia is infection. The disease process may progress to produce bleeding within the brain and other vital organs. In acute leukemia, the onset is rapid and death occurs within a few months unless treated aggressively with chemotherapy. Acute lymphocytic leukemia is the form common in children. Typically it is approximately 30% into its course before it is diagnosed. Acute myelogenous leukemia is more common in adults. Both acute forms are ultimately fatal, but long-term remissions in the childhood form, and approximately 50% cures are now being reported.

Chronic leukemia differs from acute only in that its onset is more insidious (slow), and its course is more prolonged. The median survival rate is 3 to 4 years. Often the first symptoms are a general malaise (vague discomfort, feeling "bad") and weight loss. Anemia, fatigue, and greatly enlarged spleen and lymph nodes are typical symptoms. Chronic myelogenous leukemia is almost always associated with a chromosome irregularity known as the Philadelphia chromosome. Chronic myelogenous leukemia is characterized by two distinct phases: the chronic phase, which is insidious, lasting an average of 3 to 4 years; and the eventual acute phase, an immature cell crisis, lasting only a few weeks or months before death occurs.

Diagnosis can be confirmed initially by blood studies in addition to typical clinical findings. Differentiation of type and positive identification of acute or chronic forms is possible through cellular and chromosomal analysis of bone marrow aspirates. The bone marrow sample can be withdrawn through a large-gauge needle introduced into the sternum or preferably the posterior superior iliac spine.

Treatment varies with the type and form of leukemia. Systemic chemotherapy is used to destroy abnormal white cells and induce a remission so that more normal function of the bone marrow will occur. The side effects of the drugs are loss of hair, nausea, vomiting, gouty arthritis, and a number of other complications. Some success has been achieved with bone marrow transplants among siblings, particularly twins. This procedure is especially indicated in treatment of children and younger adults. Before the marrow is given, the patient is medicated with large doses of drugs to completely suppress the body's ability to react to foreign material. Total bone radiation treatments are used to induce marrow aplasia (lack of function) and aid in lowering the body's resistance to the transplant. Approximately 500 to 750 mL of bone marrow is removed from the pelvic bones of the donor. The marrow is processed and then given to the recipient intravenously. To prevent contact with any microorganisms, the patient is placed in a reverse isolation unit. The patient is in an extremely vulnerable state, and a prolonged hospital stay is inevitable. Barring complications, which are numerous, chances for recovery are good.

Murmur. The abnormal sound of blood flowing through a heart valve can be heard with a stethoscope and is known as a **murmur.** The murmur is named for the valve which is "leaking." The mitral valve is the one most frequently affected and the gurgling or swishing sound is called a mitral murmur. Murmurs are further identified as systolic or diastolic. This classification specifies whether the sound is heard during the contraction or relaxation phase of the heartbeat.

Valve damage that results in murmurs can be caused by rheumatic fever, an inflammatory disease which follows a streptococcal infection. The valves may become inflamed and in time thicken and develop scar tissue. Hence the valves lose their flexibility and no longer close completely.

Endocarditis is another condition that may lead to valve damage. As previously discussed, bacteria circulating through the heart collect on the valvular surfaces causing the growth of vegetation and resulting in ulceration and death of some tissue. In its damaged state, the valve is no longer capable of normal function. Preexisting valve damage from rheumatic fever, especially of the mitral valve, is quite common in endocarditis. Artificial valve replacement may be indicated to alleviate the problem.

Myocardial Infarction (MI). A complication of coronary artery disease that results from occlusion (partial or complete) of the artery causing myocardial tissue destruction. It is characterized by severe, crushing pain, which radiates through the chest to the neck and jaw and down the left arm. It is not relieved by rest, as with angina, and is accompanied by nausea, perspiration, a change in blood pressure, hypo- or hypertension, and dyspnea. MIs are one of the leading causes of death in the United States. Mortality is high when treatment is delayed; approximately 50% of patients die within an hour after symptoms develop.

Predisposing factors include sedentary life-style, stressful occupation, obesity, cigarette smoking, hypertension, aging, positive family history, and elevated levels of cholesterol and triglycerides in the blood. An attack can often be precipitated by a heavy meal, physical exertion, or exposure to cold weather.

Treatment of MI is directed at relieving the pain with strong analgesic drugs, such as meperidine (Demerol) or morphine and administering extra oxygen to maintain an adequate supply to the tissues. It is important to prevent complications. Heart rhythm must be stabilized to prevent arrhythmia, which can lead to con-

gestive heart failure. Complete bed rest must be enforced to decrease cardiac workload and a possible additional infarction. **Anticoagulant** drugs are given to reduce the tendency to develop a thromboembolism.

Severe complications may occur in the damaged ventricular area in addition to the systemic threat of embolism and heart failure. Unusual and potentially lethal conditions may develop. The ventricular septum may rupture, causing a circulatory defect in which blood flows between the ventricles. The ventricular wall may weaken due to necrosis following infarction. The wall may develop an aneurysm, leading to a ventricular rupture.

The patient who survives an MI will be faced with a lengthy recovery period. Life-styles may need to be altered and dietary and smoking habits changed. An exercise rehabilitation program must be initiated and adhered to, to promote optimum recovery and maintenance of a healthy state.

Phlebitis. This localized inflammation of a vein causes an alteration in the epithelial lining, which is predisposing to the formation of a thrombus. **Phlebitis** can occur in deep or superficial veins (see thrombophlebitis).

Sickle Cell Anemia. This is a congenital anemia occurring primarily among blacks, about 1 in 10 of whom carry the abnormal gene. When two carriers have children, there is a 25% chance that each child will have the disease. When two persons with the disease **sickle cell** anemia have children, all children will have the disease. If only one has the disease and the other is normal, all children will be carriers of the trait.

Sickle cell anemia is characterized by red blood cells with a hemoglobin defect in their molecular structure that causes the cells to become sickle-shaped. Cells of this shape cannot pass easily through blood vessels and tend to interfere with circulation.

Symptoms are tachycardia, cardiomegaly, cardiac murmurs, chronic fatigue, unexplained dyspnea, chest pain, enlarged liver, jaundice, pallor, swollen joints, aching bones, and leg ulcers. These symptoms begin after about 6 months of age, when the protective excess amounts of hemoglobin present at birth are exhausted.

The most common feature of the disease is a painful crisis, which usually appears first at about age 5. Sickled red blood cells become tangled, causing blood vessel obstruction and a lack of oxygen to the tissues, with possible destruction of the involved area. This tissue infarction causes severe pain to the affected area. Usual sites are the lungs, liver, bones, and spleen. The spleen, particularly, is affected so frequently that the resulting damage and scarring cause it to shrink and cease functioning. A crisis usually lasts from 4 days to several weeks and recurs cyclically.

Diagnosis can be made from a positive family history and the typical clinical features. It is confirmed by a blood smear that shows the sickled cell structure. At present, research has failed to discover a means to prevent the sickling alteration. Treatment focuses on alleviating the symptoms of the disease and on transfusions with packed red cells when an aplastic crisis occurs (depression of bone marrow activity and destruction of RBCs).

The disease produces long-term complications, such as delayed puberty and a tendency toward delayed growth. If the patient survives to adulthood, the body is described as spider-like, with a narrow trunk and long extremities, curved spine, elongated skull, and barrel-shaped chest. Premature death may result from repeated infarctions within vital organs or from an infectious process. The most successful treatment may be prevention through genetic counseling of persons known to be carriers. Information is provided to allow individuals to arrive at informed decisions regarding the conception and birth of children.

Stasis Ulcer. This is a secondary condition resulting from chronic venous insufficiency, a lower extremity trauma, or a skin irritation. The most common site of **stasis ulcers** is the ankle at the internal malleous area. Stasis ulcers develop following deep vein thrombophlebitis which destroys the valve structures. Communicating veins in the affected area fail to compensate for the damaged vein. The venous pressure increases, causing fluid to enter the interstitial tissues and produce edema. The tissue swelling leads to fibrosis and skin discoloration from blood entering the subcutaneous tissues. The poor condition of the skin and the inadequate circulation from the area lead to a breakdown of the surrounding tissues, Figure 4–104.

Treatment of small ulcers involves elevation of the affected extremity, warm soaks, bed rest, and the use of drugs to counteract infection. When the swelling subsides, pressure is applied by a sponge rubber dressing or an Unna's boot (zinc gelatin boot). Large stasis ulcers not responding to treatment may require removal of the ulcer site followed by a skin graft.

Thrombophlebitis. This is an acute condition in which the lining of the vein wall becomes inflamed and a thrombus forms. **Thrombophlebitis** can develop within small superficial veins and is usually self-limiting. DVT can affect small or large veins. When there is an alteration of the vein lining, platelets begin to collect at the area. The platelet fibrin catches red blood cells, white blood cells, and additional platelets, forming a blood clot. The thrombus enlarges rapidly, particularly if the blood flow is slow, causing an inflammation which becomes fibrotic. The enlarging clot may completely fill the vein opening, occluding the vessel, or it may break loose, becoming an embolus.

DVT usually results from lining damage, but it can also follow accelerated blood clotting and a slow, reduced flow of blood. Conditions that precipitate thrombophlebitis are prolonged bed rest, trauma, childbirth, surgery, and the use of oral contraceptives.

Symptoms of deep thrombophlebitis include severe pain, fever, chills, and possibly edema, with discoloration of the affected extremity. When superficial veins are involved, visible and palpable signs may include heat, swelling, tenderness, redness and discoloration, and induration (hardening) along the affected portion of the vein.

Treatment is directed toward preventing complications, controlling the development of thrombi, and relieving the dis-

FIGURE 4–104 Stasis ulcer and gangrene (From Burke, *Human Anatomy and Physiology in Health and Disease*, 3d ed. Copyright 1992, Delmar Publishers Inc.)

comfort. The patient is maintained on bed rest, with the affected extremity elevated to aid circulation. Warm, moist soaks are applied to the affected area. Medication is given to relieve pain, and frequently anticoagulants are used to reduce the blood's clotting ability. Antiembolism stockings (tight-fitting, elastic, knee- or thigh-length hose) are indicated to assist the return of blood from the legs to the heart. Individuals who are prone to develop thrombophlebitis should avoid prolonged periods of sitting or standing, especially with little movement, to help eliminate pooling of blood in the lower extremities. When sitting, the legs should be resting on a support that does not cause pressure to interfere with return circulation.

Varicosities. Veins which become dilated, twisted, and inefficient are known as **varicose** veins. The condition usually results from weakness of the valves in the saphenous vein and its branches, which permits blood to leak backward due to incomplete closure. As the blood accumulates, the veins become dilated, the valve is no longer capable of reaching across the opening of the vein, and the situation becomes worse. This stasis (stagnation) of blood is often the result of occupations requiring long periods of standing or of other factors interfering with circulation, such as pressure against the veins during pregnancy.

Symptoms include a feeling of heaviness, night leg cramps, aching, and a feeling of fatigue. With deep vein involvement, edema may accumulate in the feet and ankles, often associated with the discoloration that precedes stasis ulcers. Superficial varicosed veins can often be seen or palpated behind the knees or on the medial surface of the calf. Varicosed veins are not to be confused with the tiny purplish red surface veins seen on the skin of most adults. These are commonly referred to as spider veins and are evidence of increased venous pressure. They are often associated with varicosities.

Treatment for mild to moderate varicosities includes an exercise program to improve circulation; use of antiembolism stockings; attention to sitting position; and the elimination of tight-fitting or constricting clothing such as girdles, garters, elastic bands of clothing, and knee-high or thigh-high hose. More severe varicosities may require injection of a sclerosing agent into small venous areas to scar and harden the vein. Larger involvement will necessitate surgical ligation (tying off) of the involved vein from its branches and stripping the vein from the leg.

Complete Chapter 4, Unit 8 in the workbook to help you meet the objectives at the beginning of this unit and therefore achieve competency of this subject matter.

U N I T   9
The Immune System

OBJECTIVES ....

Upon completion of this unit, you will meet the following terminal performance objectives by verifying knowledge of the facts and principles presented through oral and written communication at a level deemed competent by the instructor or employer.

1. Relate the origin and maturation of blood cells.
2. List the organs of the immune system and identify their locations.
3. Explain how the immune system differentiates between "self" and "nonself."
4. Differentiate between the roles of B cells and T cells.
5. Discuss the three types of T cells describing their roles.
6. Tell how NK cell action differs from phagocytic action.
7. Discuss complement and what it does.
8. Explain what causes an inflammatory response.
9. Differentiate between antibody-mediated and cell-mediated immune response.
10. Tell how immunizations and vaccines work.
11. Explain how the AIDS virus destroys the immune system.
12. Identify ways to acquire the AIDS virus.
13. List four high-risk behaviors to avoid.
14. Discuss how an allergen causes an immune response.
15. Explain how cancer develops and what might be some causative factors.
16. Identify the characteristics of a cancerous cell.
17. List the six factors that interfere with or prohibit immune response.
18. Discuss eight diagnostic procedures used to determine the presence of cancer.
19. Discuss the three major methods of treating cancer.
20. Discuss 10 new investigative treatments for cancer.
21. Discuss chronic fatigue syndrome, its symptoms and treatment.
22. Discuss how lupus erythematosus affects the immune system and the major body organs it may effect.
23. Differentiate between discoid, systemic, and drug-induced lupus.
24. Identify the general and suggestive symptoms of lupus.
25. Discuss how lupus is treated.
26. Discuss how rheumatoid arthritis may be connected to the immune system.
27. Describe the beginning and eventual symptoms of rheumatoid arthritis.
28. Spell and define, using the glossary at the back of the text, all the words to know in this unit.

WORDS TO KNOW ....

abstinence
acquired immunodeficiency syndrome (AIDS)
allergens
allergies
anaphylaxis
antibody
antibody-mediated
antigen
antigen–antibody complex
autoimmune
autologous
basophil
benign
biopsy
cancerous
carcinoembryonic antigen
carcinogensis
carcinoma
cell-mediated
chemotherapy
clone
complement
corticosteroids
cytotoxic
debilitating
desensitization
discoid
eosinophils
extracellular
heterosexual
histamine
homosexual
humoral
hyperthermia
immune

immunoglobulin
immunosuppressed
interferon
interleukin (IL)
intracellular
lupus erythematosus
lymphocyte
lymphokine
macrophage
malignant
metastasis
monoclonal
monokine
monocyte
monogamous
mutation
neoadjuvant
neoplastic
neutrophils
oncogenes
opportunistic
permeable
phagocyte
prostaglandin
psychoneuroimmunology
radiation
Raynaud's phenomenon
remission
retrovirus
sarcoma
suppressor
syndrome
thymus
transmission
vaccine
virus

The **immune** system is not a true body system, but rather a function of the white blood cells of the circulatory system.

Because of its essential role in the health and well-being of humans and the severity of the consequences when it fails, however, it is considered to be of sufficient significance to warrant individual emphasis.

The immune system is the body's way of defending itself against the environment of microbes in which we live. There are several **antigens** (foreign materials) in the environment that are capable of causing an immune response, such as a virus, a bacterium, a fungus, a parasite, or even only a portion or product of these organisms. Tissues or cells from another individual in transfusions or organ transplants are also "foreign" as are the proteins we eat until they are properly processed by the body. Particles in the air or foods we eat, which cause reactions, are also antigens but are called **allergens.** One's own cells, which become malignant, are likewise targeted as "different."

The body's first line of defense against disease is the protective barrier of the skin and the mucus secreted by the mucous membranes. While they are intact, antigens on their surfaces cannot enter. Various body secretions provide bactericidal components, such as acid in the gastric juice, lysozme in tears and saliva, and certain "normal" bacteria that control potential pathogenic bacteria and fungi in the vagina and intestines. The immune system is composed of billions of cells and an even greater number of protein molecules known as **antibodies** and **complement,** which can be directed toward foreign invaders.

Scientists have made great progress in understanding the function of the many components of the immune system, but a great deal still remains a mystery. The immune response is an unbelievably complicated interaction between cells, antibodies, and proteins against antigens and allergens. Recently, it has been recognized that the brain and nervous system also have an effect on the immune system. A new science, **psychoneuroimmunology,** is researching the connection between the brain, behavior, and immunity.

This unit introduces the basics of immunity—the cells, their function, the process of developing immunity, and the destruction of antigens. There are great numbers of immune cells. Some are for general defense, others are highly specific, but to be most effective they must work together. They can communicate through direct contact or chemical messengers. When an antigen appears, the specifically matched cells are stimulated to undergo mitosis and multiply rapidly to destroy the invader. When the attack has succeeded, another message stops the activity. A look at some of the diseases resulting from ineffective or inappropriate immune response and how science is using its knowledge of the immune system to try to control their outcome will prove most interesting.

Origin of Cells

To understand immunity, it is necessary to learn about the structure and function of its component parts. In the last unit, it was stated that cells within the blood are of three types—red, white and platelets. The leukocytes (white cells) were identified as playing a vital role in defending the body. It is

these cells in cooperation with protein molecules that are responsible for immunity.

All blood cells originate in the bone marrow and initially develop from stem cells, Figure 4–105. They progress through stages on their way to maturity. Erythrocytes (RBCs) develop from erythroid stem cells and mature in the bone marrow. White blood cells (WBCs) which become the granulated **eosinophils, neutrophils** and **basophils,** develop from myeloid stem cells. One type of agranulocyte, the **lymphocyte,** develops from a lymphocyte stem cell into two major classes, B cells that mature in the bone marrow and T cells that mature in the **thymus.** Mononuclear phagocyte stem cells become the **monocytes,** which circulate in the blood then enter into the tissue to become **macrophages. Phagocytes** are cells that engulf and destroy antigens. Several cells have this capability, mainly the monocytes and macrophages. Neutrophils are also phagocytic but in addition carry granules with potent chemicals to destroy microorganisms. They are key players in acute inflammatory reactions. Eosinophils and basophils, also granulated cells, release their chemicals to effect cells or microbes in their environment.

Organs of the Immune System

The organs of the immune system are located throughout the body and are generally known as lymphoidal organs because they are where lymphocytes develop, grow, or perform their functions. These organs include the bone marrow, the thymus, lymph nodes, spleen, tonsils, adenoids, appendix, and clumps of lymphoid tissue in the small intestine called Peyer's patches, Figure 4–106, page 106. The blood and lymphatic vessels are also considered to be lymphoid organs. When the B and T lymphocytes leave the bone marrow and thymus they travel throughout the body in the blood and lymphatic vessels. All along the lymphatic vessels are clusters of lymph nodes. Each node contains specialized compartments that store large numbers of B and T cells as well as others that are capable of trapping antigens to present to the T cells for destruction, Figure 4–107, page 180.

The spleen likewise provides a place for antigen destruction to occur. It also has compartments for different types of cells. As the lymph flows around the cells and through the body, it carries the lymphocytes, macrophages, and antigens to the lymph nodes where the antigens are filtered out and shown by the macrophages to the immune cells to be destroyed. Then the lymphocytes and other immune cells go back into circulation to search for more foreign materials, gradually working their way back to the lymphatic vessels and nodes and another cycle is completed.

Cell Markers

Basic to the immune system is the ability of cells to distinguish between self and nonself. Immune cells are also able to remember previous encounters and react accordingly. All body cells carry molecules that are encoded by a group of genes contained in a specific chromosome known as the *major*

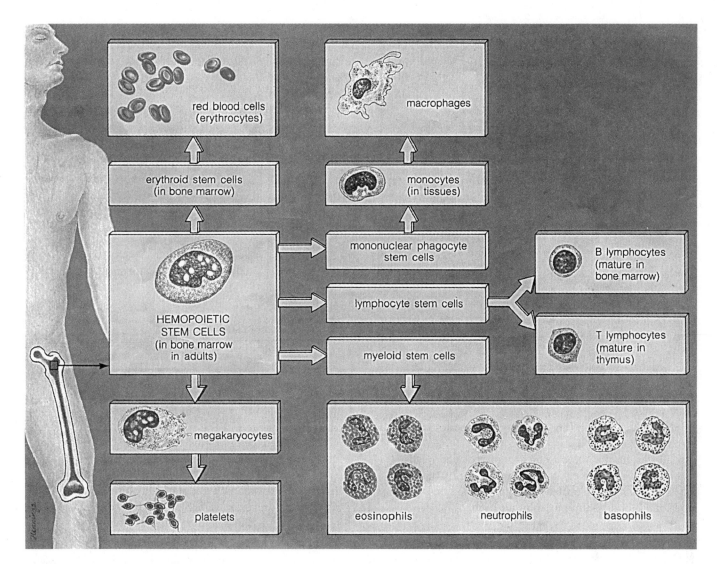

FIGURE 4–105 Origin of cells (From Starr & Taggart, *Biology, The Unity and Diversity of Life,* 5th ed. Copyright 1989, Wadsworth, Inc. Reprinted by permission of the publisher.)

histocompatibility complex (MHC). This allows immune cells to recognize and communicate with each other. The body's immune defenses do not normally attack cells carrying this "self" marker. But when they meet molecules carrying foreign markers, they move quickly to destroy them. Any substance capable of triggering an immune response is considered to be an antigen. An antigen announces its foreignness by carrying perhaps several hundred different kinds of characteristic shapes called *epitopes,* which stick out from its surface. The immune system is capable of recognizing millions of nonself molecules or it can produce molecules and cells that can match to and counteract against each one.

Lymphocytes

Lymphocytes are the small white cells charged with immunity functions. Both B cells and T cells are able to recognize specific antigen targets. When B cells are maturing, they go through two stages of development beginning before birth and lasting for the first few months of an infant's life. Each

immature cell inserts numerous molecules of one specific kind of antibody into its cytoplasmic membrane. Antibodies belong to a family of large molecules known as **immunoglobulins,** which are protein substances that have two areas on their surface to uniquely match the surface of an antigen molecule. Scientists have identified nine distinct classes of human immunoglobulins (Ig). IgG coats microorganisms to speed up the uptake by other immune system cells. IgM is very effective in killing bacteria. IgA is concentrated in body fluids to guard the entrances of the body. IgE is effective against parasites but also is the "problem" in allergies. IgD is found in the membranes of B cells and is thought to regulate the cell's activities.

When B cells come into contact with antigens, they undergo a second change. When the combining site of a B cell's surface "fits" one of the variety of antigen's shapes, they join and are changed into an **antigen-antibody complex.** The antibody can then perform its duty or cause the antigen to stick to other antigens forming clumps so the large macrophages can destroy large numbers of them at one time.

Organs of the Immune System

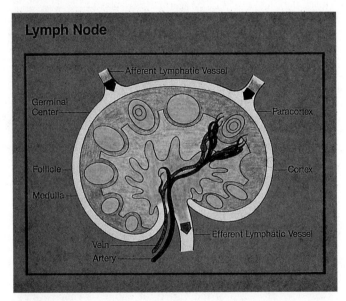

Tonsils and
Adenoids

Thymus

Lymph
Nodes

Spleen

Peyer's
Patches

Appendix

Lymph
Nodes

Bone
Marrow

Lymphatic
Vessels

FIGURE 4–106 Organs of the immune system (Courtesy of the National Cancer Institute.)

Lymph Node

Afferent Lymphatic Vessel

Germinal
Center

Paracortex

Follicle

Cortex

Medulla

Vein

Artery

Efferent Lymphatic Vessel

FIGURE 4–107 Lymph node. T cells concentrate in the para-cortex, B cells in and around the germinal centers, and plasma cells in the medulla. (From Starr & Taggart, *Biology, The Unity and Diversity of Life,* 5th ed. Copyright 1989, Wadsworth, Inc. Reprinted by permission of the publisher.)

After B cells have undergone antigen–antibody complex, they begin to divide, rapidly producing many clone cells with the same antibody. Later the cells divide into memory, or plasma, cells, Figure 4–108. The memory cells go to the lymph nodes to stand by for the next same antigen invasion while the plasma cells continue to secrete millions of identical antibody molecules.

Complement System

Antibodies may change their shape slightly when they bind with antigens. This change will expose two regions called complement-binding sites. Complement is a group of about 20 *inactive* enzyme proteins normally present in the blood. When one complement protein meets an antibody–antigen complex, it will *activate* and begin a chain reaction of attracting the others. The consequences are the creation of lethal chemicals to attract the phagocytes to the scene, coat the target cell to make it more recognizable, or destroy the antigen by puncturing its membrane. In this way, antibodies and the complement system work together to destroy antigens by **antibody-mediated** response also known as **humoral** immunity. This type of immunity is the resistance to disease produced by antibodies, Figure 4–109, page 182.

The events set off by antibody-mediated response and other chemicals help to develop an inflammatory response. When complement proteins begin to act, basophils and mast cells are also activated. Both cells release the substance called **histamine,** which dilates blood vessels and makes the vessel walls more **permeable.** This slows down the rate of flow and allows fluid to seep into the surrounding tissues. The result is localized warmth, redness, and swelling. The complement proteins and other factors in the fluid can easily leave the blood vessels and attract the phagocytes to fight the intruders.

T cells, in contrast to B cells, interact directly with their targets in what is called cellular immunity, or **cell-mediated** response. T cells function in two major ways. Some are vital to the operation of other cells. B cells cannot make antibodies against most substances without a regulatory T cell assistance. One type of cell is known as the helper T and is identifiable by the T4 cell marker. Helper T cells are essential for activating B cells and other T cells as well as the natural killer (NK) cells and macrophages. A subset of T cells acts to turn off or "suppress" these cells. **Cytotoxic** (killer) T cells act directly on infected or malignant cells, as well as any other body cell that has a target antigen and an MHC marker. These cells usually carry the T8 marker and are called killer T cells (refer to Figure 4–108). One type can attach tightly to its target, secrete perforin and other chemicals, which make holes in the cell membrane, destroying it before it can reproduce. Unfortunately, killer cells can also cause rejection of tissue and organ transplants because of nonself markers.

Cytokines

Cytokines are nonantibody proteins that regulate the immune response. One type are **lymphokines,** which are secreted by T cells, and the **monokines,** produced by monocytes and

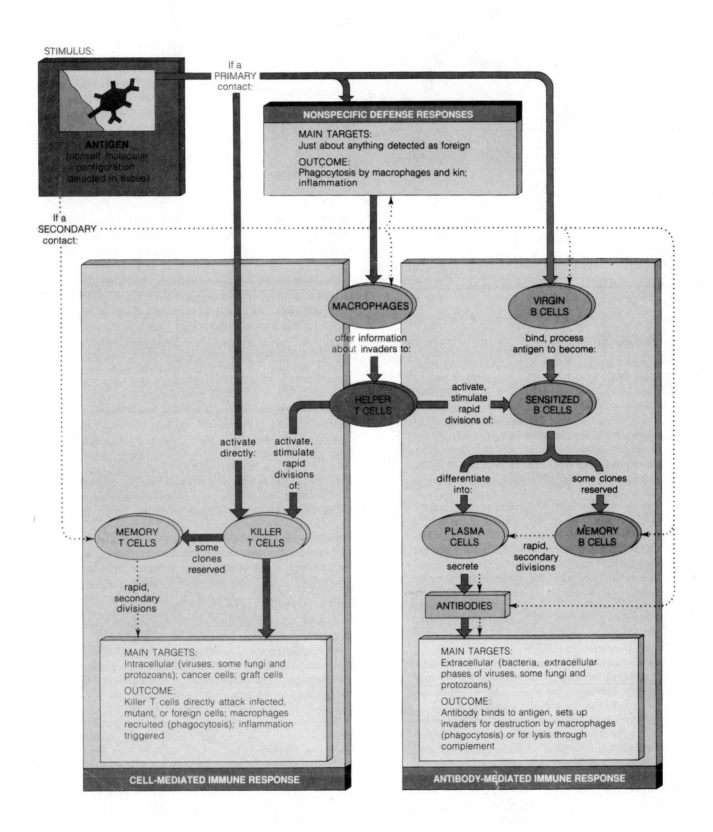

FIGURE 4–108 The development of B cells in antibody-mediated immune response and T cells in cell-mediated immune response (From Starr & Taggart, *Biology, The Unity and Diversity of Life,* 5th ed. Copyright 1989, Wadsworth, Inc. Reprinted by permission of the publisher.)

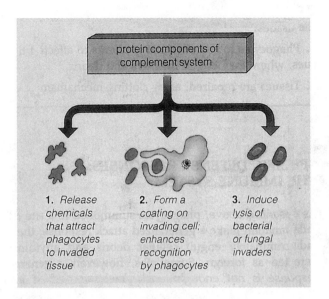

1. *Release chemicals that attract phagocytes to invaded tissue*

2. *Form a coating on invading cell; enhances recognition by phagocytes*

3. *Induce lysis of bacterial or fungal invaders*

FIGURE 4–109 Function of proteins in the complement system (From Starr & Taggart, *Biology, The Unity and Diversity of Life,* 5th ed. Copyright 1989, Wadsworth, Inc. Reprinted by permission of the publisher.)

macrophages. These substances are diverse and potent chemical messengers. Lymphokines bind to specific receptors on target cells and set off other actions, such as involving other cells and substances, encouraging cell growth, and stimulating macrophages. Two other cytokines are lymphotoxin from lymphocytes and tumor necrosis factor from macrophages. Both of these cytokines kill tumor cells. Many cytokines have been renamed as **interleukins (IL)**, which means "messengers between leukocytes." IL-1 from macrophages helps to activate B and T cells. IL-2 is produced by antigen-activated T cells and promotes rapid growth of mature B and T cells and the development of different types of T cells. There are three other types of interleukins.

Natural Killer (NK) Cells ....

Natural killer cells (NK) are another type of deadly lymphocytes that contain granules filled with potent chemicals. They get the name "natural" because they do not need to recognize a specific antigen to kill a cell. They target tumor cells and protect against a wide variety of microbes. In AIDS, this killer cell's activity is deactivated. NK cells, like killer T cells bind to their targets and deliver a lethal burst of chemicals to produce holes in the target cell's membrane leading to its destruction.

Immune Responses ....

The immune response system has two branches, one resulting from B cell activity, antibody-mediated immune response and one resulting from T cell activity, cell-mediated immune response (review Figure 4–108). The response can also be primary, the first encounter with the antigen, or a secondary response with subsequent encounters. In primary antibody-mediated response, an antigen enters the body and goes unde-

tected past "virgin" B cells until it meets one with matching antibody sites. The B cell connects (becomes sensitized) and processes the antigen, displaying its fragments bound to its MHC molecule to attract helper T cells. When the sensitized B cell and the helper T combine, interleukins are released, which cause the cell to begin mitosis. At the same time, other similar antigens have been engulfed and displayed by the macrophages. Helper T cells bind with the macrophages, and interleukins are secreted. The secretion of interleukin stimulates the helper T cells to mature and secrete lymphokines to cause a rapid growth and division of the B cells. This produces a group of **clones** that release identical antibodies to bind with more antigens to be recognized and destroyed. Some of the B cells convert to memory B cells and go to lymphoidal tissues.

The immunoglobulins get other cells and substances involved. IgM and IgG activate macrophages and the complement system. IgE stimulates mast cells to release histamine. IgA causes secretions in the first line of defense in the saliva, tears, lungs, and intestines to protect the body's entrances. IgD works in the cell's membranes to regulate activity. A full primary immune response requires 5 to 6 days to develop.

Antibody-mediated responses act against bacteria and **extracellular** viruses, fungi, and parasites. It *cannot* react to an invader already within a cell's cytoplasm, only those in circulation or attached to a cell's surface.

In a secondary response, the reaction is much faster, only 2 to 3 days. This is possible because leftover clonal lymphocytes with memory are able to attack the antigen. Once one of the cells meets the same antigen, mitosis is immediate and large numbers of appropriately matched cells and antibodies are produced.

Primary response of T cells in cell-mediated response has already been described. The action is direct and quick. After the initial contact with an antigen, some T cells will also develop memory and are held in reserve for subsequent invasions. Cell-mediated immune responses attack **intracellular** viruses, fungi and protozoans, cancer cells, and transplant tissue cells. T cells will destroy any cell with an MHC marker and a target antigen.

Killer cells that cause rejection of organ transplants do so because the MHC markers of the donor cells are not identical self-markers unless from an identical twin. Individuals who are to receive organs are usually given drugs to destroy the killer T cells to prevent rejection but that leaves the recipient without the ability to have a full immune response to other invaders and can lead to death from infections, such as pneumonia.

Both antibody-mediated and cell-mediated immune responses are controlled reactions. When the "battle" is won, binding sites are saturated with antibodies, and the **suppressor** T cells stop the attack. Without this feedback, immune reactions would go out of control.

There is a recognition of a connection between nutrition, mental and emotional health, and physical activity to the status of the immune system. There also seems to be a significance in the appropriate amounts of zinc, iodine, fats, sugars, and fiber. Some vitamins appear to reduce chronic stress, which is an immune depressor. The personality, coping style, quality of life, exercise, support of loved ones, and optimism, to name a few, all appear to greatly influence the effectiveness of the components of the immune system.

The following material is taken from a presentation by Elaine Glass, RN, MS, OCN; clinical nurse specialist in medical oncology and hematology at The Arthur G. James Cancer Hospital and Research Institute. She explains the functions of the components of the immune system and relates them to the familiar roles of a police and military force. She also interjects the emotions and activities that affect the action of the components. This provides a good summary of the immune system.

COMPONENTS OF THE IMMUNE SYSTEM
AGRANULOCYTES
A. Macrophages/Monocytes
The cop on the beat
Monocytes circulate in the blood; macrophages infiltrate the tissues. They engulf antigens and summon other cells to analyze them.
(Stress causes release of cortisol that renders the macrophage unresponsive.
Exercise increases endorphins [natural brain analgesic] which may increase macrophage activity.)
B. Lymphocytes
A collective label for T and B immune cells
1. T CELLS
Involved in the cellular immune system response. Mature in the thymus gland.
  a. Helper T cell
  The detective
Identifies the antigens trapped by macrophages or monocytes and stimulates other cells to destroy them. Does not attack or destroy by itself.
  b. Activated helper T cell
Helps destroy identified antigens by producing interleukin-2, which stimulates other helper and killer T cells to multiply.
  c. Killer T cell
  SWAT team member
Destroys cells that have been invaded by antigens. They can trigger a process that punctures a cell membrane and destroys it before the invading virus inside has a chance to grow.
  d. Natural killer T cell
  Rambo or a vigilante
Attacks cancerous or virus-infected cells without previous exposure to the antigen. NKs are stimulated by interferon. They can recognize artificial antigens created in a lab to which humans have never come into contact.
(In one study, patients with a lot of support from their "significant others" and doctors, had higher levels of NK cells.)
  e. Suppressor T cell
  The police chief
Slows down or stops other immune cell activity after antigens are destroyed.
2. B CELLS
Produces antibodies against antigens; involved in the humoral immune response.
  a. Plasma cell

The army sergeant
Descends from B cells to produce antibodies. They make thousands of antibodies per second.
  b. Antibodies
  The foot soldiers
Proteins that neutralize antigens and destroy other cells where the antigen has invaded.
    1) IgG
The most common protein antibody in the blood and tissue spaces where it coats antigens speeding their uptake by other immune cells.
    2) IgM
A protein antibody that circulates in the bloodstream in star-shaped clusters, very effective in killing bacteria.
    3) IgA
A protein antibody in body fluids (tears, saliva, respiratory and digestive tracts) to guard body entrances.
(College students who watched a video of Mother Theresa had higher levels of IgG and A than students who watched a video that did not stimulate positive emotions.)
    4) IgE
A protein antibody that attaches itself to mast cells and basophils. When it encounters its matching antigen, it stimulates the cell to pour out its contents. It provides protection by coating bacteria and viruses.
    5) IgD
A protein antibody that inserts itself into the membrane of the B cell to regulate the activation of the cell.
  c. Complement
  Flying Aces
A series of 20 proteins that circulate in the blood in an inactive state until they are triggered by contact with antigen–antibody complexes or by contact with the cell membrane of an invading organism.
3. MEMORY CELLS
T cells = Police chief with a history on the force
B cells = Army sergeant with a history in the service
T and B cells that have been activated by an antigen and continue to circulate within the body, ready to attack an antigen if it reinvades. (These cells are the basis of how vaccines work.)

GRANULOCYTES
A group of immune cells filled with granules of toxic chemicals that enable them to digest microorganisms.
A. Neutrophil
Like cop on beat but more heavily armed.
A circulating WBC that destroys foreign matter and cell debris by phagocytosis, by digesting cellular membranes, and by releasing chemotactants and pyrogenic substances that cause fever.
B. Basophil
A firefighter
A circulating WBC that is responsible for allergy symptoms by releasing heparin, histamine, bradykinin, and serotonin from its granules, to cause vasodilation and permeability.

C. Eosinophil

A circulating WBC that can digest microorganisms, especially parasites, and assists in allergic reactions by detoxifying some of the inflammation-inducing substances to prevent the spread of the local inflammatory process.

D. Mast cells

Special member of police force that is armed with chemicals

Special cells found in tissues that contain granules of chemicals that produce redness, warmth, and swelling (allergy symptoms).

CYTOKINES

All nonantibody proteins that regulate the immune response. Cytokines produced by T cells are called *lymphokines.* Cytokines produced by macrophages/monocytes are called *monokines.*

A. Lymphokines

A number of proteins produced by T cells

1. GM-CSF

Granulocyte-macrophage colony-stimulating factor stimulates the growth of neutrophils, eosinophils, and macrophages. It increases the ingestion of bacteria and the killing of tumors coated with antibody. It activates mature granulocytes and macrophages.

2. Interferons

A class of lymphokines with important immunoregulatory functions, especially improving the activities of macrophages and NK cells. Exercise may increase the production of interferon.

a. Alpha (IFN-α)

Is produced by leukocytes in response to viral infections. It also increases NK activity and the numbers of cytotoxic T cells, and starts the tumoricidal activity of macrophages.

b. Beta (IFN-β)

Its activity is similar to IFN-a

c. Gamma (IFN-γ)

Is produced by T and NK cells. It (1) activates killer T cells; (2) increases the ability of B cells to produce antibodies; (3) keeps macrophages at the site; (4) assists them in digesting bacteria and cancerous cells they engulf. IFN-γ also regulates other lymphokines, increases NK activity, and starts the production of T cell suppressor factor.

(Interferon is now produced synthetically and is being used as an anticancer drug. It has shown promise in the treatment of some types of malignancies.)

3. IL-2 (Interleukin-2)

Is produced by helper T cells and NK cells, which stimulates other helper, killer, and suppressor T cells to multiply. It starts cytokine production by T cells and monocytes. It improves NK cell activity.

4. IL-3

Is produced by activated T cells. It is a growth factor for mast cells and most bone marrow progenitor (after stem) cells.

5. IL-4

Is called B cell growth factor, causes B cells, mast cells and resting T cells to multiply. It increases toxicity of killer T cells and macrophages. It is produced by helper T cells.

6. IL-5

Is produced by activated T cells. It is an important factor in the final differentiation of eosinophils and activated B cells. It increases IgA, IgM, and IgE development and secretion. It begins the appearance of IL-2 receptors on B cells.

7. SIRS

Soluble immune response suppressor is released by suppressor T cells and may slow down immune cell activity.

B. Monokines

Proteins produced primarily by monocytes

1. G-CSF

Granulocyte colony-stimulating factor stimulates the growth and activity of neutrophils. It is produced by monocytes and some other nonblood cells.

2. M-CSF

Macrophage colony-stimulating factor stimulates the growth and activity of macrophages. It is also produced by monocytes and other nonblood cells.

C. Other Cytokines

(Produced by both lymphocytes and macrophages/monocytes)

1. IL-1

Is produced by macrophages, T cells, granulocytes, and NK cells. It activates helper T cells and raises the body's temperature. (Fever increases immune cell activity). It stimulates the production of lymphokines and activates macrophages to immobilize cancer cells. It starts the differentiation of stem cells and activated B cells and increases the number of activated B cells. Exercise may increase IL-1 production.

2. IL-6 (BCDF)

Is called B cell differentiation factor, which causes some B cells to stop dividing and to start making immunoglobin and antibodies. Improves the differentiation of killer T cells. Is produced by helper T cells, monocytes, and fibroblasts. It also stimulates the production of platelets.

3. TGF-β

Tumor growth factor-beta is produced by T cells, macrophages, and tumor cells. It suppresses T and B cell growth and differentiation and antibody secretion.

4. TNF-B

Tumor necrosis factor-B, also known as lymphotoxin, is produced by B cells, T cells, mast cells, and macrophages. It makes some cells more vulnerable to lysis by NK cells.

5. TNF

Tumor necrosis factor is produced by monocytes, activated macrophages, NK cells, and mast cells. It can kill tumors or retard their growth. It causes some tumors to bleed and die. It stimulates the production of lymphokines and activates macrophages.

By now you are probably amazed at the complexity and function of the immune system. The previous outline of the duties of its components causes one to wonder how all that coordinated effort ever gets accomplished. And yet, so much more is not understood.

To give an overall picture of what happens during an immune process, Elaine outlines the following, which is demonstrated with a series of cartoon slides:

Immune System Surveillance Process

1. A macrophage (or complement protein, NK cell, or memory cell) recognizes an antigen.
   (A cop begins to struggle with an alien.)
2. Helper T cells bind to the macrophage and become activated by the cytokine, IL-1, which also causes fever.
   (The detective sees the cop and alien struggling and calls for help.)
3. Activated helper T cells produce a lymphokine, IL-2, which stimulates other helper and killer T cells to multiply.
   (Help arrives, detectives, SWAT team, and a few army sergeants.)
4. Helper T cells also secrete a lymphokine, IL-4, which causes B cells to multiply.
   (The detective decides more army personnel are needed and calls in the troops. The army comes marching in.)
5. Helper T cells also secrete a lymphokine, IL-6, which causes some B cells to stop dividing and start making antibodies.
   (The sergeant calls the foot soldiers into duty.)
6. Helper T cells also produce the lymphokine interferon, which activates killer T cells, increases the ability of B cells to produce antibodies, and keeps macrophages at the site and assists them in digesting the cells they engulf.
   (The detective calls out words of encouragement to the SWAT team, the sergeants and the street cops.)
7. Killer T cells destroy the cells where antigens have invaded.
   (The SWAT team member nails an alien inside a phone booth.)
8. Antibodies neutralize the antigen and destroy other cells that have also been infected.
   (A foot soldier punches out an alien.)
9. Complement proteins, triggered by antigen–antibody complexes, or the cell membranes of some invading microorganisms:
   (The flying aces come into the action.)

   - Cause chemotaxis of macrophages and neutrophils to the area. *(An ace calls in the street cop.)*
   - Increase phagocytosis of macrophages and neutrophils. *(The street cops look mean and ugly.)*
   - Activate basophils and mast cells to release immobilizing chemicals and other products that increase inflammation. *(The firefighters and cops with chemicals soak the aliens.)*
   - Change the invader's cell surface, causing them to stick together. *(The aliens get stuck.)*
   - Attack the invader's structure and make it inactive. *(The aces crop-dust the aliens.)*
   - Rupture the invader's cell membrane. *(The ace's gunner blows a hole through the alien.)*

10. Suppressor T cells halt the immune response after the antigen is destroyed.
    (The police chief enters the scene and halts the action once the aliens are destroyed.)

11. Memory T and B cells are left in the blood and lymph system to defend against another attack.
    (The detectives and the army sergeants have the alien's ID in case future attacks occur.)

Figure 4–110, page 186, illustrates a portion of the B and T cell activities.

Elaine points out that study is just beginning on the connection between the brain and immunity. Scientists have discovered the brain produces over 50 neuropeptides that have receptors on WBCs which can affect the cell's activity. For example, people who feel hopeless have sluggish macrophages. Laughter increases NK activity, lymphocyte proliferation, migration of monocytes, and the production of IL-2 and IgA. It would seem we have the power to improve our own immune system if we can learn how.

Immunization

With the knowledge of immune reactions, it is easy to understand how immunizations (shots) and vaccinations provide protection against antigens. The smallpox **vaccine,** for instance, is deliberately introduced into the body in a state that causes only minor reaction but is sufficient for the body to produce an antigen–antibody complex and eventually memory cells against the disease. Other examples of purposeful antigen introduction are measles, mumps, diphtheria, and pertussis given routinely to infants and children and tetanus toxoid given to selected individuals.

Vaccines are often given in initial and "booster" doses to provide additional memory cells and antibodies for a longer period of time. These methods provide *active immunity* because the recipients make their own immunity. Another form is known as *passive immunity* and is given to people already exposed to a disease, such as tetanus. Antibodies from another source are injected into the person to provide a temporary immunity to counter the immediate attack of pathogens. This immunity is short-lived.

Diseases and Disorders

The following diseases are illustrative of what happens when the immune function for some reason fails to operate properly.

Acquired Immunodeficiency Syndrome (AIDS). The beginning of **acquired immunodeficiency syndrome** (AIDS) in the United States is well documented. Between October 1980 and May 1981, five young, previously healthy **homosexual** men were treated for a pneumonia caused by a parasite, *Pneumocystis carinii.* They were treated at three different hospitals in Los Angeles. Doctors and health care professionals were curious because usually *P. carinii* pneumonia occurred only in **immunosuppressed** patients, especially those receiving cancer therapy. At the same time, a rare and unusual blood vessel malignancy called Kaposi's sarcoma was being diagnosed with increasing frequency in young homosexuals in California and

Activation of B Cells to Make Antibody

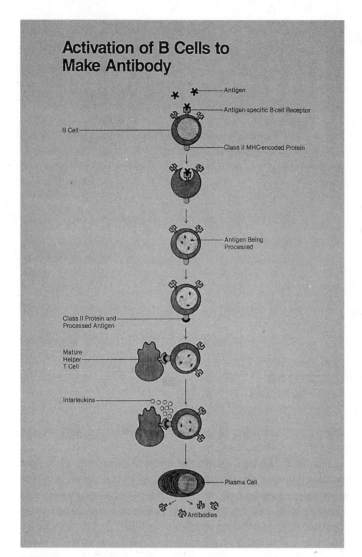

Activation of T Cells

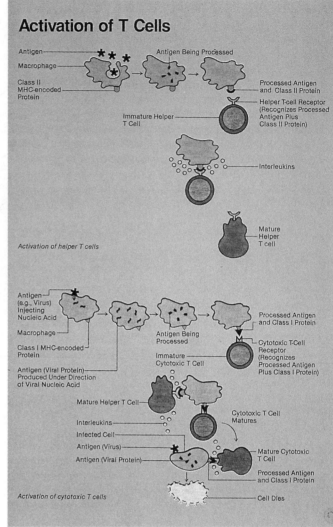

FIGURE 4–110   B cell and T cell function (Courtesy of the National Cancer Institute.)

New York. By July 1981, 26 cases of Kaposi's sarcoma had been diagnosed. Seven of these men also had serious infections; four had *P. carinii* pneumonia. These cases were an early indication of an epidemic of a previously unknown disease. Later it was called the acquired immunodeficiency syndrome, AIDS. Because of the nature and severity of the disease, the United States Department of Health and Human Services began a surveillance program to track cases, collect data, and prepare information for the medical community and the general population. The Center for Disease Control (CDC) in Atlanta, Georgia, maintains vital statistics and publishes frequent reports on the incidence among the population, modes of transmission, race/ethnicity, sex and age of infected, and case-fatality rates.

AIDS is an infectious disease caused by the human immunodeficiency **virus** (HIV), which renders the body's immune system ineffective. The virus has been found in many body fluids but survives well only in those with numerous WBCs such as blood, semen, and vaginal secretions. The virus invades the helper T cells and macrophages, hiding within their membranes. Since both stimulate one another at different times in the immune response, when the helper Ts are "disabled" they

do not cause the macrophages to act, which results in the diversion of B cell antibody production and the absence of NK cell formation. HIV is a **retrovirus;** therefore, its genetic material is RNA instead of DNA. Its core is wrapped in a lipid envelope from the host helper T cell membrane. Once inside the host, an enzyme uses the viral RNA as a "pattern" for making DNA and inserts it into the host's chromosome.

From 2 weeks to 3 months following infection and thereafter, antibodies to several HIV proteins can be detected in the body, BUT, they do not eliminate the infected cells. Several variations of the disease are possible. Some individuals remain well but are still carriers and capable of infecting others. Some people will develop a less serious disease than AIDS called AIDS-related complex (ARC). Persons with ARC will present a set of less severe clinical symptoms than those with AIDS. The symptoms include loss of appetite, weight loss, fever, night sweats, skin rashes, diarrhea, fatigue, lack of resistance to infection, and swollen lymph nodes. Unfortunately, these are also signs of many diseases.

The virus stays in the cells for months to years. At some time, the body makes a secondary response and the infected cells are activated. They copy their new DNA with the viral RNA and new virus particles are assembled. They form "buds" on the helper T cell membrane and separate, and the cell is destroyed. This process continues until the helper T cells are depleted and the body cannot mount an immune response. Even though its effects are devastating, the virus is fragile outside the body and cannot survive. It is easily destroyed by alcohol, hydrogen peroxide, Lysol, heat of 132°F (56°C) for 10 minutes, or a solution of 1:10 household bleach.

Symptoms of AIDS include:

- Unexplained fatigue
- Unexplained weight loss of 10 to 15 pounds in less than 2 months
- Unexplained fever, chills, and night sweats for more than 2 weeks
- Unexplained swollen lymph glands or nodes
- Unexplained diarrhea or bloody stools for more than 2 weeks
- Unexplained persistent dry cough (not from smoking), shortness of breath, or difficult breathing
- Creamy white patches on the tongue or mouth that cannot be scraped off

Without an intact immune system, **opportunistic** infections, those not likely to cause disease normally, are contracted. The most common are *P. carinii* pneumonia and Kaposi's sarcoma. AIDS patients also develop other forms of pneumonia, meningitis, encephalitis, esophagitis, persistent diarrhea, and skin inflammation. These are often resistant to treatment. About 60% of AIDS patients have neurological symptoms, including motor problems, inability to concentrate, memory loss, and progressive mental deterioration. It is believed to be caused by brain infection or cancer.

AIDS is diagnosed from careful assessment of the symptoms and the presence of opportunistic diseases. No blood test verifies the disease. Two types of AIDS tests can be helpful, however. The ELISA (enzyme-linked immunosorbent assay) test is an AIDS antibody indicator. It can detect antibodies the body has developed to fight the AIDS virus but NOT the virus itself. A positive test may not mean you are infected because some false results do occur. A follow-up test called the Western blot indirect and another called IFA (indirect immunofluorescent assay) are used to confirm a positive ELISA. A negative test, on the other hand, is also not conclusive. There may not have been enough time to develop antibodies since becoming infected. Once infected, a person remains so throughout life, capable of transmitting the virus to others even though it may take years to begin to show the classical symptoms of AIDS.

Diagnosis of AIDS has been difficult at best. Prior to 1987, the working definition included primarily the classical symptoms of the syndrome and the absence of other known diseases. With the development of the blood tests, diagnosis was somewhat more reliable, yet still not exact. Since 1993, the additional presence of any of four specific clinical findings has been considered to be diagnostically significant for a diagnosis of AIDS:

- Severe HIV-related immunosuppression (refers to a very low T-cell count with confirmed HIV infection)
- Pulmonary tuberculosis
- Recurrent pneumonia
- Invasive cervical cancer

As a result of this new interpretation, previous data were adjusted to reflect additional cases due to the new criteria. This caused some additional numbers to be added to former totals. In some instances, this may have caused the underestimation of future numbers by experts.

Because of the great delay of time between infection and development of symptoms, currently hundreds of thousands of people are unaware they have the virus and are spreading the disease among the population.

The incidence of AIDS among the population increases daily. In 1993, it was estimated that well over 1 million people (adults, adolescents, and children), in the United States were infected with the AIDS virus and assumed capable of spreading it to others. Of this number, it is believed over 200,000 will develop ARC. (Estimation is difficult because it may take as long as 10 years to develop symtpoms.) Scientists predict 20% to 30% of the infected people will develop an illness meeting the definition of AIDS within a five-year period. The total number of people in the United States known to have AIDS as of June 1993 was 315,390, with 194,334 (about 61.6%) having died of the disease. With no cure, the others are also expected to eventually die.

AIDS is not transmitted by casual contact. Even family members have not developed the disease from sharing food, dishes, towels, toothbrushes, or kissing each othaer. Health care workers, however, must take precautions in caring for AIDS patients. The virus has been found in tears, saliva, urine, and other body secretions, but there is no evidence that the virus is transmitted by fluids other than blood, semen, vaginal secretions, and breast milk. It may be that concentrations of the virus are not sufficient in other body fluids. But because of the severity of the consequences, activities known as *universal precautions* must be taken to protect oneself (see Chapter 3). Through the use of aseptic procedures, gloves, and care with syringes and needles to avoid accidental puncture, contracting the virus can be prevented.

A lot of controversy has surfaced recently regarding mandatory testing of health care providers for the AIDS virus. People are afraid they may contract the disease from their physician or dentist. Two cases in particular have caused this concern: One was a hospital OB/GYN resident who later developed and died from AIDS. Of the 1100 patients he had treated, nearly half have been tested and none have contracted the disease. The other was a dentist. He had infected five of his patients, presumably from suffering injury to his hands while providing dental care, which caused his blood to come into contact with open areas in the patients' mouths. Health care professionals have argued that the risks of them acquiring the virus from caring for patients far exceeds the danger of patients acquiring the disease from them. Prior to 1990, about 12 cases had developed among health care workers; 7 from needle sticks, 1 from contaminated blood coming into contact with an open wound, 2 from providing prolonged unprotected personal care, 1 from accidentally splattering blood into the mouth, and 1 from blood contact with severely chafed hands. As of June 1993, that number has increased to 37 known infected on the job. Of this number, 14 were clinical laboratory technicians and 13 were nurses, both occupations with risks from continual contact with blood and body fluids. This is extremely low incidence among nearly 7 million health care and related (eg: housekeeping) workers. The use of universal precautions is essential to controlling the spread of the disease.

According to data from the Centers for Disease Control, there are about 7000 health care workers who have AIDS. Of that number, 761 are physicians and 1539 are nurses. All persons, health care providers and patients who know they have the virus should reveal their condition to others who might be at risk from contact. Because of the implications upon the practice of physicians and dentists, it presents a very real dilemma which has ethical and legal implications.

AIDS is primarily acquired by two main ways:

■ Having sexual intercourse (oral, vaginal, or anal) with an infected person, male or female
■ Sharing drug needles and syringes with an infected person. (A drop of blood from an infected person left in the needle will infect the next user.) One research team tested known IV drug users in a northeastern city and discovered all were HIV-positive.

The virus can also be transmitted in other ways. Another group of infected individuals are the newborns who acquired the virus from their mothers during pregnancy or at the time of birth and through breast milk afterward. About one-third of the babies born to HIV-positive mothers will become infected. Most babies with AIDS have been born to women who are IV drug users, prostitutes or are a sexual partner of an IV drug user. Women who have had sex with someone in the high-risk group should consult a physician before beginning a pregnancy.

A small number of infected people are hemophiliac men, their sexual partners, and other transfused patients who have acquired the virus in donated blood, especially prior to 1985 when blood banks began testing for the virus.

It is also possible to acquire AIDS from previously used needles with ear piercing or tattooing. The use of a new needle and separate inks for each person would eliminate this concern. Another area requiring surveillance and screening for antibodies are sperm obtained from sperm banks and organs used in transplant operations.

Information presented in the following tables was obtained from publications titled *HIV/AIDS Surveillance,* issued in April 1991 and July 1993, by the U.S. Department of Health and Human Services, Public Health Service Centers for Disease Control, Division of HIV/AIDS. Table 4–4 Shows the number of adult and adolescent cases of AIDS by exposure category and sex for April 1990 to March 1991 as compared to July 1992 to June 1993, along with the cumulative total as of June 1993. The number in parentheses reflects the percentage of total cases represented by this exposure route. By reviewing the statistics, one can observe that homosexual contact is the primary source of infection for males, with intravenous drug use being second. Primary exposure category for females is intravenous drug use, with heterosexual contact being a close second. Heterosexual statistics include opposite sex contact from prostitutes, partners who are IV drug users, partners with hemophilia, and persons

TABLE 4–4

Adult and Adolescent Cases of AIDS by Exposure Category and Sex During April 1990 to March 1991 and July 1992 to June 1993, with Current Cumulative Totals

| | Males | | | | Females | | | | Cumulative Total | |
| | April 1990 March 1991 | | July 1992 June 1993 | | April 1990 March 1991 | | June 1992 June 1993 | | June 1993 | |
Exposure Category	Cases	Rate	Cases	Rate	Cases	Rate	Cases	Rate	Cases	Rate
Men who have sex with men	23,726	(63%)	41,029	(57%)					172,085	(55%)
IV drug use	7,610	(20%)	16,267	(22%)	2,397	(48%)	5,685	(46%)	73,610	(24%)
Men who have sex with men and inject drugs	2,275	(64%)	4,636	(6%)					19,557	(6%)
Heterosexual contact	1,122	(3%)	2,991	(4%)	1,745	(35%)	4,556	(37%)	21,873	(7%)
Hemophilia/Coagulation disorders	317	(1%)	866	(1%)	7	(0%)	24	(0%)	2,762	(1%)
Receipient blood transfusion, components or tissue	504	(1%)	651	(1%)	333	(7%)	456	(4%)	5,733	(2%)

from Pattern II countries (some areas of Africa and the Caribbean). Other unusual and unidentified risks, not included in the table, make up the remaining percentages.

AIDS can be prevented by practicing personal measures to protect oneself. The disease is contracted primarily through contact with an infected person's blood, semen, or vaginal secretions. The virus enters through the vagina, penis, rectum, or mouth (in oral sex). The safest life-style is sexual **abstinence** or a faithful **monogamous** relationship between uninfected partners. If absolute certainty is not known, then precautions must be taken.

1. Avoid high-risk sexual activities. Behaviors that may cause you to acquire the virus are clear:
   ■ Having unprotected sex, homosexual or heterosexual, with an HIV-infected person; oral, vaginal, or anal
   ■ Using IV drugs and sharing needles
   ■ Having many sexual partners; risk increases with number of partners
   ■ Having other sexually transmitted diseases, such as gonorrhea, syphilis, or genital herpes
2. Use a latex condom *properly* to maintain a barrier to the transmission of the virus. It must stay intact and be in place from the beginning to the end of vaginal, anal, or oral sex. The use of a spermicide provides additional protection. The condom must be carefully removed and disposed of properly. Condoms must never be reused.

Unfortunately, no vaccine, antitoxin, or drug "cures" AIDS. The current best line of treatment is a drug called zidovudine (formerly AZT). It boosts the immune system to stay stronger. Many patients cannot tolerate the side effects and bone marrow toxicity. Another drug, dd I, has been released by the government and is being used to treat patients with advanced AIDS who are rapidly deteriorating or with those patients who cannot tolerate zidovudine. Experimental agents include another drug dd C, interferon, IL-2, and vaccines. Often, supportive measures to help control the symptoms of AIDS are all that can be offered the patient.

AIDS must be of concern to everyone. The full impact of the virus is yet to come. It is anticipated that mental disturbances due to the virus's effect on the brain will develop even in the carriers over time. Economically, the cost of care to AIDS patients will strain the health care delivery system. Currently the cost per patient can range from $50,000 to $150,000 or more. With known cases in 1993 exceeding 300,000, at an average cost of $100,000 each, this represents a $30 billion expenditure. AIDS is preventable. The best line of defense is education for prevention. Everyone must become personally responsible for eliminating the transmission of AIDS.

Incidence is usually reflective of population and the presence of large cities within a state, but from reviewing the figures, it is apparent this is not always true. Table 4–5 shows the number of cases and the rate of incidence per 100,000 population during April 1990–March 1991 and June 1992–1993. It is clear, that the *rate* is a better indicator of the extent of the disease among a given population. The higher the rate, the greater the chance of acquiring the AIDS virus.

Another interesting look at AIDS incidence is shown in Table 4–6. The 12 top metropolitan areas in the US with the highest rate per 100,000 population have been listed. The Table also shows the total number of cases for two time periods plus the total cumulative cases to date. Again, the higher the rate within a population, the greater the chance of acquiring AIDS or knowing someone who is infected.

Other data giving information about the increased incidence and the ultimate outcome of the disease shows:

■ Overall fatality rates for adolescents and adults since records have been kept is 61.7% of the 310,680 AIDS cases reported.
■ Rates for children under 13 show 53.3% of the 4,710 cases have died.
■ The incidence of infection in 1983 was only 1,964 people;

TABLE 4–5

Adult, Adolescent, and Children AIDS Cases and the Annual Rates per 100,000 Population in the 10 States with the Highest Rate of Incidence for July 1992 to June 1993 as Compared to April 1990 to March 1991

State	April 1990 March 1991		July 1992 June 1993		Cumulative Total Cases
	Cases	Rate	Cases	Rate	
1. District of Columbia	746	(122.9)	1,083	(183.6)	4,890
2. New York	7,871	(43.8)	14,099	(77.8)	60,570
3. Florida	4,746	(36.7)	8,765	(64.4)	30,786
4. California	7,683	(25.8)	15,402	(49.7)	58,016
5. New Jersey	2,502	(32.4)	3,482	(44.7)	17,255
6. Delaware	89	(13.4)	305	(44.0)	763
7. Connecticut	428	(13.0)	1,444	(43.8)	4,071
8. Maryland	997	(20.9)	2,058	(41.7)	6,726
9. Nevada	214	(17.8)	541	(39.6)	1,537
10. Texas	3,267	(19.2)	6,223	(35.1)	22,091

TABLE 4–6

Cases of AIDS and Rate per 100,000 Population in the 12 Top Metropolitan Areas in the U.S. During July 1992 to June 1993 as Compared to April 1990 to March 1991, and Accumulative Totals as of June 1993

Metropolitan Area	April 1990 March 1991		July 1992 June 1993		Accumulative Totals as of June 1993
	Cases	Rate	Cases	Rate	Cases
1. San Francisco, CA	2,155	(134.4)	3,862	(235.3)	16,254
2. New York, NY	6,674	(78.1)	11,798	(137.9)	52,238
3. Miami, FL	1,323	(68.3)	2,068	(102.3)	9,026
4. West Palm Beach, FL	419	(48.5)	837	(92.0)	2,896
5. San Juan, P.R.	1,122	(70.3)	1,645	(87.7)	6,475
6. Jacksonville, FL	260	(28.7)	813	(84.6)	2,013
7. Fort Lauderdale, FL	1,034	(82.4)	1,080	(81.9)	4,948
8. Jersey City, NJ	382	(69.1)	421	(76.0)	2,754
9. Newark, NJ	993	(54.4)	1,283	(70.6)	7,038
10. Orlando, FL	320	(29.8)	850	(64.8)	2,183
11. Tampa St. Petersburg, FL	488	(23.6)	1,314	(61.6)	3,581
12. Houston, TX	1,329	(40.2)	2,160	(60.8)	8,624

however, 1,826 (93%) of those have died during the past 10 years. Children under age 13 diagnosed during the same year numbered 75 with 71 (95.5%) having died as of June 1993.

- In 1992, 57,023 adult and adolescent cases were reported with 33,399 having died during the year. There were 649 children under age 13 diagnosed with 346 having died during the year.
- Seventy-four percent of all diagnosed males and females are between the ages of 25 and 44.

A March 26, 1992 news release from Louis W. Sullivan, M.D., secretary of US Department of Health and Human Services, was alarming. It included the following statements:

- Over a million Americans are currently infected with HIV; this represents about 1 in every 100 adult males and about 1 in every 800 adult females.
- Another person is infected about every 13 minutes
- During 1992 alone, over 50,000 Americans were infected and as many as 40,000 will die as a result of AIDS
- The number of *reported* AIDS cases just surpassed 315,000; the epidemic is increasing. It took 8 years to reach the first 100,000, only two years to reach the second.
- AIDS is now the third leading cause of death among adults 25–44.

Dr. Sullivans predictions proved to be underestimated in one area and overestimated in another. Final data for 1992 showed 57,622 adults, adolescents, and children were diagnosed and 33,745 died. The reported total accumulative number of AIDS cases by the end of 1992 was 299,153.

AIDS must be prevented. To obtain a free brochure, materials and confidential AIDS counseling, call the toll-free National AIDS Hotline (1-800-342-AIDS).

Allergies. Sometimes the immune system can damage instead of protect the body. A secondary response to a normally harmless substance is seen in **allergies** and may actually damage tissues. About 15% of human beings are predisposed to become sensitive to dust, animal dander, certain food, pollen, insect stings, drugs, and other substances. When exposed to the sensitive allergens, the antibody IgE is produced, resulting in allergic symptoms. Other factors, such as emotional state, air pressure or temperature change, and infections can either trigger or complicate allergic reactions. With each additional exposure to the allergen, IgE antibody is produced and becomes attached to the mast cells or basophils, which in turn release histamine and **prostaglandins,** Figure 4–111. The histamine causes the mucous membranes to

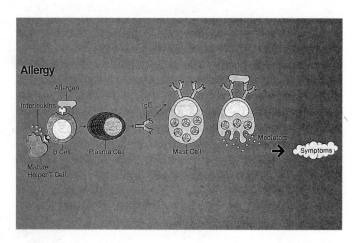

FIGURE 4–111 Response to allergens (Courtesy of the National Cancer Institute.)

secrete and capillaries to become more permeable. Prostaglandins constrict smooth muscle in some organs, such as the bronchioles of the lungs. The two initiate a local inflammatory response. With hay fever or asthma, for example, there is sneezing, runny nose, congestion and difficult breathing.

Exaggerated reactions to allergens can be life-threatening. For instance, some people are very sensitive to bee stings and certain drugs. The histamine and prostaglandins cause extensive bronchial constriction, mucous production, and excessive capillary permeability. Breathing is difficult and extensive loss of blood plasma drastically lowers the blood pressure leading to circulatory collapse and death. This reaction is known as **anaphylaxis** and the situation is called *anaphylactic shock.*

Diagnostic tests to confirm allergies consist of blood counts to determine eosinophil numbers (increase denotes allergy); chest X ray to determine congestion and perhaps focal atelectasis (mucous plugs with asthma); and pulmonary function test to evaluate lung condition. Often there is a family history of sensitivity. A series of skin tests can identify allergic substances (see Chapter 8).

Treatment consists of eliminating contact with allergens and other causative factors as much as possible. **Desensitization** to specific allergens may be helpful. By injecting minute amounts of the allergen intradermally and gradually increasing the amount, the body can be urged to produce IgG antibodies, which circulate and bind with the allergen prohibiting its interaction with IgE. In addition, antihistamines, bronchial dilators, antibiotics for secondary infection and sometimes corticosteroids, are helpful.

Cancer. Cancer is a large group of diseases characterized by uncontrolled growth and spread of abnormal cells. Cancer cells might arise at any time as a result of **mutations** induced by an event, such as viral infection (especially the Epstein–Barr virus that causes infectious mononucleosis), irradiation, chemicals, genetic predisposition, diet, and immunological factors. The malignant transformation of cells is known as **carcinogenesis.** A *carcinogen* is anything that is capable of causing cancer. **Radiation** is the most dangerous because it damages the DNA, which could lead to abnormal cells. Other known carcinogenic substances are asbestos, vinyl chloride, chemicals in polluted air, and cigarettes. Cancers of the colon seem related to dietary causes, such as a high-protein and fat intake; liver tumors may arise from nitrate additives.

A cancer cell is one that has begun reproducing erratically at a rapid rate and continues to grow until it interferes with surrounding cells and the function of tissues. Normal cells have a built-in mechanism that permits controlled division. Tumor cells do not, and continue to divide as long as growth conditions are favorable. Some of the tumors are "clonal," meaning all their cells are genetically identical to the parent cell. Tumor cells that divide but stay in one place forming a mass are known as **benign.** Tumor cells that spread into surrounding tissue and migrate to other organs are said to be malignant. To be considered a **malignant** cell, it must have certain characteristics:

- Profound abnormalities in the plasma membrane (absence or change in surface proteins)
- Extreme changes in the cytoplasm
- Abnormal growth and division; proteins formed that cause extensive growth of capillaries to service the mass
- Loss of capacity to hold cells in the parent tissue

With the change in membrane proteins, cells do not "know" each other and fail to bind together as tissues. This allows cells to travel from the primary site through the blood and lymph to start new secondary growths in other tissues. This process is known as **metastasis.**

Cancers can be classified according to their cellular origin. Malignant tumors from epithelial tissues are known as **carcinomas,** those from connective, muscle, or bone tissue are called **sarcomas.** Cancer cells are also called **neoplastic:** they are larger than normal, divide quickly, and serve no useful purpose.

Theoretically, the body develops cancer cells continuously, but the immune system recognizes them as foreign and destroys them. The cellular response causes T cells to become sensitized to the antigen (cancer cell). The sensitized T cells release lymphokines to destroy the antigen and transform some T cells into killer T cells. At the same time, the plasma cells release antibodies, and the complement system activates to destroy the cell. The difficulty arises from opposing immune factors, the "blocking antibody," which actually enhances tumor growth by protecting cells from immune destruction. Factors that prohibit immunity are

- Aging cells that begin to err in copying their genetic material, causing mutants that the aging immune system fails to recognize
- A decrease in antibodies and lymphocytes due to cytotoxic drugs or steroids
- Stress, which stimulates production of *cortisol,* a lymphocyte destroyer
- Severe systemic infection, which depresses the immune system
- Cancer itself causes suppression of the immune system and eventual exhaustion of a response
- Increased infection due to radiation, toxic drug therapy, and bone marrow depression, which interferes with leukocyte production

Some scientists believe that the mutated cell's surface markers either did not change (still say "self"), are disguised, or even are released and cause immune fighters to follow them instead of destroying the cell.

Diagnostic Procedures. Currently diagnostic procedures from simple to complex include thorough medical history, physical examination, X rays, computerized axial tomography (CAT) scans, magnetic resonance imaging (MRI), and **biopsy** of the suspected tissue. A more recent blood test **carcinoembryonic antigen** (CEA), a tumor marker, can detect malignancies involving the large intestine, stomach, pancreas, lungs, breast; and sometimes sarcomas, leukemias, and lymphomas. CEA presence above a certain level indicates suspicion or confirmation if higher. The test is also used to determine tumor extent, degree of treatment response, and tumor recurrence, but it is not organ-specific. A similar new test is specific. Prostate-specific antigen is capable of measuring the presence and extent of disease in the prostate gland. This is possible because the specific antigen markers have been identified. Ultrasound, a probe used to produce images on a screen, is being used rectally to view the prostate gland to increase early detection of occult (before suspected, hidden) cancer.

Genetic researchers have identified genes in tumor cells call **oncogenes.** Their activity is associated with the transformation of normal to cancer cells. This is beneficial in predicting which family members are likely to be at risk, due to similar genes.

Treatment.   Treatment consists primarily of three major therapies: surgery, radiation, and **chemotherapy** (potent drugs), either individually or in combination. The choices depend upon the type of cancer. If the tumor is contained within an organ, such as the uterus or prostate, surgical removal is indicated, usually followed by chemotherapy. When cancer affects bone marrow or the lymphatic system, which is spread throughout the body, however, chemotherapy becomes the principal method. Unfortunately, chemotherapy and radiation cannot distinguish between regular and **cancerous** cells, so both are destroyed. In some instances with leukemia, surgery in the form of a bone marrow transplant, as described in the previous unit, may be an option. Then the patient's old bone marrow is purposely destroyed before new marrow is transplanted. Several new techniques and treatments are being investigated and tried:

- Taxol, a new drug which is extracted from the bark of yew trees. In clinical trials it has been effective in the treatment of ovarian cancer.
- **Neoadjuvant** chemotherapy, given to shrink the cancer before surgery has been successful in treating certain types of cancers.
- IL-2 stimulates cells to fight cancer directly. It is being researched for use in kidney cancer and melanoma.
- The use of a patient's own bone marrow, **autologous** bone marrow transplant, removes a portion of the marrow before treatment, saves it, and later gives it back to the patient. This eliminates the need for donor matching and makes it possible to give the patient larger doses of chemotherapy and radiation. Obviously, this will not work if the bone marrow is the source of the cancer.
- The use of heat, **hyperthermia,** to increase body temperature. It is known that heat of 45°C (113°F) kills cancer cells and a temperature of 42° to 43°C (107.6° to 109.4°F) makes the cell more susceptible to the effects of radiation. Studies are being conducted to see if hyperthemia can increase the effect of radiation and chemotherapy.
- Immunotoxins are antibodies that are targeted against cancer cells and can be coupled with toxins, drugs, or radioactive substances and delivered directly to the cancer cell.
- New immune therapy is being researched and is in the experimental state. This form of treatment uses the body's immune system to direct its effects to the cancerous cells.

Some therapy stimulates the immune mechanisms to produce additional antibodies and lymphocytes. It can be directed specifically to a particular tumor antigen or nonspecifically to multiple antigens. Stimulation also helps combat the immunosuppressive effects of cancer and its treatments.

- Interferons are lymphokines produced by leukocytes following viral infections. They improve the activity of macrophages and NK cells. Interferon can be administered to patients and has been shown to be effective with certain cancers but not universally beneficial as hoped.
- Perhaps the most exciting immune therapy is **monoclonal** antibodies. Scientists implanted specific cancer cells (antigens) into a mouse, Figure 4–112. The mouse made antibody-producing plasma cells specific to the antigens, which were then extracted from its spleen and fused with a malignant plasma cell. These new "hybrid" cells multiplied rapidly in a culture producing the same antibodies as the mouse cells. These clone cells will continue indefinitely making the same identical antibody, therefore the name "monoclonal" antibody.

Monoclonal antibodies may be effective for use as passive immunization for flu and hepatitis B. Theoretically, they can

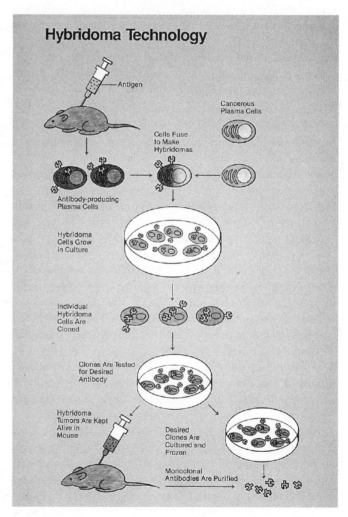

FIGURE 4–112   Producing monoclonal antibodies (Courtesy of the National Cancer Institute.)

be cloned for various diseases. With cancer, the hope is to attach highly toxic drug molecules to the antibodies so they can be specifically targeted to the cancerous cell and avoid damage to healthy cells. Scientists have since devised human monoclonal antibodies that eliminate the recipient's reaction to mouse proteins. Uses for these engineered antibodies are just beginning to be tested, but the future looks promising.

Monoclonal antibodies are also being used in radioimmunology. The antibodies are *radiolabeled* (treated) with a radioactive substance specific for certain tissues. The cells "take up" the substance and can be detected by scanning equipment. This makes it possible to determine the location and size of a tumor.

Surgeons at The Ohio State University Medical Center pioneered the use of a small hand-held scanner called a Neoprobe during surgery. The scanner connects to a monitor that produces audible beeps and digital readouts of radiation levels. Patients, primarily with colon cancers, are given radiolabeled antibodies over a specified period just before surgery. On the day of surgery, external probe counts are taken and recorded over the heart, liver, and perineal areas. When the abdomen is opened, probe counts are taken and recorded at the tumor site(s), lymphatic drainage areas, and any identifiable metastatic sites. Then appropriate resection (removal) of all identifiable disease is completed. The abdomen is again scanned with the probe to locate any other areas of radioactive concentration that may have been missed. If found, they are first biopsied and the specimen sent immediately for frozen section evaluation. If tumor is verified, further resection is carried out.

The use of the Neoprobe has helped surgeons locate disease that was neither visible nor palpable. It is capable of finding minute segments of the tumor as well as ruling out suspicious areas, which prove to be nonmalignant, that could have been unnecessarily removed. This process, known as "second look surgery," is also being used in rectal, primary breast, and pancreatic cancer surgery.

Another researcher funded by the American Cancer Society is studying the chemicals in the cells that are required to begin the mitosis process. If these can be isolated, blocked, labeled with chemotherapy, and targeted toward cancer cells, they can be prevented from completing division to multiply. The researcher is studying drugs that will block the chemical changes.

Hopefully, more effective means of treatment and even cures will soon be discovered to control this devastating disease. Currently the outlook for some patients is guarded at best. The following data were obtained from *Cancer Facts and Figures—1993,* a publication of the American Cancer Society. Note the estimates for incidence and deaths by cancer site, Figure 4–113, and the increase in 5-year survival by site and race, Figure 4–114, page 195. It is plain that the odds are still poor for survival from cancers of the esophagus, stomach, liver, pancreas, and lungs.

In 1992, it was estimated that about 1,130,000 people were diagnosed as having cancer. In addition, over 600,000 people developed cancer in situ, basal, or squamous cell skin cancer. About 520,000 died, or about 1400 per day. One of every five

deaths from all causes is cancer. The rate per 100,000 people has been increasing. In 1930, it was 143 people; in 1940, it was 152; by 1950 the rate had risen to 158 and has remained at 171 since 1984. The major cause of this increase is cancer of the lung, ironically, the major one that could be drastically reduced by doing just one thing—stop smoking. Cigarette smoking is responsible for 84% of lung cancer cases and 30% of all cancer deaths. About 76 million Americans now living will eventually have cancer, about one in three, at the present rate. Cancer will strike in three of every four families. A study from the National Cancer Institute put overall costs for cancer at $104 billion in 1990: $35 billion for direct medical costs, $12 billion for lost productivity, and $57 billion for mortality costs. The cost for detection activities, mammograms, Pap smears, and colorectal screening adds another $3 to $4 billion to the overall costs.

KNOW THE SEVEN WARNING SIGNALS OF CANCER

1. Change in bowel or bladder habits
2. A sore that does not heal
3. Unusual bleeding or discharge
4. Thickening or lump in breast or elsewhere
5. Indigestion or difficulty in swallowing
6. Obvious change in wart or mole
7. Nagging cough or hoarseness

IF YOU OR SOMEONE YOU KNOW HAS A WARNING SIGNAL, SEEK MEDICAL ADVICE

The most effective means of dealing with cancer is prevention first and early detection second. The following information from the American Cancer Society identifies factors to avoid and actions to follow to increase the odds against its development.

PREVENTION

AVOID THOSE FACTORS THAT MIGHT LEAD TO THE DEVELOPMENT OF CANCER (PRIMARY PREVENTION)

SMOKING   Cigarette smoking is responsible for 90% of lung cancer cases among men and 79% among women— about 84% overall. Smoking accounts for about 30% of all cancer deaths. Those who smoke two or more packs of cigarettes a day have lung cancer mortality rates 15 to 25 times greater than nonsmokers.

SUNLIGHT   Almost all of the more than 600,000 cases of basal and squamous cell skin cancer diagnosed each year in the United States are considered to be sun-related. Epidemiologic evidence shows that sun exposure is a major factor in the development of melanoma and that the incidence increases for those living near the equator.

IONIZING RADIATION   Excessive exposure to ionizing radiation can increase cancer risk. Most medical and dental X rays are adjusted to deliver the lowest dose possible without sacrificing image quality. Excessive radon exposure in homes may increase risk of lung cancer, especially in cigarette smokers. If levels are found to be too high, remedial actions should be taken.

CANCER INCIDENDCE AND DEATHS BY SITE AND SEX—1992 ESTIMATES

CANCER INCIDENCE BY SITE AND SEX*

PROSTATE 132,000	BREAST 100,000
LUNG 102,000	COLON & RECTUM 77,000
COLON & RECTUM 79,000	LUNG 66,000
BLADDER 38,500	UTERUS 45,500
LYMPHOMA 27,200	LYMPHOMA 21,200
ORAL 20,600	OVARY 21,000
MELANOMA OF THE SKIN 17,000	MELANOMA OF THE SKIN 25,000
KIDNEY 16,200	PANCREAS 14,400
LEUKEMIA 16,000	BLADDER 13,100
STOMACH 15,000	LEUKEMIA 12,200
PANCREAS 13,900	KIDNEY 10,300
LARYNX 10,000	ORAL 9,700
ALL SITES 565,000	ALL SITES 565,000

*Excluding nonmelanoma skin cancer and carcinoma in situ.

CANCER DEATHS BY SITE AND SEX*

LUNG 93,000	LUNG 53,000
PROSTATE 34,000	BREAST 46,000
COLON & RECTUM 28,900	COLOR & RECTUM 29,400
PANCREAS 12,000	PANCREAS 13,000
LYMPHOMA 10,900	OVARY 13,000
LEUKEMIA 9,900	UTERUS 10,000
STOMACH 8,000	LYMPHOMA 10,000
ESOPHAGUS 7,500	LEUKEMIA 8,300
LIVER 6,600	LIVER 5,700
BRAIN 6,500	BRAIN 5,300
KIDNEY 6,400	STOMACH 5,300
BLADDER 6,300	MULTIPLE MELANOMA 4,500
ALL SITES 275,000	ALL SITES 245,000

FIGURE 4–113 Estimates of cancer incidence and deaths by site and sex (From American Cancer Society, *Cancer Facts & Figures*—1992, Reproduced with permission.)

NUTRITION AND DIET   Risk for colon, breast, and uterine cancers increases in obese people. High-fat diets may contribute to the development of cancers of the breast, colon, and prostate. High-fiber foods might help reduce risk of colon cancer. A varied diet containing plenty of vegetables and fruits rich in vitamins A and C may reduce risk for a wide range of cancers. Salt-cured, smoked, and nitrite-cured foods have been linked to esophagus and stomach cancer.

ALCOHOL   Oral cancer and cancers of the larynx, throat, esophagus, and liver occur more frequently among heavy drinkers of alcohol especially when accompanied by cigarette smoking or tobacco chewing.

SMOKELESS TOBACCO   Use of chewing tobacco or snuff increases the risk of cancer of the mouth, larynx, throat, and esophagus and is a highly addictive habit.

ESTROGEN   Estrogen treatment to control menopausal symptoms increases the risk of endometrial cancer. Including progesterone in estrogen replacement therapy, however, helps to minimize this risk. Consultation with a physician will help each woman to assess personal risks and benefits.

OCCUPATIONAL HAZARDS   Exposure to several different industrial agents (nickel, chromate, asbestos, vinyl chloride, etc.) increases the risk of various cancers. Risk from asbestos is greatly increased when combined with cigarette smoking.

ACTIONS TO DIAGNOSE A CANCER OR PRECURSOR AS EARLY AS POSSIBLE (SECONDARY PREVENTION/EARLY DETECTION).

BREAST CANCER DETECTION   The American Cancer Society recommends that screening mammography begin by age 40. Women age 40–49 should have mammography every 1–2 years, depending on physical and mammographic findings. Women age 50 and older should have mammograms yearly. The ACS recommends the monthly practice of breast self-exam (BSE) by women 20 years and older as a routine good health habit. Clinical examination of the breast should be done every 3 years from ages 20–40 and then every year.

COLORECTAL   The American Cancer Society recommends three tests for the early detection of colon and rectal cancer in people without symptoms. A digital rectal examination by a physician during an office visit, should be performed every year after the age of 40; the stool blood test is recommended every year after 50; and the proctosigmoidoscopy examination should be carried out every 3 to 5 years, based on the advice of a physician.

PAP TEST   For cervical cancer, women who are or have been sexually active, or have reached age 18, should have an annual Pap test and pelvic examination. After a woman has had three or more consecutive satisfactory normal annual examinations, the Pap test may be performed less frequently at the discretion of her physician.

TRENDS IN SURVIVAL BY SITE OF CANCER, BY RACE
Cases Diagnosed in 1960-63, 1970-73, 1974-76, 1977-80, 1980-87

	WHITE					BLACK				
	RELATIVE 5-YEAR SURVIVAL					RELATIVE 5-YEAR SURVIVAL				
SITE	1960-63[1]	1970-73[1]	1974-76[2]	1977-80[2]	1981-87[2]	1960-63[1]	1970-73[1]	1974-76[2]	1977-80[2]	1981-87[2]
All sites	39	43	50	51	53*	27	31	39	39	38
Oral cavity & pharynx	45	43	55	54	54–	–	–	35	34	31
Esophagus	4	4	5	6	9*	1	4	4	4	6*
Stomach	11	13	14	16	16*	8	13	16	16	17
Colon	43	49	50	53	58*	34	37	46	48	47
Rectum	38	45	49	51	55*	27	30	41	37	44
Liver	2	3	4	3	5	–	–	1	3	5
Pancreas	1	2	3	2	3*	1	2	2	5	4
Larynx	53	62	66	67	68	–	–	59	58	54
Lung & bronchus	8	10	12	13	13*	5	7	11	12	11
Melanoma of skin	60	68	80	82	82*	–	–	69†	51‡	70
Breast (female)	63	68	75	75	78*	46	51	63	63	63
Cervic uteri	58	64	69	68	68	47	61	63	62	57
Corpus uteri	73	81	89	86	84*	31	44	62	56	56
Ovary	32	36	36	38	39*	32	32	41	40	36
Prostate gland	50	63	67	72	76*	35	55	58	62	63*
Testis	63	72	79	88	93*	–	–	77†	73†	94
Urinary bladder	53	61	74	76	79*	24	36	48	55	59*
Kidney & renal pelvis	37	46	52	51	53	38	44	49	57	52
Brain & nervous system	18	20	22	24	24*	19	19	27	28	33
Thyroid gland	83	86	92	92	94	–	–	87	92	94
Hodgkin's disease	40	67	71	73	77*	–	–	68	73	74
Non-Hodgkin's lymphoma	31	41	47	49	51*	–	–	48	49	45
Multiple myeloma	12	19	24	25	26*	–	–	27	32	28
Leukemia	14	22	34	36	36*	–	–	31	30	29

Source: Cancer Statistic Branch, National Caner Institute.

[1]Rates are based on End Results Group data from a series of hospital registries and one population-based registry.

[2]Rates are from the SEER Program. They are based on data from population-based regietries in Connecticut, New Mexico, Utah, Iowa, Hawaii, Atlanta, Detroit, Seattle-Puget Sound and San Francisco-Oakland. Rates are based on follow-up of patients through 1988.

*The difference in rates between 1974-76 and 1981-87 is statistically significant (p<0.05).

†The standard error of the survival rate is between 5 and 10 percentage points.

‡The standard error of the survival rate is greater than 10 percentage points.

– Valid survival rate could not be calculated.

FIGURE 4–114 Cancer 5-year survival rates by site and race (From American Cancer Society, *Cancer Facts & Figures*—1992, Reproduced with permission.)

Chronic Fatigue Syndrome (CFS).

This **debilitating** disorder was officially recognized and reported in 1984 by two doctors near Lake Tahoe, Nevada. It was officially declared a disease in 1988. The CDC started a surveillance program costing $1.5 million to track the frequency and impact of the disorder. They also established the following guidelines to help physicians diagnose the condition.

■ Persistent overwhelming fatigue for at least 6 months, that does not go away with rest
■ Low-grade fever
■ Sore throat or swollen lymph nodes or both
■ Headaches
■ Lingering fatigue after levels of exercise that would normally be easily tolerated
■ Unexplainable muscle weakness or pain
■ Pain in joints without swelling
■ Forgetfulness, irritability, confusion, inability to concentrate, depression, sensitivity to light, and impaired vision
■ Sleep disturbances

Patients experience varying levels of ability to perform activity from profound fatigue to being completely bedridden. CFS affects twice as many women as men, particularly between 25 and 45 years old. Children and senior citizens have also been diagnosed, however.

The disorder begins suddenly like the common flu, but the CFS symptoms last for 3 to 4 years. Only about 15% to 20% seem to recover fully; 5% are homebound or bedridden.

The cause of the disorder appears to be genetically predisposed. About 79% to 80% of CFS patients have allergies. Current theories suggest that a virus, bacterium, allergen, or environment chemical enters the body but does not set off the normal immune response to fight the invasion. Instead, the system continues to make symptom-producing chemicals. A second theory suggests that some unidentified organism weakens the immune system, allowing normally dormant viruses to become activated. This theory is supported by the presence of high levels of antibodies to Epstein–Barr virus and others.

Physicians still do not know much about the disorder; some deny its existence because it cannot be detected by a blood test. Diagnosis requires a thorough physical examination and laboratory tests to rule out other conditions with similar symptoms.

Treatment consists of analgesics for pain, antihistamines for allergic symptoms, antidepressants to improve sleep and reduce fatigue. Patients should avoid emotional and physical stress and have good nutrition. Exercise must be appropriate. Psychological counseling may be required to help a patient deal with the changes caused by CFS.

Lupus Erythematosus. **Lupus erythematosus** is a chronic disease of unknown cause in which striking changes occur in the immune system. It causes inflammation of various parts of the body. It can involve only a few body organs or cause serious life-threatening problems. Lupus can affect the skin, joints, kidneys, lungs, heart, nervous system, and other body organs and systems.

In lupus, the usually protective antibodies are produced in large quantities but react against the person's own normal tissue; therefore, it is called an **autoimmune** disease. There are three main types of lupus:

1. Cutaneous, or **discoid,** lupus, which is confined to the skin and causes a persistent flush of the cheeks or disklike lesions on the face, neck, scalp and other areas exposed to ultraviolet light. The rash is usually scaly and red but not itchy. If not treated, scarring may result, and if on the scalp, bald spots may occur.
2. Systemic lupus erythematosus (SLE) inflames the organs of the body. Some persons also have skin and joint involvement, others, skin and lungs or kidneys and blood. The disease is characterized by periods of **remission** when few if any symptoms are evident and other periods of active disease and symptoms.
3. Drug-induced lupus can be caused by certain medications and is similar to SLE. The most common offenders are hydralazine for hypertension and procainamide for cardiac arrhythmia. The symptoms fade when the drugs are stopped.

The incidence of SLE in the United States is approximately 500,000 people. SLE effects women nine times more often than men, most frequently during the childbearing years. Lupus is more common in blacks, Asians, and certain Indian tribes. About 16,000 new cases are diagnosed each year.

General symptoms of beginning lupus are

fever	loss of appetite
weight loss	nausea and vomiting
headache	easy bruising
fatigue	hair loss
swollen glands	edema
depression	

Suggestive symptoms of lupus include

A rash over cheeks and bridge of nose	Discoid lupus lesions
	Ulcers inside mouth
Rashes developing after being in the sun	Pleurisy
	Anemia
Arthritis in two or more joints	**Raynaud's phenomenon** (fingers turn white or blue in the cold)
Seizures	
Bald spots	

Diagnosis is made on the strength of symptoms and blood tests showing low cell counts. Urine is checked for protein, RBCs, and WBCs. A specific antibody test ANA (antinuclear antibody) looks for antibodies to the nuclei of cells. Over 99% of people with lupus will have a positive test; however, only 33% of people with a positive ANA have SLE.

Treatment of SLE consists of assuring patients they can live near-normal lives. Limits on activities are dictated by the disease. Patients are encouraged to rest when needed but otherwise engage in normal employment and exercise. Sun exposure should be avoided at peak hours (10:00 A.M. to 2:00 P.M.), otherwise as tolerated. Sunscreens of at least SPF 15 are advisable. No medication has been developed to cure lupus. Joint and muscle pain is controlled with antiinflammatory and analgesic drugs, such as aspirin, ibuprofen, Naprosyn, and Tylenol. During flare-ups or if major organs are involved, steroids, such as prednisone, are often used to suppress inflammation. The steroid also interferes with the proliferation and interaction of the cells in the immune system and causes T cells to gather in the lymph nodes, which removes them from concentrating at the inflammation sites. The drugs chloroquine and hydroxychloroquine sulfate (Plaquenil) (antimalarials) are valuable in managing the skin lesions and also help control arthritis symptoms.

Many new treatments are being tested, several dealing with self-antigens, immunoreplacement therapy, and even plasmapheresis (the removal of blood plasma, and hence antibodies). It is believed that with further understanding of the immune system, an effective treatment of lupus will be discovered.

Rheumatoid Arthritis. This chronic systemic inflammatory autoimmune disease affects the joints and surrounding muscles, tendons, ligaments, and blood vessels. It affects women three times more often than men. It occurs primarily between the ages of 20 and 60 with a peak onset period between 35 to 45. This disease was discussed in the unit on the skeletal system; however, it is believed there is a connection to the immune system. Recent findings suggest a link to genetic defects, which cause the cells to display a specific cell marker. Patients may also have an autoantibody known as *rheumatoid factor,* which locks onto the body's own IgG molecule as if it were an antigen. These antigen–antibody complexes seem to be deposited on the synovial membranes of the joints and are the targets of the inflammatory response.

When the complement system is activated, the macrophages gather at the joint. The inflammatory response dilates the blood vessels, and fluid accumulates in the joint cavity. The cells of the membrane proliferate in response, thickening the joint membrane and causing more swelling. These events continue in cycles and result in the destruction of the joint.

The symptoms develop insidiously, then become localized in joints, usually bilaterally. The affected joints stiffen following inactivity, swell, and may show beginning signs of deformity. They eventually become tender, painful, hot and enlarged, have marked deformities, and decreased function.

Treatment consists primarily of salicylates to reduce inflammation. Corticosteroids (prednisone), antiinflammatory agents (such as ibuprofen), gold salts, and antimalarial drugs may prove helpful. Patients need periods of rest during the day and 8 to 10 hours of sleep every night. Activities, such as range-of-motion exercises, application of heat during chronic episodes, and ice packs with acute phases, may be helpful. Advanced disease may necessitate total joint replacement or joint fusion to relieve pain.

Complete Chapter 4, Unit 9 in the workbook to help you meet the objectives at the beginning of this unit and therefore achieve competency of this subject matter.

U N I T   1 0

The Digestive System

OBJECTIVES

Upon completion of this unit, you will meet the following terminal performance objectives by verifying knowledge of the facts and principles presented through oral and written communication at a level deemed competent by the instructor or employer.

1. Define digestion.
2. Name the raw materials required for a healthy body.
3. Trace the pathway of food through the alimentary tract.
4. Describe the structures of the mouth and the digestive processes that occur there.
5. Explain the process of swallowing.
6. Describe how the esophagus propels food toward the stomach.
7. Describe the structure and function of the stomach.
8. Describe the structure and function of the small intestine.
9. Tell why the duodenum is such a vital link in the digestive system.
10. List the functions of the liver, including the portal circulation connection.
11. Describe the role of the gallbladder and its association with the liver.
12. Describe the location and function of the pancreas.
13. Explain how and where nutrients are absorbed.
14. Name the sections of the colon and describe its function.
15. Describe the function of the rectum.
16. Describe the structure and function of the anal canal.
17. Describe 11 diagnostic examinations of the digestive tract.
18. Discuss 26 disorders of diseases or the digestive system.
19. Spell and define, using the glossary at the back of the text, all the words to know in this unit.

WORDS TO KNOW

alimentary canal	hernia
anal	herniorrhaphy
anus	hiatus
appendectomy	hydrochloric acid
appendicitis	ileocecal
ascending	ileostomy
bile	ileum
bolus	impaction
cardiac sphincter	incontinent
cecum	insulin
cholecystectomy	intestine
cholelithiasis	jaundice
chyme	jejunum
cirrhosis	liver
colitis	mesentery
colon	mouth
colostomy	nausea
common bile duct	pancreas
constipation	pancreatitis
Crohn's disease	paralytic ileus
cystic	peptic
defecate	peristalsis
descending	polyp
diarrhea	proctoscope
digestion	pruritus ani
digestive	pyloric
diverticulitis	rectum
duodenum	saliva
emesis	salivary glands
enzyme	sigmoid
esophagus	sigmoidoscopy
fecal	spastic colon
fissure	stenosis
fistula	stomach
flatus	stool
gallbladder	tongue
gastric	transverse
gastrointestinal (GI)	ulcer
gastroscopy	varices
hemorrhoidectomy	vermiform appendix
hemorrhoids	villi
hepatic	villous adenoma
hepatitis	vomit

The **digestive** system is the group of organs that changes food eaten into a form that can be used by the body's cells. The system is also known as the **gastrointestinal (GI)** tract or system, and the connecting chain of organs is sometimes referred to as the **alimentary canal.** The digestive process can be divided into four phases: *ingestion, digestion, absorption,* and *elimination.* Food which is consumed is acted on by various mechanical and chemical means as it progresses through the body. Each organ, whether main or accessory, plays an important role in physically or chemically altering the composition of the food, selectively absorbing the elements, or eliminating the remains.

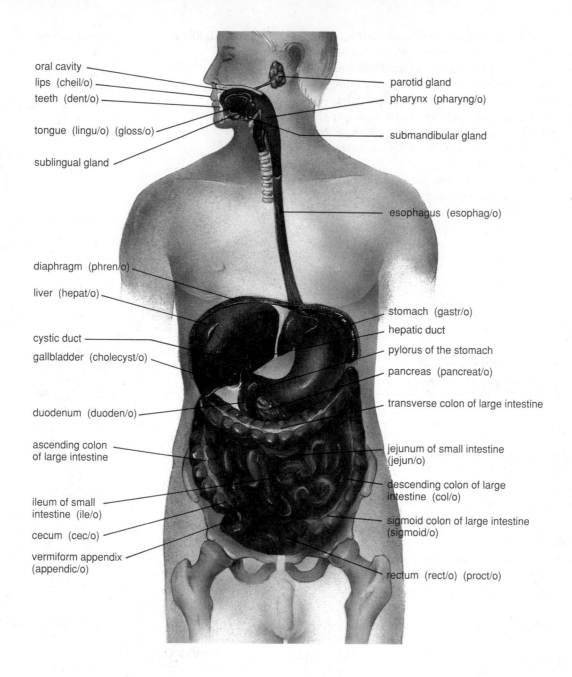

oral cavity
lips (cheil/o)
teeth (dent/o)
tongue (lingu/o) (gloss/o)
sublingual gland

parotid gland
pharynx (pharyng/o)
submandibular gland

esophagus (esophag/o)

diaphragm (phren/o)
liver (hepat/o)
cystic duct
gallbladder (cholecyst/o)
duodenum (duoden/o)
ascending colon
of large intestine
ileum of small
intestine (ile/o)
cecum (cec/o)
vermiform appendix
(appendic/o)

stomach (gastr/o)
hepatic duct
pylorus of the stomach
pancreas (pancreat/o)
transverse colon of large intestine
jejunum of small intestine
(jejun/o)
descending colon of large
intestine (col/o)
sigmoid colon of large intestine
(sigmoid/o)
rectum (rect/o) (proct/o)

FIGURE 4–115   The digestive system (From Smith, *Medical Terminology, A Programmed Text*, 6th ed. Copyright 1991, Delmar Publishers.)

The main organs of the system are those through which the food passes. These organs form a continuous tube from the entrance to the exit of the body. They are the mouth, pharynx, esophagus, stomach, small intestine, and large intestine. As important as these organs are, it is the accessory organs which play a major role in the digestive process. In the mouth there are the teeth, salivary glands, and tongue. The liver, gallbladder, and pancreas have access to the small intestine, Figure 4–115.

_____ is the activity performed by the organs of the digestive system and is defined as the process by which food is broken down, mechanically and chemically, in the gastroin-

testinal tract and converted into an absorbable form that can be used by the cells of the body. This process cannot occur within the digestive system alone. As with all body functions, an interrelationship of systems is required to achieve the desired results. Digestion requires cooperation from the nervous system, the muscular system, the circulatory system, and the endocrine system.

The human body can be compared to an engine that needs appropriate fuel to operate. The energy we need to function must come from the foods we eat. The right fuel will not only supply the body with energy, but also provide the materials necessary to build and repair the body so that it can operate efficiently. If the wrong fuel is used too often, the machine will eventually break down.

The human body can manufacture the appropriate fuel if it receives an adequate supply of the right raw materials, mainly carbohydrates, proteins, fats, minerals, vitamins, water, and roughage. All these raw materials are available from the basic food groups and should be eaten daily.

Carbohydrates supply about two-thirds of the energy calories needed each day. Fats are also an excellent source of energy; in fact, an ounce of fat yields about three times the calories of an ounce of carbohydrate. Unfortunately, the body does not waste excess energy-producing calories but stores them instead. Therefore, when all the calories eaten are not used for energy, they are stored as excess body tissue we may not desire.

Proteins are obtained primarily from plant and animal sources but are not stored by the body. It is especially important that they be eaten daily because they are the main ingredients needed to build and repair cells and tissue.

Other raw materials required for a healthy body are vitamins and minerals. Vitamins are regulating chemicals needed for growth and control of body activities. For instance, the chemical that becomes vitamin D must be absorbed by the body and then become activated in the skin by contact with the sun. The body needs vitamin D to absorb and use calcium. Calcium and another mineral, phosphorus, are needed by the body for the muscles, nerves, and blood as well as the teeth and bones. The formation of red blood cells requires iron and copper. We have already learned that the combination of an iron pigment and a protein forms the hemoglobin of the red blood cells, which enables them to attract O_2 and CO_2 as they move through the body.

All the raw materials the body needs are altered by the digestive system to provide the essential elements necessary for good health. The various stages in this process will become clearer by tracing the pathway of food through the alimentary canal.

The Mouth

Food enters the body through the **mouth.** It is held in the oral cavity while the initial digestive process is begun. Teeth break up food into small pieces to make it easier to swallow and also to prepare it for more effective action by digestive enzymes. "Baby" teeth are called *deciduous* and begin to appear at about 6 months of age. They are gradually exchanged for permanent teeth beginning at about age 6 years. Different teeth have specific duties to perform. The incisors bite food with their sharp edges. The canines (or cuspids) are pointed to puncture and tear. The premolars (or bicuspids) and the molars are for grinding and crushing, Figure 4–116. The **tongue** aids in the process by moving the food around within the mouth, bringing it into contact with the teeth. The tongue is a muscle and can alter its shape to reach all areas of the mouth. The surface of the tongue contains the taste buds, located within the papillae projections.

The **salivary glands** excrete the fluid known as **saliva.** It is released from three pairs of glands: the parotid, the submandibular, and the sublingual, Figure 4–117, page 201. Certain foods cause the glands to excrete profusely, often producing some discomfort, as when eating something sour. The disease called mumps is the inflammation of the parotid glands. A virus causes the glands to enlarge and become painful. With mumps, mastication (chewing) causes great discomfort, because the muscle action squeezes the swollen glands.

Saliva contains an **enzyme** called ptyalin. This chemical begins the breakdown of carbohydrates into sugar. Saliva also provides moisture that enables the taste buds to perceive the sensations of sweet, sour, bitter, and salty. In addition, saliva aids in cleansing the teeth by washing away food particles that might allow bacteria to grow. The presence of saliva in the oral cavity keeps the surfaces moist and flexible, which aids in the production of speech.

The combination of mashed food substances and saliva is called a **bolus.** When it has been mixed well and contains sufficient moisture, it can be easily swallowed. For this to occur several muscles must work together. The tongue presses upward and backward against the palate (roof of the mouth) while the muscles in the cheeks help in the formation of a chute to direct the bolus toward the back of the mouth and into the pharynx, Figure 4–118, page 201. At this point, the bolus could go in three different directions: into the nasal cavity, down and forward into the trachea, or down into the **esophagus.**

The directing of the bolus is accomplished by a complex combination of "lids" and muscles, which operate automatically. As the bolus is swallowed, it raises the soft palate, closing off the nasal cavity. At the same time, the epiglottis, a cartilage lid attached at the top of the larynx, moves across the opening into the larynx when the tongue pushes the bolus against the palate. At the moment of swallowing, the larynx moves upward against the epiglottis to close the opening. Usually, this reflex action works perfectly, but when the timing is slightly off, food may enter the larynx, triggering the cough reflex (to remove the material). We say, "It went down the wrong pipe."

The Esophagus

Once food is swallowed, its movement through the body is maintained by the smooth, involuntary muscle action called **peristalsis.** The esophagus has two layers of involuntary muscles. The inner layer forms circles around the esophagus, and the outer layer runs longitudinally along its approximately 10-inch length. When food enters the esophagus, the muscles alternately contract and relax, squeezing the bolus. Together they create the peristaltic "milking action," which moves the bolus to the **stomach.** The whole process only requires about 5 seconds. Because peristaltic action moves material in one direction only, and this process does not depend on gravity, it is possible to drink a glass of water while standing on your head.

central incisor (7-8 years)
lateral incisor (8-9 years)
cuspid (9-10 years)
first premolar, or bicuspid (10-12 years)
second premolar, or bicuspid (10-12 years)
first molar (6-7 years)
second molar (12-13 years)
third molar (17-25 years)

upper teeth

third molar (17-25 years)
second molar (12-13 years)
first molar (6-7 years)
second premolar, or bicuspid (10-12 years)
first premolar, or bicuspid (10-12 years)
cuspid (9-10 years)
lateral incisor (8-9 years)
central incisor (7-8 years)

lower teeth

A. PERMANENT TEETH

central incisor (7-9 months)
lateral incisor (9-11 months)
cuspid (18-20 months)
first molar (14-16 months)
second molar (24-26 months)

upper teeth

second molar (24-26 months)
first molar (14-16 months)
cuspid (18-20 months)
lateral incisor (9-11 months)
central incisor (7-9 months)

lower teeth

© Richardson 1983

FIGURE 4–116 Permanent teeth and Deciduous (From Fong, *Body Structures and Functions*, 8th ed. Copyright 1993, Delmar Publishers Inc.)

The Stomach ....

The upper opening to the stomach is controlled by a circular muscle called the **cardiac sphincter.** As the peristaltic wave approaches, the sphincter dilates, allowing the food to enter. Once the food is inside, this one-way "gate" closes to prevent its escape.

The stomach is a 10-inch-long, J-shaped organ constructed of three layers of strong muscle tissue, Figure 4–119. It lies just beneath the diaphragm. The inner lining of the stomach is thick and full of folds called *rugae*. Because muscle tissue is elastic and the folds in the lining can straighten out, the stomach is capable of expanding. It can hold about half a gallon of food and liquid.

Once the material has entered the stomach, the muscular layers begin to contract. A circular layer, a longitudinal layer, and an oblique layer work together in a strong rhythmic motion to break up the food into tiny particles. The stomach continues the

ACCESSORY PAROTID GLAND

PAROTID BLAND (MAIN BODY)

STENSON'S DUCT

WHARTON'S DUCT

SUBMANDIBULAR GLAND

SUBLINGUAL GLAND

FIGURE 4–117   Salivary glands (From Anderson & Burkard, *The Dental Assistant.* Copyright 1978, Delmar Publishers, Inc.)

digestive process that began in the mouth. The churning action is prolonged and made more difficult by poorly chewed food.

The mechanical digestive process is assisted by a chemical process. The stomach lining is formed of mucous membrane, whose glands secrete mucus. The stomach lining also has about 35 million **gastric** glands, which secrete **hydrochloric acid** and several enzymes. As the stomach contents are being kneaded, acid and enzymes are secreted by the gastric glands and thoroughly mixed into the bolus. One enzyme (rennin) curdles milk. Another enzyme (lipase) splits certain fats, and pepsin digests the milk curds from the rennin. The hydrochloric acid unites with protein to form another chemical, which in turn is split by the pepsin.

Since hydrochloric acid burns holes in most things it touches, you may wonder why it doesn't destroy the stomach. This is because the lining also secretes small amounts of ammonia, which is capable of counteracting normal amounts of the acid. When a sufficient amount of excess acid is present for a sufficient length of time, however, an **ulcer** (open sore) will develop, usually along the posterior wall near the pylorus. An ulcer in the stomach is known as a gastric (stomach), or **peptic,** ulcer.

The partially digested food in the stomach is changed into a semiliquid state called **chyme** in 3 to 5 hours. Liquids, on the other hand, pass through the stomach in a matter of minutes. Of the solid foods, carbohydrates are digested first, proteins second, and fats last. When the consistency of the chyme

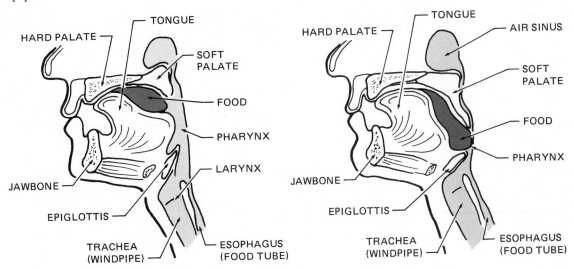

HARD PALATE

TONGUE

SOFT PALATE

FOOD

PHARYNX

LARYNX

JAWBONE

EPIGLOTTIS

TRACHEA (WINDPIPE)

ESOPHAGUS (FOOD TUBE)

HARD PALATE

TONGUE

AIR SINUS

SOFT PALATE

FOOD

PHARYNX

JAWBONE

EPIGLOTTIS

TRACHEA (WINDPIPE)

ESOPHAGUS (FOOD TUBE)

FIGURE 4–118   The process of swallowing

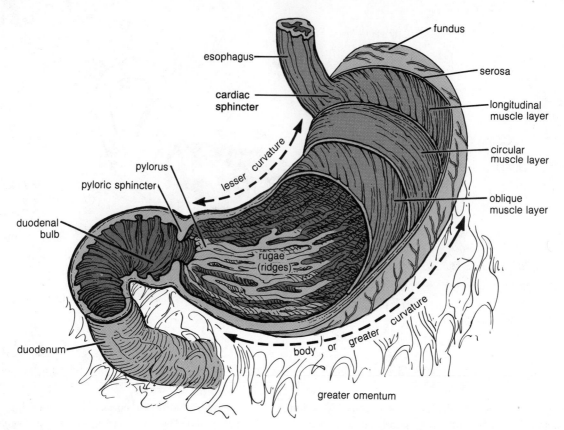

FIGURE 4–119   Parts of the stomach (Copyright by Richardson. From Fong, *Body Structures and Functions*, 8th ed. Copyright 1993, Delmar Publishers Inc.)

is right, the **pyloric** sphincter, at the end of the stomach, allows the chyme to spurt through the sphincter into the small **intestine.**

Because of the two sphincters, food is held in the stomach until it is properly prepared to leave. But occasionally when you suffer from **nausea** and **vomit,** it is obvious the material did not go in the right direction. This action is accomplished by the contraction of the abdominal muscles, forcefully squeezing the stomach as it is pushed downward by the diaphragm. With this pressure and reverse peristaltic waves, the contents of the stomach are forced out, and **emesis** (vomiting) occurs.

The Small Intestine ....

The small intestine is a tube about 1 inch in diameter and about 20 feet in length. It completes the digestive process and absorbs the nutrients from the chyme.

The small intestine is divided into three sections. The first is a C-shaped segment, about 9 inches long, called the **duodenum** (see Figure 4–119). Since this area receives the highest concentration of acid from the stomach, it is especially prone to the development of ulcers. An ulcer in this area is called a duodenal ulcer.

The next segment, the **jejunum,** is about 8 feet in length. The last segment, about 12 feet long, is called the **ileum.** The jejunum and ileum are suspended in the abdominal cavity by the **mesentery,** a fan-shaped fold of tissue which is attached to the posterior abdominal wall.

The ileum is reduced to about half an inch in diameter by the time it joins the large intestine in the right lower quadrant of the abdomen. The junction is marked by a sphincter called the **ileocecal** valve, which allows the chyme to enter the **cecum** (first segment of the large intestine) but prohibits anything from returning to the ileum. (Refer to Figure 4–124, page 206.)

The small intestine completes the digestive process with the aid of accessory organs and intestinal juice secreted by the glands of the small intestine.

The Liver and Gallbladder   The **liver** is the largest gland in the body. It lies below the diaphragm in the upper right quadrant of the abdomen, extending into the upper left quadrant, Figure 4–120. The liver is a vital organ performing several functions for the body. It secretes **bile** at a rate of over a pint a day, and the bile is continuously excreted through bile passages to the bile duct. Unconcentrated liver bile is a bitter, yellow-orange liquid that is required to digest fats. Bile is composed primarily of water and contains pigment from red blood cells that have been destroyed (carried to the liver from the spleen in the portal vein). The pigment is changed in the intestines and excreted in **fecal** material, giving it its yellow-brown color. The iron from the destroyed cells is reabsorbed into the body.

The liver also stores glycogen, a form of glucose (carbohy-

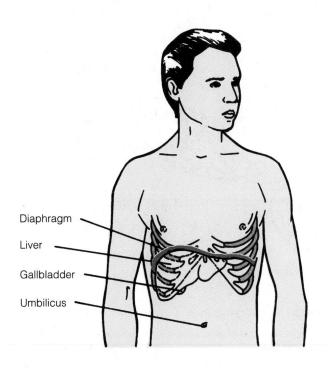

FIGURE 4–120 The liver and gallbladder

Diaphragm

Liver

Gallbladder

Umbilicus

drate). When the body needs additional blood sugar, it changes the glycogen back to glucose and releases it. In addition, the liver processes proteins from amino acids and either burns fats as fuel or stores them. The liver performs the life-essential service of manufacturing fibrinogen, prothrombin, and other substances required for the process of clotting blood. Antibodies to counteract certain disease organisms are produced in the liver. Also, toxins (poisons) that have been absorbed from the intestine, inhaled, injected, or otherwise taken into the body are circulated in the blood to the liver, where for the most part they are rendered harmless. The liver is also an important storage area for blood and body fluid, because of its large size.

The liver receives blood from two separate systems. It receives arterial blood for its own support and preservation from the hepatic artery. It also receives blood from the portal vein that conveys absorbed nutrients and other substances from all the abdominal organs for processing.

The **gallbladder** is a small sac attached to the underside of the liver, Figure 4–121. Its sole purpose is the concentration and storage of bile. When the body needs bile to digest food, the gallbladder releases the concentrated bile to supplement that being currently produced by the liver. Concentrated bile is very bitter and is green-yellow in color. The gallbladder empties its contents via the **cystic** duct. The cystic duct from the gallbladder and the **hepatic** duct from the liver combine to form the **common bile duct.** This combined duct empties the bile directly into the duodenum to be added to the chyme during the digestive process. The duodenum is a very vital segment of the digestive system. Not only does it receive chyme from the stomach and bile from the liver and gallbladder, but as we will soon see, it also receives pancreatic juices from the pancreas.

Obstruction of the bile ducts by **cholelithiasis** (gallstones) is not uncommon. Bile contains certain mineral salts that can become crystallized into "stones" in the gallbladder, perhaps from poor drainage or extended storage. Frequently the stones will be expelled into the cystic duct where they become lodged, causing pain, an inadequate supply of bile, and frequently requiring surgical removal. If the stone reaches the common bile duct before becoming lodged, a much more serious situation results. Now neither the gallbladder nor the liver can empty its bile. The liver maintains its production, but now the bile is absorbed into the bloodstream, producing the yellow discoloration of the sclera, mucosa, and skin known as **jaundice.** The gallbladder itself may become infected or filled with stones and nonfunctional. Periodic "gallbladder attacks" will usually prompt a **cholecystectomy** (surgical removal of the gallbladder). The hepatic duct and the common bile duct must remain for the liver to function, however.

A new surgical procedure to remove cholelithiasis has revolutionized the way cholecystectomies are performed. The procedure is accomplished with the use of three laparoscopes inserted into the abdomen. One is placed in the RUQ, one at the umbilicus, and one in the midupper abdomen. One scope serves as the light source, another to supply air to manipulate tissues, and one through which the operation is performed. The gallbladder and its contents, if any, are excised and removed through the operative scope. Following surgery, only a few sutures are required to close the small abdominal openings. Previous surgery resulted in a long incision extending down the right side of the abdomen and a considerably uncomfortable postoperative period. The new laparoscopic surgery has shortened recovery to 2 weeks or less from about 6 weeks.

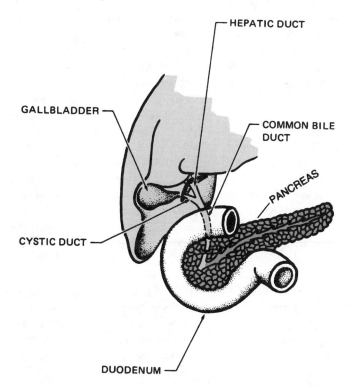

HEPATIC DUCT

GALLBLADDER

COMMON BILE DUCT

PANCREAS

CYSTIC DUCT

DUODENUM

FIGURE 4–121 The gallbladder and cystic, hepatic, and common bile ducts on the undersurface of the liver

FIGURE 4–122 The duodenum and pancreas. A window has been cut in the anterior wall of the duodenum to show the openings of the common bile duct and the pancreatic ducts into the lumen of the duodenum.

The Pancreas

The **pancreas** lies behind the stomach, with its head in the curve of the duodenum, Figure 4–122. The pancreas, like the liver, is a gland but it secretes substances in two different ways. Functioning as an *exocrine gland* (secreting through ducts), the pancreas secretes pancreatic juice via the pancreatic duct directly into the duodenum. The three powerful enzymes in pancreatic juice react chemically on all three types of nutrients to break them down for absorption into the bloodstream. Most of the chemical changes that occur in the intestinal tract are due to pancreatic juices, which are probably sufficient to digest all foods by themselves. If pancreatic juice is absent, serious digestive problems occur.

Functioning as an *endocrine (ductless) gland,* the pancreas also secretes directly into the bloodstream a substance called **insulin.** This function will be covered in Unit 12, The Endocrine System.

It should be clear now why the duodenum is such a critical segment of the digestive tract. Since it receives products from four organs—stomach, liver, gallbladder, and pancreas—it is a vital connective link. When ulceration occurs or a tumor develops in this area, it may interfere drastically with the digestive process. Involvement of the duodenum is a cause for concern.

The Absorption Function

When all the digestive juices and enzymes have been added and the chyme passes into the jejunum, digestion has progressed to the point where absorption of some nutrients and other substances can begin. Absorption is a vital function of the small intestine, occurring primarily in the jejunum and gradually decreasing toward the end of the ileum.

Absorption is accomplished through millions of microscopic structures known as **villi,** Figure 4–123. The villi project from the lining of the major part of the small intestine. These fingerlike structures serve a dual purpose. First, they continuously swing back and forth, keeping the chyme thoroughly mixed with the digestive juices. Second, each projection is equipped with blood capillaries and a lacteal (intestinal lymphatic capillary) from the lymphatic system. The external cells of the villi absorb the nutrients, minerals, and water from the chyme. Some fats and all carbohydrates and proteins, in the form of sugar and amino acids, are absorbed into the capillaries of the villi, to be sent by way of the portal vein to the liver. Here, the products are processed and released into the body or stored in reserve. Many fats are absorbed into the lacteals of the lymphatic system, to be processed through the lymph nodes and eventually returned to the circulatory system for distribution.

The Large Intestine

With digestion completed and the useful nutrients and other substances absorbed from the chyme, the waste products, any undigestible material, and the excess water are sent on to the large intestine through the ileocecal valve. The large intestine is only about 5 feet long, but it is approximately 2 inches in diameter. The **colon,** as it is also called, frames the abdomen, Figure 4–124.

The large intestine absorbs the excess liquid from the chyme through capillaries in the lining. There are no villi in the large intestine. The absorbed water, plus some salts and proteins, are later filtered out of the blood by the kidneys to be eliminated in the urine. The remaining fibrous waste materials are formed into semisolid feces to be eliminated through the **rectum.**

The Cecum and Appendix

When material leaves the ileum it enters a small, pouchlike segment of the colon called

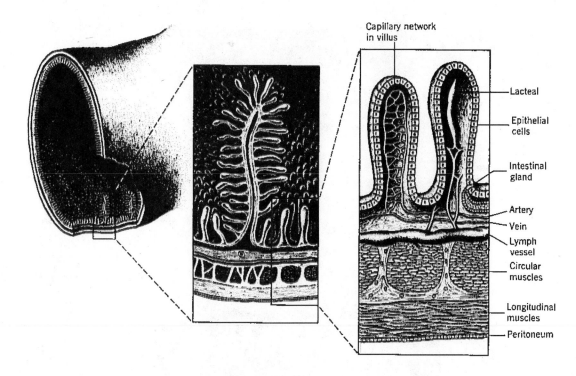

FIGURE 4-123 A magnified view of the inner lining of the small intestine, showing the villi with blood and symphatic capillaries for the absorption of the products of digestion (From Burke, *Human Anatomy and Physiology in Health and Disease*, 3d ed. Copyright 1992, Delmar Publishers Inc.)

the **cecum.** A small projection, the **vermiform appendix,** extends from the cecum. The appendix is a blind worm-shaped structure about the size of the little finger. It tends to fill easily but drain rather slowly. Occasionally, a substance causes irritation to the lining, resulting in a painful, inflammatory process known as **appendicitis.** If it persists or progresses, a surgical procedure called an **appendectomy** is indicated.

The Ascending, Transverse, and Descending Colon

The large intestine is divided into **ascending, transverse,** and **descending** sections as a means of identification. The ascending section joins the cecum at the level of the ileocecal valve and continues upward along the right side of the abdomen to the hepatic flexure (bend at the liver). It is generally a little larger in diameter than the descending section. The upper right corner, the hepatic flexure, lies in front of the right kidney and behind the right lobe of the liver. The transverse section begins at the hepatic flexure and extends in a loop across the abdominal cavity to a point below the spleen, the splenic flexure (bend at the spleen). The center section is attached to the mesentery but can move freely. Both the hepatic and splenic flexures are firmly attached to the rear of the abdominal wall with the splenic attachment being slightly higher.

The descending section begins at the splenic flexure and extends downward along the left side of the abdomen until it reaches the edge of the pelvic cavity. This section is somewhat smaller in diameter. It is firmly anchored to the abdominal posterior wall to maintain its position.

The Sigmoid, Rectum, and Anal Canal After the large intestine enters the pelvic cavity, it makes two bends suggestive of an S and is therefore labeled the **sigmoid** section of the colon. The sigmoid section extends from the left iliac crest over and back to join the rectum. The rectum is 6 to 8 inches long. It serves as a collecting area for the remains of digestion. When enough material is accumulated, sensors are activated, and the urge to **defecate** is felt.

The **anal** canal is a narrow passageway about an inch long, extending from the rectum to the **anus** (opening from the body). Both ends of the anal canal are controlled by sphincter muscles. The internal anal sphincter is an involuntary muscle. When defecation occurs, the nerve endings in the rectum are stimulated to contract and the internal sphincter is relaxed, allowing the fecal material to enter the anal canal. The external anal sphincter is a voluntary muscle and can be consciously controlled to prevent the rectum from emptying when it is inappropriate. It is unwise to make a habit of delaying defecation unnecessarily, however, as this tends to a lessening of the urge, which can result in **constipation.**

When a patient's condition interferes with the ability to control the anus, as in a stroke with paralysis, and the rectum empties whenever the nerve impulse is triggered, the patient is said to be **incontinent** of feces. This situation can be extremely embarrassing to a patient who is still capable of being aware of this occurrence. The opposite problem is often the result of prolonged or serious illness causing a loss of muscle tone so that the patient is too weak to expel the contents of the rectum. This results in material becoming more and more solid

FIGURE 4–124   The large intestine (Adapted from Fong, *Body Structures and Functions*, 8th ed. Copyright 1993, Delmar Publishers Inc.)

as fluid content is lost and the mass becoming of such size that it cannot be expelled. This condition in known as a fecal **impaction.** The best solution is manual breakup of the mass followed by an enema to irrigate the rectum and remove the material. A patient may attempt to remove the impaction by taking a laxative. Laxatives work either by increasing the rate of passage through the tract, therefore reducing the water absorption time, or by stimulating the secretion of fluid into the tract. Whatever type of laxative is employed, the results will not help an impaction but only cause an uncontrollable flow of liquid **stool** around the mass.

The proper function of the digestive system is essential to health. If raw materials cannot be digested and absorbed, the patient will starve. If waste products are not adequately removed, toxins may accumulate and cause illness and even death. This vital function requires a total of about 36 hours from the mouth to the anus. Of course, this time period is influenced by the type of foods eaten and the rate of the peristaltic action.

Diagnostic Examinations ....

A great many studies can be done on blood to determine the function of the digestive organs. Also chemical analysis can be performed on secretions withdrawn by catheter from the stomach or small intestine. Six other types of examinations will be discussed here, however, because they are so frequently used in diagnosis.

■ Cholecystography—An X-ray examination of the gallbladder following oral administration of a contrast medium. The patient is instructed to take the tablets, one at a time, 5 minutes apart, about 2 hours after dinner the evening before the examination is scheduled. After the tablets are taken, the patient must refrain from any food or drink. The medium is digested and absorbed by the small intestine and sent to the liver by the portal vein. The liver processes the blood, excreting the medium in the bile. The gallbladder concentrates the bile. X rays taken 12 to 14 hours after ingestion of the pills will show the gallbladder filled with the medium. If a fatty substance is then given to the patient to eat or drink, the gallbladder should contract and empty bile into the duodenum. This study allows the physician to determine if the gallbladder is functioning properly. A nonfunctioning gallbladder will neither absorb nor empty the dye properly. The presence of cholelithiasis or obstruction of the bile ducts can be determined.

- Colonoscopy—An examination to view the entire large intestine using a flexible fiberoptic scope. It is indicated in patients with complaints of diarrhea, constipation, bleeding, or lower abdominal pain. It is usually indicated following negative or inconclusive results from barium enema studies or sigmoidoscopy examination. Preparation for the examination is like that for sigmoidoscopy. The patient is positioned on his or her left side, and the scope is guided and advanced through the large intestine. The physician may insert air to distend the walls of the intestine to facilitate passage. Manipulation of the abdomen also assists with insertion as well as the repositioning of the patient to facilitate passage through the splenic and hepatic flexures. It is possible to obtain tissue samples and secretions through the scope to provide cytology studies. Polyps can also be snared and electrocautery can be performed through the instrument.

- Gastrointestinal series (X rays)—Radiological studies of the GI tract are indicated for a wide variety of reasons and concentrated on various portions of the system.

  Barium swallow—If the condition or function of the esophagus is in question, the patient may be asked to drink a radiopaque liquid called barium while the action of the esophagus is observed by fluoroscope. This test is known as a barium swallow. It aids in diagnosing condition, such as hiatus hernia, diverticulosis, and varices. It also detects strictures, tumors, ulcers, and functional disorders. The barium swallow is usually included as part of the more complete GI series.

  Upper GI series—A barium swallow is performed initially to evaluate the esophagus. Then 16 to 20 ounces of additional barium are drunk as the progress of the medium is observed by fluoroscope. X-ray films are taken at specific times to permit further evaluation. The stomach is compressed to ensure that the barium coats the entire lining. As the barium enters the small intestine, the radiologist manipulates the abdomen to obtain distribution of the barium throughout the bowel loops. The patient is rotated to several positions to record pertinent areas. Spot films may be taken at 30- to 60-minute intervals until peristalsis carries the barium to the ileocecal valve.

  An upper GI series is not painful, but the chalky taste and consistency of barium are unpleasant. Preparation for the test may require a 2- to 3-day diet of low-residue foods before the examination. All oral intake must stop at least 8 hours before the test is scheduled. The patient must also refrain from smoking. Both a laxative and a cleansing enema may be ordered the evening before the procedure to be certain the tract is empty.

  An upper GI series aids in the diagnosis of gastric ulcers, tumors, strictures of the sphincters, inflammation of the lining, motility irregularities, duodenal ulcers, tumors, filling defects, and the like. Following the exam, another laxative may be ordered to aid in removal of the barium from the intestines. Retained barium may cause constipation, obstruction, or fecal impaction.

  Lower GI series—To permit viewing of the entire large intestine, the barium mixture is administered as an enema. The medium outlines the interior wall of the colon for detection of mucosal changes, tumors, polyps, ulcerated sites, diverticulitis, and structural irregularities. The patient must be carefully prepared with a restrictive, low-residue diet for about 2 days, followed by liquids only the day before examination. A cathartic (strong laxative) is ordered the afternoon preceding the test and the colon is thoroughly emptied with tap water enemas until no more fecal material is expelled.

  A barium enema of 1000 to 1500 cc is administered through a tube inserted into the rectum. This tube is often capable of being inflated with a balloon-like section to aid in retention of the medium until the examination is completed. As the medium is instilled, the filling is observed by fluoroscope. The patient is rotated on the X-ray table to assist the flow of the barium. The patient is placed on the left side to fill the descending, on the back to fill the transverse, and on the right side to fill the ascending colon. Periodic X-ray films are taken.

  When the procedure is completed, the balloon is deflated and the tube is removed. The patient is instructed to expel as much barium as possible. An additional X ray may be taken to record the ability of the colon to empty.

- Gastroscopy/Esophagogastroduodenoscopy—Viewing of the esophagus, stomach, and upper duodenum through a flexible scope which is lighted by fiberoptics. This permits observation of the inside of the organs without an exploratory operation. If an unusual area or growth is seen, a biopsy (small piece) can be removed through the scope. The procedure is also used to remove small foreign objects, obtain cells from the lining, and, with the attachment of a camera, to photograph suspicious areas for later study.

  The patient is prepared by spraying the back of the throat with local anesthetic to block the gag reflex and given a sedative to produce drowsiness. The patient must be awake to swallow the scope. As it is passed into the patient, air is instilled to expand the pathway or flatten out folds. Water may also be instilled to wash off the lens and is removed, along with the air and any other secretions, by suction.

  The examination is especially helpful in diagnosing tumors, ulcers, structural abnormalities, damage from ingested chemicals, and esophogeal varices.

- Nuclear medicine study—Scanning of structures, such as the liver or spleen, is made visible by radioactive materials. A special camera or scanning device may be used to screen the liver for disease processes, infarcts, cysts, tumors, and organ size. The patient is given an intravenous injection of a radioactive material which the body will absorb in the cells of the liver. The scanner is positioned above the patient and passes slowly back and forth in a descending pattern over the area being examined. The resulting pictures outline the organ and indicate irregularities in its composition. A gamma camera is capable of producing images instantly without the scanning procedure.

Similar studies are accomplished with different types of equipment. Computerized axial tomography studies (CAT scans) are multiple X-ray beams passed into tissue to be interpreted and reconstructed by a computer into a three-dimensional picture on a screen. This type of study can be done on the liver, the ducts, and the pancreas.

- Occult blood test—When bleeding from the intestinal tract is not visible because of the small quantity, it can be detected through analysis of the feces. Visible blood in the stool has a characteristic coloration that suggests the approximate location of the bleeding. Basically, the nearer the bleeding site is to the rectum, the brighter red the blood. Dark maroon stool is an indication of bleeding in the ileum or jejunum. Bleeding from the stomach or esophagus will be acted on by gastric juices, which cause it to turn black, resulting in a tarry-looking stool. Occult blood studies are frequently used to identify bleeding associated with colorectal malignancy.

- Proctoscopy—An examination of the lower rectum and anal canal through a 3-inch-long **proctoscope.** It is preceded by a digital examination to determine anal sphincter condition. The proctoscope permits detection of hemorrhoids, polyps, fissures, fistulas, and abscesses. The patient may need an enema if fecal material is obstructing the view.

- **Sigmoidoscopy**—An examination to view the lower portion of the sigmoid and rectum through a 10- to 12-inch sigmoidoscope. A longer flexible fiberoptic scope is capable of manipulation into the descending colon. A digital examination to determine anal sphincter condition precedes insertion of the scope. The patient is examined, preferably on a special jackknife table, otherwise in the less comfortable knee-to-chest position. Sigmoidoscopy aids in the diagnosis of inflammation, infection, or ulcerative conditions. It also permits viewing of tumors, polyps, and other disease processes. Biopsy through the scope permits confirmation of a diagnosis without surgery. The patient must be prepared for the examination with an enema administered a short time before. Soap or other irritants must not be added to the water because they may affect the appearance of the lining.

- Ultrasound—Ultrasonography uses high-frequency sound waves directed toward the liver, gallbladder, or pancreas. The waves create echos of varying degrees, which are changed into patterns of dots on a screen. The patterns reveal the size, shape, and position of the organ being studied. Ultrasonography is especially useful when liver and gallbladder functions are impaired and the use of contrast media is ineffective.

Disorders and Diseases ....

Anorectal Abscess and Fistula. This localized infection is due to a collection of exudate in the soft tissue adjacent to the anus or rectum. It is characterized by a throbbing, painful lump, which makes sitting, coughing, or similar activities very uncomfortable. The abscess may be initiated from within the rectum due to a sharp object in the feces, such as a piece of seashell or bone, penetrating the surrounding tissue. Because the feces contain bacteria, an infection develops and an abscess results. The exudate may develop an escape route into the rectum, anal canal, or skin surface, which will periodically relieve the pain and excess pressure. Such a tract is known as a **fistula.** Surgical intervention is indicated to correct the condition by incision and drainage of both the abscess and the tract.

Occasionally, an abscess occurs without a fistula. It may appear on the surface of the perineum as a large, firm, red mass, with or without a yellow center. This abscess requires incision to promote drainage and eventual expression of the solid core of material. The application of heat by sitting in a tub of warm water aids in the drainage process and relieves discomfort.

Appendicitis. An acute inflammation of the appendix probably is due to an obstruction of the intestinal lumen. When obstruction occurs, an inflammatory process begins and leads to infection, thrombosis, destruction of tissue, and eventually perforation of the appendix. On rupture, the infectious material spills into the abdominal cavity and initiates peritonitis, a serious complication. If left untreated, it is fatal.

Symptoms of appendicitis begin with generalized abdominal pain that later localizes in the lower right abdomen at a site known as McBurney's point. Increased tenderness, anorexia, nausea, vomiting, and rebound tenderness (produced by slowly compressing abdomen over site then suddenly releasing the pressure) occur. A slight fever may be present. A moderately elevated white blood cell count (12,000–15,000) in addition to the physical findings supports the diagnosis. The sudden cessation of symptoms is an indication of infarction or rupture.

The only effective treatment for appendicitis is surgical removal, an appendectomy. When appendicitis is suspected, abdominal heat, enemas, or laxatives must never by administered because of the risk of causing perforation. Usually pain medication is avoided to prevent masking of the symptoms. Positioning patients on their right side with the knees flexed will usually help to reduce the discomfort.

Cirrhosis. This chronic disease of the liver causes destruction of the liver cells. The destruction leads to impaired blood and lymph circulation and interferes with the life-preserving functions of the liver. The most frequent cause of **cirrhosis** is malnutrition associated with alcoholism. Other causative factors are hepatitis or the suppression of bile flow due to a disease of the ducts.

Early symptoms include a variety of GI tract signs, such as lack of appetite, indigestion, nausea, vomiting, constipation, and **diarrhea.** Later, nosebleeds, bleeding gums, and anemia may develop. The liver becomes enlarged, jaundice is present, and ascites (collection of fluid) occurs within the abdomen. Because the disease interferes with portal circulation, hypertension occurs in the portal system causing esophageal varices that eventually rupture and bleed.

Various blood tests support the diagnosis of cirrhosis, but

positive confirmation can be obtained through a liver biopsy. A liver scan will detect abnormal thickening and a mass. Treatment consists of measures to prevent further damage or complications, and dealing with the underlying cause. Dietary changes, supplemental vitamins, rest, and appropriate exercise are indicated. Extra care is required when prescribing drugs because the damaged liver may not be able to process them. Alcohol must be prohibited. It is also important to avoid contact with infections. Mortality is high, with many patients dying within 5 years of diagnosis.

Colitis. This inflammation of the colon causes tenderness and discomfort. It may be acute, occurring as the result of a bacterial invasion, or chronic, associated with allergy, emotional stress, or other diseases. (See ulcerative **colitis.**)

Colostomy. This is an artificial opening of the colon, allowing fecal material to be excreted from the body through the abdominal wall. **Colostomies** are classified according to the portion of the colon involved; for example, transverse colostomy. The terms *single* and *double barrel* tell whether only the proximal loop is involved or both the proximal and distal loop. A colostomy can also be temporary or permanent. If a disease process could improve if the colon were not constantly irritated by passing feces, then a temporary colostomy is indicated. By surgically providing for the fecal material to empty through an opening in the colon before reaching the affected area, the area is allowed to rest and heal. After an adequate period, surgery is performed to reattach the ends of the colon.

A colostomy is also indicated when an obstructive growth process, such as a tumor, prohibits the passage of feces. When the growth is close to the end of the rectum, there may not be enough healthy tissue remaining to which a segment of the colon can be attached. There may also be evidence that removal of the affected area, even if possible, would be to no advantage. In these cases a colostomy will be performed, in order for elimination to occur until the disease process results in death.

The colostomy patient has a major emotional as well as physical adjustment to make. The alteration in body image may be difficult to accept. The thought of fecal material being expelled into a pouch attached to the abdomen may be very unappealing. Consider also that there is no control over the expulsion of **flatus** (gas) or stool, and it is easy to understand the new patient's rejection. With time, diet control, and the use of irrigation, however, a colostomy can be regulated so that its emptying is at the patient's convenience. Support groups of colostomy patients provide emotional and physical assistance to help new ostomy patients adjust to their changed life-style.

Constipation. This condition is characterized by dry, hard, infrequent bowel movements. To have normal elimination of body wastes, three things are necessary: a proper diet (including bulk), adequate fluid intake, and exercise. When one or more of these elements is missing, constipation is likely to occur. Other contributing factors are habitual disregard of the impulse to defecate and the chronic use of laxatives or enemas,

which dulls the impulse stimulation. Constipation is common among the elderly, persons with paralysis, and the chronically ill or bedridden, due to lack of activity.

Treatment varies with the cause and condition of the patient. If possible, increasing the dietary bulk, fluid intake, and amount of exercise will usually solve the problem. Prompt response to the urge to defecate is necessary. Normally, a person's body will establish a routine schedule given the opportunity. The habitual use of laxatives and enemas must be stopped. The use of bulk-forming products and glycerin suppositories can be substituted until new bowel habits are learned.

Crohn's Disease. This is an inflammation of any portion of the GI tract, most common in the terminal ileum. The inflammation involves all layers of the intestinal wall leading to edema, ulceration, narrowing, and the formation of abscesses and fistulas. Symptoms vary according to the location of the disease. An acute episode often causes appendicitis-type complaints of pain, cramping, and tenderness in the right lower quadrant with flatulence, nausea, fever, and diarrhea. Bloody stools are also possible. Chronic disease is characterized by diarrhea of four to six stools daily, marked weight loss, weakness, and difficulty in coping with everyday stress. The exact cause of **Crohn's disease** is unknown. Some feel it is caused by allergies or immune disorders, obstruction of the lymphatics, or infection.

Diagnosis is made after positive blood tests showing increased white blood cells, decreased hemoglobin, and other specific abnormalities. Barium enema studies showing segments of stricture separated by normal bowel known as *string signs* supports the diagnosis. Sigmoidoscopy, which reveals patchy areas of inflammation, helps to differentiate Crohn's disease from ulcerative colitis.

Treatment is mainly symptomatic and may include dietary supplements, steroids to reduce the inflammation, and the use of antibacterial agents. Most important are changes in life-style to obtain more rest and dietary adjustments to eliminate contributing agents. The ingestion of fruits and vegetables must be restricted with intestinal stenosis (narrowing). Surgery may be necessary if certain conditions develop, such as a fistula, bowel perforation, hemorrhage, or obstruction. With extensive disease of the colon, a colectomy with ileostomy may be required (see Ileostomy).

Diarrhea. This condition is characterized by frequent, liquid stools. It can be very serious in infants and small children due to the excessive loss of body fluid. Diarrhea can be caused by a bacterial, viral, or amebic organism. It can also result from a poor diet, toxic substances, foods (such as prunes) that stimulate peristalsis, or an irritated colon. Basically, diarrhea occurs because the chyme is moved too rapidly through the colon without sufficient time for the water to be absorbed. When the lining is inflamed, as with colitis, rapid peristalsis occurs as soon as material reaches the affected area. In addition, the lining secretes excess mucus to counteract the irritating material. This response results in a liquid stool with shreds of mucus.

Diarrhea can also result from nervousness or anxiety. Again, the peristaltic action is stimulated, and the waves move rapidly. Diarrhea is best treated by providing an adequate intake of liquids and taking care of the underlying cause. Medication to slow down peristalsis is helpful, but it will not treat the underlying cause.

Diverticulosis. This is the presence of bulging pouches in the wall of the GI tract where the lining has pushed into the surrounding muscle. The sigmoid colon is the most common site, but diverticuli can occur anywhere from the esophagus to the anus. They are believed to be caused by a high degree of internal pressure and an area of weakness in the intestinal wall. There is a theory that lack of roughage in the diet permits the bowel lumen (opening) to narrow, resulting in higher pressure developing during defecation. The disease is much less common in nations where more natural food and fiber are eaten.

Diverticulitis develops when undigested food mixes with the bacteria normal to the tract and collects in a diverticular sac, forming a hard mass. The mass shuts off the blood supply to the thin-walled sac, followed by inflammation, possibly perforation (a hole), abscess, or hemorrhage.

Symptoms of diverticulitis include irregular bowel movements, lower left abdominal pain, nausea, flatus, low-grade fever, and an increase in WBCs. Chronic diverticulitis may result in fibrosis and adhesions (tissues growing together) that severely limit or obstruct the lumen. Symptoms progress from constipation to ribbon-like stools, diarrhea, distention (swelling up) of the abdomen, nausea, vomiting, pain, and abdominal rigidity.

Treatment initially consists of preventing constipation and combating infection. A liquid diet, antibiotics, and one medication to soften the stool and another to relieve pain and relax muscle spasms are called for. When conservative measures fail, the affected colon section may need to be removed.

Esophageal Varices. Dilated, tortuous veins in the lower section of the esophagus are called esophageal **varices** and are the result of hypertension within the portal vein. The blood flowing through the portal system in the liver meets with resistance due to cirrhosis, a tumor, thrombosis, or occlusion of the veins. As a result, blood backs up to the spleen causing it to enlarge, and the blood flows through other veins. The number of platelets decreases, and the other veins dilate. This results in fluid entering the abdominal cavity causing ascites. With the veins dilated and therefore thinner, and the number of platelets reduced, hemorrhage occurs readily and is often the first sign of the condition. Often massive hemorrhage occurs, producing bloody emesis and stools.

Treatment is limited. To control bleeding, a tube may be inserted into the esophagus to put pressure against the bleeding site. In addition, iced salt water may be instilled into the tube. A drug may be given to control bleeding temporarily. Surgical bypass procedures to correct venous flow may cause from 25% to 50% mortality, and the patient may still die eventually from liver complications instead of hemorrhage. Blood transfusions are also temporary measures. At best, the patient can be kept comfortable until the inevitable massive hemorrhage or coma from liver damage occurs.

Fissure of the Anus. An anal **fissure** is a crack or tear in the lining of the anus, usually the result of passing large, hard stools that stretch the lining beyond its capacity. Symptoms of acute fissure are a burning pain and a few drops of blood on the toilet tissue or underwear. The fissure may develop a swelling at the lower end known as a *sentinel pile*. This protrusion may ulcerate, resulting in painful anal sphincter spasms.

A fissure may heal completely or become chronic due to partial healing and retearing. Later, scar tissue develops in the area, narrowing the passageway. Since the anus must stretch each time stool is passed, healing is difficult.

Treatment consists of digital dilation to prevent stricture, a low-residue diet, stool softeners, adequate liquid intake, hot sitz baths, and a local medication for pain. A chronic condition will require surgical excision of the scar tissue, providing two fresh surfaces that can heal by a gradual regrowth of tissue. Fissures can be prevented by drinking plenty of fluids (eight glasses of water a day), eating a proper diet, and passing stool promptly when indicated.

Gastroenteritis. An inflammation of the stomach and intestines, this term may be applied to such conditions as intestinal flu, traveler's diarrhea, and food poisoning. The inflammation usually subsides within a couple of days and poses no threat to persons in good general health. The very young, the elderly, and the generally debilitated, however, are at risk due to the loss of intracellular fluid.

Gastroenteritis is characterized by fever, nausea, abdominal cramping, diarrhea, and vomiting. It is treated with bed rest, increased fluid intake, and diet. Antibiotics may be indicated for the person at risk, as well as intravenous fluids to combat dehydration. Medication may be needed to control vomiting and diarrhea.

Hemorrhoids. The anal canal and the lower portion of the rectum contain vertical folds of mucous membrane called anal and rectal columns. The veins in the mucosa of the folds frequently become dilated, resulting in internal or external **hemorrhoids.** Hemorrhoids can result from long periods of sitting or standing, diarrhea, constipation, vomiting, coughing, hepatitis, alcoholism, loss of muscle tone, pregnancy, or anorectal infections. Any condition that increases portal pressure, such as pregnancy or hepatitis, or that leads to a trapping of blood in the veins, as when stool is being expelled, interferes with the return flow of blood. As more blood enters the veins, it causes dilation, and the veins bulge into the anal canal or protrude to the outside, resulting in hemorrhoids. With protrusion comes the possibility of developing a thrombosis. The blood may become trapped externally, forming a painful, hard lump. Once this occurs, it will probably need to be incised to remove the clotted blood.

Treatment of mild to moderate hemorrhoids involves regulating bowel habits; limiting sitting time on the toilet; increasing intake of water, raw vegetables, fruits, and fiber; and applying local heat. When swelling and discomfort persist, with pain and bleeding on defecation, additional treatment is indicated. A sclerosis agent can be injected into internal hemorrhoids, which causes scar tissue to develop, thus reducing the dilation. More severe involvement requires surgical removal of the dilated vein and the surrounding stretched mucosa in a procedure called a **hemorrhoidectomy.**

Hepatitis. This three-stage viral infection of the liver results in cell destruction, which causes jaundice, hepatomegaly (enlarged liver), and loss of appetite. **Hepatitis** occurs in three forms called type A (infectious), type B (serum), and a type non-A, non-B hepatitis that is being called type C. All three types are found throughout the world. Type A tends to be self-limiting and rather benign. Type B is extremely contagious and has a higher mortality rate. Type C is the mildest of the three. Type A is also highly contagious and is usually transmitted by the fecal–oral route, meaning organisms from sewage, human, or animal wastes get into the food chain. It is usually transmitted through ingestion of food, water, or milk that has been contaminated, and from seafood taken from contaminated water. Type B is usually transmitted parenterally (other than by mouth). Health care workers are especially prone to it, due to contact with human secretions and feces. Universal precautions are indicated when caring for all patients to prevent acquiring or spreading the disease. Like AIDS, hepatitis B can be acquired through sexual intercourse and contaminated needles, including ear piercing and tattooing. It can also be passed from mother to newborn during delivery. But it can be spread by more casual contact through cuts in the skin and in saliva.

In most patients, involved cells will repair themselves leaving little damage, and in the case of type A hepatitis only, confers a lifelong immunity. When other disorders are present, such as congestive heart failure, diabetes, severe anemia, cancer, and advanced age, complications are more likely, and the prognosis is poor.

Hepatitis produces a variety of additional symptoms, which appear suddenly with type A; type B and C symptoms are insidious. Clinical features of stage one include: fatigue, malaise, headache, anorexia (lack of appetite), sensitivity to light, sore throat, cough, nausea, vomiting, frequently a fever of 100° to 101°F (37°–38°C), and possibly liver and lymph node enlargement. These symptoms occur during the preicteric (before jaundice) stage and disappear when jaundice begins. About 6% to 10% of adults and 25% to 50% of children become chronic carriers. These individuals are infectious and can develop potentially fatal complications due to liver degeneration and cancer.

The second, icteric, stage has begun once the urine becomes dark, the stool is clay-colored, the sclera and skin yellow, and a mild weight loss has occurred. The liver remains enlarged and tender, and the spleen and cervical nodes swell. The jaundice may continue for 1 to 2 weeks. Then liver enlargement subsides, but the fatigue, flatulence (intestinal gas), abdominal tenderness, and indigestion continue. The third stage, posticteric, usually lasts for 2 to 6 weeks. Full recovery requires 6 months.

Complications may develop leading to a chronic hepatitis, which occurs in benign or active forms. The active, known as chronic aggressive hepatitis, has about a 25% fatality rate due to liver failure from cell destruction.

Diagnosis is made based on history that reveals recent exposure to drugs, chemicals, a jaundiced person, or a recent blood transfusion and the presence of typical symptoms. Blood tests revealing hepatitis B antigens and the presence of B antibodies confirm type B hepatitis. Antigens are present only in the early phase of the disease, so a false negative result may occur if the blood is drawn too late.

Presence of the antibody (anti-HAV) indicates type A hepatitis. If these antigens and antibodies are absent, but the patient still exhibits appropriate symptoms, then type C hepatitis is confirmed.

A vaccine has been developed to prevent hepatitis B and is recommended for the following groups of people:

- Newborns
- IV drug users
- Health workers
- Individuals living with an infected person
- Sexually active homosexuals
- Heterosexuals with multiple partners
- Recipients of certain blood products
- Children born to immigrants from regions where hepatitis B is common, such as Southeast Asia
- Infants born to infected women. (Up to 90% of children born to infected mothers become infected and suffer a high death rate.)
- Travelers spending more than 6 months in an area with high incidence

The main problem with the vaccine is it requires three shots over an 8-month period and costs approximately $120 in the United States. Many of the targeted groups of people, except for health care workers and infected mothers, are difficult to reach. It is interesting to note several developing countries are immunizing newborns and others at a cost of about $1.

There is no specific treatment nor cure for hepatitis B. Patients are expected to rest and eat small meals with highcalorie and high-protein content. Medication to help relieve nausea and vomiting may be necessary. An effort is made to determine the source of infection or contagion. Hepatitis is one of several contagious diseases that are to be reported to the local public health department.

Health care workers should protect themselves from suspected or confirmed disease by wearing gloves to handle body secretions or draw blood. Hospitalized patients are isolated, with strict techniques utilized to prevent the spread of the disease.

Hernia (Hiatus). The protrusion of an internal organ through a natural opening in the body is known as a **hernia,** or rupture. One form of hernia involves a defect in the diaphragm that allows a portion of the stomach to move up into the chest cavity through the opening for the esophagus. It is called a **hiatus,** or **hiatal,** hernia. There are three types of hiatal hernias: sliding, which is most common; rolling, or paraesophageal (alongside the esophagus); and mixed, which is a combination of

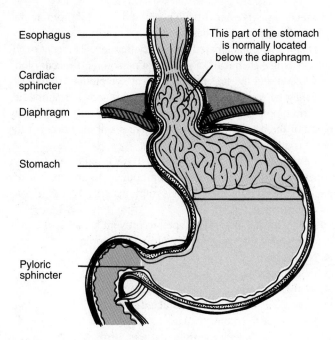

Esophagus

Cardiac
sphincter

Diaphragm

Stomach

Pyloric
sphincter

This part of the stomach
is normally located
below the diaphragm.

FIGURE 4–125   Hiatal hernia

both. This condition is found in up to 50% of the population over 50 years old. If no symptoms occur, no treatment is required.

In all forms of hiatal hernia, some portion of the stomach, the end of the esophagus, or both slips through the diaphragmatic opening, Figure 4–125. In a paraesophageal hernia, a portion of the stomach "rolls" through the opening into the chest but causes few symptoms except a feeling of fullness in the chest and angina-like pain. This type of hernia needs surgical repair. A sliding hernia may cause symptoms, such as heartburn, from 1 to 4 hours after eating, which is often aggravated by reclining and occasionally results in regurgitation or vomiting; chest pain, caused by the reflux (return) of gastric juices; distention and spasms of the stomach; difficulty swallowing, due to inflammation of the esophagus, or an ulcer. The most serious symptom is severe pain and shock, which result from *incarceration* (when a large portion of the stomach is trapped above the diaphragm cutting off circulation to that part of the organ). Since strangulation leads to tissue death, immediate surgery is indicated.

Conservative treatment for uncomplicated hiatal hernia involves medication to strengthen the esophageal sphincter muscle, using gravity to decrease the reflux of gastric juices, and a diet of small, frequent, bland meals. Other helpful measures include waiting at least 2 hours after eating to lie down, eating slowly, and avoiding spicy foods, fruit juices, alcohol, and coffee. Smoking is discouraged because it stimulates the production of gastric acid.

Hernia (Inguinal).   The wall of the abdominal cavity has normal openings through which blood vessels or other body structures pass. For example, the male's spermatic cords pass through the inguinal rings of the lower abdominal wall to reach the testes, which are external to the body. When the surrounding

structure of fibrous tissue, the fascia, becomes weak, it allows a loop of small intestine to protrude through the ring, following the path of the spermatic cord. This type of hernia is called an inguinal hernia, and it often extends into the scrotum when the patient stands. Diagnosis of a smaller hernia can be made on manual examination of the inguinal ring while the patient is asked to cough. If the examiner feels something touch the examining finger, the patient has a hernia.

A protruding hernia can usually be reduced, or pushed back into place. Some patients may wear a device called a truss, which exerts pressure directly over the herniated opening, to hold the protruding mass inside the cavity. Occasionally, the mass cannot be reduced and will remain in the hernial sac. It is then possible for additional intestine to enter the sac or the contents to become twisted or trapped, interfering with the circulation of blood to the intestine. This condition is referred to as a *strangulated hernia* and requires a surgical procedure known as **herniorrhaphy** as quickly as possible. The procedure replaces the contents of the sac within the abdominal cavity and closes the opening.

Hernias can be the result of weak abdominal muscles due to a congenital condition or the natural process of aging. Hernias can also develop from increased abdominal pressure due to heavy lifting, pregnancy, obesity, or straining.

Other types of hernias are femoral, which occurs where the femoral artery exits the abdomen to the legs; umbilical, involving the structure around the umbilicus; and incisional, in an area of previous surgery.

Ileostomy.   This surgical opening of the ileum allows the chyme of the small intestine to empty through the abdominal wall. An **ileostomy** is similar to a colostomy except that the chyme is liquid and highly caustic to the skin due to the digestive juices. The patient with an ileostomy has no control over its function and must wear an ostomy appliance (collection bag) attached to a donutlike disk that perfectly surrounds the stoma (mouth or opening). A protective adhesive creates a watertight seal. A belt attached to the disk supports the device. A permanent type of bag may be attached, which must be emptied and cleaned periodically. Disposable plastic bags can also be used. Some disposable types incorporate a deodorizing material; the permanent type requires instillation of a deodorizer.

The patient with an ileostomy must accept a great alteration in body image and function. The passing of flatus and the gurgling of liquid stool being expelled occurs without warning and cannot be controlled. Most patients who have had ileostomy surgery feel better off than before surgery. Many had extensive ulcerative colitis with much pain, bleeding, and excessive, sudden, and frequent diarrhea, and were in poor physical condition from the debilitating effects of the disease. The removal of the diseased colon necessitates the ileostomy. Other patients may have been affected by Crohn's disease, which causes inflammation, scarring, and near or complete obstruction of the bowel. These patients experienced pain, nausea, fever, cramping, bleeding, and diarrhea, occurring four to six times a day. The freedom from pain and relative increase in control over excretion are often considered to make an ileostomy worthwhile. Many times, these patients have been nearly confined to their homes because of their weakness and the characteristics of the disease. With an ileostomy they can regain fairly good health and live a nearly normal life.

Oral Cancer. The mouth should be examined for oral cancer every time a visit is made to a dentist for routine cleaning and examination. It should also be inspected by the physician as part of a physical examination. People who do not visit a dentist or physician frequently should observe their own mouths for the following oral cancer warning signals:

- Swelling, lump, or growth anywhere in or about the mouth
- White scaly patches inside the mouth
- Any size sore that does not heal
- Numbness or pain anywhere in the mouth area
- Repeated bleeding in the mouth without cause

Any of these signals should be examined by a physician or dentist. Oral cancer can result in a disabling and disfiguring condition when areas are excised. If the tongue is involved, speech and the process of eating become difficult.

Pancreatitis. This is inflammation of the pancreas, which occurs in both acute and chronic forms. The most frequent predisposing factors are alcoholism, trauma to the pancreas, reaction to certain medications, and pancreatic carcinoma. It may also develop as the result of a duodenal ulcer. **Pancreatitis** progresses in an unusual manner. The enzymes normally produced and excreted into the pancreatic duct remain and digest the pancreatic tissue. If the cells that produce insulin are destroyed, the condition will be complicated by diabetes.

Mild pancreatitis is characterized by epigastric pain not relieved by vomiting. A severe attack causes extreme pain, persistent vomiting, a rigid abdomen, and rales (noisy, ausculated breath sounds) at the lung bases with pleural fluid on the left side. Tachycardia may occur, and a fever of from 100° to 102°F (38°–39°C) with cold, perspiring extremities. Rapidly progressing pancreatitis can cause massive hemorrhage, which results in shock and coma. Mortality is as high as 60% when there is tissue destruction and hemorrhage.

The complicated treatment consists of methods to decrease pancreatic secretions and relieve pain while maintaining adequate fluids. Shock is treated vigorously by replacing electrolytes and proteins IV to prevent death. After the emergency passes, IVs containing electrolytes and proteins that do not stimulate the pancreas are continued for 5 to 7 days. This may be followed by tubal feeding if the patient is unable to take enough nutrients by mouth. In extreme cases, a pancreatectomy, the removal of the pancreas, may be indicated.

Paralytic Ileus. A physiological intestinal obstruction, a **paralytic ileus** usually occurs in the small intestine. Peristalsis is either drastically reduced or totally absent. This results in severe abdominal distention and distress, frequently accompanied by vomiting. The condition is often precipitated by manipulation of the bowel during abdominal surgery or the

paralyzing effects of the anesthesia. The ileus usually disappears after 2 to 3 days. If it continues for more than 48 hours, it may be necessary to insert a weighted tube into the small intestine to remove the accumulated fluids and gas. Medication to stimulate colon action may be given.

Peptic Ulcer. This encircled lesion in the mucous membrane lining of the stomach, lower esophagus, duodenum, or jejunum is caused by contact with gastric juices, especially hydrochloric acid. Predisposing factors include long-term overproduction of secretions due to emotional stimulation; damage from chemical irritants (alcohol and aspirin); stimulation of secretions by tobacco; reflux (backflow) of bile into the stomach through a relaxed pylorus; and an overactive vagus nerve, increasing secretions that damage the duodenum.

Gastric (stomach) peptic ulcers are often associated with older men who are undernourished and chronic users of aspirin and alcohol. Duodenal peptic ulcers account for approximately 80% of peptic ulcers. They often become chronic, recurring after a time of remission. About 10% of these patients will require surgical treatment.

Duodenal peptic ulcers cause heartburn, epigastric pain that is relieved by food, a weight gain (due to extra eating), and a strange feeling of bubbling hot water in the back of the pharynx. Attacks occur whenever the stomach is empty or after drinking alcohol, juice, or coffee. Complications that may develop with either type of ulcer are perforation, hemorrhage, and pyloric obstruction.

Treatment consists of diet, drugs, rest, and informed patient cooperation. Medications are used to reduce gastric secretions, with antacids to help neutralize the acidity. Sedatives and tranquilizers are given for gastric ulcers. Drugs that inhibit the vagus nerve are used for duodenal ulcers. Surgical cutting of the branches of the vagus nerve may be indicated to correct excess secretion. Partial removal of the diseased portion of the stomach may be required as a final measure.

Polyp. This is a mass of tissue that results from an overgrowth of upper epithelial cells of the mucosal membrane of the GI tract. There are five varieties, some hereditary, others of common adenoma structure. Most are benign, but **villous adenoma** and hereditary polyps show a tendency to become malignant. Most types develop in adults over 45 years old. Predisposing factors are age, heredity, diet, and infection.

Polyps are difficult to diagnose because they are almost always asymptomatic. They are usually discovered accidentally during a rectosigmoidoscopy or lower GI series X ray. The most common symptom is rectal bleeding. The structure of the polyps varies from small lesions covering the surface of the rectum or sigmoid to large lesions attached by long, thin stalks. The type of polyp determines its physical characteristics.

Treatment consists of surgical removal often by electrocautery, especially if benign and pedunculated (on a stalk). If they are villous adenomas, which are invasive and therefore malignant, treatment usually involves abdominoperineal resection (removal of the colon and rectum, including the area around the anus), with a resulting permanent ileostomy. Each type of polyp is dealt with in relation to its current state or its tendency to become malignant.

Pruritus Ani. This is itching of the area surrounding the anus, often associated with irritation and burning. The main contributing factors for **pruritus ani** are harsh, vigorous rubbing with soap and a washcloth; poor hygiene; spicy foods; anal skin tags (small pieces of suspended extra skin); excessive perspiration; a systemic disease, such as diabetes; the use of perfumed or colored toilet paper; coffee, alcohol, or food preservatives; a fungus or parasitic infection; an anorectal disease such as fissure, fistula, or hemorrhoids; and certain skin cancers.

Classical symptoms are itching after a bowel movement or at night. Scratching can cause reddened, weeping skin or thickened, leathery, darker tissue.

Treatment consists of removing the underlying cause, such as a rectal tag, and eliminating irritants to the skin such as soaps, powders, and colored tissue. The area should be kept clean and dry. Witch hazel applied on wiping pads or cotton balls is soothing. Steroid creams aid in reducing inflammation and controlling itching.

Pyloric Stenosis. This narrowing of the pyloric sphincter interferes with the emptying of the stomach. **Stenosis** can be caused by scar tissue developed during healing of a gastric ulcer. It can also be a congenital condition in infants. The sphincter is enlarged and often cartilagenous, causing a narrowing of the opening, which results in the dilation of the stomach. Forceful vomiting will develop by the third week after birth and lead to a serious dehydration problem.

Congenital stenosis often corrects itself in time if the vomiting is not so intense as to require surgical correction. In adult stenosis, the patient may be able to alter the diet and use medication for some time; however, surgical correction will probably be required eventually.

Spastic Colon. This common condition is characterized by alternating periods of constipation and diarrhea. A **spastic colon** is a functional disorder, often associated with stress. It can also be caused by physical conditions, however, such as diverticulitis, food poisoning, cancer of the colon, and eating certain irritants such, as raw fruits or vegetables.

The condition is characterized by lower abdominal pain, which is relieved by expelling flatus or stool, and the occurrence of diarrhea during the daytime. This pattern alternates with constipation or normal function. Sometimes the stool contains mucus.

Treatment consists of therapy to relieve symptoms such as counseling for stress, dietary restriction of known irritant foods, rest, heat to the abdomen, and the use of sedatives for a short time.

Ulcerative Colitis. An inflammatory disease, often chronic, that affects the mucosa of the colon. It usually begins in the sigmoid and rectum, extending upward to involve the whole colon. The small intestine is seldom involved. The disease produces congestion followed by edema, which makes the mucosa fragile. As the lining breaks down, ulcers are formed, which eventually develop into abscesses. The disease can be confined to one area and be known as segmented colitis, or it can spread throughout the colon. Severe colitis may cause a perforation of the colon, which can result in a life-threatening infection called peritonitis, as well as toxemia (blood poisoning).

Ulcerative colitis primarily affects young adults, mostly female. Predisposing factors are a family history of colitis, a bacterial infection, overproduction of enzymes that damage the mucous membrane, emotional stress, an autoimmune reaction, and allergic reactions to some foods.

The prime symptom of ulcerative colitis is recurrent bloody diarrhea, often containing exudate and mucus. The frequency and intensity will vary with the extent of the disease. Other symptoms include weight loss, weakness, anorexia, nausea, vomiting, irritability, and abdominal pain. The disease leads to other complicating conditions, such as anemia, coagulation defects, liver damage, arthritis, loss of muscle mass, hemorrhoids from frequent stools, and stricture due to no solid stool, perforated colon, and toxemia.

Treatment consists of controlling inflammation, maintaining nutrition and blood volume, and preventing complications. Patients are usually placed on bed rest, IV fluid replacement, and a clear liquid diet. Drug therapy is used to control the inflammatory process and combat infection. Severe involvement may necessitate antispasmotics and pain medication to relieve the cramping and discomfort. If the patient fails to respond to medical treatment and the symptoms become intolerable, surgical resection (removal) of the colon is indicated, with an ileostomy as previously described. Patients who develop colitis before age 15, which persists for at least 10 years, are especially prone to colorectal cancer. Figure 4–126 illustrates some of the disease conditions of the colon and may help in the visualization of their characteristics.

Complete Chapter 4, Unit 10 in the workbook to help you meet the objectives at the beginning of this unit and therefore achieve competency of this subject matter.

FIGURE 4–126 Common conditions of the colon (Courtesy of Marion Merrell Dow, Inc.)

U N I T   1 1

The Urinary System

OBJECTIVES ....

Upon completion of the unit you will meet the following terminal performance objectives by verifying knowledge of the facts and principles presented through oral and written communication at a level deemed competent by the instructor or employer.

1. Explain the three main functions of the urinary system.
2. Identify the organs of the urinary system and describe their physical characteristics.
3. Explain how the urinary system functions with other systems.
4. Describe the interior structure of the kidney.
5. Name the parts of a nephron and explain how each part functions.
6. Describe the process of dialysis and name two types.
7. Discuss the likelihood of success with a kidney transplant.
8. List the two main categories of diagnostic examination and give examples, explaining briefly how each test is performed and for what purpose.
9. Describe 10 diseases or disorders of the urinary system.
10. Spell and define, using the glossary at the back of the text, all the words to know in this unit.

WORDS TO KNOW ....

anuria
bladder
Bowman's capsule
calculi
calyces
calyx
catheterization
cortex
cystitis
dialysis
dribbling
dysuria
elimination
excretion
fistula
frequency
glomerulonephritis
glomerulus
graft
hematuria
hemodialysis
hesitancy
hilum
intravenous pyelography (IVP)
kidney

lithotripsy
medulla
nephron
nephrotic syndrome
nocturia
oliguria
peritoneal
polycystic kidney disease
polyuria
ptosis
pyelonephritis
renal
renal failure
residual
retention
secretion
stricture
suppression
uremia
ureter
urethra
urgency
urinary
urinary meatus
urine
void

The **urinary** system removes nitrogenous waste products, certain salts, and excess water from the blood and eliminates them from the body. At the same time, it evaluates the body's acid–base balance and selectively reabsorbs the elements needed to maintain the proper ratio.

The urinary system performs three main functions. The first is **excretion,** the process of removing waste products and other elements from the blood. The second is **secretion,** by which it produces **urine.** The third is **elimination,** or emptying of the urine from its bladder storage.

The major work of the system is performed by two organs called the **kidneys,** Figure 4–127. The well-being of the human body depends heavily on the function of the kidneys. When waste products are not removed from the blood, they build up, producing potentially fatal toxicity. After the kidneys have performed their functions, the waste material, urine, is carried through the **ureters,** one for each kidney, to temporary storage in the **bladder.** When an adequate amount has been accumulated, the bladder expels the urine through the **urethra,** eliminating it from the body.

As we have said before, no system can function by itself. The urinary system is no exception. Waste products and other substances that are filtered out of the blood must first have been ingested, digested, and absorbed by the digestive system into the circulatory system, to be delivered in the blood to the kidneys. The peristalsis of the muscular system moves the urine through the ureters. The nervous system, in cooperation with a muscular sphincter, controls elimination. The respira-

tory system and the urinary system cooperate to control the body's acid–base balance and the amount of fluid retained. Pulmonary action influences the amount of O_2–CO_2 exchange as well as the amount of fluid loss through respiration. Hormones from the endocrine system also influence the amount of urine excreted. And the integumentary system works in close relationship with the urinary system to remove or retain body fluid as required. Once again it is apparent that the body is a complex, interdependent organism.

The Kidneys

The kidneys are shaped like lima or kidney beans. Each kidney is about $4\frac{1}{2}$ inches long, from 2 to 3 inches wide, and about an inch thick, and weighs about $\frac{1}{4}$ pound. The kidneys are located on each side of the vertebral column, high up on the posterior wall of the abdominal cavity, between the muscles of the back and the parietal peritoneum that covers the abdominal organs. Because they are not within the area occupied by the organs, the kidneys are said to be retroperitoneal (behind the peritoneum). The left kidney is slightly higher than the right, which is displaced by the liver. Normally, a heavy cushion of fat helps keep the kidneys in their proper position. A condition known as **ptosis** (dropping) occurs in very thin persons due to an inadequate fatty cushion.

Externally the kidney is covered with a tough, fibrous capsule. The concave border has a notch called the **hilum** through which the **renal** (kidney) artery enters and the renal vein and renal pelvis of the ureter exits. Internally the kidney is divided into two section: an outer layer, the **cortex,** and an inner, the **medulla,** Figure 4–128. The medulla is divided into triangle-shaped wedges called renal pyramids with bases toward the cortex and "tops," or renal papillae, emptying into cavities called **calyces** (singular, **calyx**). The pyramids have a striated (striped) appearance; the cortex appears smooth. The cortex extends inward between the pyramids in sections called renal columns.

The Nephrons

The life-preserving service of the kidney is performed by microscopic units called **nephrons.** Each kidney has over 1 million of these units, which altogether contain roughly 140 miles of filters and tubes. Each minute, the kidneys filter over 1000 cc of blood, producing about 60 cc of urine per hour. In an average day, a person takes in 2500 cc of fluid ($2\frac{1}{2}$ qt) and generates another 300 cc (10 oz) of water, which is formed by the cells in the process of combining oxygen and other materials. About 1500 cc ($1\frac{1}{2}$ quarts) is eliminated as urine each day. Additional fluid is lost through feces and respiration. Some moisture is also lost through the skin, especially when perspiring. Despite the amount of liquid consumed, the kidneys maintain a constant amount of fluid in the body's tissues, excreting the excess as urine. The concentration of the urine is in direct relationship to the amount of liquid consumed.

The process by which the nephrons produce urine is complex. The nephron is a peculiarly shaped structure resembling

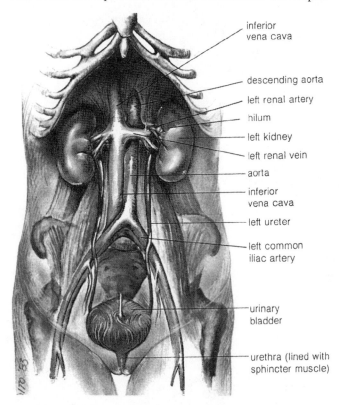

inferior
vena cava

descending aorta

left renal artery

hilum

left kidney

left renal vein

aorta

inferior
vena cava

left ureter

left common
iliac artery

urinary
bladder

urethra (lined with
sphincter muscle)

FIGURE 4–127 The urinary system (From Fong, Body Structures and Functions, 8th ed. Copyright 1993, Delmar Publishers Inc.)

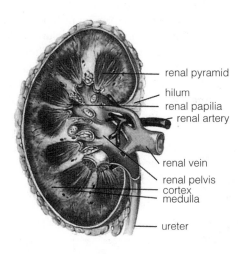

FIGURE 4–128 Cross section of the kidney (From Fong, *Body Structures and Functions,* 8th ed. Copyright 1993, Delmar Publishers Inc.)

a funnel with a long, twisted tail, Figure 4–129. The top of the funnel is a double-walled hollow capsule called the **Bowman's capsule.** Each capsule contains a cluster of about 50 capillaries called the **glomerulus.** The Bowman's capsule

and the glomerulus together are known as the renal corpuscle.

Blood enters the glomerulus by way of an afferent arteriole, flows through the glomerular capillaries, and leaves through the efferent arteriole. The efferent arteriole branches into capillaries that surround the renal tubule. The capillaries come back together in tiny veins, which join a branch of the renal vein.

Beyond the Bowman's capsule is a twisted section of tubule called the *proximal convoluted tubule.* The capsule and this section of tubule descend into the medulla and are called the *loop of Henle.* This loop has a straight descending and ascending limb, but when it returns to the cortex it changes into another twisted section called the *distal convoluted tubule.* Several distal tubules join into a straight collecting tubule, which empties into the calyx.

Filtration and Reabsorption. Filtration is the first process in the formation of urine. Blood enters the capsule by way of the afferent arteriole, carrying waste products, water, salt, urea, and glucose. The arteriole divides, forming approximately 50 glomerular capillaries. Because so many capillaries are emptied by a single efferent arteriole, blood pressure increases significantly. This higher pressure forces the fluid to leave the blood by filtration and enter Bowman's capsule at the rate of about 125 mL a minute. This equals a rate of 60,000 mL (60 L, or 56.8 qt) in an 8-hour period.

By a reabsorption process, 99% of the filtrate is returned to the bloodstream. Not only fluid but also useful substances, such as glucose, vitamins, amino acids, electrolyte salts, and bicarbonate ions (base) are reabsorbed. As the filtrate enters the proximal tubule, about 80% of the water is reabsorbed into the sur-

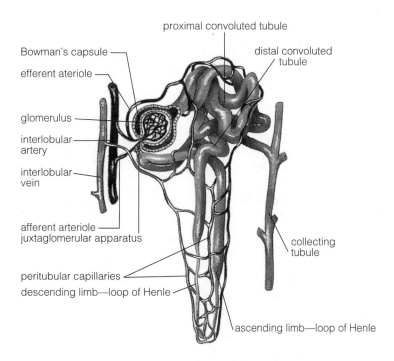

FIGURE 4–129 A nephron unit and related structures. (The collecting tubules, which are not microscopic, give the pyramids of the medullary portion of the kidney a striated appearanced. As shown, there are some collecting tubules in the cortical portion of the kidney.) (From Burke, *Human Anatomy and Physiology in Health and Disease,* 3d ed. Copyright 1992, Delmar Publishers Inc.)

FIGURE 4–130 The ureter, renal pelvis, and calyces

sium ions, and drugs. The elements are selectively secreted to maintain the body's acid–base balance.

Urinary Output. Anything that increases the volume of blood in the capillaries increases the output of urine; conversely, the urine output decreases with a lessening of blood volume. For example, a large fluid intake increases the volume of blood and the output of urine. Hemorrhage or dehydration decreases blood volume and urine output.

Another factor regulating secretion is the amount of solutes in the filtrate. Again considering the diabetic, when there is an increase in the amount of glucose, it spills over into the urine, increasing the urine volume eliminated because more liquid is allowed to pass through to dilute the glucose content.

The functional capacity of the healthy kidney is so great that removal of one kidney poses no problem to the body in removing liquid wastes.

The Ureters

The urine secreted by the nephrons drops out of the collecting tubules into the calyces, then enters the renal pelvis and continues down the ureters into the urinary bladder, Figure 4–130. The ureters begin with a widened upper portion, continuing as a long, slender, muscular tube approximately 10 to 12 inches in length. Peristaltic waves, at a rate of one to five a minute, move the urine down the ureter to enter the lower posterior wall of the bladder. Because of the solutes in urine, some persons tend to form renal **calculi** (stones). As the calculi form in the renal pelvis, they are washed into the ureter by the urine. When a stone is large enough to become lodged in the ureter, severe pain results. Frequently, removal of the stone may be required if it cannot be passed into the bladder. (See Renal Calculi in Diseases and Disorders.)

The Urinary Bladder

The bladder is a collapsible bag of muscular tissue lying behind the symphysis pubis. The lining has many folds, giving it the ability to expand. The bladder serves as a reservoir for urine, collecting approximately 250 cc before the urge to **void** (urinate) is felt. The capacity of the bladder is two to three times this amount, and in instances of **retention** (inability to empty the bladder), may be in excess of 1000 cc. In such instances, urine must be removed by inserting a catheter through the urethra into the bladder to relieve the distention and discomfort. This procedure is known as **catheterization.**

The Urethra

The urethra is a tube leading from the bladder to an exit from the body. In the female, it is a straight tube about 1½ inches in length. It opens externally between the clitoris and the vagina within the folds of the labia minora. The opening is called the **urinary meatus.** Only urine passes through the female urethra. In the male, the urethra is about 8 inches long, extending internally from the bladder down through the prostate gland

rounding peritubular capillaries along with other substances the body needs to maintain a proper balance. For example, the filtrate contains glucose, which is normally completely reabsorbed. When levels exceed normal limits, however, the selective cells lining the tubules no longer reabsorb glucose but allow it to remain in the tubule to be eliminated in the urine. The term used to describe the limit of sugar reabsorption is the *threshold.* Passing this level is referred to as *spilling over the threshold.* Patients who have diabetes spill sugar frequently and therefore test its presence in their urine to determine the need for additional insulin.

A final reabsorption takes place in the distal tubule. The remaining 10% to 15% of water may be reabsorbed depending on the body's need. The process is controlled by a hormone that acts upon the nephron.

Secretion. The secretion function of the nephron moves substances directly from the blood in the peritubular capillaries into the urine in the distal and collecting tubules. The substances secreted directly are ammonia, hydrogen ions, potas-

and out through the penis to the meatus. The male urethra also serves as a passageway for semen.

A circular muscle sphincter within the urethra permits voluntary control of bladder function. This control, however, requires an intact nerve supply and motor area of the brain. Involuntary emptying of the bladder is known as *incontinence*.

Other medical terminology commonly used to describe urinary output includes **anuria,** an absence of urine; **dysuria,** pain or discomfort associated with voiding; **hematuria,** blood in the urine; **nocturia,** having to urinate at night; **oliguria,** a scanty urinary output; and **polyuria,** excessive urination. Descriptive words used to clarify symptoms are **dribbling,** the involuntary loss of drops of urine; **frequency,** the necessity to void often; **hesitancy,** difficulty in initiating urination; and **urgency,** the sudden need to void.

Dialysis ....

Dialysis is the mechanical process of removing waste products from the blood normally removed by the kidneys. Basically it is a process for purifying blood by passing it through thin membranes and exposing it to a solution which continually circulates around the membranes. The solution is called *dialysate.* Substances in the blood pass through the membrane into the lesser concentrated dialysate in response to the laws of diffusion. This is called **hemodialysis.**

The term *artificial kidney* is often used to refer to the kidney dialysis unit. The part of the unit that actually substitutes for the kidney, however, is a glass tube approximately 8 inches long and about 1½ inches in diameter. The tube, called the dialyzer, is filled with thousands of minute hollow fibers attached firmly at both ends, Figure 4–131. Blood from the patient

FIGURE 4–131 Dialyzer

FIGURE 4–132 Hemodialysis unit

flows through the fibers, which are surrounded by circulating dialysate. The dialysate can be individualized for each patient to provide the appropriate levels of sodium, bicarbonate, and other substances. These cross the membrane and enter the blood. At the same time, extra water and waste products leave the blood to enter the dialysate.

The patient is connected to the dialysis unit by means of needles and tubing that take blood from the patient, circulate it through the machine and return it to the patient. New programmable dialysis management systems, as seen in Figure 4–132, can monitor blood pressure; allow variable control of solution substances; adjust temperature, flow, and filtration rate of the blood; and preset the length of treatment time, plus other functions, all automatically. (On the system pictured, the dialyzer is located just left of center; it has black ends with tubing attached to both ends.)

A **fistula** (opening between an artery and vein), or a **graft** (vein inserted between an artery and a vein) is surgically constructed in the patient to provide a site for inserting the large needles required in dialysis, Figure 4–133, page 220. The fistulas and grafts are artificial veins that can withstand repeated

ARTERIOVENOUS FISTULA

ARTERIOVENOUS VEIN GRAFT

FIGURE 4–133 Hemodialysis sites

needle insertions. They lie just under the skin surface and require 2 to 4 weeks for a graft and 8 to 12 weeks for a fistula to completely heal before they can be used. There is considerable amount of pressure within the blood vessels, which could rupture new sites.

The initial site is the nondominant forearm, usually at the radial artery. When this begins to fail, sites are constructed at the brachial artery, then in the dominant arm, and finally grafts at the femoral artery in the groin area. Artificial veins last from 3 to 5 years. Some patients who have had a graft constructed from one of their own veins have had unusually successful sites for as long as 10 years, but this is not the norm. Since dialysis occurs so frequently, the multiple needle insertions not

only affect the grafts or fistulas but the overlying skin as well. When too much damage has occurred, the site is no longer usable. The patient must learn to care for the site and protect it from damage. This is truly the lifeline for the patient with renal failure. Nothing, such as tight clothing or elastic cuffs, must constrict the site area. The patient is not allowed to sleep on the involved arm. Women cannot have purse straps across the forearm. Care must be taken when carrying any objects in the arms, such as grocery bags, boxes, firewood, books, and similar articles, that could damage the site.

Since the rest of the patient's life depends on dialysis, access to a machine becomes critical. Most patients are assigned to dialysis centers for periodic treatment. Equipment can be obtained for home dialysis, however, when the patient and the family are willing to assume the responsibility. Patients usually require dialysis two to three times per week, for 3 to 5 hours each time.

An alternative to hemodialysis is continuous ambulatory **peritoneal** dialysis, Figure 4–134. Instead of an artificial dialyzer to cleanse the blood, the patient's own peritoneal membrane is used (the peritoneum covers the abdominal organs and lines the abdominal cavity). The dialyzing solution is introduced into the peritoneal cavity where it comes into contact with blood vessels. The solution enters through a catheter permanently implanted into the abdomen. The solution tubing is aseptically attached and approximately 2 L of dialyzing solution are infused by the process of gravity by suspending the bag at shoulder level. Then the empty bag is rolled up and placed around the waist under the clothing. The solution attracts the waste products and water from the blood and they are suspended in the solution. After approximately 4 to 6 hours, the bag is unrolled, placed lower than the abdomen, and the waste-bearing dialyzing solution is drained out. Another fresh bag is infused and the dialysis continues. The exchange process of draining the solution and infusing fresh solution requires from 30 to 45 minutes. This is repeated about every 4 to 6 hours during the day and for an 8-hour period at night.

FIGURE 4–134 Peritoneal dialysis. (a) Infusion of the solution. (b) Rolled empty solution container is hidden under clothing.

Another form of peritoneal dialysis is called *automated peritoneal dialysis*. This is more acceptable to some individuals because the dialysis is accomplished during 6 to 8 hours every night while they sleep. This is especially well suited for children. The patient can completely control peritoneal dialysis, permitting greater freedom of activity; however, solution exchanges approximately four times daily do create some inconvenience.

The main complication of peritoneal dialysis is peritonitis, an inflammation of the peritoneum from accidental contamination of the tubing when connecting and disconnecting solutions. Users of the method must be meticulous in performing the procedure. Peritonitis is painful and can cause scarring of the peritoneum, making it no longer useful for dialysis. Peritonitis can be fatal.

Many considerations must be weighed when dialysis becomes necessary. Routine procedures, such as taking medications, for example, must be timed after dialysis to prevent removing them from the bloodstream. For additional information about this life-prolonging procedure, contact your local branch of the National Kidney Foundation, inquire at a dialysis center, or consult your physician.

Kidney Transplant

The transplantation of body organs is always at risk of recipient rejection; however, the kidney appears to be fairly successfully transplanted. Transplantation is indicated in cases of prolonged chronic debilitating disease and renal failure involving both kidneys. It is usually done following an extended period on dialysis waiting for a compatible organ.

The demand exceeds the supply for healthy organs. In addition, blood and other cellular structure must "match" to ensure the greatest probability for a functioning transplanted organ. There is an anticipated percentage of success within immediate family members. A twin provides the greatest likelihood, with a brother or sister, parent, or child providing decreasing percentages of success in that order. The surgical procedure itself is well established and presents virtually no concern as far as the success of the transplanted kidney. The patient, however, is almost always in a state of relatively poor physical condition due to the effects of the extended illness. This status plus the tendency of the body to reject a "substance" that is foreign and not of the same cellular structure sometimes results in the organ not surviving in its new host. The use of drugs to control the body's natural defensive mechanism of rejection increases the rate of success. Research into new and more effective drugs is a continuing process.

Diagnostic Examinations

Several procedures and tests are used to determine the physical characteristics of the urinary system and assess its function. Analysis of the blood can determine levels or uric acid and the amount of urea nitrogen present. Urinalysis (analysis of the urine) can determine presence of blood cells, bacteria, acidity level, specific gravity (weight), and physical characteristics, such as color, clarity, and odor.

■ Noninvasive procedures—Procedures that attempt to evaluate function deal with urinary output. An intake–output measurement involves keeping a record of all fluid, or food that melts to liquid, that is consumed, along with all urine or other fluid loss, be measured or estimated. For example, emesis would be measured; perspiration estimated as slight, moderate, or profuse; diarrhea indicated as to frequency; and any other loss, such as bleeding; drainage through a stoma, or excessive respiratory activity, evaluated. Hence, intake is compared to output to evaluate fluid balance within the body.

A 24-hour urine test collects all urinary output, from a specified hour one day until the same time the next day, in a special container under specific conditions (see Chapter 7). Urine can be collected by various methods, depending to some degree on the purpose for collection. A routine specimen, preferably the first of the morning, is simply voided into a clean container. A clean catch specimen, usually for culture purpose, pregnancy determination, or microscopic examination, involves specific cleaning of the meatal area and catching the specimen midstream in a sterile container.

An X ray or plain film of the abdomen may be taken to determine size, shape, and position of the urinary organs. It may also indicate the presence of calculi. This is usually referred to as a KUB (kidney, ureters, and bladder) series.

The kidney is also frequently examined by ultrasound to detect abnormalities or to clarify findings from other tests. It is a safe, painless procedure that can be used especially in cases where sensitivity to the radiological opaque materials prohibits other tests. Examinations for kidney function that use a contrast medium are of little value when there is renal failure. Ultrasound, however, can be used to at least view the structure of the kidney in these instances.

■ Invasive procedures—Another means of collecting a urine specimen is to withdraw it directly from the bladder through a catheter into a sterile container by strict aseptic (sterile) technique.

One of the most common diagnostic procedures is an X-ray series called **intravenous pyelography (IVP)**. The patient is required to fast (no food or water) for approximately 10 hours beforehand. A laxative or cleansing enema removes from the colon any fecal material that might obscure the urinary organs. A contrast medium is injected into a vein, usually at the antecubital space of the arm. After a period of time, a film is taken to demonstrate the function, location, and position of the kidneys, as determined by the presence of the dye. Subsequent films outline the ureters and bladder as the dye is processed by the system. The film is taken at specific intervals to assess the efficiency of the kidney function. Because the contrast medium is iodine-based, it is extremely important to determine if the patient has an allergic response to iodine or seafood before the injection.

Cystourethroscopy is an examination using lighted instruments inserted into the urethra and bladder to view the interior surfaces. A local anesthetic (sometimes a general) is given. Then the urethroscope is inserted into a lubricated sheath. As the scope and sheath are inserted, the interior of the urethra is observed. The scope is then advanced into the bladder. The urethroscope is withdrawn and the cystoscope inserted through the sheath to view the interior of the bladder. A solution is instilled to distend the bladder lining for observation and to make the ureteral openings visible. At this point, based on findings, other procedures can be performed, such as catheterization of the kidney(s) by inserting a catheter up through the ureter(s); biopsy of a tumor; or removal of calculi in the bladder. It may be possible to crush larger calculi with an instrument and irrigate the pieces out through the scope. When examination of the bladder is completed, the cystoscope is withdrawn and the urethroscope reinserted. Both the scope and the sheath are slowly withdrawn while the neck of the bladder and the interior of the urethra are examined.

Other standard procedures performed initially during cystourethroscopy are obtaining a sterile specimen for culture and sensitivity testing and measuring the amount of **residual** urine left in the bladder after the patient has voided, just prior to the examination.

Other X-ray examinations can be performed in connection with endoscopic examinations. When a catheter is inserted into the ureters and passed into the pelvis of the kidney, any urine present can be removed and a radiopaque medium instilled. This procedure, known as *retrograde ureteropyelography,* is especially useful for viewing the renal structure when poor kidney function prohibits an IVP procedure. The structure of the ureters can be seen by an additional dye injection as the catheter is withdrawn.

Fluoroscopy as well as X-ray films aid in determining abnormalities. A delayed film, 15 to 20 minutes following instillation of the dye, can be taken to check for retention indicative of urinary stasis (stagnation). If an obstruction of the kidney is observed, it can be located by the film to be corrected. When an obstruction prohibits urinary function, the catheter may be left in position temporarily to ensure adequate drainage. A kidney can be severely, if not permanently, damaged in a relatively short time if pressure from urine builds up due to the inability to drain.

Diseases and Disorders ....

Cystitis. This inflammation of the bladder usually results from an ascending organism introduced through the meatus. The most common cause in women is *Eschervichia coli* (E. coli) from the rectum, which is carried to the meatus by improper cleansing following defecation. Women should be instructed to always cleanse from front to back when washing, wiping, or drying the perineal area. **Cystitis** can also be caused by organisms from the vagina or a sexual partner. Women are far more prone to infection than men, presumably because the urethra is so short. Also the prostatic fluid in the male acts as an antibacterial shield.

Symptoms of cystitis are frequency, dysuria, spasms of the bladder, nocturia, and often fever and hematuria. Nausea, vomiting, chills, tenderness over the bladder area, and lower-back pain may occur. A frequent complaint is sharp, stabbing pain when voiding, especially at the end of the stream. This discomfort, together with the urge to void small amounts frequently, prompts the patient to seek medical help.

Diagnosis is confirmed by clinical characteristics and the presence of organisms in the urine in excess of normal amounts. Cystitis is treated with antibiotics sufficient to sterilize the urine. Usually, medication is given for approximately 5 days. A culture of the urine after 3 days should show no organisms. If bacterial resistance to a certain medication has developed, the drug of choice will need to be changed. The sensitivity studies performed on the urine culture will identify appropriate alterations.

Urinary tract infections (UTI) are particularly common in patients with neurogenic bladders. The problem stems from the loss of innervation to the bladder, which can cause incontinence, residual retention, spasticity, or flaccidness. Bedfast patients or those confined to wheelchairs are especially susceptible. The use of indwelling catheters to deal with incontinence or the inability to void frequently results in UTI due to the direct entrance route for bacteria into the bladder.

Glomerulonephritis. This inflammation of the glomerulus of the nephron occurs in both acute and chronic forms. Acute **glomerulonephritis** (AGN) always follows a streptococcal infection, usually of the respiratory system. It affects boys ages 3 to 7 most frequently, but can strike either sex at any age. Up to 95% of children and 70% of adults recover fully, with the remainder developing chronic renal failure. AGN results from a collection of antibodies from the streptococcal infections, which become entrapped in the glomeruli membranes. The entrapment causes interference in the glomerular function, damaging the membrane and resulting in the loss of its ability to selectively filter solutes. Red blood cells and protein molecules are allowed to filter out and the filtration rate drops. Uremic poisoning may result. (See Uremia.)

AGN usually begins from 1 to 3 weeks after an untreated throat infection. Symptoms include moderate edema, protein in the urine, hematuria, oliguria, and fatigue. Hypertension may develop due to retention of sodium or water from the decreased glomerular filtration rate. Diagnosis is made following a detailed history and clinical assessment. Laboratory findings confirm elevated electrolytes, BUN (blood urea nitrogen), and creatinine in the blood as well as red and white blood cells, and protein in the urine. A throat culture may show a streptococcal organism.

Treatment consists of bed rest, fluid and salt restriction, and correction of the electrolyte imbalance. Diuretics (water pills) may be used to reduce the accumulation of cellular fluid. At this time the use of antibiotics is controversial. The course of AGN usually resolves in about 2 weeks.

Chronic glomerulonephritis is a slow, progressive disease that results in scarring and sclerosing of the inflamed glomeruli, gradually leading to renal failure. Unfortunately, sufficient symptoms are not produced to cause early clinical investigation. The first symptoms are proteinuria (protein in the urine), hematuria, and a specific form of a urine cast. By the time it is diagnosed, chronic glomerulonephritis is usually irreversible. Occasionally, the chronic form follows AGN, but most frequently it is an insidious disease precipitated by other primary renal disorders or systemic syndromes.

The chronic stage can be asymptomatic for many years, suddenly becoming progressive and producing hypertension, proteinuria, and hematuria. In the later stages, uremic symptoms occur, such as nausea, vomiting, pruritus, dyspnea, fatigue, mild to severe edema, and anemia. Severe hypertension may cause enlargement of the heart, congestive heart failure (CHF), and eventually renal failure.

Treatment consists of measures to treat the symptoms only, such as a diet to restrict sodium, antihypertensive drugs, correction of the electrolyte imbalance, reduction of edema, and prevention of cardiac failure.

Nephrotic Syndrome (Nephrosis). This noninflammatory disease involving the glomerular membrane allows a large number of protein molecules to leave the blood and enter the urine. As a result, large amounts of water accumulate in the body, causing generalized dependent edema. This often leads to pleural effusion, swollen external sex organs, and ascites (fluid within the abdomen). **Nephrotic syndrome** occurs most often in children, but adults can contract the disease as well.

The underlying cause of the disease is usually glomerulonephritis (75% of the cases). The remaining 25% are associated with diabetes; circulatory diseases such as sickle cell anemia, CHF, and renal vein thrombosis; toxins that affect the nephrons, such as mercury, bismuth, or gold; allergic reactions; and systemic infections, such as tuberculosis. Symptoms range from the dominant clinical feature of edema to hypotension, especially on standing, lethargy, fatigue, lack of appetite, pallor, and depression.

Diagnosis can be confirmed with consistently elevated proteinuria over a 24-hour period, the presence of characteristic fatty casts and oval fat bodies in the urine, and increased serum cholesterol levels with decreased albumin levels.

Treatment consists of correcting the underlying cause whenever possible. Supportive treatment involves a high-protein diet, restrictive sodium intake, diuretics for edema, and antibiotics to combat infection. Some favorable results have occurred with the use of corticosteroids, but they are limited to specific uses.

Polycystic Kidney Disease. An inherited disorder, **polycystic kidney disease** is characterized by bilateral, grapelike clusters of fluid-filled cysts. The presence of the cysts greatly enlarges the size of the kidney externally and also compresses the nephrons inside, eventually replacing the functioning renal tissue. The disease appears in an infantile form, which results in stillbirth or early newborn death. Occasionally, an infant will survive for about 2 years before developing renal failure. The adult form has an insidious onset, usually apparent between ages 30 to 50. The deterioration of the

kidney is slower but is nevertheless fatal unless treated by dialysis.

Symptoms of the infantile form include a pointed nose, small chin, floppy low-set ears, and folds in the inner eyelids. The kidneys become huge bilateral masses between the bottom of the ribs and the top of the ileum and are symmetric, firm, and dense. Usually there is evidence of CHF and respiratory distress. Adult polycystic disease initially presents nonspecific symptoms, such as hypertension, polyuria, and UTI. Eventually additional symptoms appear relating to enlarged kidney masses, such as lumbar pain, widened body, and a swollen, tender abdomen. As the disease advances, the patient develops recurrent hematuria, life-threatening bleeding from cyst rupture, proteinuria, and pain due to ureteral spasm from the passing of clots or calculi. After approximately 10 years, the insufficiency of the kidney results in failure and uremia.

Polycystic disease is not curable but it can be managed, to a certain degree, by controlling hypertension and urinary infections. Treatment is like that for any chronic, destructive kidney disease, and includes dialysis.

Pyelonephritis. One of the most common kidney diseases, acute pyelonephritis is caused by bacteria that normally inhabit the intestines. The bacteria typically spread from the bladder up the ureters and into the pelvis, causing the development of colonies of bacteria within 24 to 48 hours. **Pyelonephritis** may also result from urinary stasis, the inability to empty the bladder completely, or urinary obstruction due to strictures, tumors, or enlarged prostate in males.

Symptoms associated with pyelonephritis include urgency, dysuria, burning during urination, nocturia, and hematuria. The urine may have an ammoniac or fishy odor and is usually cloudy in appearance. Other common symptoms include fever of 102°F (39°C) or higher, chills, lack of appetite, flank pain, and fatigue. The symptoms generally develop rapidly and may subside within a few days. A residual bacterial infection may recur at a later time, however.

Diagnosis is confirmed by urinalysis, which shows sediment containing leukocytes and possibly a few red blood cells. Culture reveals a significant population of bacteria. Specific gravity is below normal due to the temporary inability to concentrate urine. Treatment consists of antibiotics determined by culture and sensitivity tests. A course of treatment is usually 10 to 14 days even though urine becomes sterile after 2 to 3 days.

Reculturing is done 1 week after treatment and periodically for the next year to observe for residual infection, Mechanical problems causing urinary stasis, such as strictures, "dropped" bladder (positioned so that it cannot totally empty), or tumors should be corrected.

Renal Calculi. Kidney calculi (stones) are formed from chemicals in the urine forming crystals that stick together. They may be as small as a grain of sand or as large as a golf ball. Small stones pass out of the kidney with the urine. Some that are larger become caught in a ureter where they cause severe pain. Still others may pass into the bladder where they continue to enlarge and will again cause pain if they get washed into the urethra and become lodged.

Kidney stones affect primarily young to middle-aged adults, with men being affected four times as often as women. The condition tends to recur. The causes of calculi formation are not always clear; however, certain factors seem to contribute to their development.

- Drinking too little fluid
- Chronic UTIs
- Blockage of the urinary tract
- Prolonged limited activity
- Misuse of certain medications
- Certain genetic and metabolic diseases
- Specific foods in certain susceptible people

Symptoms of renal calculi are

- Severe pain, starting suddenly in the kidneys or lower abdomen moving to the groin area. It may last for minutes or hours alternating with periods of relief.
- Nausea and vomiting
- Burning and frequent urge to urinate
- Chills, fever, and weakness, probably from infection
- Cloudy or foul-smelling urine
- Blood in the urine
- Blocked urine flow

Diagnosis is made based on symptoms, X rays (such as KUB or IVP), and ultrasound. Once size and location are determined then an appropriate course of action can be selected. About 90% can be passed without requiring special treatment or surgery. Often increasing fluids and a specific medication to dissolve the stone is sufficient. Calcium-containing stones, the most common type, however, cannot be dissolved.

The simplest treatment is chosen first. Many stones, if in the bladder or ureters, can be removed through the ureterocystoscope either directly or following crushing or breaking up with laser or sound waves. Stones in the kidney may still be removed through a scope inserted through the side into the kidney proper to remove stones whole or break them up by crushing, sound waves, or other methods and allowing them to pass normally in the urine within a few weeks.

A relatively new method of stone removal is called extracorporeal shock-wave **lithotripsy** (ESWL). Shock waves (high-energy pressure waves) similar to sonic booms generated by aircraft are produced outside the body by an electrical spark. The patient, in a disposable swimsuit, is positioned and strapped into a hydraulic chair. IV sedation is given to make the patient comfortable. The chair is lowered into a tank of warm water and the shock wave-producing device is positioned to focus on the stone. The waves travel through the water and the body without damaging living tissue.

It takes about 2000 shock waves to break up the average stone and requires about 1 hour to complete the treatment. Most describe the shock feeling as a slapping or tapping sensation. Patients are fitted with headphones to listen to music while the procedure is being done. About an hour after the treatment, most patients are allowed to leave. The remaining small fragments of the stone can be easily passed in the urine. It may take several weeks to completely pass all the fragments.

Most patients experience some abdominal discomfort with or without bruising on the abdomen or back. Frequent urination with burning and slight tinge of blood is common. Patients are instructed to collect passed stone fragments for analysis and to see their urologists as a follow-up to be certain there is no kidney blockage from the fragments.

Occasionally people do not qualify for ESWL due to stone location or one of the following:

- Weight in excess of 295 pounds
- Height over 6 foot 6 inches
- Involved kidney has little or no function
- Uncontrolled urinary infection
- Cardiac pacemaker or severely irregular heartbeat
- It is the urologist's opinion that another form of treatment is more appropriate

If no other method can be used, the stone will be removed by surgical incision into the kidney. This is now considered the final choice to solve the problem because of the risks involved with any major surgical procedure and the length of recovery time required.

Renal Failure (Acute and Chronic). A critical illness, acute renal failure results in the sudden cessation of kidney function. **Renal failure** may be caused by an obstruction, inadequate circulation, or damage to the nephrons. Effective medical treatment usually can overcome the problem. If not, however, it will progress to uremia and death. Failure due to bilateral obstruction is usually associated with calculi, blood clots, tumors, strictures, an enlarged prostate, or urethral edema. Inadequate blood flow results from low blood pressure, as well as volume, in the arteries, which eliminates the force required for the kidney to filter out water and solutes from the blood. This can result from shock, embolism, hemorrhage, loss of fluid due to burns, congestive heart failure, and arrhythmias. Nephron damage, which may cause failure, can result from acute glomerulonephritis, sickle cell anemia, bilateral renal vein thrombosis, acute pyelonephritis, renal myeloma (tumor), or toxic substances.

Symptoms initially apparent are oliguria and azotemia (nitrogenous products of protein metabolism in the blood). Without filtration the waste products and excess solutes quickly collect in the blood, resulting in severe electrolyte imbalance, acidosis, and uremia, which interfere with the function of the other body systems. A vast number of other symptoms develop, listed here by body system and in ascending order within the system: gastrointestinal: anorexia, nausea, vomiting, hematemesis (bloody vomitus); nervous: headache, drowsiness, confusion, convulsion, coma; integumentary: dryness of the skin, pruritis, pallor, uremic frost (powdery white crystals of urea on the skin); circulatory: hypotension initially, then hypertension, cardiac rhythm irregularities, CHF, edema, anemia, pulmonary edema; respiratory: Kussmaul's respirations (fast, deep respirations, over 20 per minute and usually sounding labored, resembling sighs). Fever and chills, indicators of infection, are an expected complication.

Diagnosis of renal failure is confirmed by blood test findings of greatly elevated quantities of urea, nitrogen, and creatinine and urine samples with casts, protein, and altered specific gravity. Additional verification with diagnostic examinations such as KUB, IVP, and retrograde pyelography may be indicated.

Treatment consists of a high-calorie diet that is low in protein, sodium, and potassium. Fluids are controlled. Dialysis may be required.

Chronic renal failure occurs as an end result of the progressive loss of kidney function. Symptoms do not develop significantly enough to warrant investigation until almost 75% of glomerular function is gone. The remaining normal nephrons gradually deteriorate, causing symptoms of renal failure and other system involvement.

Chronic failure can be the result of many preexisting conditions, such as chronic glomerular disease, chronic infections, obstructions, endocrine diseases, vascular diseases, and chronic overdose of toxic agents. Signs and symptoms initially are related to the loss of sodium, which causes hypotension, dry mouth, listlessness, fatigue, and nausea. Later the patient will begin experiencing mental dullness and confusion. Symptoms increase as more nephrons fail. Muscular irritability results from potassium retention and eventually changes to weakness.

Additional system involvement is similar to that described with acute failure, but a few specific differences do occur with the slower progressive course. Children with chronic failure show stunted growth patterns due to endocrine abnormalities. Infertility and amenorrhea (lack of menses) in women, impotence in men, and impaired carbohydrate metabolism also result from improper endocrine action. The skeletal system develops a mineral imbalance that results in bone pain due to parathyroid hormone imbalance. This in turn allows the minerals to be withdrawn from the bones, causing fractures. Calcifications develop in the brain, eyes, joints, myocardium, and blood vessels.

Diagnosis is made in the same manner as for acute renal failure. Treatment is almost exclusively dependent on dialysis to eliminate or decrease the effects of the disease. Other treatment is required for the complications developed in the other body systems. Long-term dialysis also requires specific physical as well as psychological therapy. Patients must be meticulous in their personal care. The skin must be clean and lotions applied to combat dryness and itching. Good oral hygiene is a must to alleviate bad breath and counteract excessive dryness and bad taste. Diet is extremely critical and requires individual adjustments in relation to dialysis. Daily records of intake and output aid in determining fluid status. If urine is not being excreted, fluid builds up within the body's tissues. Dialysis removes this fluid causing the patient to express feelings of being "wrung out."

Stricture. Narrowing of a passageway interferes with the movement of substances through its interior. For example, the **stricture** of a ureter interferes with the flow of urine to the bladder. A more common stricture occurs in the urethra, particularly in male children. It may be a congenital abnormality or, in either sex, the result of scarring following infection.

Symptoms of urethral stricture are indicative of a decreased passageway, such as a small urine stream and prolonged urination time. Stricture of a ureter may not be evident until distention occurs due to the buildup of pressure, or until kidney stones develop from urinary stasis. Complete stricture of a ureter will destroy the function of the affected kidney.

Urethral strictures can be readily treated by dilation to open up the narrowed passageway. Increasingly larger dilators are inserted into the urethra to stretch the constricted area. The procedure often needs to be repeated periodically to maintain patency (openness), especially with the growing child.

Suppression. This term is used to describe the complete failure of a natural secretion or excretion. In the context of the urinary system, it refers to the failure of the kidneys to secrete urine. When anuria occurs, catheterization is indicated to determine if urine is present in the bladder but cannot be expelled. The absence of bladder urine indicates no production by the kidneys. Therefore the patient has **suppression.**

Uremia. This term describes the presence in the blood of products normally found in the urine. It is a toxic condition leading to coma and death if not treated. As previously described, it can be the end result of many acute and chronic kidney diseases. Any condition which renders the kidney unable to regulate the chemical composition of the blood by excretion of waste products causes the wastes to accumulate, slowly building to a toxic level. When renal failure exists, **uremia** is inevitable. Dialysis is the only substitute for kidney function, except for surgical transplantation of another kidney.

Complete Chapter 4, Unit 11 in the workbook to help you meet the objectives at the beginning of this unit and therefore achieve competency of this subject matter.

U N I T   1 2
The Endocrine System

OBJECTIVES ....

Upon completion of the unit you will meet the following terminal performance objectives by verifying knowledge of the facts and principles presented through oral and written communication at a level deemed competent by the instructor or employer.

1. Differentiate between endocrine and exocrine glands and give an example of each.
2. Give examples of body functions affected by hormones.
3. Name and locate the nine glands discussed in the unit.
4. Describe the structure and function of the pituitary, thyroid, parathyroid, adrenal, pancreas, and thymus glands.
5. Describe the hormones and functions of the pineal body and the gonads.
6. Explain the hormone secretion abnormalities that cause

gigantism, dwarfism, acromegaly, goiter, tetany, diabetes, cretinism, Cushing's syndrome, and myxedema.

7. Describe the interrelationship of the hormonal secretions.
8. Identify the diagnostic examinations used to confirm diabetes, thyroid function, pregnancy, and Cushing's syndrome.
9. Describe briefly the symptoms, characteristics, and the usual course of action of five endocrine disorders presented in the unit.
10. Spell and define, using the glossary at the back of the text, all the words to know in this unit.

WORDS TO KNOW ·····························

acromegaly	hormone
adrenal	hyperglycemia
adrenaline	hyperthyroidism
adrenocorticotropic hormone (ACTH)	hypoglycemia
aldosterone	hypothyroidism
cretinism	islets of Langerhans
Cushing's syndrome	luteinizing
diabetes mellitus	myxedema
dwarfism	ovary
endocrine	parathyroid
epinephrine	pineal body
estrogen	pituitary
exocrine	progesterone
exophthalmia	puberty
gigantism	testes
glycosuria	testosterone
goiter	tetany
gonad	thymus
gonadotropic	thyroid
	thyroidectomy

The **endocrine** system is a group of glands that secrete substances directly into the bloodstream. Endocrine glands are ductless; in other words, their secretions do not drain into the body by way of a duct but are secreted directly into the capillaries of the circulatory system. Glands secreting substances through ducts are **exocrine** glands. The liver secretes bile through the hepatic duct; therefore it is an exocrine gland. Similarly, the pancreas secretes pancreatic juices by way of a duct into the duodenum, so it is an exocrine gland. The pancreas, however, also secretes insulin directly into the blood, which also makes it an endocrine gland.

The secretions from endocrine glands are called **hormones.** A hormone is a complex chemical which influences and controls body functions. Hormones are chemical messengers that cause changes which persist for a considerable time in the activity of other glands or organs. Examples of body functions affected by hormones are growth and development, metabolism, the composition of the blood and bones, sexual maturity, and the function of all endocrine glands.

Nine glands or groups of glands will be discussed: the **pituitary, thyroid, parathyroids,** pancreas (introduced in Unit 10, The Digestive System), **adrenals, ovaries, testes, thymus,** and the **pineal body,** Figure 4–135. Each gland performs a specific function. The hyper- or hypoactivity of the gland causes changes in the body, often altering its appearance, always altering its function, even to the point of death in specific hormonal crises. Hormones either stimulate or inhibit glandular function to maintain homeostasis. See Table 4–7, page 229, for a summary of the glands and their functions.

Pituitary Gland ·····························

The pituitary gland is considered to be the "master" gland of the body, secreting a large number of hormones that affect other glands, growth, and development.

The gland is attached by a thin stalk to the undersurface of the brain. It is so vital to the body that it is protected within a bony cradle deep within the skull. It sits in a bony depression of the spheroid bone of the skull, called the *sella turcica,* behind the bony orbits of the eyes at about the level of the bridge of the nose. This tiny gland, not much larger than a pea, secretes nine known hormones.

The pituitary is constructed of a large anterior and a small posterior lobe, each producing specific hormones. A thin sheet of tissue lies between the two lobes. The production of pituitary hormones is under the control of the hypothalmus of the brain by way of a feedback mechanism that senses the level of all hormones available to the body and the need for hormones to be released in response to stimuli.

Anterior Lobe   The hormones of the anterior lobe are as follows:

■ Growth hormone (GH)—Essential for normal growth of the body's tissues, affects the length of long bones and therefore height. Insufficient production during childhood results in **dwarfism,** whereas overproduction produces **gigantism,** Figure 4–136. Overproduction in adulthood will produce a condition known as **acromegaly,** which is characterized by overgrowth of cartilagenous and connective tissue resulting in a bulky appearance, protrusion of the eyebrow area, enlargement of the hands and feet, and deformation of the features, Figure 4–137.
■ Thyrotropin, the thyroid-stimulating hormone (TSH) — Increases the growth and activity of thyroid cells to produce thyroid hormone.
■ **Adrenocorticotropic hormone (ACTH)**—Stimulates the cortex of the adrenal gland.
■ Melanocyte-stimulating hormone (MSH)—Increases skin pigmentation.

The following three **gonadotropic** hormones control the development of the reproductive system in both males and females, including the female menstrual cycle. If production

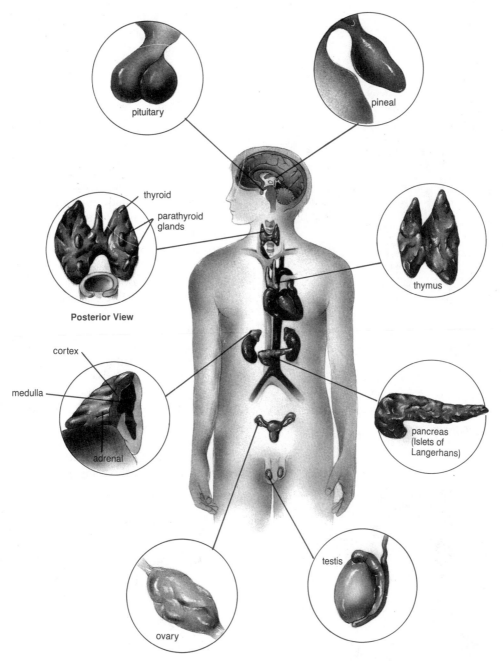

FIGURE 4–135 The endocrine system (From Burke, *Human Anatomy and Physiology in Health and Disease*, 3d ed. Copyright 1992, Delmar Publishers Inc.)

fails before **puberty,** sexual maturity will not occur. If it fails after puberty, secondary sexual characteristics regress.

- Follicle-stimulating hormone (FSH)—Enlarges the graafian follicle of the ovary to the point of rupture and stimulates the follicle to produce estrogen in the female. FSH stimulates the production of the sperm in the male.
- **Luteinizing** hormone (LH)—In the female causes the ruptured ovarian follicle to become a corpus luteum that in turn secretes the hormone progesterone. Interstitial cell-stimulating hormone (ICSH) in the male stimulates the interstitial cells in the testes to produce testosterone.

- Prolactin (PR)—Responsible for breast development and the production of milk.

Posterior Lobe　The hormones of the posterior lobe are as follows:

- Oxytocin—Stimulates the contractions of the uterus, especially during childbirth; it also is responsible for the flow of milk from the breast.
- Vasopressin, or the antidiuretic hormone (ADH)—Acts on the kidney tubule cells to concentrate urine and conserve

water within the body. It also stimulates the smooth muscles of blood vessels to constrict.

FIGURE 4–136 The effect of growth hormone—a giant, a dwarf, and a normal-sized person (From Anthony, C.P., and G. Thibodeau, *Textbook of Anatomy and Physiology*. St. Louis: C.V. Mosby, Reproduced with permission.)

Thyroid Gland...

The thyroid gland has two lobes, one on each side of the larynx, with a connecting central section called the isthmus, Figure 4–138. It is located in front of the upper portion of the trachea in the lower part of the neck. The gland is encased in a capsule of connective tissue.

The thyroid gland produces three hormones: thyroxine (T_4), triiodothyronine (T_3), and thyrocalcitonin. Thyrocalcitonin causes calcium to be stored in the bones to reduce the level of calcium in the blood. The other two hormones strongly affect metabolism, which influences both the physical and mental activity necessary for normal growth and development. When thyroid activity is below normal it is called **hypothyroidism,** indicating a decrease in the basal metabolic rate. An overactive thyroid is called **hyperthyroidism** and indicates an increased metabolic rate.

The thyroid gland requires iodine to form the thyroid hormones. Iodine is obtained by eating vegetables grown in soil containing iodine, seafood, or food seasoned with iodized salt. Lack of the element causes the thyroid gland to enlarge because of the feedback mechanism. When the pituitary receives information that the level of thyroid hormones is too low it sends out TSH to stimulate the thyroid cells. The cells in turn enlarge, trying to increase output, and eventually enlarge the entire gland. An enlarged thyroid gland is commonly known as a **goiter.**

FIGURE 4–137 Acromegaly (From Chaffee, E. E., and Lytre, I.M. *Basic Physiology and Anatomy*, 4th ed. Philadelphia: J.B. Lippincott, Co., 1980.)

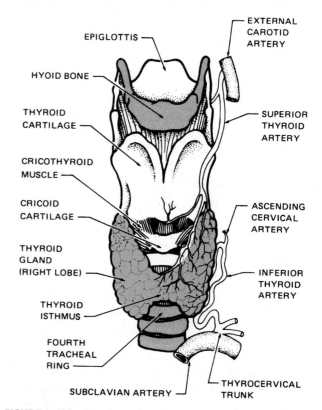

EPIGLOTTIS

HYOID BONE

THYROID CARTILAGE

CRICOTHYROID MUSCLE

CRICOID CARTILAGE

THYROID GLAND (RIGHT LOBE)

THYROID ISTHMUS

FOURTH TRACHEAL RING

SUBCLAVIAN ARTERY

EXTERNAL CAROTID ARTERY

SUPERIOR THYROID ARTERY

ASCENDING CERVICAL ARTERY

INFERIOR THYROID ARTERY

THYROCERVICAL TRUNK

FIGURE 4–138 The thyroid gland

TABLE 4–7
Endocrine Glands

Gland	Location	Hormone	Principal Effects
PITUITARY Anterior lobe	Undersurface of the brain in the sella turcica of the skull	Growth hormone (GH)	Normal growth of body tissues
		Thyroid stimulating hormone (TSH) (thyrotropin)	Stimulates growth and activity of thyroid cells to produce thyroid hormone
		Adrenocorticotropic hormone (ACTH)	Stimulates the cortex of the adrenal gland
		Melancocyte-stimulating hormone (MSH)	Increases skin pigmentation
		Follicle-stimulating hormone (FSH)	Stimulates the maturity of the graafian follicle to rupture and to produce estrogen in the female. In the male it stimulates the development of the testes and the production of sperm
		Luteinizing hormone (LH) Interstitial-cell stimulating hormone (ICSH)	Causes the development of the corpus luteum, which then secretes progesterone in the female. ICSH in the male stimulates the interstitial cells of the testes to produce testosterone.
		Prolactin (PR)	Develops breast tissue and stimulates secretion of milk from mammary glands
Posterior lobe		Oxytocin	Stimulates contraction of uterus, especially during childbirth; causes ejection of milk from mammary glands
		Vasopressin or antidiuretic hormone (ADH)	Acts on cells of kidney tubules to concentrate urine and conserve fluid in the body. Also acts to constrict blood vessels.
THYROID	Lower portion of the anterior neck	Thyroxine (T_4) and triiodothyronine (T_3)	Increases metabolism; influences both physical and mental activity; promotes normal growth and development
		Thyrocalcitonin	Causes calcium to be stored in bones; reduces blood level of calcium
PARATHYROID	Posterior surface of thyroid gland	Parathormone	Regulates exchange of calcium between the bones and blood
ADRENAL Medulla	Superior surface of each kidney	Adrenaline (epinephrine)	Increases heart rate, blood pressure, and flow of blood; decreases intestinal activity
		Aldosterone (mineral corticoid)	Controls electrolyte balances by regulating the reabsorption of sodium and the excretion of potassium
Cortex		Glucocorticoids	Affect the metabolism of protein, fat, and glucose, thereby increasing blood sugar
		Sex hormones (androgens)	Govern sex characteristics, especially those that are masculine
PANCREAS	Behind the stomach	Insulin	Essential to the metabolism of carbohydrates; reduces the blood sugar level
		Glucagon	Stimulates the liver to release glycogen and convert it to glucose to increase blood sugar levels
THYMUS	Under the sternum	Thymosin	Reacts upon lymphoid tissue to produce T lymphocyte cells to develop immunity to certain diseases
PINEAL BODY	Third ventricle in the brain	Melatonin	Controls onset of puberty
OVARIES	Female pelvis	Estrogen	Promotes growth of primary and secondary sexual characteristics
		Progesterone	Develops excretory portion of mammary glands; aids in maintaining pregnancy
TESTES	Male scrotum	Testosterone	Develops primary and secondary sexual characteristics; stimulates maturation of sperm

FIGURE 4–139 Hyperthyroidism with exophthalmia (From DeGroot, *The Thyroid and Its Diseases*, 4th ed. New York: John Wiley & Sons, Inc. 1975.)

A person who has hypothyroidism feels fatigued, has low blood pressure and pulse rate, often a subnormal temperature, and may be overweight due to decreased metabolism. The hyperthyroid patient is nervous, restless, and irritable, with heart rate above normal and elevated blood pressure. The patient may lose weight despite a good appetite. Occasionally the eyes protrude dramatically in a condition called **exoph-thalmia,** Figure 4–139.

Treatment of hypothyroidism is relatively simple: the thyroid hormone is taken orally as a supplement. Hyperthyroidism may initially be treated with supplemental iodine to prohibit or control gland enlargement. With progressive disease, it may be necessary to remove part or all of the gland or limit its function by radiation. The surgical removal of the thyroid is called a **thyroidectomy.**

A thyrotoxic crisis or thyroid storm is the extreme clinical development of hyperthyroidism. It produces a greatly accelerated metabolism, severe nervous system malfunction, overheating, and heart failure. The situation is precipitated by stress or a severe infection and is usually fatal. The vigorous use of antithyroid drugs can frequently prevent the complication from occurring.

Parathyroid Glands.............................

The parathyroid glands, usually two pairs, are embedded on the posterior surface of the thyroid gland. Their number and size vary greatly, but normally they resemble grains of wheat. The parathyroids are responsible for regulating the calcium content of the blood. The parathyroid hormone, or parathormone, cooperates with vitamin D to balance the level of calcium in the blood by stimulating the bones to release stored calcium and phosphate into the circulation.

Hyperparathyroidism results in increased levels of calcium in the blood, which causes lethargy and the excretion of large quantities of calcium salts in the urine, leading to the formation of kidney stones. The condition leads progressively to decalcification of the bones and is usually associated with a tumor of one of the glands. Decalcified bones are prone to pathological fracture.

Hypoparathyroidism is dramatically demonstrated by a condition known as **tetany,** an uncontrollable twitching of the muscles of the body. This results from hyperirritability of the nervous system in response to the lowered concentration of calcium throughout the body. The condition is easily treated by the addition of calcium. Hypoparathyroidism occurs following damage to or accidental removal of the parathyroids during a thyroidectomy.

Adrenal Glands (Suprarenal).....................

The adrenal glands sit atop each kidney, hence the additional name of *suprarenal.* Each gland is contained in a fibrous capsule and is composed of two parts, each of which acts separately. The outer glandular tissue is called the *cortex,* and the inner tissue is referred to as the *medulla.*

The principal hormone of the medulla is **adrenaline,** also called **epinephrine.** Another hormone, norepinephrine, has a similar action on the body. Together they are considered to be the "flight or fight" hormones because of their effects in emergency situations. The hormones cause an increase in the heart rate, blood pressure, and flow of blood, and a decrease in intestinal activity. The adrenal medulla is considered to be nonessential to life.

The cortex of the adrenal gland, however, is essential to life. The cortex produces steroid hormones in three categories: mineral corticoids, glucocorticoids, and sex steroids. The mineral corticoids, of which **aldosterone** is the principal one, control electrolyte balances through regulating the reabsorption of sodium in the kidney tubules and the excretion of potassium. The glucocorticoids affect the metabolism of protein, fat, and glucose. They stimulate the liver to convert protein into glycogen and then break it down into glucose, thereby increasing blood sugar level. This change is seen when the body is subjected to stressful situations. The hormone level is increased, which in turn accelerates the conversion process to allow the body to cope.

The sex steroids govern certain sexual characteristics, especially those that are male. These steroids are referred to as *androgens.* Excessive secretions cause the virilization and development of masculine secondary sex characteristics in the female and immature male, Figure 4–140. A mature female's voice will deepen, a growth of beard will appear, menstruation will become irregular, and sterility will result.

FIGURE 4–140 Effects of excess androgens on a young female (Adapted from Anthony, C.P., Thibodeau, G. *Textbook of Anatomy and Physiology,* 11th ed. 1983. St. Louis, C.V. Mosby Co. Courtesy Dr. William McKendree Jeffries, Case Western Reserve University School of Medicine, Cleveland, Ohio.)

Pancreas

The pancreas is a dual-function organ. It has an exocrine function, producing pancreatic juices excreted by way of the pancreatic duct into the duodenum to become part of the digestive juices. It is also an endocrine gland. The hormone *insulin* is secreted by the B cells of the **islets of Langerhans,** often called beta cells, Figure 4–141. They are one of four cell types, A, B, C, and D, located in the pancreas. It is known that the A cells secrete glucagon, but the exact function of this substance is uncertain. It may stimulate the liver to release glycogen, converting it to glucose to raise the blood sugar level.

Insulin is necessary for the metabolism of carbohydrates. With reduced islet function, the level of blood sugar rises to an abnormal amount and is referred to as **hyperglycemia.** Conversely, an abnormally low level of blood sugar is known as **hypoglycemia.** When excess glucose is present in the blood, it is excreted in the urine, a finding known as **glycosuria.** Hyperglycemia and glycosuria are the two outstanding characteristics of **diabetes mellitus.**

The exact function of insulin and its relationship to diabetes are not clearly understood. It is believed that insulin makes it possible for the cells to use the glucose present in the body tissues. Without the ability to burn glucose, it cannot be changed into energy and is therefore passed on to the kidneys for excretion. Insulin is also required for the metabolism of fat and protein.

Thymus Gland

The thymus gland is a two-lobed structure, located under the sternum. It is composed primarily of lymphoid tissue and enclosed in a fibrous capsule. The thymus is fairly large during childhood, but begins to disappear with the onset of puberty, becoming a small mass of connective tissue and fat in adulthood. It appears to produce a hormone known as thymosin, which is believed to react on lymphoid tissue to produce T lymphocytes and develop immunity against certain diseases.

Pineal Body

The pineal body is a small mass of tissue attached by a slim stalk to the roof of the third ventricle in the brain. The pineal body is believed to produce a substance called melatonin. This substance combines with a hypothalamic substance to delay puberty until the normal time.

Gonads (Testes and Ovaries)

The ovaries in the female and the testes in the male are called the **gonads,** or sex glands. The ovaries are located in the pelvic cavity, one on each side of the uterus. The testes are located outside the body of the male, suspended in the scrotum. Both gonads secrete hormones that control the development of secondary sex characteristics.

In the female, the ovaries secrete **estrogen,** which reacts on the lining of the uterus, promotes growth and development of the primary and secondary sex organs, and maintains them

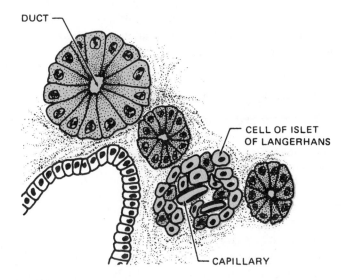

FIGURE 4–141 Pancreatic structure

throughout adult life. Estrogen also affects the release of other hormones from the pituitary. Another hormone, **progesterone,** is also secreted by the ovaries. It affects the uterine lining as well as the development of the secretory portion of the breasts. It aids in maintaining pregnancy.

In the male, the testes produce a hormone known as **testosterone.** This hormone develops the primary male sexual characteristics as well as the secondary characteristics of a deep voice, muscular development, and body hair distribution. It stimulates maturation of sperm cells.

The gonads are the organs of fertility and reproduction in both sexes. The maturity of the organs and the proper balance of hormonal secretions creates the desire for and ability to engage in sexual activity.

Interrelationship of the Glands ....

As stated previously, hormonal secretion is regulated by a feedback mechanism. When the hormone is present or the substance produced by the effect of that hormone on another gland or organ is present, further secretion is affected. For example, the parathyroids increase secretion of parathormone to raise the serum calcium level to be withdrawn from the bones. When the serum level rises, a negative feedback message is signaled, and the secretion of parathormone is decreased. A more complicated feedback involves both positive and negative action. For example, the pituitary gland secretes TSH, which causes the thyroid gland to increase the production of hormones. When the appropriate level is reached, TSH secretion is inhibited—a negative feedback. The hypothalamus produces a thyrotropin-releasing hormone (TRH), which is stimulated by low levels of thyroid hormone. Therefore, when the level again drops, the hypothalmus secretes TRH, which stimulates the pituitary to release TSH, which in turn stimulates the production of the thyroid hormones—a positive feedback mechanism.

In the next unit, the interrelationship of the pituitary and the ovary will be discussed to explain how this complex balance prepares the female for pregnancy and then either sustains that hormonal state or allows it to alter, all in response to the feedback mechanism.

Diagnostic Examinations ....

A great variety of diagnostic tests can be performed on blood and urine, which either measure the amount of specific hormones present in the body or measure the effectiveness of their function. A few of the more common tests are

- Blood sugar, frequently measured after fasting (FBS)—To assess the function of the pancreas, including insulin production and utilization.
- T_3 and T_4—To measure the level of the thyroid hormones.
- Urine human chorionic gonadotropin (HCG) (pregnancy test)—To measure the presence of a hormone secreted by the placental cells

- Glucose tolerance—To measure the body's ability to process a large dose of glucose. Multiple blood and urine samples are taken at specific intervals following ingestion.

There are also specific tests measuring hormone levels in the blood to aid in confirming diagnoses, such as

- ACTH, FSH, LH, and TSH—When acromegaly or dwarfism is suspected.
- FSH, LH, estrogen and testosterone—When sex organs fail to develop properly.
- ACTH, cortisol—When Cushing's syndrome (chronic excessive glucocorticoids) is suspected.
- PTH—When hypo- or hyperparathyroidism is suspected.

Scanning Tests   The thyroid gland is probably the one most frequently scanned.

- Radioactive iodine uptake test—An oral dose of radioactive iodine is given to the patient. After intervals of 2, 6, and 24 hours, an external detector (scintillation counter) measures the amount of the original dose that is present in the gland. Thyroid function can be determined by the gland's ability to absorb and retain iodine.
- Thyroid scan—The thyroid gland is viewed by a scintiscanner camera following either an oral or IV dose of a radioactive iodine. The scan is indicated by discovery of a palpable nodule or mass, enlarged thyroid gland, or asymmetric goiter. The camera is capable of photographing the isotopes, which identify the size of the gland, position, and uniformity of absorption. A nodule with poor or no uptake capability shows as a "cold spot," suggesting a possible malignancy. A "hot spot" indicates a hyperfunctioning nodule, possibly a toxic nodular goiter. A total gland picture that shows little uptake is indicative of hypothyroidism; an enlarged gland showing uniformly increased uptake is indicative of hyperthyroidism.

Diseases and Disorders ....

Cretinism.   This condition results from serious lack of the thyroid hormone thyroxine beginning in the early stages of life. **Cretinism** is characterized by lack of mental and physical growth resulting in mental retardation and a characteristic dwarflike appearance, Figure 4–142, page 233. If thyroid replacement is initiated early enough, a degree of normal development may be achieved, but once cretinism has developed, total normal development is not possible. An infant born without thyroid hormones of its own must be treated within a few weeks to prevent irreversible mental retardation.

Cushing's Syndrome.   This disorder is characterized by a group of symptoms that result from the hypersecretion of glucocorticoids from the adrenal cortex due to excess ACTH production. **Cushing's syndrome** may also be directly related to a tumor of the cortex of the adrenal gland. Symptoms include hypertension, obesity, weakness of the muscles, and a tendency to develop bruises. Typical characteristics result from the rapid deposit of body fat: a deposit of fat between the shoulders, referred to as "buffalo hump," and a rounded face referred to as "moon face," Figure 4–143, page 234. Purple streaks develop in the skin, called striae (stretch marks). The trunk becomes obese, yet the arms and legs are slender.

The excess amount of glucocorticoids, which metabolize protein into glycogen and then into glucose, results in a "steroid diabetes" with hyperglycemia and glucosuria. The urinary system is affected by the hormone imbalance and excretes excessive amounts of potassium, which results in hypokalemia. The lack of potassium results in muscular weakness. Muscle mass slowly wastes away. The decreasing amount of bone minerals results in pathological fractures.

Treatment is related to the underlying cause. If there is an adrenal tumor, then the adrenal gland must be removed. If both adrenals are removed, replacement steroid therapy must be instituted. If the adrenals are being stimulated because of a pituitary tumor, then the pituitary gland must be irradiated or removed. Afterwards rigorous hormone therapy would be required to replace all the pituitary's secretions. Many drugs, some experimental, are used to suppress adrenal function and destroy adenocortical cells.

Diabetes Mellitus. A chronic disease of insulin deficiency or resistance, diabetes mellitus interferes with the metabolism of carbohydrates, proteins, and fats. Insulin in the blood "carries" glucose into the cell to be used for energy or stored as glycogen. It also stimulates the formation of proteins and free fatty acid storage. Without sufficient insulin being secreted by the pancreas, the body's tissues do not have access to essential nutrients for fuel or storage.

The cause of diabetes is unknown, but the following factors contribute to its development:

- Heredity—There is a tendency among family members.
- Weight—Weight plays an important role because obesity causes resistance to insulin. Eighty percent of all diabetics are overweight when diagnosed.
- Pregnancy—Pregnancy adds extra demands on the body. Increased levels of estrogen and other hormones antagonize insulin. Women who deliver large babies or have repeated miscarriages may be diabetic.
- Physical trauma or emotional stress—Crisis, emotional tension, a major illness, or physical trauma from surgery or an accident can lead to development of diabetes because of prolonged elevation of stress hormones raising demands on the pancreas.
- Virus—Certain cases of insulin-dependent diabetes are viral in origin.

FIGURE 4–142 (Top) Cretinism of a 16-year-old female due to lack of thyroid hormone. (Bottom) Same female after two years of treatment with thyroid extract. (From Anthony, *Textbook of Anatomy and Physiology,* 6th ed. 1963, St. Louis, C.V. Mosby Co; Courtesy Dr. Edward E. Beard.)

FIGURE 4–143 Cushing's syndrome from excessive glucocorticoids. (a) Preoperatively. (b) 6 months postoperatively (Adapted from Anthony, C.P., and Thibodeau, G. *Textbook of Anatomy and Physiology,* 11th ed. 1983, St. Louis, C.V. Mosby Co. Courtesy Dr. William McKendree Jeffries, Case Western Reserve University School of Medicine, Cleveland, Ohio.)

Diabetes mellitus affects an estimated 5% of the U.S. population or approximately 12 million people. About one-half are unaware they have diabetes.

There are two forms of diabetes: a juvenile (or insulin-dependent) diabetes mellitus (IDDM), and a mature-onset (or noninsulin-dependent) form (NIDDM). IDDM usually occurs before age 30. The patient is thin and requires insulin support therapy and diet control. NIDDM occurs most frequently among obese adults and responds to diet with or without oral hypoglycemics or insulin.

Signs and symptoms of diabetes include fatigue, due to the lack of energy production, and hyperglycemia, because the glucose cannot be utilized. The elevated glucose level in the blood causes fluid to be withdrawn from the body's tissues. The excess fluid in the blood causes polyuria and dehydration of the cells. The diabetic patient is frequently thirsty and has dry mucous membranes. The lens of the eye becomes affected by deposits of sugar and edema, which results in visual difficulties. Characteristically, glycosuria is present, as the body tries to eliminate excess glucose from the blood. This wasting of sugar causes the weight loss and hunger of the IDDM patient.

There are many long-term effects of diabetes. Patients are prone to myocardial infarction and stroke and deteriorating disease of the retina and nerves. It contributes to renal failure, peripheral vascular disease, and blindness. Approximately 50% of patients who have had myocardial infarctions and

75% who have had cerebrovascular accidents are also diabetic. It also interferes with resistance to organisms, which may result in skin and bladder infections because the glucose content of the epidermis and urine are conducive to bacterial growth. Diabetic retinopathy results from circulatory changes in the retina of the eye in the poorly controlled diabetic. In patients who have had diabetes for 20 or more years, 80% develop retinopathy. It is the leading cause of adult acquired blindness.

Treatment begins with a strict diet, planned to meet the nutritional needs of the individual patient and to control the blood sugar level. When diet alone is inadequate, insulin injections or the use of an oral hypoglycemic drug are indicated. Injections may be necessary only once a day, using a long-acting insulin; when control is more difficult, a regular insulin, injected at specific times, may be used. Diabetic patients are taught to evaluate their glucose level by performing a urine test for sugar or a finger stick for blood analysis. The amount of the insulin injected is based on the findings. Hypoglycemic drugs are taken orally to aid in the metabolism of sugar. Oral therapy is usually adequate only for NIDDM patients.

The glucose level of the blood can be affected by circumstances other than food or insulin. For example, the diabetic will require either less insulin or more food when engaging in a high level of physical activity. Adjustments are also required with illness. A patient who has diarrhea or vomiting requires less insulin. Pregnancy, the use of contraceptives, a fever, and periods of stress, all influence the diabetic's need for supplemental insulin or hypoglycemic therapy.

Diabetic patients must be encouraged to maintain their optimal level of health. They must guard against injury, especially to the lower extremities, because of the difficulty of healing. They must use extreme caution when cutting toenails and must never try to remove corns or calluses themselves. Diabetics frequently suffer amputations as a result of infection from an injury that would not heal or from the loss of peripheral circulation, which causes tissue death.

Patients should be encouraged to visit an ophthalmologist regularly to detect the possibility of retinal changes. Blindness will result from uncontrolled diabetes. The physician must be alert to signs of cardiovascular complications as well as urinary tract involvement. Cerebral vascular disease, coronary artery disease, and renal failure due to vascular deterioration in the kidney are not uncommon.

Graves' Disease. This condition, caused by the overproduction of the thyroid gland, is the most common form of hyperthyroidism. The thyroid gland enlarges, the patient becomes nervous; has an intolerance to heat; loses weight; sweats; and may have diarrhea, tremors, and palpitations. The increased thyroxine may also cause difficulty in concentrating because of the accelerated cerebral functioning. Mood swings and emotional instability may occur. The cardiovascular system is also affected and results in tachycardia, increased cardiac output and blood volume, cardiomegaly, and possibly atrial fibrillation (especially in the elderly). The patient may experience dyspnea and an array of musculoskeletal symptoms ranging from weakness and fatigue to localized or generalized paralysis. The dominant feature of exophthalmus may also be present.

The patient can get into serious difficulty if the hyperthyroidism escalates into a thyroid storm. The symptoms persist and others develop, such as hypertension, extreme irritability, vomiting, high fever, delirium, and eventually coma.

Myxedema. This condition is caused by hyposecretion of the thyroid gland in adulthood. Clinically, **myxedema's** characteristics are in relation to the degree of hypothyroidism. If it is mild, the patient will probably complain of forgetfulness, dry skin, and an intolerance for cold. With more severe myxedema, the decreased metabolism and vital functions will become more evident. Decrease in heat production (because of decreased metabolism) causes a marked intolerance for cold. There is a noticeable weight gain. The motor function and reflex actions are slowed. The voice becomes low and husky. A characteristic yellowish discoloration of the skin, called *carotenemia,* results from reduction in the conversion of carotene to vitamin A. Levels of cholesterol are increased and may also produce atherosclerosis. Since cardiac function is depressed, the myocardium becomes flabby and weak. Protein and certain electrolytes accumulate in the tissue spaces, causing edema. Myxedema patients have a characteristic drowsy appearance, with puffiness about the eyes, Figure 4–144. There is a marked degree of fatigue and weakness. The temperature, pulse, respiration, and blood pressure are all below normal.

Treatment consists primarily of thyroid hormone replacement to a level necessary to maintain normal balance.

Diagnosing, treating, and maintaining hormonal balance in patients with endocrine gland malfunctions is an involved and challenging endeavor because of the hormone interactions. What may appear to be a simple overproduction by the thyroid may actually be a pituitary malfunction, a failed hypothalamus, or an inhibitor that did not cause the pituitary to stop secreting a thyroid stimulant. Many possibilities must be considered to explain the symptoms presented by a patient with endocrine dysfunction.

Complete Chapter 4, Unit 11 in the workbook to help you meet the objectives at the beginning of this unit and therefore achieve competency of this subject matter.

FIGURE 4–144 Myxedema (From Burke, *Human Anatomy and Physiology in Health and Disease,* 3d ed. Copyright 1992, Delmar Publishers Inc.)

U N I T   1 3

The Reproductive System

OBJECTIVES ....

Upon completion of this unit, you will meet the following ter-minal performance objectives by verifying knowledge of the facts and principles presented through oral and written com-munication at a level deemed competent by the instructor or employer.

1. Differentiate between sexual and asexual reproduction.
2. Describe the differentiation of reproductive organs.
3. Explain how sperm are able to fertilize an egg.
4. Describe male prenatal development.
5. Name the male sex organs and describe their location and function.
6. Explain how pituitary hormones affect the functions of the testes.
7. Identify the male secondary sex characteristics.
8. Trace the pathway of sperm from production to expulsion.
9. Name the components of semen.
10. Describe four diseases and disorders of the male reproduc-tive system.
11. Name the female sex organs and describe their location and function.
12. Explain the interaction of pituitary hormones with the ovaries and other organs.
13. Identify the female secondary sex characteristics.
14. Describe the maturation and release of an ovum.
15. Compare the internal and external sexual organs of the male and female.
16. Describe the phases of the menstrual cycle and the pur-pose of menstruation.
17. Explain how fertilization occurs.
18. Discuss the events occurring during each trimester of pregnancy as they relate to the woman and the embryo and then the fetus.
19. Discuss the events that occur in the three stages of labor.
20. List eight reasons for practicing contraception.
21. Identify 10 contraceptive methods, stating their relative effectiveness.
22. Describe eight diagnostic tests of the female reproductive system.
23. Describe 20 diseases or disorders of the female reproduc-tive system.
24. Identify the characteristics of eight sexually transmitted diseases.
25. Spell and define, using the glossary at the back of the text, all the words to know in this unit.

WORDS TO KNOW ....

ablation	labia majora
abortion	labia minora
amniotic	ligation
areola	mammary glands
Bartholin's glands	mammogram
benign hypertrophy	mastectomy
bulbourethral glands	menarche
cervical	menopause
cervix	menorrhagia
cesarean	menstruation
chlamydia	mons pubis
circumcision	myometrium
clitoris	nonspecific urethritis
coitus	os
colposcopy	ovarian
conceive	ovulation
conception	ovum
contraception	Papanicolaou (Pap) smear
contraction	penis
corpus luteum	perineum
cryptorchidism	phimosis
dilation and curettage (D&C)	placenta
dysmenorrhea	pregnancy
ectopic	prolapse
effacement	prostate
ejaculation	prostatectomy
ejaculatory duct	rectocele
embryo	reproductive
endometrium	retroflexed
epididymis	retroverted
episiotomy	salpingo-oophrectomy
erectile	scrotum
fallopian tubes	semen
fertilization	sperm
fetus	spermatazoan
fibroid	suprapubic
foreskin	syphilis
gamete	transurethral
genital herpes	trichomoniasis
genitalia	trimester
gonorrhea	uterine
graafian follicle	uterus
gynecology	vagina
hydrocele	vaginal
hymen	vaginitis
hysterectomy	vas deferens
hysteroscopy	vasectomy
impotence	vulva
inguinal canal	womb
inguinal hernia	zygote

The **reproductive** system consists of the organs that are capable of accomplishing reproduction, the creation of a new individual. All living organisms reproduce, some very simply by an asexual method, or without the need of sexual contact. An example of asexual reproduction is one of the simplest forms of life, a single cell. In binary fusion, a cell divides into two cells by simple cleavage. In mitosis, a single cell rearranges its chromatin into chromosomes and then divides into two cells (the method by which human cells reproduce). Both methods require that the "parent" become the "children"; therefore both parent and child cannot exist at the same time.

Sexual methods of reproduction are found in most multi-celled forms of life, including humans. The methods may vary, but certain characteristics are usually common to all. In each species, there are sexes, namely a male and a female. Each sex has special sex glands, or gonads, which produce sex cells (**gametes**). In humans, the union of the male gamete (a **spermatozoan**) with the female gamete (an **ovum**) forms a new one-celled structure called a **zygote.** The zygote then undergoes mitosis repeatedly to form a new individual.

In Unit 1, the cell was described as having 46 chromosomes, or 23 pairs. Each chromosome has a partner of the same shape and size. One pair of chromosomes are the sex chromosomes. In the female, both chromosomes in the pair are X chromosomes, but in the male, one is an X and one is a Y. When the gonads produce the ovum and spermatozoan cells, the number of chromosomes is reduced to 23 (one-half). When the two cells unite as fertilization occurs, the new cell, a zygote, will again have 46 chromosomes. If the spermatozoan carries an X chromosome, the embryo will develop female characteristics. If it carries a Y chromosome the embryo will develop as a male.

The reproductive organs are the only organs in the human body which differ between the male and female, and yet there is still a significant similarity. This likeness results from the fact that male and female organs develop from the same group of embryonic cells. For approximately 2 months, the embryo develops without sexual identity. Then the influence of the X or Y chromosome begins to make a differentiation.

Differentiation of Reproductive Organs

The gonads of the embryo begin to evolve into the sexual organs of the female at about the tenth or eleventh week of pregnancy. The ovaries of the embryo develop high in its abdomen from the same type of tissue as the testes. The testes, however, evolve from the medulla of the gonad, and the ovaries develop from the cortex. Figure 4–145 illustrates how the undifferentiated external **genitalia** develop into fully differentiated structures. In the male, the tubercle becomes the glans **penis,** the folds become the penile shaft, and the

swelling develops into the **scrotum.** In the female, the tubercle becomes the **clitoris,** the folds the **labia minora,** and the swelling the **labia majora.**

Internally, there is also a similarity of structures. The embryonic müllerian ducts degenerate and the wolffian ducts become the **epididymis, vas deferens,** and **ejaculatory duct** in the male. In the female, the wolffian ducts degenerate and the müllerian ducts develop into the **fallopian tubes,** the **uterus,** and the upper portion of the **vagina.** It is believed that the presence of the testes in the male is the differentiating factor in the development. Without the androgens (male hormones) from the testes, a female develops. With the androgens, a male develops. Another substance called the müllerian inhibitor works in partnership with the androgens to produce sex differentiation.

Male Reproductive Organs

When the zygote contains a Y chromosome, a male child will develop. About the seventh or eighth week of pregnancy, the testes begin to develop within the abdominal cavity at about the level of the ileum of the pelvis bone. The sex of the fetus is evident by about the fourth month.

During the eighth and ninth months of pregnancy, the testes move from the abdomen through the **inguinal canal** into the external pouch called the scrotum, Figure 4–146, page 239. After the testes pass, the canal closes to prevent the descent of other structures into the scrotum or the return of the testes into the abdomen. When a loop of small intestine descends through the canal due to improper closure or later in life due to relaxed inguinal structures, it in known as an **inguinal hernia,** Figure 4–147, page 239.

If the testes fail to descend or if they return to the abdomen, a condition known as undescended testicle (unilateral or bilateral) exists, which must be corrected or sterility will result. An undescended testicle is known medically as **cryptorchidism.** The testes normally produce sperm, but sperm cannot be produced or survive in the internal heat of the body. It is this characteristic that necessitates the location of the testes outside the body.

The scrotum, which contains the testes, has another function as well, which is to regulate the temperature of the testes' environment. Sperm are most effectively produced at temperatures 1.5° to 2°C below body temperature. To maintain this difference, the scrotum contains many sweat glands that perspire profusely to dissipate heat. The scrotum also has cremasteric muscles, which can contract to draw the testes closer to the body and increase the temperature or relax to lower them away from the body and reduce it.

Testes The testes, or testicles, are the primary sex organs of the male. They are of equal size, oval in shape, about 2 × 1 × 1½ inches in size, and are suspended in the scrotum, with the left testis usually somewhat lower than the right. A testis has two functions, to produce sperm and to secrete testosterone, the

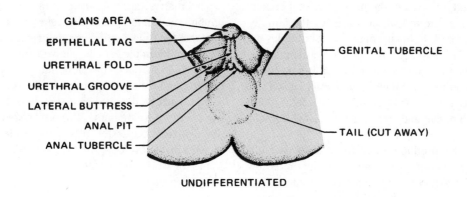

GLANS AREA
EPITHELIAL TAG
URETHRAL FOLD
URETHRAL GROOVE
LATERAL BUTTRESS
ANAL PIT
ANAL TUBERCLE

GENITAL TUBERCLE

TAIL (CUT AWAY)

UNDIFFERENTIATED

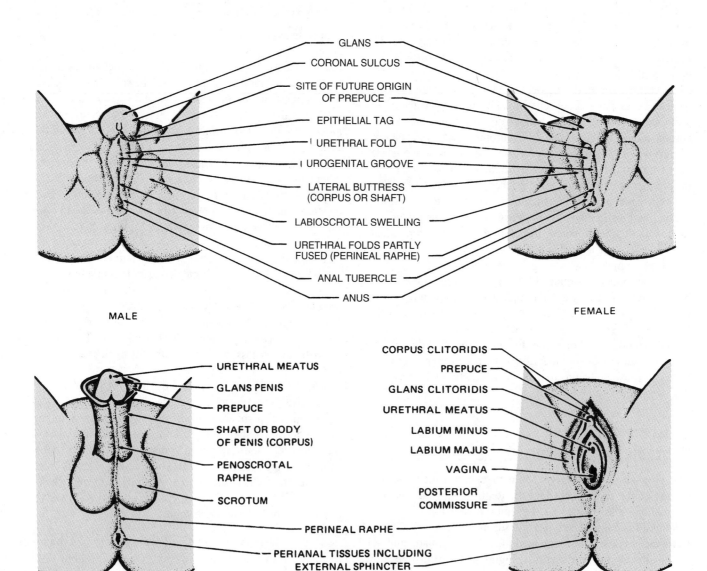

GLANS
CORONAL SULCUS
SITE OF FUTURE ORIGIN OF PREPUCE
EPITHELIAL TAG
URETHRAL FOLD
UROGENITAL GROOVE
LATERAL BUTTRESS (CORPUS OR SHAFT)
LABIOSCROTAL SWELLING
URETHRAL FOLDS PARTLY FUSED (PERINEAL RAPHE)
ANAL TUBERCLE
ANUS

MALE

FEMALE

URETHRAL MEATUS
GLANS PENIS
PREPUCE
SHAFT OR BODY OF PENIS (CORPUS)
PENOSCROTAL RAPHE
SCROTUM

CORPUS CLITORIDIS
PREPUCE
GLANS CLITORIDIS
URETHRAL MEATUS
LABIUM MINUS
LABIUM MAJUS
VAGINA
POSTERIOR COMMISSURE

PERINEAL RAPHE
PERIANAL TISSUES INCLUDING EXTERNAL SPHINCTER

FULLY DEVELOPED

FIGURE 4–145 Sexual differentiation before birth

FIGURE 4–146 The descent of the testes

male hormone. These functions begin to occur about age 10 when the hypothalamus releases a hormone that initiates puberty. The hormone stimulates the anterior pituitary gland, which then releases the gonad-stimulating hormones to effect change in the testes.

Male gonadotropic hormones secreted by the pituitary are FSH (follicle-stimulating hormone) and ICSH (interstitial cell-stimulating hormones). FSH causes sperm to develop in the male and ova to mature in the female, a very similar function.

Sperm Production. Sperm develop and mature in microscopic tubes in the testes known as *seminiferous tubules,* Figure 4–148, page 240. FSH stimulates the production of sperm in the cells that line the tubules. There are about 300 sections of coiled tubules which, if uncoiled, it is estimated, would extend over a mile. As the sperm develop, they are released into the tubules to start their journey from the testes. Sperm formation in an adult male requires about 74 days to maturity. The function normally begins to develop at about age 12, and the first mature sperm are ejaculated at about age 14.

Testosterone. As sperm are developing, ICSH is causing the interstitial cells in the network of structures around the tubules to secrete testosterone. Testosterone aids in the maturing of sperm and also causes many changes in the male body as the

hormone circulates in the bloodstream. These changes are referred to as the development of secondary sex characteristics, Figure 4–149.

In the male, secondary sex characteristics are

1. Longer and heavier bone structure
2. Larger muscles
3. Deep voice
4. Growth of body hair
5. Development of the genitalia (external sex organs)
6. Increased metabolism
7. Sexual desire

Epididymis, Vas Deferens, and Seminal Vesicles

The epididymis is a coiled structure about 20 feet in length. It is shaped like a half-moon and sits with its head on top of the testes and its tail extending down the side to join the vas deferens, Figure 4–150, page 241.

After sperm are produced in the tubules they pass into the epididymis where a small number are stored. The sperm mature in the epididymis for about 18 hours. The fluid secreted by the epididymis adds to the volume of ejaculant.

The vas deferens serves as the passageway for sperm to exit the body from the epididymis. On each side, one vas deferens

— INTESTINE

FIGURE 4–147 Inguinal hernia

SEMINIFEROUS TUBULE

INTERSTITIAL CELLS

FIGURE 4–148 *The production of sperm in the seminiferous tubules and the secretion of testerone by the interstitial cells*

The seminal vesicles are a pair of convoluted tubes lying posterior to the bladder. They also empty into the ejaculatory duct. The vesicles secrete a fluid that contains fructose, a simple sugar, which provides nutrition for the sperm. The fluid makes up a major portion of the ejaculant. The ejaculatory duct is a short straight tube that passes through the **prostate** gland to join the urethra.

Prostate Gland, Bulbourethral Glands, and Urethra

The prostate gland is a doughnut-like pyramidal structure with the urethra extending through its center, Figure 4–151. The gland is positioned just beneath the bladder. It produces secretions that are drained through tiny tubules into the prostatic section of the urethra. The fluid secreted is alkaline in nature. Its addition to the ejaculant stimulates sperm motility and the preserves their life by neutralizing the acidity of the vagina. The prostate is also constructed of muscular tissue that contracts during ejaculation to empty the **semen** (ejaculant fluids and sperm) into the urethra to be propelled from the body.

The **bulbourethral glands** lie beneath the prostate and empty their contents into the urethra. The fluid the glands secrete aids in the movement of sperm as well as making the normally acid male urethra alkaline just prior to ejaculation. The secretions may also serve as a lubricant for intercourse. Bulbourethral glands are sometimes called Cowper's glands.

Semen The combined secretions from all the glands and ducts along with the sperm is called the seminal fluid, or semen. Approximately 3.5 mL of total fluid is expelled per

joins one epididymis extending upward for about 45 cm through an inguinal canal to the base of the urinary bladder. Each vas joins with a duct from a seminal vesicle to form a common ejaculatory duct, Figure 4–151, page 242.

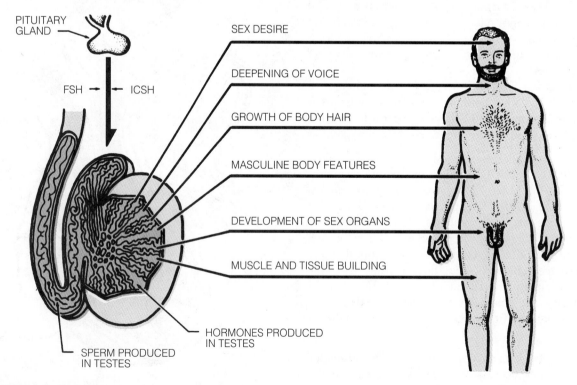

PITUITARY GLAND

FSH → ← ICSH

SEX DESIRE

DEEPENING OF VOICE

GROWTH OF BODY HAIR

MASCULINE BODY FEATURES

DEVELOPMENT OF SEX ORGANS

MUSCLE AND TISSUE BUILDING

HORMONES PRODUCED IN TESTES

SPERM PRODUCED IN TESTES

FIGURE 4–149 *Secondary sex characteristics of the male*

VAS DEFERENS

EPIDIDYMIS

SEMINIFEROUS TUBULES

SCROTUM

FIGURE 4–150 Seminiferous tubules, epididymis, and vas deferens

orgasm (series of rhythmic muscular contractions). Semen is composed of

■ Fluids from the testes and epididymis containing about 350 million sperm (5%)
■ Fluid secreted by the seminal vesicles (30%)
■ Fluid secreted by the prostate gland (60%)
■ Fluid secreted by the bulbourethral glands (5%)

Penis
The penis is constructed of three columns of sponge-like **erectile** tissue surrounded by a layer of subcutaneous tissue and covered with skin. The distal end of the penis enlarges to form the glans. A circular fold of skin that extends down over the glans is called the prepuce, or **foreskin.** A number of small glands in the foreskin secrete a waxy, odoriferous substance called smegma onto the glans. A **circumcision** (surgical removal of the foreskin) is performed on most male infants to prevent accumulation of the smegma. It has also been observed that circumcised men have a lower incidence of cancer of the penis and that women married to circumcised men have a lower incidence of cancer of the cervix. Circumcision is also indicated to correct **phimosis,** a narrowed opening of the foreskin, which prohibits its retraction over the glans. Phimosis also contributes to the accumulation of smegma. Many men also feel that sexual sensations are heightened when the glans is not covered or restricted by the foreskin.

Erection and Ejaculation
The urethra extends down the length of the penis, opening at the urinary meatus of the glans. The urethra serves two purposes, to empty urine from the urinary bladder and to expel semen. Sexual intercourse becomes possible due to the columns of erectile tissue in the penis. When a male is sexually aroused, nerve impulses cause the erectile tissue to engorge with blood, which makes the erectile tissue increase in size and become firm. Blood entering the dilated arteries squeezes the veins against the penile structures, prohibiting venous return.

After stimulation of the glans results in maximum stimulation of the seminal vesicles, impulses are sent to the ejaculatory center and orgasm occurs. Orgasm is the result of muscular contractions from the vas deferens, seminal vesicles, ejaculatory ducts, and prostate gland. Secretions produced and stored in these structures, along with the sperm, are forcefully expelled through the urethra after which the engorgement gradually subsides.

Vasectomy
Vasectomy is a simple surgical procedure to prohibit the ejaculation of sperm and effect sterilization of the male. It has become a popular means of birth control. The procedure involves making a small incision in each side of the scrotum near the attachment to the body. The vas deferens on each side is grasped, and a loop is withdrawn through the incision. The physician ties off the duct in two places and removes a piece of the duct between the ties. The cut ends may be turned back and sewn. The ends are placed back in the scrotum, and the small incision is closed with sutures. The procedure can be performed in the physician's office under local anesthesia or in a hospital outpatient clinic. It is a much simpler means of sterilization than the surgery required to perform a similar procedure on a female.

Vasectomy does not interfere with the ability to have intercourse. The sperm are still produced but there is no place for them to go. The testosterone is an endocrine function so it is not altered. Most men report as much or more sexual activity after as before their surgery. The only negative factor is that the procedure is likely to be permanent. Recently, success at restoring fertility has been achieved by surgical repair in about one out of five attempts. The patient may, however, have developed autoantibodies toward his own sperm and may no longer be fertile.

Testicular Self-Examination.
The American Cancer Society recommends that men perform routine testicular self-examination (TSE) as a means of early identification of testicular cancer. The testicle is the most common site of cancer in men from 29 to 35 years of age. It tends to occur primarily in men from 20 to 40 years of age. The society recommends monthly TSE beginning at 15 years of age (see Chapter 6).

Diseases and Disorders of the Male Reproductive System ....

Epididymitis.
This is an infection of the epididymis and is a common infection of the male reproductive tract. It may

FIGURE 4–151   Longitudinal section of the male reproductive system (From Creager, *Human Anatomy and Physiology.* Copyright 1983, Wadsworth Publishing Co. Reprinted with permission.)

spread to the testicle, causing *orchitis* (inflammation of the testicle). The causative organism is usually staph or strep and generally follows urinary or prostatic infections. Other causes include trauma, gonorrhea, or syphilis. The primary symptom is intense pain with swelling in the groin and scrotum. Other symptoms include fever, malaise, and a characteristic waddle when walking.

Treatment consists of bed rest, elevation of the scrotum on towel rolls, and ice to relieve pain and swelling. A broad-spectrum (inclusive) antibiotic and pain medication are indicated. Therapy must be initiated immediately, especially if there is bilateral involvement, because of the threat of sterility.

Hydrocele.   The presence of an excessive amount of normal fluid within the structures of the scrotum is called **hydrocele** and may occur following injury or inflammation or may develop as a result of the aging process. It is usually caused by excess production of fluid, lack of reabsorption, or blockage of the circulatory process. If the excess fluid that collects causes discomfort, it may be necessary to aspirate the liquid to temporarily relieve the situation. Surgical correction is indicated with continued involvement.

Impotence.   This is an inability to have or sustain an erection to complete intercourse. Primary **impotence** refers to the patient who has never had an erection. Secondary impotence refers to the patient who is currently impotent but has had

intercourse in the past. Transient periods of impotence are not considered a dysfunction and probably occur in half the adult male population. The incidence of impotence increases with age.

Impotence is approximately 80% psychogenic in origin. The usual causes are anxiety, fear of failure, depression, parental rejection, and previous traumatic sexual experiences. Occasionally, impotence may result from stress. Interpersonal factors, such as insufficient knowledge of sexual function or lack of communication with one's partner, may cause impotence. Organic dysfunction may result from a chronic illness, such as diabetes, renal failure, or cardiopulmonary disease. Spinal cord trauma, the effects of alcohol, or the results of certain drug therapy may also cause organic dysfunction.

Treatment of impotence consists primarily of sexual therapy to reduce the anxiety and usually involves both partners. The type of therapy chosen depends on the specific cause of the dysfunction. Most often it involves improving communication, reevaluating attitudes toward sex, restricting sexual activity, and encouraging attention to the physical sensations of touching. Patients with organic impotence need to develop alternative means of sexual expression. Some patients may benefit from surgically inserted inflatable penile implants. Such implants can be operated by the patient to effect an erection by releasing fluid from a reservoir to distend the implant. A noninflatable type provides a constant state of firmness. Because of the negative connotation of the word *impotent,* some physicians and sex therapists are now using the term *erectile dysfunction* to identify the occurrence.

Prostatic Hypertrophy. This enlargement of the prostate gland common in men over age 50 may be caused by inflammation, a tumor, nutritional disturbances, or a change in hormonal activity. In nonmalignant, **benign, hypertrophy,** the prostate may enlarge sufficiently to constrict the urethra, making it difficult to empty the bladder. Surgery may then be indicated to remove the obstructive gland. A malignant prostate is one of the most common forms of cancer found in men.

Symptoms of hypertrophy vary with the extent of involvement. Usually the initial symptoms are reduced force and size of urinary stream, difficulty in starting a stream, dribbling, a feeling of incomplete voiding, nocturia (having to void at night), and frequent urination. As the hypertrophy increases, symptoms become more pronounced, and eventually hematuria and retention may develop. Diagnosis of hypertrophy can be confirmed by a digital examination to palpate the prostate through the rectal wall, Figure 4–152.

Treatment of benign hypertrophy of the prostate will be conservative until the gland squeezes the urethra and interferes with voiding. Sitz baths, prostatic massage, and fluid restriction (for a short time) can be used, with the addition of antibiotics if an infection develops due to urine retention. Prostatic congestion may benefit from regular sexual intercourse. Conservative therapy is usually only temporary, with a more permanent surgical solution required to effectively relieve urinary retention and other symptoms.

A **prostatectomy** (removal of the prostate) can be performed by different methods. A **suprapubic** (above the pubis bone) is indicated with a large prostate or advanced malignancy. An incision is made through the pubic area, and the total gland is removed. Another common method is the **transurethral** prostatectomy (TUR). In this procedure, a resectoscope is inserted into the urethra, and the prostate is approached through an incision in the wall of the urethra, Figure 4–153. A wire loop with electrical current removes a segment of the gland, thereby interrupting the integrity of the prostate and prohibiting its constricting action.

When hypertrophy is due to malignancy, symptoms are the same and unfortunately are not apparent before the disease is in the advanced stages. A rectal examination that identifies a small, firm nodule would be the first finding. Physical examinations of men over age 40 should always include a routine prostatic screening examination. There is a 5-year survival rate in 70% of the patients without metastasis and in less than 35% after metastasis. The usual site of a fatal secondary involvement is bone. Typically, primary prostatic cancer spreads along the ejaculatory ducts, in the space between the seminal vesicles.

Treatment is determined by clinical assessment, expected life span, the stage of the disease, and tolerance for the therapy. Usually, patients are older men with complicating conditions of hypertension, diabetes, or heart disease. Normally radiation, a

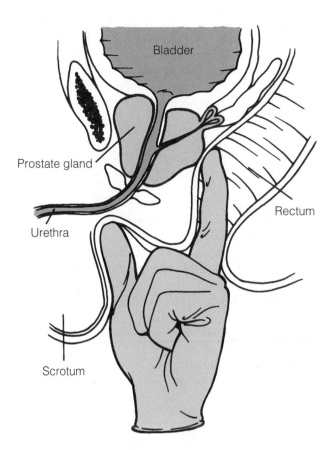

FIGURE 4–152 Digital examination of the prostate gland

prostatectomy, an orchidectomy (removal of testes to reduce hormone production), and oral doses of female estrogen are used alone or in combinations, according to the stage of the involvement, to arrest and control the malignancy, Favorable results are obtained from high doses of radiation. Not only does the cancer go into remission but the associated metastatic skeletal pain, if present, is also relieved.

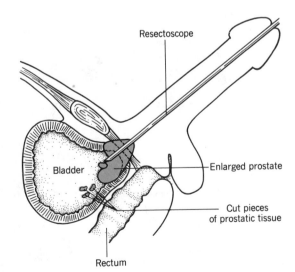

FIGURE 4–153 Transurethral prostatectomy (From Burke, *Human Anatomy and Physiology in Health and Disease,* 3d ed. Copyright 1992, Delmar Publishers Inc.)

Female Reproductive Organs ....

Since the similarity in function of the male and female reproductive organs is another indication of their common origin, a comparison will be made, when appropriate, as each organ or structure is presented. The order of presentation will be, as with the male, from the formation of the sex cell to its exit from the body.

Ovaries The embryonic gonadal tissue that is to become the ovaries begins to develop about the tenth or eleventh week of pregnancy. The ovaries of the fetus develop high in the abdominal cavity near each kidney, but descend to the pelvis as the time for delivery nears. Ovaries are small, almond-shaped glands measuring about $1\frac{1}{2} \times 1 \times \frac{1}{4}$ to $\frac{1}{2}$ inch, Figure 4–154. They are supported by the ligaments, which attach to the uterus and tubes to ensure their position near the fimbriated (fringe-like projections) ends of the fallopian tubes. These two organs play a significant role in the life of every female. They have two main roles: to produce the sex cell, (the ovum), and to secrete hormones. These functions parallel the role of the testes in the male.

It is estimated that at birth the ovary has between 200,000 and 400,000 primary **graafian follicles** (podlike structures), which contain immature ova. Many follicles never mature and degenerate by puberty. During the reproductive life of a female, about 375 will develop and mature, releasing an ovum. By age 50, most of them have disappeared.

The ovaries are the primary sex organs of the female. When the female is about age 8, the pituitary gland begins to send hormonal messages that puberty is approaching. Within a few years, the messages get stronger, and the pituitary hormone causes the ovaries to begin releasing estrogen into the blood. Estrogen affects the development of the sex organs, such as the fallopian tubes, the uterus (or **womb**), and the vagina, causing them to increase in size and maturity, Figure 4–155, page 245.

Estrogen also produces secondary sex characteristics, which alter the shape and appearance of the female body, Figure 4–156, page 245. In the female, secondary sex characteristics are

1. Broadening of the pelvis, making the outlet broad and oval (to permit childbirth). (The male pelvic outlet is oblong and narrow.)
2. The epiphysis (growth plate) becomes bone, and growth ceases. In the absence of estrogen, females continue to grow, becoming several inches taller than normal
3. Development of softer and smoother skin
4. Development of pubic hair in a flat upper border pattern
5. Deposits of fat in the breasts and development of the duct system
6. Deposits of fat in the buttocks and thighs
7. Sexual desire

In addition to physical changes, two physiological functions begin to occur, namely **ovulation** and **menstruation.** Ova are produced in the germinal epithelium layer of the ovary, Figure 4–157. There a "nest" of cells undergoes change, with some cells forming a wall around a liquid-filled cavity. Other cells join to thicken one area of the wall. This structure is known as a primary follicle. One of the inner cells will become the ovum. Under the continued influence of FSH and LH from the pituitary, the follicle and ovum mature. Additional fluid collects within the follicle, and it begins to resemble a blister. The follicle moves toward the surface of the ovary and develops a small protrusion called a stigma.

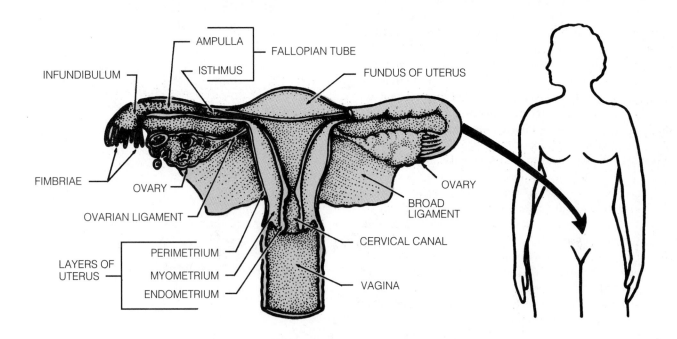

FIGURE 4–154 Female internal reproductive organs

FUNDUS

CERVIX

VAGINA

EXTERNAL
GENITALIA

| BIRTH | 1-10 YR. | PUBERTY | ADULT | ADULT PAROUS | POST-MENOPAUSE |

FIGURE 4–155   Development and maturity of the uterus, vagina, and external genitalia

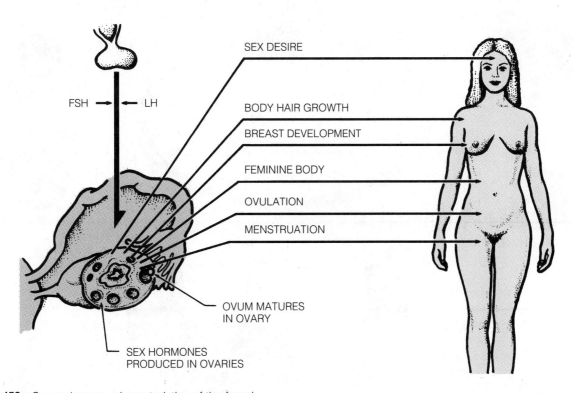

FSH →   ← LH

SEX DESIRE

BODY HAIR GROWTH

BREAST DEVELOPMENT

FEMININE BODY

OVULATION

MENSTRUATION

OVUM MATURES
IN OVARY

SEX HORMONES
PRODUCED IN OVARIES

FIGURE 4–156   Secondary sex characteristics of the female

The maturing follicle, called a graafian follicle, produces estrogen, which in turn stimulates the pituitary to release increasing amounts of FSH and LH. When maturity has been achieved and the amount of LH is high, the stigma disintegrates, allowing the follicle to rupture and release the egg into the surrounding area. This action is known as ovulation. At this point, the follicle undergoes change to provide support to the ovum. Under the influence of LH, the follicle fills with a yellow material and begins to function as a temporary endocrine gland, secreting a hormone called progesterone. The follicle is now called a **corpus luteum** (yellowish body).

The high levels of FSH and LH act as a feedback mechanism to prevent the pituitary gland from secreting FSH to mature an additional follicle. The corpus luteum continues to secrete estrogen and progesterone, which prepare the uterus for reception of a fertilized ovum. If fertilization does not occur, the ovum will pass from the body through the vagina, and the corpus luteum, after 10 or 12 days, degenerates and becomes inactive, causing a sharp decline in the hormonal level. This decline stimulates the pituitary to again begin releasing FSH and LH, and the cycle starts again.

Fallopian Tubes

The fallopian tubes extend about 4 inches from the superior lateral surface of the uterus and are attached to the broad ligament, see Figure 4–154. The vas deferens and ejaculatory ducts of the male can be compared to the fallopian tubes of the female. The ducts provide a passageway for sperm as the fallopian tubes provide a passageway for the ovum to reach the uterus.

The fallopian tubes are constructed of four layers, including a muscle layer and ciliated mucosal layer. The distal ends of the tubes expand into funnel-shaped openings with many finger-like projections (fimbriae). Upon ovulation it is believed the fimbriae move the ovum toward the opening of the tube. At the same time, the muscular layer of the tube contracts to produce a vacuum within the tube, and the cilia beat to create a current moving towards the uterus.

The ovary and fallopian tubes lie close together but are not connected. An ovum may be lost within the surrounding abdominal space. Occasionally, sperm will locate and fertilize such an ovum, which will then attach itself to a nearby structure and develop into an abdominal pregnancy. At term, surgical removal of the baby is necessary because no outlet for delivery exists.

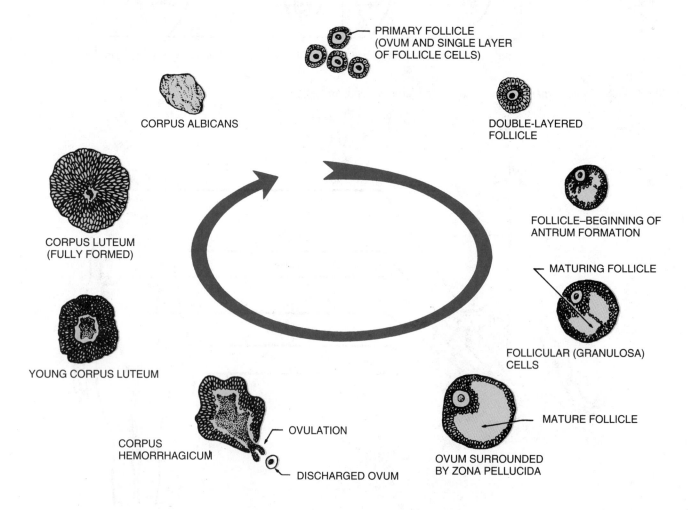

FIGURE 4–157 The life cycle of an ovarian follicle and the ovum

Normally, **conception (fertilization)** takes place in the outer third of the fallopian tube. Upon union, the two cells begin to multiply. The corpus luteum causes secretions to be released from glands within the mucosa of the tubes. The secretions provide nutrition for the new zygote, which must now move into the uterus within 3 to 7 days for implantation and development. The opening of the tube narrows in the isthmus section, however, to about 1 mm in diameter near the entrance to the uterus. If the zygote is unusually large or slow, or if there is any constriction of the tube, the zygote may not be able to pass through the opening, and an **ectopic** (abnormal location) tubal pregnancy develops. Since there is no space for growth, pain and discomfort will develop within a few weeks. Surgical removal of the embryo is imperative to prevent rupture of the tube.

Uterus   The uterus is a thick-walled, hollow, muscular organ lying within the pelvis, behind the urinary bladder, and in front of the rectum. It is shaped like an upside-down pear, measuring, before pregnancy, about 3 x 2 x 1 inch, Figure 4–158. The uterus is divided into three parts: the fundus, or rounded upper portion where the fallopian tubes are attached; the body, or middle and main portion; and the **cervix,** or narrowed section that opens into the vagina. The cervix has an internal and an external os (opening), with the cervical canal between them. The cavity within the uterus is a small triangular opening.

The uterus has three layers within its walls. The innermost is called the **endometrium.** The structure of the endometrium changes considerably in response to the influence of hormones, as will be discussed under menstruation. The **myometrium** is made up of three layers of muscle fibers running circularly, longitudinally, and diagonally. The outer layer consists of the serous membrane, which covers most of the body and fundus of the uterus.

The uterus has a great capacity for expansion. During pregnancy, its thick walls stretch and thin out until the fundus touches the diaphragm. Even at this great overextension, the powerful uterine muscles are still able to contract forcefully to produce labor and delivery. In addition, the uterus is flexible in its position, being easily moved in all directions. It is pressed posteriorly when the bladder fills and anteriorly when the rectum is full.

Certain uterine positions are considered to be abnormal, however. When the uterus is horizontal, at right angles to the vagina, it is in its normal position, Figure 4–159. When only the body is tilted posteriorly and the cervix is still in its normal position, the uterus is said to be **retroflexed,** Figure 4–160. When the entire uterus tilts posteriorly, either moderately or markedly, it is said to be **retroverted.** When the supporting structures become weakened, the uterus may **prolapse** (drop) from its normal position. The extent of prolapse is specified as first-, second-, or third-degree. Once the prolapse passes the introitus (vaginal opening), the uterus and a portion of the vagina are exterior and it is considered to be a third-degree prolapse.

Vagina   The vagina is a collapsible muscular tube lined with mucous membrane, which is arranged in folds. The

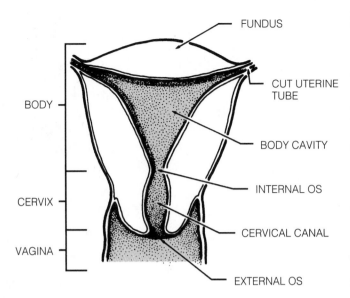

FIGURE 4–158   The uterus

walls of the vagina lie in contact with each other. The posterior wall is 3 to 4 inches long. The anterior wall extends about 2½ or 3 inches to the cervix. The vagina is capable of great expansion. It serves as the passageway for menstruation, an organ of sexual intercourse, and the birth canal for delivery of an infant.

Behind the vagina and anterior to the rectum is a rectouterine pouch—a space called the cul-de-sac (or pouch of Douglas). Infection occasionally develops in this area and necessitates draining. A surgeon can make an incision through the vaginal wall, eliminating the need for abdominal surgery. This is also the area where abdominal ectopic pregnancies usually occur. Though rare, this type of ectopic pregnancy occurs because the fertilized ovum goes out the open end of the fallopian tube instead of descending into the uterus. It falls naturally by gravity into the cul-de-sac.

Near the outlet of the vagina is a muscular sphincter that can be detected when inserting tampons or upon examination. The sphincter will maintain a tampon within the vagina and provides a "snugness" for sexual intercourse. The vaginal canal is kept moist by secretions from the uterus and by droplets of mucoid material from the vaginal walls.

Up to this point, all the structures discussed have been internal. Whereas the external genitalia of the male are quite visible, those of the female are practically hidden from sight. Many authorities recommend that a woman become familiar with her genitalia by making a thorough examination using a mirror and a good light. It is almost inevitable that you will be assisting with the examination of female patients, and it would be to your advantage to be aware of the structures.

The vagina opens onto the surface of the body at the **perineum,** posterior to the urinary meatus and anterior to the anus, Figure 4–161. The external opening is partially covered by folds of mucous membrane called the **hymen,** which border the edges prior to intercourse. Occasionally, the hymen is

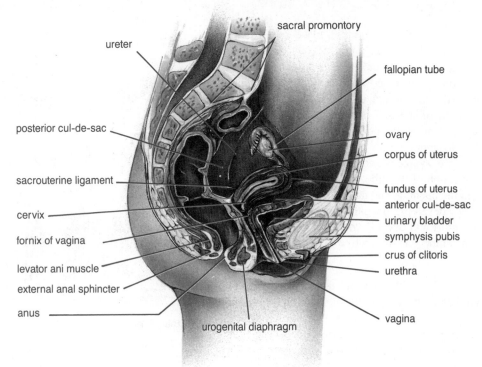

FIGURE 4–159 Female internal reproductive organs with uterus in normal position (From Burke, *Human Anatomy and P{hysiology in Health and Disease,* 3d ed. Copyright 1992, Delmar Publishers Inc.)

thicker than normal or covers the entire opening (imperforate hymen). The tissue must be removed prior to menstruation when imperforate. It occasionally requires surgical removal (hymenectomy) to permit intercourse when the narrowing tissue cannot be stretched naturally.

Vulva

The **vulva** is the area of the female external sexual structures. The large pad of fat that is covered with course hair on the mature female and overlies the symphysis pubis is known as the **mons pubis.** The labia majora (large lips) are a pair of rounded folds of skin on each side of the vulva and are continuous with the mons pubis. The labia are covered with hair on the exterior surface but with pigmented smooth skin on the inner surface. The labia are composed mainly of fat and numerous

glands. The labia majora develop in the female from the same embryonic tissue that becomes the scrotum in the male.

The labia minora (small lips) lie within the labia majora and come together anteriorly in the midline continuous with the prepuce which covers the glans of the clitoris. The labia minora are covered with mucous membrane that is continuous with the lining of the vagina. The female labia minora develop from the same embryonic tissue as the male penile shaft.

The term *vestibule* is used to denote that portion of the vulva that lies inside the labia minora and posterior to the clitoris. It contains the opening to the urethra and the vagina. The ducts to the vestibular glands (**Bartholin's glands**) open at the base of the labia minora. They secrete a fluid which serves as a lubricant for **coitus** (intercourse). Posteriorly the labia minora

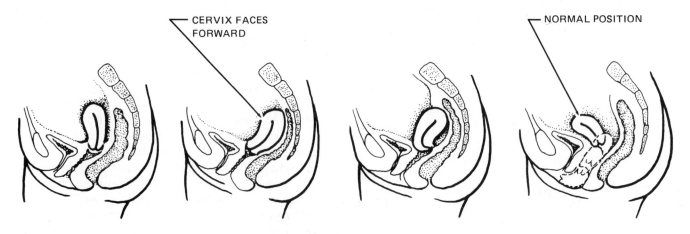

FIGURE 4–160 Abnormal uterine positions

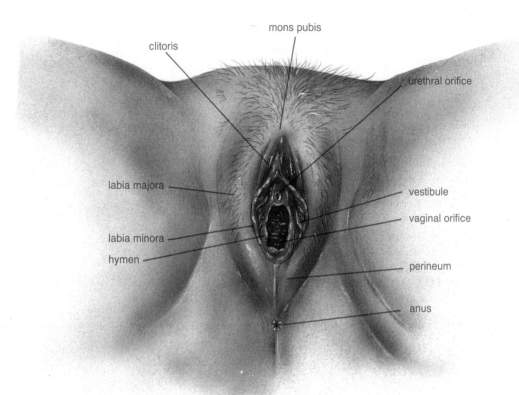

FIGURE 4–161 Female external genitalia (From Burke, *Human Anatomy and Physiology in Health and Disease,* 3d ed. Copyright 1992, Delmar Publishers Inc.)

are connected by a thin piece of tissue called the fourchette, which is just posterior to the vaginal opening. The fourchette is destroyed by the birth of the first child.

Clitoris   The clitoris is a rounded mass composed of two small columns of erectile tissue. The clitoris develops in the female similarly to the glans and penis of the male, except that the urethra does not descend through its interior. The clitoris and the glans penis are very sensitive and provide for heightening of sexual excitement. The clitoris becomes enlarged and engorged with blood and is involved in the orgasmic response to sexual arousal.

Perineum   The perineum is identified in two different manners. Some physicians consider the entire pelvic floor as the perineum and apply the term to both male and female. But in **gynecology** (the study of female diseases), the perineum refers to the area posterior to the vaginal introitus and anterior to the anus. In the male, the perineum in this sense is posterior to the scrotum and anterior to the anus. The perineal area is composed of muscles that form a sphincter for the vestibule. During childbirth, the perineum must stretch adequately to permit the delivery of the infant. If it appears the tissue might be torn, the physician will surgically cut the perineum to avoid a ragged tear. This procedure is known as an **episiotomy.** Following delivery, the straight, clean cut is sutured (sewn closed). When the repair heals, the perineum is much smoother, with less scar tissue, than if torn tissue had healed.

Mammary Glands (Breasts)   The mammary glands are secondary sexual structures that develop and function only in the female. The breast consists of lobes separated into sections by connective tissue, somewhat like the structure of a grapefruit half. Each lobe has several lobules composed of connective tissue with grapelike clusters of secreting cells (alveoli) embedded in the tissue. The glandular clusters are drained by minute ducts that unite into a single duct for each lobe for a total of about 15 to 20 in each breast, Figure 4–162. The ducts are arranged like the spokes of a wheel, meeting at the nipple. Here they enlarge slightly to form small reservoirs. The main ducts exit on the surface of the nipple through tiny openings.

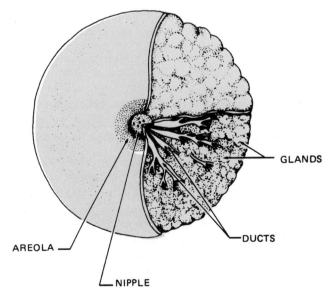

FIGURE 4–162   The structure of the breast

Fatty tissue is deposited around the surface of the gland, between the lobes and beneath the skin. A darkened area called the **areola** surrounds the nipple. The color of the areola varies from pink in light blonds and redheads to brown in brunettes. A pink areola will turn brown early in pregnancy and regress somewhat after delivery, but will not return to pink. About 3 days after delivery, the glands begin to secrete milk due to hormonal stimulation from the pituitary. The hormone prolactin stimulates the production of milk, and oxytocin causes it to be ejected in response to the infant's suckling.

Menstruation   When the ovum is not fertilized and therefore the uterine structures prepared for reception of the embryo are not needed, the lining deteriorates and is discharged from the body in the process called menstruation. Menstruation begins at **menarche** (first cycle) and ends with **menopause** (last cycle). A complete cycle is approximately 28 days in length. If menarche occurs at age 13, the female will experience approximately 455 cycles over the following 35 years. A 28-day cycle is based on a lunar month, not a calendar month; therefore, there are 13 cycles (lunar months) per year.

The menstrual cycle is a result of the interaction of hormones and the endometrium of the uterus. Normally, menstruation is interrupted only by pregnancy or severe illness. The interrelated effects of the hormones and their effects on the sex organs are illustrated in Figure 4–163, page 251. The menstrual cycle can be divided into four phases, each characterized by hormonal, ovarian, and uterine changes.

Phase I—The Follicular Phase.   Beginning about day 5 in the cycle (counting from the first day of menstruation), the pituitary secretes high levels of FSH to stimulate the ovarian follicles. One follicle ripens an egg and brings about ovulation, at the same time secreting estrogen. About day 10, the pituitary begins to secrete LH in large amounts to react on the follicle. As the estrogen increases, the FSH slows down. The follicle continues to move its maturing egg toward the ovarian surface. At the same time, the endometrium of the uterus has been stimulated by the high level of estrogen and grown a thick lining in preparation for receiving a fertilized egg. This change in the lining in known as *proliferation.*

Phase II—Ovulation.   The follicle releases the matured ovum. Estrogen is at a high level; FSH is reduced just prior to ovulation. The high level of estrogen stimulates the release of LH by the pituitary, which causes the follicle to rupture about day 14 in the cycle. The endometrium has continued to grow a thick lining.

Phase III—The Luteal Phase.   After the egg is released, the empty follicle undergoes a rapid change due to the influence of LH. It becomes a glandular mass of cells called the corpus luteum and begins to release progesterone as well as estrogen. The progesterone reacts on the glands in the endometrium to begin secreting a nourishing substance for the egg. The corpus luteum continues to secrete progesterone for about 12 days, until approximately day 26 of the cycle. As the level of progesterone rises, LH is inhibited and the LH level falls. When LH

drops, the corpus luteum degenerates, causing the levels of progesterone and estrogen to decline sharply.

Phase IV—Menstruation.   With hormonal support gone, the lining buildup in the uterus begins to slough off (shed), causing menstruation from day 1 to 5. The excess endometrium and a small amount of blood pass out through the cervix. Estrogen and progesterone levels are low, but the FSH level is rising to start the next cycle, preparing the uterine lining and the next ovum for the opportunity of pregnancy.

Fertilization ....

The miracle of reproduction begins with fertilization. In the process of sexual intercourse, **sperm** at the rate of about 360 million per **ejaculation** are deposited into the female vagina. From here the microscopic sperm begin an incredible journey toward a single female ovum, which will normally be in the outer one-third of one of the fallopian tubes. The ovum must be fertilized within 24 hours after expulsion from the ovary, or fertilization will have to be postponed until the next ovum is ready in approximately 1 month.

The sperm travel at a rate of about 1 to 5 millimeters per minute; their course seems to be in a straight line but in a random direction. Studies on humans are difficult to do, but some research has been conducted. In one study, it was found that sperm deposited in the vagina of a woman just prior to surgery had migrated through the fallopian tubes by 30 minutes later. This finding could not be explained based on sperm motility alone. It is hypothesized (suggested) that intercourse or artificial insemination causes the release of a hormonal substance that increases uterine contractions, propelling sperm toward their destination.

The ovum is considerably larger than the sperm, yet it is still only about 1/125 of an inch in diameter, Figure 4–164, page 252. When the sperm reach the egg, they surround its outer surface attempting to enter. Only the strongest sperm are able to survive the acidity of the vaginal secretions to attack the protective corona radiata that surrounds the ovum. In repeated attacks, the sperm release an enzyme called hyaluronidase, which gradually breaks down the ovum's protection. Eventually, an exposed area of membrane will allow one spermatozoan to penetrate the ovum. The head and middle of the sperm enter the ovum while the tail drops off outside. Immediately, the membrane becomes sealed against additional sperm. The nucleus of the sperm moves to combine with the ovum nucleus, and a zygote is formed. At this time, the traits which are inherited, as well as the sex of the new individual, are determined and cannot be altered. The father has determined the sex, but the other characteristics are contributed by both parents. At this point, conception has occurred.

Following fertilization, the zygote begins the journey to the well-prepared uterus, arriving about 6 days after ovulation. There it implants itself in the thick wall and a change in the menstrual cycle begins. At this point, phase III is at about day 20. The endometrium is at its peak. The levels of estrogen and progesterone are high. LH and FSH are low due to the feedback of adequate amounts of hormones; this is preventing

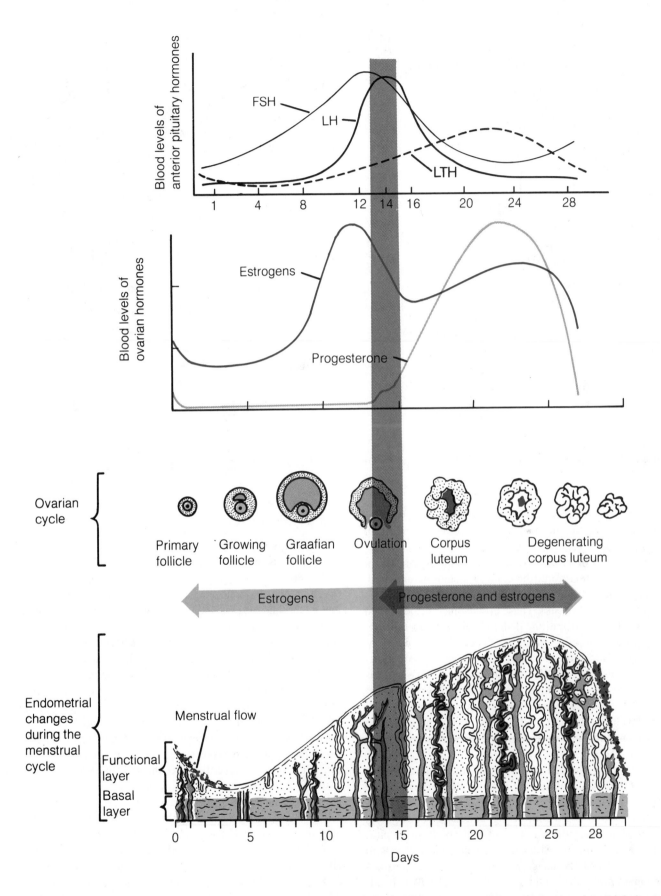

FIGURE 4–163 Menstrual cycle illustrating the levels of pituitary and ovarian hormones, ovarian cycle, and endometrial changes (From Burke, *Human Anatomy and Physiology in Health and Disease,* 3d ed. Copyright 1992, Delmar Publishers Inc.)

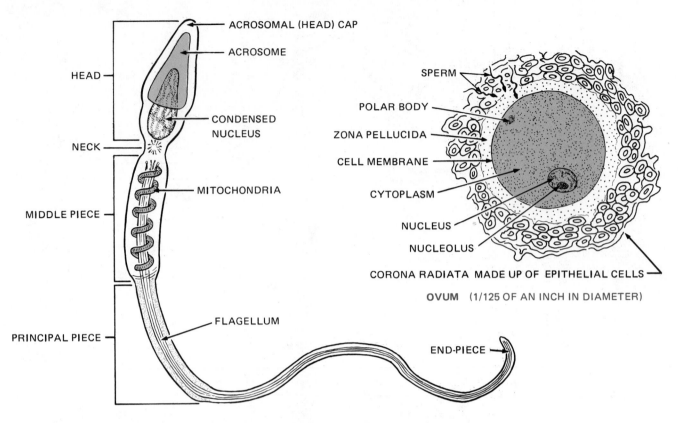

ACROSOMAL (HEAD) CAP

ACROSOME

HEAD

CONDENSED NUCLEUS

NECK

MIDDLE PIECE

MITOCHONDRIA

FLAGELLUM

PRINCIPAL PIECE

SPERM

POLAR BODY

ZONA PELLUCIDA

CELL MEMBRANE

CYTOPLASM

NUCLEUS

NUCLEOLUS

CORONA RADIATA MADE UP OF EPITHELIAL CELLS

OVUM (1/125 OF AN INCH IN DIAMETER)

END-PIECE

SPERM (1/500 IN., IN LENGTH)

FIGURE 4–164 Sperm and ovum (Copyright by Richardson. From Fong, *Body Structures and Functions,* 8th ed. Copyright 1993, Delmar Publishers Inc. Used with permission.)

stimulation of new follicle maturity. The secretions from the fallopian tubes and the uterine glands are providing nutrition for the embryo.

The high level of progesterone inhibits the myometrium from contracting; therefore, the embryo cannot be expelled. Progesterone also stimulates development of the ducts of the **mammary glands** (breasts). These effects must be continued to maintain the implantation. If the corpus luteum fails, so does the production of progesterone. Therefore, the developing **placenta** (afterbirth) secretes a hormone, human chorionic gondadotropin (HCG), which maintains the corpus luteum during the early stages of pregnancy. This is the hormone that is detectable on urine pregnancy tests. As the embryo develops, the placenta begins to secrete progesterone and estrogen, and the corpus luteum degenerates and disappears.

The placenta maintains its high level of hormone output throughout pregnancy. When the time for delivery nears, the placenta decreases production of progesterone, which allows the myometrium to begin contracting, and labor begins. With progesterone diminished, the release of prolactin from the pituitary can occur. Prolactin stimulates the mammary glands to produce, for the first few days, *colostrum,* a thin nutritious liquid, and later, milk. The continued production of milk depends on stimulation from the regular suckling of the infant or the removal of milk by pumping.

Pregnancy

About 36 hours after fertilization occurs, the zygote begins to grow from its one-celled beginning. It is almost beyond comprehension to realize that everything necessary to the formation of a new life, the bones, muscles, blood vessels, the brain, all the organs, and the skin and hair are all contained in one microscopic cell. In addition, the life-support system of the placenta and umbilical cord and the protective membranes and **amniotic** fluid, also develop from this single cell. By about day 6, the small cluster of cells firmly implant within the uterine wall and it enters the embryonic period (8 weeks) of development when most of the major organ systems are formed at an amazing speed. The group of cells arrange themselves into three layers from which the various organs are formed. One layer, the *ectoderm,* becomes the nervous system, skin, hair, and parts of the eye. The *endoderm* layer becomes the digestive and respiratory systems. The skeletal, muscular, connective tissue, reproductive, and circulatory systems develop from the *mesoderm* layer.

The **embryo** develops from the head down which explains why in Figure 4–165 the head is so large compared with the rest of the body. By the end of the tenth week of **pregnancy,** all systems are completed, even to nails on the fingers. Many of the organs begin limited function by the seventh week. After 8 weeks, the embryo is called a **fetus.** By week 12 the sex can be determined and the fetus is about 4 inches long and weighs about ⅔ ounce. This marks the end of the first **trimester,** or one-third the total pregnancy period.

It is obvious the fetus has a lot of growing to do, and it does so rapidly. By week 14, movement can be felt and by week 18, the heartbeat is detectable with a stethoscope. By now the pregnancy is about half-way. A fetus must be carried past the next several weeks to survive. If born in week 23, a little past 5 months, it will weigh less than 2 pounds and has a 1 in 10,000 chance or surviving.

By the twentieth week, the fetus opens its eyes and by week 24, it can hear sounds from inside the uterus. The movements are very vigorous by now and there are periods of sleep and wakefulness as the second trimester ends.

During the last trimester, the fetus adds greatly to its size. By the end of the seventh month, it has assumed a head-down position and if born would have over a 50% chance of survival. The odds increase to about 95% at 8 months when weight reaches 5 pounds to 99% at full term 9 months with average weight being 7 ½ pounds and a length of 20 inches.

The pregnant woman also undergoes body changes during pregnancy. Initially the first sign is a missed menstrual period. This is a time of joy for couples who have been trying to **conceive** but may be less than welcome to others. Another early sign is breast tenderness due to the stimulation of hormones. Some women will experience "morning sickness" especially for the first 6 to 8 weeks. Usually there is more frequent urination, fatigue, and the need for additional sleep. By the sixth to eighth week, pregnancy can be detected by manual pelvic examination and the bluish hue of the formerly pale pink cervix. Once pregnancy is confirmed, the woman is usually interested in the expected delivery date. It is calculated using Nagele's rule which states: take the first day of the last menstrual period, subtract 3 months, and add 7 days plus a year. For example, if the first day of the last period was September 1, 1992 the expected day of delivery would be June 7, 1993. Remember, this is only the "expected" date. Babies have a habit of being born when they are "ready." On a percentage basis, 39% are born within 5 days of the projected date and another 55% are within 10 days. The rest obviously are either early or late.

It is important to confirm pregnancy early so that good prenatal care is started. Proper nutrition, vitamin supplements, and exercise are extremely important. It is also critical to the health and welfare of the fetus that the mother refrain from the use of tobacco, alcohol, and drugs, all of which cause problems, such as low birth weight, drug addiction, and birth defects. The added dangers from AIDS, hepatitis, or the effects of genital

FIGURE 4–165 Changes in the body size of the embryo and fetus during development in the uterus (From Burke, *Human Anatomy and Physiology in Health and Disease,* 3d ed. Copyright 1992, Delmar Publishers Inc.)

herpes from an infected mother can be deadly. Every pregnant woman should consider it her responsibility to do everything possible to ensure the birth of a healthy baby. A child born with any condition that could have been prevented must suffer throughout its lifetime and probably succumb to an early death.

Other symptoms experienced with pregnancy develop as the weeks pass. Usually there are psychological changes, such as the stereotypes of "being radiant," happy and having "cravings," such as for dill pickles at unusual times of the day. The symptoms of depression and fatigue are also common, however. In general, the symptoms are influenced by the attitude toward the pregnancy. If there are marriage conflicts or economic problems, or it's an unwanted pregnancy, it can hardly be a time of joy and anticipation.

As the pregnancy continues, the morning sickness disappears and edema of the hands, face, feet, and legs appears. There may also be constipation due to pressure on the rectum. Urinary frequency is universal due to the bladder being limited in its expansion. As the third trimester progresses, the size of the uterus causes shortness of breath and indigestion because of pressure from displaced organs and the uterus against the lungs and stomach. Hemorrhoids are common due to the constipation and pressure on the blood vessels of the rectum.

Weight gain continues throughout pregnancy. Most physicians prefer to establish a set amount of permissible gain. The total weight of the baby (7½ pounds), placenta (1 pound), enlarged uterus (2 pounds), enlarged breasts (1½ pounds), and additional fat and water (about 6 pounds) add up to about 18 pounds, so 20 pounds is sometimes the recommended amount of gain. Excess weight causes complications such as hypertension, increased stress on the heart, and the problem of weight to be lost after delivery.

The Birth Process

The beginning of the birth process is usually signaled by a show of bloody mucus. This is from the mucous plug that was in the cervix to protect the fetus from organisms in the vagina. There may also be a slow leak or a gush of the amniotic fluid. Irregular **contractions** of the uterus will begin and stimulation from prostaglandin may initiate labor.

Labor is divided into three stages. The first begins when uterine contractions become regular and proceeds through cervical dilation and **effacement** (thinning out). The cervix must dilate to about 10 centimeters (4 in.) in diameter before the baby can be delivered. Contractions increase in frequency and intensity until they become very strong, uncomfortable, and exhausting. First-stage labor varies between as little as 2 to as long as 24 hours; 12 to 15 hours is average for a first pregnancy.

The second stage of labor begins with complete dilation and the entrance of the head (or another part) into the vagina. Continued contractions and bearing down by the woman push the baby through the vagina until it is visible at the entrance; this in known as *crowning* (if it is a head presentation). Strong contractions and pushing force the head through the vaginal opening, then the baby rotates to the side so the shoulders can be

TABLE 4–8
Apgar Scoring System

Sign	0	1	2	Rating 1 min	5 min
Heart rate	Not detectable	Below 100	Over 100		
Respiratory effort	Absent	Slow, irregular	Good, crying		
Muscle tone	Flaccid	Some flexion	Active motion of extremities		
Reflex irritability (response to flick on sole)	No response	Grimace, slow motion	Cry		
Color	Blue, pale	Body pink, extremities blue	Completely pink		
			TOTAL		

Scoring system developed by Dr. Virginia Apgar

delivered. The rest is easily passed, and the second stage is completed.

The baby is suctioned to remove mucus from its mouth and nose, and crying begins to inflate the lungs. The baby's body function changes dramatically. For the first time it must breathe on its own to take in oxygen and begin to circulate its own blood. It changes from a bluish color to a healthy skin tone within a couple of minutes. As soon as baby's condition is satisfactory, the umbilical cord is clamped, tied, and cut.

To help assess a newborn's condition, a universally accepted evaluation technique called the Apgar scoring system is used. Observation of the newborn is made at one and five minutes following delivery. The ratings are entered on a chart and the scores totaled. A score of 10 is considered the best possible condition. A score of 7 to 9 is considered adequate, and no treatment is required. A score of 4 to 6 indicates close observation and some intervention, such as suctioning, is necessary. A score below 4 requires immediate intervention and continued evaluation. Table 4–8, is an example of the Apgar scoring system.

The third state of labor begins with the detachment of the placenta from the uterine wall and the *afterbirth* (placenta and its membranes) are expelled. Usually a few more contractions are required to accomplish this stage. After it has emptied, the muscles of the uterus maintain a level of contraction to close off open blood vessels and control bleeding.

In some cases, such as inadequate pelvic outlet, breech presentation (other than head), large baby, ineffective labor, or the development of a serious complication, the baby may need to be removed by **cesarean** section. This involves cutting through the abdomen and into the uterus to remove the baby and the afterbirth. About 10% of all deliveries are cesarean. Repeated pregnancies may be delivered normally; however, if there are structural problems, then as the old saying goes, "once a cesarean, always a cesarean."

Contraception

The authors acknowledge that some religious and ethnic groups oppose birth control and this text does not ignore that issue; however, this subject matter is presented factually, from a clinical viewpoint, as information required for practice as a medical assistant. As the word implies, **contraception** is literally "against" conception. Several reasons may be given to avoid pregnancy.

- Avoid health risks to the woman. A woman in poor health may not survive a pregnancy.
- Spacing pregnancies. Some women are very fertile and conceive every year or less. The infant death rate is reported to be 50% higher at 1-year intervals than at 2 or more years.
- Avoid having babies with birth defects. Some women have chromosome defects or are genetic disease carriers (or married to carriers) and choose not to risk pregnancy.
- Delay pregnancy early in marriage to allow a time for adjustment to avoid additional stress in the new relationship and establish a strong marriage.
- Limiting family size. It is sometimes a personal decision and other times a reality of limited resources.
- Avoid pregnancy among unmarried couples. Single parenthood is difficult.
- Permit the woman to develop a successful career with planned pregnancies to integrate motherhood. A career can be useful if the woman is left to raise the child alone.
- Curbing population growth. The concern over worldwide food supply and supportive environment prompts some to promote contraception. It is anticipated the population will double between 1960 and the year 2000, only 40 years. Each successive doubling time becomes shorter.

Several methods to prevent conception and their relative percentage of effectiveness are listed in Table 4–9. Selection is usually made by the woman in consultation with her doctor. The cost, ease of use, degree of effectiveness, and likelihood of side effects, must be taken into consideration when selecting a method.

Diagnostic Tests of the Female Reproductive System

- **Colposcopy**—An examination of the cervix using a colposcope. It is used to rule out cancer when there are questionable Pap smear results prior to performing a biopsy. Often cell structure may be temporarily altered by antibiotics, yeast infections, and other reasons which might give a false positive Pap smear. The cervix is cleansed with a solution of acetic acid and the scope introduced. The cervix can then be viewed through the colposcope which magnifies the mucosa making cellular structure visible.
- Diaphanogram—A study that uses light and sound waves and the detection of malignancy of the breast. Diagnostic accuracy is similar to mammography and it can be repeated as often as desired without patient risk from radiation. Diaphanography uses infrared light, which is directed through the breast and photographed. Dense tissue shows as darker areas on the film, healthy tissue is translucent, fluid cysts are bright spots, benign tumors are red, and malignant growths are dark brown or black. The test is not always reliable, because certain structures may be falsely interpreted; therefore it is not used very often.
- **Hysteroscopy**—A hysteroscope is inserted vaginally into the uterus. It is connected to a monitor that permits viewing of the endometrium. By using instruments through the scope it is possible to do a biopsy of suspicious areas and remove polyps and fibroid. It is possible to take photographs or make a videotape for documentation of findings.
- **Mammogram**—An X ray of the breast for the detection of malignancy. A mammogram is indicated whenever there are palpable breast masses, breast pain, or nipple discharge. The film can also help differentiate between benign breast disease or breast malignancy. The American College of Radiologists recommends a single baseline mammogram for all women between ages 35 and 40. All women over age 50 should have an annual mammogram. Women at risk require earlier and more frequent examinations. Risk-related factors are fibrocystic disease; history of breast, uterine, ovarian, colorectal, or salivary gland cancer; or a family history of breast malignancy.
- Maturation index—A means of determining hormonal level by examining the percentage of certain types of cells in scrapings taken from the lateral vaginal walls.
- **Papanicolaou's (Pap) smear** (test)—A routine examination done on secretions removed from the cervix and upper vagina to determine the presence of cancerous cells.
- Pregnancy test—Conducted on a first voided morning urine specimen to determine presence of the hormone human chorionic gonadotropin (HCG), which is produced by the developing placenta at the onset of pregnancy.
- Ultrasonography—A test for malignancy. A transducer is used to focus a beam of high-frequency sound waves through the skin into the breast. Sound waves bounce back echos, which are displayed on a computer screen for diagnosis. Ultrasound can detect tumors less than $\frac{1}{4}$ inch in diameter and can distinguish between cysts and solid tumors. It is anticipated that ultrasonography will eventually replace mammography in breast cancer screening programs.

Diseases and Disorders of the Female Reproductive System

Abortion (Miscarriage). This is the spontaneous (unforced) or induced (therapeutic) loss of a pregnancy of less than 20 weeks' gestation. A spontaneous **abortion** usually results from one of three factors: (1) *fetal:* defective implantation or development of the embryo (most common cause); (2) *placental:* premature sep-

TABLE 4–9
Different Methods of Preventing Conception

Effecive	Method	Description/Comments
100%	Abstinence	Refraining from sexual intercourse; absolutely most effective
100%	Sterilization	Tubal **ligation** (cutting of the fallopian tubes) in the female. The cut ends can be sewn back in opposite directions or cauterized. The surgical procedure is done through a laparoscope inserted into the abdomen. The procedure is considered permanent. A vasectomy in the male is comparable to a tubal ligation, but the ends are sewn in opposite directions. The surgery is performed through a small incision at the base of the scrotum. Vasectomies are usually not reversible; however, in some instances, reconstructive surgery has been successful, especially in cases of shorter duration; sperm production is usually significantly decreased in time. Usually a second marriage and the desire for another child prompt the attempt. These methods are relatively expensive initially.
95%–99%	Birth control pills	Many different kinds are available. They are a combination of hormones that prevent ovulation; no ovum, therefore no pregnancy. Failure occurs when pills are not taken as prescribed. Side effects can be prohibitive for some women. Available only by prescription and requires regular visits to a physician. Cost is a factor to consider.
93%–99%	IUD	The intrauterine device is a small piece of plastic or coiled material inserted into the uterus to prevent implantation of a fertilized egg, presumably by providing irritation to the endometrium. Failure can occur if the device is expelled and during the first few months after being inserted. Initial insertion costs involved, and cost of removal. Side effects bother some women.
90%–99%	Diaphragm	A thin piece of dome-shaped rubber with a firm ring, which is inserted into the vagina to cover the cervix and provide a barrier to sperm. It is most effective when used in combination with a contraceptive cream placed into the dome before inserting. Failure usually results from improper insertion, a defect in the rubber, such as a hole, failure to insert before any penile penetration, or failure to maintain in place at least 6 hours following intercourse. Initial cost to examine and fit and purchase. No side effects. Requires cleaning and inspection after each use.
85%–97%	Condom	A thin sheath of rubber or latex that fits over an erect penis to catch the semen. A properly used condom is very effective. It must be unrolled onto an erect penis *before* any penetration occurs. It is important to leave about 1/2 inch of free air space at the tip (unless the condom is constructed with a tip) to catch the semen; otherwise, the force of the ejaculant may burst the condom. It must also remain in place throughout intercourse. After ejaculation has occurred, care must be taken to withdraw with the condom in place. It may require grasping with the fingers. This is the only contraceptive that also provides a level of protection against sexually transmitted diseases. It is relatively inexpensive, easy to use, and readily available. Remember, only a latex condom is also effective against the AIDS virus.
70%–75%	Spermicides	Contraceptive foams, jellies, and creams with *sperm-killing* ingredients, inserted by applicator, deep into the vagina before intercourse. It must remain for at least 6 to 8 hours afterward. Each application is good for only one act of intercourse. They should not be relied on alone as an effective contraceptive. Combined with a diaphragm or condom, they are effective. Few side effects (some report allergic reactions), easily used, and readily available. Must not be confused with lubricants such as K-Y or Lubafax, which contain *NO* spermicide.
?%	Douching	Absolutely not reliable. It only takes a couple of minutes for sperm to enter the cervix. In all reality, douching cannot be accomplished quickly enough. In fact, it may even assist sperm towards the cervix.
70%–80%	Withdrawal	This method has been practiced since Biblical times. It simply requires that the penis be withdrawn and ejaculation occur outside the vagina. It is not very effective because some sperm are deposited in the vagina before ejaculation occurs. In addition, the man may not be able to withdraw in time. It requires a lot of concentration to control. It is also not advised because it may lead to a sexual dysfunction if practiced for a prolonged period of time.
65%–85%	Rhythm	Is the practice of abstinence during an 8-day period from day 10 to 17 of the menstrual cycle when conception is theoretically possible. The method works fairly well for women who are extremely regular in their cycles and couples who can practice strong self-control. It requires a careful assessment of at least 6 months of cycles to establish ovulation days, however. If cycles vary in length, the period of abstinence must be increased to cover the longest possible period of time.

aration or abnormal implantation of the placenta; or (3) *maternal:* endometrial rejection, infection, malnutrition, trauma, drug reaction, endocrine difficulties, or blood group incompatibility. Spontaneous abortions occur in about 30% of all first pregnancies and up to 15% of all pregnancies.

Symptoms of spontaneous abortion are a pink or brownish discharge for several days followed by uterine cramping and increasing vaginal bleeding. When contractions are sufficient, the cervix dilates, and the fetus is expelled. A complete abortion includes expulsion of the fetus, placenta, and membranes, resulting in the end of cramping and minimal bleeding because the uterus contracts to close off the blood vessels. An incomplete abortion results from the retention of some or all of the placenta. If the placenta (or a portion) adheres to the uterine wall, bleeding will persist, necessitating a **dilation and curettage (D & C)** to scrape out the retained placenta and permit the uterus to close off the blood vessels.

A therapeutic abortion is one performed to preserve the mother's mental or physical health in such instances as rape, unplanned pregnancy, or an existing medical condition, such as cardiac or kidney disease.

Cervical Erosion.   Ulceration of the epithelium on a portion of the cervix usually results from chronic cervicitis. The area bleeds easily when touched during examination, and may cause intermenstrual bleeding. Erosion is treated locally by cauterization (burning) to destroy the abnormal tissue growth. Cauterizing agents used can be chemical, such as silver nitrate sticks, or electrical, such as the electrocautery. The treatment is administered through a vaginal speculum and produces immediate cramping, which subsides quickly. Vaginal discharge will increase for a few days as the tissue sloughs off.

Cervicitis.   This inflammation of the cervix is caused by an invading organism. Often the only symptoms are a purulent discharge and a tenderness of the cervix. Treatment consists primarily of antibiotics to destroy the organisms.

Cystitic Breast Disease (Fibrocystic).   This is the presence of multiple lumps within the breast tissue. The lumps may be fibrous tumors that have degenerated or cysts (sacs) containing fluid. They may occur singularly or in multiple clusters. Fibrous tumors are either round or lobular. They are usually firm, well-defined (with definite borders), freely moveable, and painless. Cysts are also round, soft to firm, elastic, well-defined, moveable, and often tender. Neither type is attached to underlying tissues or to the skin to cause signs of retraction. Treatment may include needle aspiration of cystic fluid followed by instillation of a steroid. Often the cyst will not refill. Women with fibrocystic disease are believed to be at greater risk of developing a malignancy in one of the masses.

Many women naturally have "lumpy" breasts and should not be classified as having a "disease." Young women often have dense breast tissue that feels lumpy all over. This is just a condition of being fibrocystic. Often breasts become fibrocystic as a woman ages. Only professional examination and mammography can accurately diagnose a fibrocystic condition.

Cystocele.   This bulging of the anterior wall of the vagina and the bladder into the vaginal canal, sometimes into the introitus, can be demonstrated by asking the patient to bear down or strain as the vaginal opening is observed. Cystocele appears in older women due to poor musculature from aging and the effects of childbearing. Other predisposing factors are obesity, lifting of heavy objects, instrument deliveries, and chronic coughing. The displacement of the bladder contributes to improper emptying, which results in cystitis, frequency (because some urine is always in the bladder), urgency, and incontinence, particularly stress incontinence as a result of coughing, sneezing, or laughing.

Dysmenorrhea.   This lower abdominal and pelvic pain associated with menstruation is common among young females and tends to decrease with maturity, particularly after pregnancy. **Dysmenorrhea** in women in their late 20s or early 30s may be a symptom of an organic disease such as cervical stenosis, pelvic congestion, or endometriosis. Dysmenorrhea typically begins 12 to 14 hours before the onset of the menses and lasts between 24 to 48 hours. It may be associated with headache, nausea, vomiting, fatigue, and diarrhea. Occasionally, pain may be felt in the back and upper legs.

Treatment consists of analgesics, heat, drugs to decrease uterine contractions, and the use of hormonal therapy to suppress ovulation. When discomfort has an organic cause, the underlying condition must be corrected.

Endometriosis.   The presence of endometrial tissue outside the uterus is most commonly found in the pelvic area, affecting the ovaries, ligaments, and peritoneal tissues. The cause of endometriosis is unknown, but, it is believed to be the result of the following:

- Recent surgery that opened the uterus
- Endometrial fragments expelled through the fallopian tubes at menstruation
- Alteration in the epithelium by inflammation or hormones that changes it to endometrium

The condition is characterized by dysmenorrhea, with constant pain in the lower abdomen, pelvis, vagina, and back beginning about a week before menses and lasting 2 to 3 days after onset. The degree of pain depends on the location of the endometrial tissue. Other symptoms include excessive, profuse menses when ovarian; hematuria when located in the bladder; rectal bleeding when located in the colon; and nausea, vomiting, and abdominal cramps when located in the small intestine.

Treatment consists of conservative methods in younger women, using androgens or progesterone to produce temporary remission by false pregnancy. When ovarian masses exist, they may be surgically removed. In women who no longer desire children, and conservative measures are not effective, **hysterectomy** (removal of the uterus) and bilateral **salpingo-oophorectomy** (removal of both fallopian tubes and ovaries) may be performed. The condition is not life-threatening, but pain and anemia must be controlled. Since the disease may cause sterility, childbearing should be accomplished as soon as convenient. Endometriosis generally subsides with menopause if surgery is ruled out.

Fibroids. Known technically as uterine leiomyomas or myomas, they are a common benign, smooth tumor formed of muscle cells, not fibrous tissue as suggested by the name. Usually **fibroids** do not occur singly and are located most often in the body of the uterus.

The cause of leiomyomas is unknown but it is believed they are cells that have grown into a tumor, probably stimulated by estrogen and the growth hormone, because following menopause they usually shrink in size and disappear. The primary symptom associated with leiomyomas is **menorrhagia** (excessive menstruation). Other characteristics are pain, a feeling of heaviness in the abdomen if the mass is large, discomfort from pressure against other organs, possible urinary frequency or constipation, and an irregular enlargement of the uterus. When a leiomyoma is attached to the lining by a stalk and is suspended within the uterine cavity, pain will occur due to the uterus contracting in an attempt to expel the mass. The patient is frequently anemic due to excessive bleeding. The diagnosis is usually confirmed by a D & C showing cells from leiomyoma in the scrapings from the endometrium.

Treatment depends on several factors, such as the patient's age, general health, and desire for children; the size of the tumors; and the severity of the symptoms. Small masses can be surgically removed, but a complete hysterectomy is indicated with greater involvement. The ovaries are left intact if possible to maintain hormone levels naturally. Uterine leiomyomas occur in about 20% of all women over age 35, with leiomyosarcoma (malignancy) developing in only about 0.1% of the patients.

Hysterectomy. This is surgical removal of the uterus, and is one of the most common procedures performed on female patients. It is not done on an elective or request basis but as a solution to a problem, such as endometriosis, leiomyomas, uterine rupture, or malignancy. A hysterectomy can be performed in different ways, depending on the situation. Figure 4–166 illustrates the extent of surgery. Removing the uterus through an abdominal incision is termed an abdominal hysterectomy. When the uterus is positioned appropriately, it can be removed through the vagina, termed a vaginal hysterectomy.

A recent controversial alternative procedure has been developed. It is called endometrial **ablation.** It is used in cases of excessive bleeding from the buildup of endometrium or benign fibroid. A pen-sized instrument called a resectoscope is inserted into the uterus through the cervix. The procedure removes the lining by electrical cautery using a loop or rollerball attached to the end of the scope. It requires about 20 minutes to perform, is relatively painless, avoids surgery, takes only a few days' recovery time, and is a fraction of the cost of a hysterectomy. In contrast, a hysterectomy is major surgery, requiring well over an hour to perform, approximately 6 weeks to recover, and costing between $4000 and $7000. The abla-

TOTAL HYSTERECTOMY

TOTAL HYSTERECTOMY WITH A SALPINGO-OOPHORECTOMY

FIGURE 4–166 Types of hysterectomies

tion is probably an alternative for 20% to 50% of the annual 600,000 hysterectomies done mainly to stop uncontrollable bleeding. The procedure almost always results in sterilization, which of course would also happen with a hysterectomy. There is a slight chance of perforating the uterine wall, which may then lead to a hysterectomy.

Malignancy of the Breast. This is the most common malignancy among females and the number two cause of death. It is most common in women over age 35. The cause is not known, but estrogen is believed to be in some way responsible. Other predisposing factors include a family history of breast cancer; long menstrual cycles; early menarche or late menopause; first pregnancy after age 35; race (white); socioeconomic status (middle to upper); stress; and previous cancer of the other breast, endometrium, or ovary.

Breast cancer is more common in the upper outer quadrant and in the left breast. It spreads through the lymphatic and circulatory system by way of the right side of the heart to the lungs, liver, bone, adrenal glands, kidneys, and brain. Cancer may be classified according to its location and cellular type as adenocarcinoma (from the epithelium) or Padget's disease (cancer of the nipple). In addition, most cancers are classified according to stages, to identify the amount of tumor, node, and extent of metastasis.

Specific warning signals which may indicate breast cancer are

- A lump or mass in the breast tissue
- Change in breast size or shape
- Change in appearance of the skin
- Change in skin temperature (a warm, hot, or pink area)
- Drainage or discharge from a nonnursing woman or discharge produced by manipulation
- Change in the nipple, such as itching, burning, erosion, or retraction

Pain should be investigated but is not usually an early symptom.

Diagnosis is most often made by mammography, ultrasonography, and surgical biopsy. The best and most reliable means of detecting breast cancer is through routine monthly breast self-examination (see Chapter 6). Almost all initial findings of breast cancer (over 90%) are made by the patient. Statistics indicate that 67,000 American women develop breast cancer each year and about one-half die within 5 years. If the malignancy is discovered very early, surgery can save 70% to 80% of the patients. Though uncommon, breast cancer can also occur among males. The technique for self-examination is the same but is much easier to complete.

The type of surgical treatment selected for breast cancer takes into consideration, first of all, the stage, the woman's age, and her menstrual status. These factual items alone, however, do not totally influence the medical team. They have become aware, during the course of their investigation, of the woman's fears, attitudes, and feelings about the disfigurement of her body, and will, if possible, choose the least radical method of surgery.

A lumpectomy (removal of the tumor only) can be done on a small mass when there is no evidence of lymph node involvement. The next step would be a lumpectomy and removal of axillary lymph nodes but not the breast itself. With additional breast involvement, but no node enlargement, a simple **mastectomy** would remove just the breast and no underlying muscles. A modified radical mastectomy removes the breast and axillary nodes. A radical mastectomy removes the breast, axillary lymph node, and muscles from the chest wall. Radical mastectomies are seldom performed, because of the lack of statistical data to verify their additional survival benefit.

Recent advances have been achieved in mastectomy surgery. Reconstruction of a breast mound can be provided for most patients. A prosthesis may be implanted after underlying tissues are excised with the skin and breast surface structures being maintained. The approach is determined by the extent of involvement. A mastectomy is disfiguring surgery that may alter the patient's body image drastically. Because it can affect a woman's opinion of her sexuality and her relationship with her sexual partner, numerous volunteer support groups and other services are available to assist with the problems of adjustment.

Surgical treatment is usually combined with chemotherapy and radiation in an attempt to destroy cells within other structures of the body. Hormone therapy involves the use of androgens, estrogen, progesterone, or an antiestrogen, depending on the hormone-receptive nature of the tumor.

Malignancy of the Reproductive Organs

Cancer of the other reproductive organs is all too common. *Cervical* malignancy is a common cancer of the female reproductive system. It produces no symptoms until the cancer cells penetrate through the membranes and begin to travel through the lymphatic vessels or spread directly to nearby structures. The earliest symptoms are abnormal vaginal bleeding, persistent discharge, and pain and bleeding after intercourse. Cervical cancer can be detected very early by a Pap smear before any clinical evidence is observable. For this reason, the American Cancer Society recommends that all adult women under 40 [and sexually active teens] have smears done at least every 3 years and women over 40 be checked annually. The Pap test is not a reliable diagnostic tool for uterine cancer, however, only for cervical cancer. Women at risk require more frequent evaluation.

Uterine cancer is the most common gynecologic malignancy, affecting, usually, the postmenopausal woman between ages 50 and 60. The first signs of uterine cancer are uterine enlargement and unusual premenopausal or any postmenopausal bleeding. It may begin as blood-streaked watery discharge but changes gradually to more bloody drainage. The only reliable diagnostic test is biopsy, with a follow-up D & C if the biopsy is negative. Surgery is the treatment of choice, removing all reproductive organs. Radiation, either by an implanted internal device or externally administered, is indicated before surgery if the tumor is poorly defined. Chemotherapy may be used as well as hormonal therapy with progesterone. Both cervical and uterine cancers are rated by stages from 0 to IV, with 0 being suspicious and IV-b indicating metastasis to distant organs.

Vaginal cancer is far less common, occurring primarily in women in their early to mid-50s. It occurs most often in the upper third of the vagina and, like cervical cancer, begins in the epithelial layer, then deepens. It spreads very slowly. Symptoms include vaginal discharge and bleeding, with an ulcerated, usually firm, lesion of the vagina. Diagnosis is made by the presence of abnormal vaginal cells on a Pap smear. A biopsy should be performed on any visible lesion. Involvement of the cervix must be ruled out. Lesions of the vagina are often difficult to visualize because of its physical structure and the presence of the vaginal speculum blades, which obstruct the view. Treatment of early stages may be confined to the area alone. Surgery or radiation varies according to the involvement. With extensive disease, surgical exenteration (removal of all pelvic organs) may be required, with construction of a colostomy and an ileal conduit (ureter emptying into the ileum). Radiation is the preferred treatment for vaginal cancer.

Ovarian cancer is one of the most common causes of cancer deaths among American women. Prognosis varies with the stage and type of tumor, but only about 25% of patients survive for 5 years. One type, primary epithelial, accounts for about 90% of the cases. Another form strikes children. It is more prevalent in women between 40 and 65 in higher socioeconomic groups and in single women. Ovarian cancer spreads rapidly by local extension and occasionally through the blood or lymphatics. The most common metastasis is through the diaphragm into the chest cavity. Because of its location, early diagnosis is difficult. Symptoms are confined to vague abdominal discomfort and mild gastrointestinal disturbances. With progression, urinary frequency, constipation, pelvic discomfort, and distention develop. Symptoms may be confused with appendicitis. Diagnosis requires careful evaluation, complete history, surgical exploration, and lab studies on tissue samples. Treatment generally involves aggressive surgery to remove all reproductive organs, affected lymph nodes, the omentum (the apron of tissue covering the organs), and the appendix. Chemotherapy may be beneficial in early stages, to extend the survival time. Recent therapy is resulting in prolonged remissions in some patients.

Cancer of the *vulva* accounts for 5% of gynecologic malignancies. It occurs usually among older women, most often in their mid-60s, but can occur at any age, even in infancy. Early diagnosis and treatment greatly enhance survival. A 5-year survival rate is possible in 85% of patients without lymph node involvement, 75% when removed nodes are positive. Symptoms often begin with pruritis, bleeding, and a small surface ulcer that becomes infected and painful. Diagnosis is tentatively made from abnormal cells on a Pap smear and the typical clinical findings. Firm diagnosis requires biopsy of the suspected lesion.

Treatment consists of surgery, which varies with the extent of involvement. Small, confined lesions without lymph node involvement are treated by simple vulvectomy, perhaps on only one side. With node involvement in advanced stages a radical vulvectomy is required. This involves the vulva, as well as superficial and deep inguinal lymph nodes. With adjoining tissue metastasis, it may be necessary to excise the urethra, vagina, and rectum, leaving an open perineal wound requiring 2 to 3 months to fill in and heal. If surgery is prohibited, radiation may be used to make the patient more comfortable.

Ovarian Cyst. A sac of fluid or semisolid material on an ovary, it is usually nonmalignant, small, and produces no symptoms. Common cysts include follicular and lutein types that occur in the follicle or the corpus luteum. They can occur any time between puberty and menopause, including during pregnancy.

Follicular cysts develop as a result of an overdistended follicle that fails to close off properly. They secrete excessive amounts of estrogen in response to the FSH hormone. Granular lutein cysts are enlargements of the ovaries caused by excessive accumulation of blood during the bleeding phase of the menstrual cycle. Another form of lutein cyst is usually found bilaterally and contains clear, straw-colored liquid.

An ovarian cyst may cause an acute abdomen (a sudden condition, probably requiring surgical treatment) if the ovary is twisted by the cystic mass or the cyst ruptures. Large or multiple cysts may cause pelvic discomfort, lower-back pain, and abnormal uterine bleeding.

PMS (Premenstrual Syndrome). This combination of characteristics appears from 7 to 14 days before menstruation and usually subside with the onset. It is estimated that the syndrome occurs in 30% to 50% of women, particularly between the ages of 25 and 40. The cause of premenstrual tension is unknown. For whatever reason, intravascular fluid enters the body tissues and results in secretion of an antidiurectic hor-

mone. This causes fluid retention with characteristic bloating. The tissue edema results in headaches and alterations in mood due to central nervous system changes.

Symptoms include any or a combination of the following:

- Behavioral changes, such as nervousness, irritability, fatigue, and depression
- Neurological changes, including headache, dizziness, numbness of extremities, and fainting
- Respiratory changes, including increase in colds, exacerbation (aggravation or increase) of allergic rhinitis, and asthma
- Gastrointestinal changes, such as constipation, diarrhea, abdominal bloating, and change in appetite
- General symptoms of backache, palpitations, temporary weight gain, increase in acne, or breast tenderness and enlargement

Treatment basically is symptomatic. Medication can be used to help relieve emotional symptoms as well as the physical manifestations. Many physicians prefer not to use drug therapy because the underlying cause for PMS is unknown.

Polyp. This is a growth with a slender stem attachment usually arising from the mucous membranes. Polyps of the cervix can often be visualized protruding from the external cervical os. They are red, soft, and rather fragile. If only the tip can be seen, it cannot be differentiated from a polyp of the endometrium. Depending on the location, size, and attachment, removal may be a simple office procedure or an outpatient surgical procedure.

Rectocele. This is bulging of the posterior vaginal wall, by the rectum, into the vagina. Inspection of the introitus may disclose a posterior mass, or it may be demonstrable on requesting the patient to bear down. It is most common in postmenopausal women. Contributing factors are believed to be pregnancies, prolonged labor, instrument deliveries, obesity, chronic coughing, and lifting of heavy objects. A **rectocele** of advanced degree may cause difficulty in emptying the rectum.

Sexually Transmitted Diseases ....

AIDS—Acquired Immune Deficiency Syndrome. Refer to Unit 9, The Immune System, for an in-depth look at this disease.

Chlamydia. The disease known as *chlamydia* is caused by a specialized bacterium that lives as an intracellular parasite. There are two types of bacteria, both of which are pathogenic to humans. One strain causes a type of pneumonia. The other, *Chlamydia trachomatis*, lives in the conjunctiva of the eye and the epithelium of the urethra and cervix. It is one of the most frequent sexually transmitted diseases in North America and affects between 3 and 10 million people each year. Approximately 10% of all college students are infected. It is probably present in half the patients with pelvic inflammatory disease (PID).

Symptoms do not easily lead to diagnosis. Men experience burning on urination and a mucoid discharge from the penis and are often misdiagnosed as having gonorrhea. Women experience a vaginal discharge mimicking gonorrhea and have frequent painful urination associated with urinary tract infections. When misdiagnosed, penicillin is given (for gonorrhea) or a medication for urinary infection, and the chlamydia remains unaffected. Proper treatment requires repeated doses of tetracycline or erythromycin for at least a week to destroy the organism. If left untreated, or mistreated, men usually have no lasting effect but carry the organism and infect their sexual partners. In women, the bacteria will travel up the reproductive tract, causing inflammation of the fallopian tubes and eventual scarring. Some develop severe pain; others are barely aware of the infection. The scarring can interfere with pregnancy by causing tubal implantation of the fertilized ovum due to the narrowed opening. Complete blockage may also occur, which prevents conception.

The disease, if contracted during pregnancy, will be transmitted to the baby during birth. The infant may develop conjunctivitis or pneumonia. Some evidence suggests that the infection may cause an increase in premature and still births. Two recently developed tests, which are inexpensive and quick to perform, accurately diagnose the disease. Because of its widespread incidence, many physicians routinely treat patients with symptoms and evidence of PID or gonorrhea even without positive chlamydia test results, due to the risk of sterility.

Gonorrhea. An infection caused by the gonococcus bacteria is known as **gonorrhea.** The organism is fragile and can survive only in a moist, dark, and warm area within the body. The most common sites are the vagina, penis, rectum, mouth, and throat. Since the organism dies almost immediately on exposure to air, it can be spread only by direct sexual contact.

Symptoms vary between the male and female. Men notice burning, itching, or pain on urination; a sore throat with gland involvement; discharge from the anus; or penile drainage that begins as a clear, watery fluid but changes to a thick, milky consistency. Women are usually asymptomatic, but they often develop an inflammation with a greenish yellow discharge from the cervix. Other common symptoms are similar to those experienced by men, including sore throat, anal discharge, and swollen glands. Women may also develop lower-abdominal pain, especially if fallopian tubes and other structures become involved (see PID). Diagnosis can usually be made on visual inspection but confirmation depends on a positive culture of the gonococcus organism (*Neissera gonorrhoeae*) from the discharge. Treatment is necessary; gonorrhea will not go away by itself.

Large doses of penicillin or tetracycline are required to destroy the organism. A follow-up examination after treatment is important because strains of the gonococcus organism have become so resistant to the drugs that one course may not be sufficient. Untreated or undertreated gonorrhea can continue to spread, causing much damage. Men may develop chronic urethritis, long-term urinary tract inflammation, and sterility.

Women may develop PID, which damages the reproductive organs and results in sterility.

Women who are infected with gonorrhea when giving birth pose a grave danger to the newborn. The gonococcus organism can infect the delicate tissues of the newborn's eyes and cause permanent blindness. All newborns therefore routinely receive silver nitrate solution in their eyes as part of immediate after-birth care.

Although gonorrhea can be controlled and prevented with proper education and treatment, using common sense—such as a knowledge of his or her sexual frequency with others—before engaging in sexual activity can prevent a person from becoming infected in the first place. An unfortunate consequence of the advent of the contraceptive pill and the IUD, is the diminished use of condoms, diaphragms, and foams. These chemical and mechanical barriers, especially the condom, somewhat deterred the spread of the disease.

Herpes. The virus causing herpes has two strains, type I and type II. Type I is the typical cold sore on the lip or at the edge of the nose. Type II is the form that appears on the external genitalia, mouth, or anus. Herpes is passed by direct skin-to-skin contact with your own or someone else's lesions, even 24 hours before they erupt. It is possible to spread your own herpes without being aware of its presence.

Herpes takes from 3 to 7 days to erupt. With **genital herpes,** fluid-filled vesicles appear on the cervix (primary site), labia, vulva, vagina, or perianal skin of the female. The male lesions appear on the glans, foreskin, or penile shaft. Nongenital lesions may cause complications, such as herpetic keratitis of the eye, which may lead to blindness. Vesicles are usually painless at first, but may rupture and develop into shallow, painful ulcers with edema, redness, and tender inguinal lymph nodes.

Diagnosis is made by observation and from patient history. Confirmation of type II herpes is possible from a culture of the vesicle fluid. Treatment with the usual antiviral medications is ineffective. Sulfa-based creams help reduce edema and ease discomfort. Antibacterial agents help combat secondary infections.

After lesions heal, the virus becomes dormant. It may never recur, but about two-thirds of herpes sufferers have additional attacks, some within a few months. Future recurrences decrease in frequency and severity. The best defense is a healthy, well-rested body that can fight the disease organism with its natural defense mechanisms.

Other complications demand attention. Newborns can be infected with herpes during vaginal delivery. Some infants survive, but others develop a brain infection that rapidly leads to death. If a woman has active herpes II lesions at the time of birth, a cesarean section delivery is indicated. Women with herpes genitalis also have a higher than usual rate of spontaneous abortion. One major long-term risk associated with the disease is cervical cancer; therefore, women infected with or exposed to herpes II should have a Pap smear every 6 months.

Nongonococcal Urethritis (NGU). Sometimes also called NSU, or **nonspecific urethritis,** this is usually the result of a bacterial infection. In men it causes urethral inflammation; in women, vaginitis. NGU is transmitted by sexual intercourse. Men can also develop inflammation or allergic reactions from vaginal creams, contraceptive foams, soaps, douching solutions, and deodorants used by their sexual partners.

Symptoms are similar to cystitis: burning on urination, frequency, itching (penile or vaginal), and possibly a thin discharge (penile or vaginal). Treatment is normally with tetracycline or a similar antibiotic because NGU does not respond to penicillin therapy. If untreated it may lead to complications like those associated with gonorrhea. The most serious complication is a scarred urethra, which results in problems with urination. In addition, some strains can cause birth defects in newborns whose mothers have the disease.

Differential diagnosis between NGU and gonorrhea must be made because the symptoms are similar, but the treatment is different. Confirmation is made by absence of the gonococcus from the culture of the discharge.

Pelvic Inflammatory Disease (PID).

This is any acute or chronic infection of the reproductive tract, including the cervix (cervicitis), uterus (endometritis), fallopian tubes (salpingitis), and ovaries (oophoritis). It can also involve the surrounding tissues. Early treatment is important to prevent reproductive damage, infertility, pulmonary emboli, septicemia (blood poisoning), and death.

PID is caused by an infection from aerobic or anaerobic organisms. *Neissera gonorrhoeae* is the most common aerobic organism. It can rapidly destroy the bacterial barrier of the cervical mucus. With the barrier gone, the bacteria present in the vagina can ascend into the uterus and cause infection. Uterine infection can also develop following insertion of an IUD (intrauterine device), which accidentally introduces contaminated cervical mucus into the uterus. Other factors causing PID are abortion, tubal examinations that test patency by inserting air, pelvic surgery, and infection associated with pregnancy. Organisms can enter from the bloodstream, an abscess, an infected tube, or a ruptured appendix.

Symptoms include purulent vaginal discharge, fever, and malaise (especially if gonorrhea-related). There is lower-abdominal pain, with severe pain on manipulation of the cervix and adjoining structures. PID can be treated with antibiotics to prevent progressive involvement. Culture of the drainage to identify the organism is important to be certain the appropriate drug is being used. Improper treatment will result in a chronic disease state. If the causative organism is *Neissera gonorrhoeae,* syphilis may also be present and require treatment. Bed rest, analgesics, and IV therapy may be indicated. Pelvic abscesses may develop, which require drainage. If permitted to rupture, they may cause a life-threatening situation.

Pediculosis pubis (Pubic Lice).

Little yellowish gray insects, about the size of a pinhead, can attach themselves to the moist hair roots in the pubic area of humans. They feed on the blood of their host and hop from person to person during sexual contact. It is possible, however, to get lice from contaminated towels, upholstery, clothing, or bedding, because they can survive for about a day without a supporting host. The prime symptom is an intense itching which can't be ignored. They are visible on close inspection.

Treatment is quite simple with lindane in such products as Kwell, applied to the infected area. All clothing, bedding, and linens must be washed in very hot water and detergent to destroy the nits (eggs) and lice. Nonwashable items can be drycleaned or ironed with a hot iron. Lice eggs can survive for a week, so uncleaned items must be avoided.

Syphilis.

The disease is caused by the delicate bacterial spirochete (*Treponema pallidum*) that inhabits the warm, moist areas of the genitals and rectum. The organism can be viewed by dark-field microscope examination. **Syphilis** is spread by direct sexual contact during either the primary, secondary, or early latent stages of infection. Prenatal transmission to the fetus across the placental barrier is possible, resulting in an infant with congenital syphilis. If the mother is in the primary or secondary stage, the infant will probably die before or shortly after birth. If syphilis is diagnosed and treated before the fourth month of pregnancy, the fetus will not develop the disease. Therefore, a blood analysis for syphilis is routinely performed as part of early prenatal care.

Symptoms vary according to the stage of involvement. Primary-stage syphilis begins with entrance of the organism through the mucous membrane of the genitals as the result of contact with an infected person. After 3 to 4 weeks, a lesion called a *chancre* appears at the point of entrance. It is an ulcer-like area with a raised, hard edge, which looks painful but is not. In the female it often appears on the cervix and is therefore hidden from sight and unknown. It may also develop on the vulva and be visible on examination. In the male, the usual site is the glans or corona (ridge) of the penis. It may also develop on the penile shaft or scrotum. The bacteria can also enter the mucous membranes of the mouth or rectum during nongenital intercourse, causing chancres to develop on the lip, tongue, tonsils, or around the anus.

The disease progresses through four stages. The primary-stage chancre, even if untreated, disappears within 1 to 5 weeks, giving the infected person a false sense of having healed. Actually, the disease enters an asymptomatic period during which the bacteria circulate through the body in the blood. About 1 to 6 months later a secondary stage begins. This stage is characterized by a generalized painless, nonitching rash. It is particularly distinctive because of its appearance on the soles of the feet and palms of the hands. Hair loss may occur during this stage as well as a sore throat, headache, loss of appetite, nausea, constipation, persistent fever, and pain in the bones, muscles, or joints. These symptoms could be indicative of any number of illnesses. If the disease is diagnosed accurately and treated, it can be cured without permanent effects. Without treatment, the disease again "goes away" in 2 to 6 weeks, leading to the belief that nothing is wrong, but on the contrary, a dangerous stage is approaching.

The third stage is the latent stage, which may last for years. There are no symptoms during this stage, but the organism is at work, burrowing into blood vessels, the spinal cord, the brain, and the bones. After the first year, the disease is no longer infectious except to a fetus. About 50% of those who contract syphilis move into the dangerous late, or tertiary, stage. This stage is further categorized according to the type of involvement: benign late (affecting internal organs); cardiovascular late (affecting the heart and major blood vessels); or neurosyphilis (affecting the brain and spinal cord). Cardiovascular forms can lead to death; neurosyphilis is almost always fatal.

Diagnosis is difficult by history alone, and physical examination at certain periods would be negative. A definitive blood test has been developed, however, and is used routinely for suspected infection and as a mass screening test by some states for persons seeking a marriage license. The test is known as a VDRL, named for the Venereal Disease Research Laboratory of the U.S. Public Health Service. The blood test is fairly accurate, cheap, and easy to perform; however, it does not give accurate results until 4 to 6 weeks after initial infection. About 25% of the tests will be false-negatives during the primary stage, but they are completely accurate in the secondary phase.

Penicillin is the treatment of choice for syphilis, which is relatively easily destroyed. Since some of the bacteria may survive, a large initial dose of long-acting penicillin (1.2 million units) is divided into two injections, one in each buttock. Much greater doses are required for latent, late, or congenital syphilis. A follow-up exam should be done to confirm freedom from organisms.

Trichomoniasis. This is an inflammation caused by the single-celled parasitic organism called *Trichomonas vaginalis.* It is oval in shape, with four hairlike strands protruding from it which whip back and forth to propel the organism. **Trichomoniasis** can be passed back and forth between sexual partners; therefore, treatment must involve both persons. The organism can also be transmitted by toilet seats and washcloths.

The prime and discriminating symptom is abundant, frothy, white or yellow vaginal discharge, which irritates the vulva and has a characteristic foul odor. There are usually no symptoms in the male. Diagnosis is made by placing a drop of the secretion on a slide and identifying the organism by microscope. This confirmation rules out ordinary vaginitis from female hygiene products or the presence of rectal *Escherichia coli* in the vagina. Treatment of choice is with metronidazole (Flagyl), which is taken orally. There is some controversy regarding its safety, however. If left untreated, the female may develop an inflamed cervix and urethra and exhibit abnormal Pap smears. Damaged cells of the cervix may make it more susceptible to cancer. Men develop an infected prostate, testicles, or bladder.

Vaginitis. This is an inflammation of the vaginal mucosa. There are several causes of vaginitis.

- Allergic reaction—this usually happens as a result of douche solutions, (especially those that are scented), spermicidal materials, deodorant treated tampons, or other materials inserted into the vagina. This can be treated easily by discontinuing the causative agent.

- Nonspecific—this can be the result of a pH imbalance, bacteria, and any number of other causes not meeting other categories. Treatment is determined by the etiology of the infection.
- Yeast—specifically, a type known as Candida, which is a fungus that requires glucose for growth. It is the most common form, often caused by birth control pills and may be secondary to antibiotic therapy. It also affects pregnant women twice as often as nonpregnant women, and commonly affects diabetics. Many women have yeast infections frequently and the cause is not readily known. This form of vaginitis causes intense itching and can be treated successfully with over-the-counter vaginal preparations.
- Vaginal mucosa atrophy—this occurs in menopausal women due to decreased levels of estrogen, which predisposes to bacterial infection.

Transsexualism

A transsexual is a person who believes that he or she is trapped inside the body of someone of the opposite gender. These are often the people who become candidates for sex-change operations. There are two kinds of transsexual: those with male bodies who think they are females, and those with female bodies who think of themselves as males. The majority (three to one) of transsexuals are people who have male bodies but think they are females. Surgical alteration is easier and more satisfactory in these cases. Sexual activity may not be the prime concern for transsexuals, rather it is the other gender identity that is desired.

Initially, a great deal of psychological counseling and evaluation is conducted. A true gender identification problem must exist before gender reassignment is appropriate. Physicians frequently require the individual to assume a life of the new gender for a period of about 6 months. The person must dress and live as the gender he or she wish to become, in an attempt to determine whether the person will regret having had the surgery. Problems may arise for males assuming a female roles and dress since cross-dressing is illegal in many cities and could result in arrest. Females can more easily dress and assume the role of a male.

If after psychological assessment and the new living expereince, the physician and patient determine a gender reassignment is appropriate, the process can be initiated. Initially, hormone therapy is begun. The male-to-female transsexual is given estrogen and must remain on the hormone for life. The breasts enlarge and female-pattern fat deposits develop. Prostate secretions decrease and eventually penile erections cease, which is pleasing to the individual since this was an unwanted characteristic. The next step is the surgery itself. The penis and testes are removed. The scrotal tissue is used to create external genitalia as much like a woman's as possible. Next an artificial vagina, 6 to 8 indes deep is constructed and lined with the skin of the penis so it has sensory nerve endings to respond to sexual stimulation. For about 6 months the vagina must be dilated with a plastic device so it does not close. Often the size of the Adam's apple may also be reduced if it is prominent.

The female-to-male transsexual change is more complex and generally less successful. This individual is given androgens to bring about a gradual masculinization. A beard may develop and the voice deepens. Fat deposits become more masculine, but the breasts do not disappear without surgery. A penis and scrotum are constructed from tissues in the genital area. The penis does not have erectile capability, however, and some individuals elect to have a rigid silicone implant inserted to make intercourse possible. Some choose to not have genital surgery and have only breast removal and a hysterectomy performed.

Usually individuals are very pleased with their gender reassignment and live happy lives. Society does make the change very difficult, however. All official records, such as social security, must be legally changed to show the new gender and name. Birth certificates are reissued and the original one is sealed away. If the person was married, a legal divorce might need to be obtained. At retirement age, another dilemma appears. Is the "new" female eligible for benefits at age 62 (the eligibility age for females) or at age 65 (the age for males)? Changing one's sex is, to say the least, a very complicated process.

If you should encounter a person who has undergone this change, we hope this brief discussion will enable you to understand somewhat the dynamics of such a decision and action. Perhaps you can help others to understand the dilemma such individuals face and to what extent he or she was willing to go to be satisfied with who they are.

REFERENCES

American Cancer Society. Atlanta, GA: *What You Should Know About Melanoma.* 1985; *The Decision is Yours.* 1986; *Cancer Facts & Figures.* 1992; *Open Wide.* *Facts on Testicular Cancer.* *For Men Only.* 1989.

American Medical Association. *The Wonderful Human Machine.* Chicago: American Medical Association, 1977.

Anderson, Pauline C., and Burkard, Martha R., *The Dental Assistant.* Albany: Delmar, 1987.

Anthony, Catherine Parker, and Thibodeau, Gary A. *Structure and Function of the Body,* 7th ed. St. Louis: C.V. Mosby, 1984.

Anthony, Catherine Parker, and Thibodeau, Gary A. *Textbook of Anatomy and Physiology,* 11th ed. St. Louis: C.V. Mosby, 1983.

Bates, Barbara. *A Guide to Physical Examination.* Philadelphia: J.B. Lippincott, 1974.

Burke, Shirley R. *Human Anatomy and Physiology for the Health Sciences,* 3rd ed. Albany: Delmar, 1992.

Burt, John J., and Meeks, Linda Brower. *Education for Sexuality,* 2nd ed. Philadelphia: W.B. Saunders Co., 1975.

Caldwell, Esther, and Hegner, Barbara. *Nursing Assistant,* 6th ed. Albany: Delmar, 1992.

Chlamydia: The silent epidemic. *Time* Magazine, February 4, 1985.

Ehrlich, Ann. *Medical Terminology for Health Professions,* 2nd ed. Albany: Delmar, 1993.

Fong, Elizabeth, Ferris, Elvira B., and Skelley, Esther G. *Body Structures and Functions,* 8th ed. Albany: Delmar, 1993.

Francis, Carl C., and Martin, Alexander. *Introduction to Human Anatomy,* 7th ed. St. Louis: C.V. Mosby, 1975.

Groer, Maureen E., and Skekleton, Maureen E. *Basic Pathophysiology,* 2nd ed. St. Louis: C.V. Mosby, 1983.

Guyton, Arthur C. *Basic Human Physiology,* 2nd ed. Philadelphia: W.B. Saunders Co., 1977.

Haslam, Robert H.A., and Valletutti, Peter J. *Medical Problems in the Classroom.* Baltimore: University Park Press, 1978.

Hohwald, Diane RN, CNN. Educational Coordinator, Riverside Outpatient Dialysis Center. Interview. Columbus, 1991.

Human Sexuality Supplement of *Current Health* 10 (1): (September 1983).

Hyde, Janet Shibley. *Understanding Human Sexuality.* New York: McGraw-Hill, 1979.

Kinn, Mary E. *Medical Terminology: Building Block for Health Careers.* Albany: Delmar, 1990.

Krames Communications. *Laser Eye Surgery* (pamphlet). Columbus: Grant Laser Center, 1991.

Krupp, Marcus A., et al. *Physician's Handbook,* 18th ed. Los Altos, CA: Lange, 1976.

Lithotripsy. Columbus: Ohio Kidney Stone Center, 1991.

"Lyme Disease Opens New Opportunities and New Risks for Pest Control Industry." *The Bell Report,* 8 (3). Madison, WI: Bell Laboratories, Inc., June/July 1989.

Majzesik, Cathy, RN, MS. et. al. "Radioimmunoguided Surgery in Primary Colon Cancer."
    Cancer Detection and Prevention, 14 (6). CRC Press, Inc.

Marieb, Elaine N. *Essentials of Human Anatomy and Physiology.* Menlo Park:
    Benjamin/Cummings, 1990.

Memmler, Ruth L., and Wood, Dena L. *Structure and Function of the Human Body,* 5th ed.
    Philadelphia: J.B. Lippincott, 1992.

Morris, Getta. "Lyme Disease: Summer's Scourge." *New Choices,* 31 (6). New York:
    Retirement Living Publishing Co., June 1991.

Nurses Reference Library. *Assessment.* Springhouse, PA: Springhouse, 1983.

Nurses Reference Library. *Diagnostics.* Springhouse, PA: Springhouse, 1983.

Nurses Reference Library. *Diseases.* Springhouse, PA: Springhouse, 1983.

Nurses Reference Library. *Procedures.* Springhouse, PA: Springhouse, 1983.

91 Questions and Answers About AIDS. Columbus: The Columbus Health Department
    Medical Services/AIDS Program, 1991.

Roitt, Ivan. *Essential Immunology,* 7th ed., Oxford: Blackwell, 1991.

Schindler, Lydia Woods. *Understanding the Human Immune System.* U.S. Department of
    Health and Human Services, NIH Publication No 90–529. Washington: National Cancer
    Institute, 1990.

Smith, Genevieve L., Davis, Phyllis E., and Dennerll, Jean Tannis. *Medical Terminology,* 6th
    ed., Albany: Delmar, 1991.

Starr, Cecie. and Taggart, Ralph. *Biology, The Unity and Diversity of Life,* 5th ed. Belmont:
    Wadsworth, 1989.

Taber, Clarence. W. *Taber's Cyclopedic Medical Dictionary,* 14th ed. Philadelphia: F.A.
    Davis, 1981.

The National Kidney Foundation. New York:
    CAPD, a New Alternative to Dialysis. 1990.
    About Kidney Stones. 1990.

U.S. Public Health Service. *Surgeon General's Report on Acquired Immune Deficiency
    Syndrome.*
    Understanding AIDS. HHS–88–8404.
    HIV/AIDS Surveillance Report. April 1992; June 1993.

University of California at Berkeley, School of Public Health. *Wellness Letter:*
    Hepatitis B: Despite an effective vaccine, the spread of the disease isn't slowing. Vol. 7,
    No. 8, April 1991.
    Lyme disease. Vol. 7, No. 10, July 1991.
    Preventing carpal tunnel syndrome. Vol. 7, No. 7, April 1991.
    Progress on the mystery disease (CFS). Vol. 7, No. 9, June 1991.
    Skin cancer: As the ozone layer thins, the risk of cancer goes up. Vol. 7, No. 10, July 1991.
    Why call it a disease when it's not? Vol. 7 Issue 8, May 1991.

Yoffe, Emily. "An Alternative to Hysterectomy." *Newsweek,* October 1990.

CHAPTER 5

Beginning the Database

UNIT 1
Managing Triage

UNIT 2
Medical History

UNIT 3
Mensurations

UNIT 4
Vital Signs

Establishing an accurate database is a most important duty. When you assist the physician in collection of vital information about patients, you must keep in mind that patients have feelings and empathy is essential in your communication with them. You must realize that patients may be seeing a physician for the first time, or may be fearful or anxious about what the outcome of their visit might be. Even though you must be efficient and use your time well to help patient flow run smoothly, you should not rush patient care. You should treat each patient as an individual. Gaining the patient's trust will yield better compliance in treatment.

Accuracy is extremely important in recording information. As you learn to assist with beginning the database in the following text, you will gain a better understanding of how valuable you can be to both physician and patient as a medical assistant, a most versatile health care team member.

To be a valuable employee, the clinical assistant must be proficient in many skills. Patients will ask many questions regarding their illnesses and treatments. You should be able to reply with correct and understandable information. You are also expected to be knowledgeable about office policies. And because health care costs are so high, you must perform tasks in a minimal amount of time while also conserving supplies. It is up to each medical assistant to practice the necessary skills. Patience and perseverance are necessary to reach the goal of proficiency.

You will be assisting in many procedures that are extremely personal in nature. Considering the patient's feelings and emotions will help in dealing with these delicate matters. The procedures patients must experience are sometimes painful, often discomforting, and may be embarrassing for them. You must always try to ease the patient's fears and anxieties. Always ask patients if they have any questions concerning the examination or procedure for which they are scheduled. Procedures that have become routine to you and other medical personnel may be new or at least unfamiliar to patients. Patients may be apprehensive not only about the procedure itself, but about what the physician may find. Finally, patients usually do not feel well and are not themselves. Empathy and understanding in handling patients will make tasks much more pleasant.

Patients who are intellectually impaired or developmentally disabled, hearing-impaired or deaf, vision-impaired or blind, elderly, senile, or non-English-speaking may need the undivided attention of the medical assistant during their visit and may take considerably more time than the average patient. Make appropriate adjustments in scheduling whenever necessary. Any significant information should be noted on the schedule and in the patient's chart to avoid awkward situations. Kindness and patients are important qualities to use especially with these patients. Assistance should be offered, but not imposed.

You should make an effort to speak directly to the patient, but you may also communicate necessary instructions to the person who accompanies the patient. Writing instructions down for these patients is one way to eliminate uncertainties concerning the patient's care. If the patient seems to be in need of a service that you know is available, your suggestion may be well received. Some people are unaware of community services and are grateful for advice.

Being friendly is a sure way to gain rapport with patients. Even the blind will hear a smile in your voice. All people smile in the same language.

For vision-impaired or blind patients, it is appropriate to offer to take their arm to guide them. You must also explain what is going on and describe the floor plans and furniture arrangements to help the patient feel more comfortable especially during times when you are not present.

In communicating with the deaf or hearing-impaired patient, you should speak clearly in a normal tone of voice while facing the patient so that your lips can be read. If the patient does not read lips, you can write notes to explain procedures and other important information.

Patients who have physical disabilities are usually self-sufficient and will need little if any assistance in getting around. Try to make them feel comfortable and do not dwell on their disabilities.

All of us can learn a great deal from patients who have a disability, no matter what it may be, for they have learned to accept life and make the best of it.

U N I T   1
Managing Triage

OBJECTIVES

Upon completion of this unit, you will meet the following terminal performance objectives by verifying knowledge of the facts and principles presented through oral and written communication at a level deemed competent by the instructor or the employer and will demonstrate the specific behaviors as identified in the terminal performance objectives of the procedures, observing all aseptic and safety precautions in accordance with health care standards.

1. Explain the difference between telephone and face-to-face triage.
2. Discuss how the term triage originated.
3. List symptoms which would be regarded as priority appointments or phone calls.
4. Describe how you should interview a patient.
5. Discuss ways to initiate conversation with patients and why you should converse with patients.
6. Explain what symptoms or problems should be listed on progress notes or telephone messages.
7. List all information that should be written on a patient's progress notes.
8. Explain why it is important to have accurate patient records.
9. Demonstrate the professional way to answer the office telephone.
10. Spell and define, using the glossary in the back of the text, all the words to know in this unit.

WORDS TO KNOW

conscientious	frenzy
discretion	triage
dispatch	trivial

Managing **triage** is a most delicate and essential responsibility. The screening of patients symptoms and assessing their needs is called triage. The term *triage* originated during wartime and referred to the seriousness assessment of injured soldiers' wounds and to where they should be *dispatched* for treatment. Today it is a term used in nursing and in medical facilities to determine what problem patients are being seen for and the procedures they will most likely need to have performed. This practice helps to expedite patient flow in and through the medical facility much more efficiently.

Usually the patient's complaint is given initially by telephone to the administrative medical assistant (the receptionist) for an appointment to be scheduled. Refer to the procedure in this unit that explains how to answer the office telephone professionally. In Figure 5–1, the medical assistant shows the

FIGURE 5–1 Always display a positive attitude in person and over the phone

pleasant manner which should be evident not only in person, but when speaking to anyone by phone. Scheduling is done by prioritizing the most serious problems first, physical examinations, well check-ups, consultations, follow-up care, and so forth. Emergencies must be worked in as necessary. Telephone triage is of vital importance because it involves screening all types of calls. Careful **discretion** must be practiced in handling calls because emergencies can happen at any time. There may be times when a patient requests speaking to the clinical assistant. Some patients simply feel more comfortable telling details of their problems to clinical personnel because clini-

cians are usually present during examinations and treatment. Patients are often instructed to call back with a report of their progress. It is easier for everyone if the patient speaks directly to either the physician or the clinical medical assistant regarding their condition so that the amount of information needed to relay the message isn't so great. Too lengthy a message gets complicated and could get distorted. This may be the reason that the receptionist may need you to answer a call. Because the clinical medical assistants usually know the patients better it may be easier for them to determine the nature or seriousness of a problem. Also, the clinical medical assistant can often see a break in the schedule when return phone calls can be made so that not all calls will be piled up at the end of the day. All messages, however, need to be documented. Figure 5–2 shows examples of telephone message pads which are used in medical practices. Note that there is space for the caller's full name and phone number, a brief message, action required, date, time of call, and, very importantly, the initials of the person taking the call. It is of paramount importance that all calls are answered in the order of their urgency by the end of each day. Obviously, emergency calls must be dealt with at once. Many times the physician will sort calls by seriousness. The ones that are less urgent may be given to the clinical assistant to return with the appropriate instructions and information. The physician usually makes the ones of grave nature personally. Dividing calls in this manner is an efficient way to clear up messages and provide patients with a sense of caring. Never tell patients that they will be called

---

P R O C E D U R E

Answer the Office Phone

TERMINAL PERFORMANCE OBJECTIVE: In a simulated situation, with a telephone, paper, and pen or pencil, the student will answer the telephone by the third ring, identifying the office and self. The voice must be clear, distinct, and at a moderate rate, expressing consideration for the needs and safety of the patient according to accepted medical standards.

1. Answer the phone promptly and pleasantly by the **third ring.**
2. Identify office by name (Dr. Brown's office).
3. Identify yourself by name (——— speaking) according to physician's preference.
4. Ask the caller if you can be of assistance (May I help you?).
5. Listen to the name of the caller and the reason for the call. Make a notation of the caller's name and concern. Note: a. Never ask an emergency call to wait.
   b. When it is necessary, ask the caller if you may place him or her on "hold."
   c. Always wait for a response. The caller may not be

able to hold or may wish to call back or to call again later. Always give an option.
   d. After you place a call on hold, go back and complete the call that was interrupted.
   e. Return to the line every 2 minutes to assure the person on hold that you have not forgotten her or him.
   f. Never question an angry patient. If necessary get another person to take over or answer other lines.
6. If a patient is calling to talk with the physician and your employer is busy, say, "I'm sorry, but the doctor is with a patient now. May I be of assistance?" If you cannot help, say, "May I have your telephone number so that your call may be returned?" **RATIONALE: Reassure the caller that the physician will respond.**
7. Record the caller's name and phone number. Request proper spelling of name and repeat the number.
8. Close the conversation politely (Thank you for calling). Use the patient's name.
9. Allow the caller to hang up first to ensure the conversation has been completed before replacing the receiver.

TELEPHONE MESSAGE LOG

Date _____ Time Of Call _____
Caller _____ Patient _____
Address _____ Age _____
Complaint _____
_____
Medication Taken _____ How Long Sick _____
Cough _____ Productive _____ Temp _____
Vomiting _____ Diarrhea _____
Pain _____ Location _____
Bleeding _____ How Long _____ From _____ How Much _____
Nurse Return Call _____ Doctor Return Call _____ Phone No. _____
Appointment Made _____
        and
Response or/Prescription given _____

A

PHONE MESSAGE

FOR ....

M ....

OF ....

TELEPHONE NO. ....

☐ Telephoned   ☐ Please Return Call
☐ Will Call Again   ☐ Came In
☐ Returned Your Call   ☐ Important
☐ See Me   ☐ Wants to See You

MESSAGE ....
....
....
....
....
....
....
....

DATE .... TIME .... BY ....

B

FIGURE 5–2 Telephone message forms (a) Requires minimal writing of message. (b) Brief message needs to be taken.

back unless you make sure that it is done. No matter how insignificant a problem may seem to you, the patient may be at home worrying into a **frenzy** over the situation. The fundamental rules of courtesy dictate that you should be kind and understanding with patients and follow through with what you say you are going to do. Being consistent in how you deal with calls is not only practical but necessary. When patients and the physician know that you can be counted on, you become a vital part of the health care team.

Certainly a great deal of skill in communication is essential to obtain pertinent information for assessing patients' complaints and prioritizing their needs in a timely manner. You should pay careful attention (and review as necessary) the lessons in Chapter 1, Units 1–3 regarding communication, and Chapter 2, Unit 4 which deals with human behaviors. These will be most helpful in dealing with patient responses and your perceptions of them. Even though experience is said to be the best teacher, if you are a **conscientious** medical assistant you will impart genuine empathy and caring to patients whether over the telephone or face to face. Your understanding of their needs will only be accomplished by carefully listening to their complaints.

When patients arrive for their appointments an assessment of their complaint is taken by the clinical medical assistant. This on-site triage should be performed in a private area away from others. It should never be done where other patients can see or hear what you and the patients are talking about. You must be constantly aware of your responsibility in protecting the confidentiality of patient information. Patients trust that any private and personal information disclosed to you is held in confidence. Remember that patients may tell you things they would not tell to anyone else. You must be discreet and honor the confidence they entrust to you.

Your judgment as to whom is seen next by the physician is a big responsibility. You must make sure that a patient who is suffering from a breathing disorder, or other grave illness is seen by the doctor before someone who is there for a well check-up. You must display tact and caring to all patients so that they will understand better why they must wait while emergencies are being taken care of as necessary. Remember that you will be interviewing patients face to face. Your personal perceptions in assessing situations is just as important as your verbal and listening skills.

You should politely, and with a smile, call patients in for their appointment time by using their correct name and title, for example, "We're ready to see you now, Ms. Winters. Would you follow me, please?" On the way back to the examination room you should speak to the patient in a normal tone of voice and ask how she is today. If the person is obviously very ill, you must concentrate on immediate needs and keep your conversation directed to the problem at hand. Show kindness and understanding as you offer to make the patient as comfortable as possible.

Patients who are scheduled to see the doctor for follow-up appointments or check-ups also need reassurance and encouragement. *Small talk* is a way to break the ice and help patients relax. Suggestions for small talk can be the weather, movies, sports, seasonal activities, or more appropriately, patient education topics. If you can't think of something to say, find a compliment to give the person, such as "You look so nice today, or, you look like you feel better! or, Is that a new suit?, it's such a good color on you!" Another way to initiate talking to patients it to try to remember their hobbies or special interests. Asking a patient, "How are the new puppies coming along?" makes a statement about your interest and caring. Often interests are listed as a part of the initial medical history. You make people feel important and worthwhile when you remember something personal about them. Often patients are nervous about their condition and need to have another's support to make them feel more comfortable. This is an ideal way to establish good rapport with patients. Your relationship with these patients will help them to feel that genuine concern is important in your health care team. Getting to know patients will also help you in future interactions with them. You will be better able to recognize when there condition changes both over the phone and in person. You will also be better able to detect the seriousness of the situation because you will know how these patients act when they are well and when they are sick.

Recording the complaints of the patients on their charts should be done briefly. Taking medical histories of patients is discussed in Unit 2. After the initial medical history is obtained and the patient's chart is established, the subsequent information on return visits is recorded on progress reports or notes. Figure 5–3 shows a sample format for progress notes. Progress reports are simply additional sheets of lined paper that are used for listing symptoms, examinations, and follow-up treatment of patients. This is where you will record all vital information regarding reasons for patients coming in to see the doctor, as well as all phone messages, medication refills, and every transaction relating to the patient. Be very careful to obtain the correct chart for the right patient. There are many variations in the spelling of names. There are also many families who have given the same family name to children generation after generation. Make sure that you have the correct name, age (birthdate), and address when you see that there are several of the same name in your file *before* you begin charting information.

Remember to speak clearly and directly to the person and to use a normal tone of voice. Establishing eye contact will help you assess the person's condition and help the patient listen more carefully to what you are saying. List all the symptoms and complaints in the order presented by the patient. They generally tell you the most bothersome complaint first and then the more **trivial** problems. Nothing should be left out, however, no matter how minor the problem may seem. If the person feels a complaint is important enough to mention, you should write it down. The physician will decide what should be done about all the symptoms listed.

Included in the patients' progress report along with the complaints, should be whatever remedies the patient has tried at home. List all medications, either prescription, over the counter, or home remedy. This is most helpful to the doctor in assessing the treatment for the patient.

Having all vital information available is necessary for correctly diagnosing and treating patients. Competent medical assistants who are efficient in keeping patient information current in charts are extremely valuable to physicians for it enables them to provide better care to patients.

Complete Chapter 5, Unit 1 in the workbook to help you meet the objectives at the beginning of this unit and therefore achieve competency of this subject matter.

U N I T   2
Medical History

OBJECTIVES ....

Upon completion of this unit, you will meet the following terminal performance objectives by verifying knowledge of the facts and principles presented through oral and written communication at a level deemed competent by the instructor or employer and will demonstrate the specific behaviors as identified in the terminal performance objectives of the procedures, observing all aseptic and safety precautions in accordance with health care standards.

1. Complete a medical history form.
2. Discuss the parts of a medical history form.
3. List the guidelines in regard to patient education.
4. Explain the benefits of the genogram type of medical history.
5. Spell and define, using the glossary at the back of the text, all the words to know in this unit.

WORDS TO KNOW ....

abnormalities	over the counter (OTC)
elicit	symptom
genogram	vertex

Patient's Medical History ....

Information needed for administrative purposes is obtained from the patient by the medical assistant in the receptionist's role. The clinical medical assistant then escorts the patient to a private area away from distractions to assist the patient in completing the medical history form. Keeping the patient out of earshot of others will allow the patient to answer personal questions without stress. It is up to you to reassure and put the patient at ease.

It is a common practice to ask the patient to fill out this form, but most patients will appreciate help because of terminology they may not understand or the manner in which questions are asked. In some cases the patient may be too ill or lacking in basic reading skills and will obviously need assistance. Assistance should always be offered but not insisted on. In some practices the medical history and patient information forms are mailed to a new patient before the initial visit. This is a most convenient practice because it not only gives patients adequate time to gather all the necessary information about their health history, but it helps with keeping the medical office on schedule by eliminating the time necessary for completing the sometimes lengthy form during the appointment.

Patient's Name: _____ Number: _____

Diagnosis: _____

Treatment:

Date			SUBSEQUENT VISITS AND FINDINGS
MO	DAY	YR	

FIGURE 5–3 Progress report form

This completed medical history provides the physician with vital information to assist in making decisions about the diagnosis and course of treatment for the patient. Thereafter, when the patient comes in for an appointment, This data may be used time and again as an essential reference in that patient's health care plan.

Any other information that you feel would have a bearing on a patient's treatment or condition should be noted and given to the physician prior to the patient's visit. You may make a brief note of your findings on a separate piece of paper and place it inside the patient's chart or you may tell the doctor verbally before the patient is seen. Such noteworthy messages may include for example, "patient lost her job last week," or, "patient's best friend passed away 2 days ago," or "daughter was in a terrible automobile accident last month." These situations will affect the patient's attention and whole being and must be brought to the attention of the doctor so that adjustments may be made in treatment. Persons react to such stressful situations differently. Some patients may speak openly about them; others may be overly quiet. If the physician knows of their problems beforehand, a more appropriate communication will be possible in meeting their needs.

Some medical facilities have a rubber stamp that outlines the body systems for a physical examination, or for a brief history to be taken. The outlines information is stamped on the progress notes instead of using a separate form for the medical history or physical exam.

P R O C E D U R E

Interview Patient to Complete Medical History Form

PURPOSE: To obtain important information about the patient in assessment and plan of the treatment and total care of the patient.

EQUIPMENT: Medical history form, clipboard, pen (blue, black, and red ink).

TERMINAL PERFORMANCE OBJECTIVE: Using copies of the medical history forms included in this text and a pen (blue/black ink), obtain and record a medical history from another student within a set time as specified by the instructor. *All* items should be appropriately marked. (Note: the only exception to this is in items the instructor has specified that only the physician should complete.)

1. Assemble clipboard, medical history form, and pen.
2. Escort patient to private area where you can both sit comfortably.
3. Sit opposite patient. **RATIONALE: Facing the patient allows you to establish eye contact.**
4. Ask necessary questions of patient and record answers neatly and accurately.
   Note:
   a. Speak in a clear and distinct voice so that patient can easily understand you.
   b. Give patient time to answer before going on to next question.
   c. Explain any terms that patient may not understand. **RATIONALE: Patients cannot give correct answers to inquiries they do not understand.**
   d. Avoid getting off subject. **RATIONALE: Is inappropriate, nonprofessional, and wastes time unless it is obvious that the patient needs to vent feelings.**
   e. Since the AIDS and hepatitis B viruses, as well as other dangerous diseases, have been made apparent as a serious threat to health, additional questions must be asked concerning any history of IV drug use and the patient's sexual activity to determine if further investigation should be made about the health status of that patient. This is a delicate subject and must be handled with the greatest degree of tact and diplomacy.

5. Forms have spaces to make check marks or write in answers. If further explanation is needed, use section for comments. If there is not an appropriate space to enter information, write a note on a separate sheet of paper to alert physician. For example, a recent death in the family or loss of a job are stress-inducing situations that could influence care and treatment of patient. Patients do not always mention these types of problems to physician.

6. You may be instructed to make certain notations about a patient's medical history in red ink to alert physician. **RATIONALE: The patient's chief complaint should be obvious to physician before entering examination room.**

7. When finished with form, thank patient and explain next step in examination. Ask if the patient needs to empty the bladder and if a urinalysis is to be performed as a part of the physical examination, obtain a urine specimen at this time. **RATIONALE: Having the patient empty the bladder helps to make the examination more successful and more comfortable for the patient.** Make patient comfortable by offering reading material if there will be a wait.

8. Gather all necessary forms into patient's permanent chart and give it to physician to use during examination.

The following terms are found on most medical history forms.

- Chief Complaint (CC)—Gives a description of why the patient is seeking medical attention. Asking an open-ended question, such as "What brings you here to see the doctor today?" will **elicit** an answer that will furnish you with the main reason for the office or clinic visit. The response to your question from the patient should be in quotation marks. The following are examples: (you should ask the length of time the patient has had the complaint and it should then be added if the patient does not include it in responding to your question).

CC—"I think I have the flu," past 3 days

CC—"I have pain when I urinate," 2 days' duration

CC—"I fell and twisted my left ankle this morning."

If the patient has no complaints or symptoms to list and has an appointment to see the physician for a check-up or a report of a physical examination or consultation, that should be noted on the chart as well. Examples of charting other reasons for appointments are as follows:

Patient states that he is here for a physical examination and has no complaints.

Patient says that she is here for her annual Pap test; reports that she has no physical complaints.

Patient said that this visit is for a routine check-up and that he feels fine.

It is recommended that you write exactly what the patient complains of in the patient's own words. If there are several chief complaints, you should make a list of the **symptoms.**

- Present Illness (PI)—A detailed description of the patient's chief complaint, including what the patient has done for the symptoms, if it has helped or not, how long it has been since the symptoms first occurred, and if the patient has ever experienced the symptoms before. Any medications the patient is taking to relieve the symptoms should be listed, whether prescription, **over the counter (OTC),** or home **remedy**.
- Review of Systems (ROS)—A systematic review of all body systems to detect any problems the patient may not yet be aware of.
- Past History (PH) or Past Medical History (PMH)—Includes usual childhood diseases (UCHD), major illnesses, surgeries, allergies, injuries, immunizations, and medications that the patient has taken, past and present.
- Family History (FH)—Past and present health of the patient's biological mother, father, and siblings; if they are deceased, the cause and their age at the time.
- Personal/Sociocultural History (PSH)—Refers to a profile of the patient's personal life history. It includes the patient's self-concept, role relationships, coping patterns, and life-

style. Risk factors are also identified. This is most helpful to the physician in planning treatment programs for patients. (Confidentiality must be practiced in regard to the information disclosed by patients to all health care professionals.)

Medical history forms vary with the type of practice. Some forms are short; others are quite extensive and time-consuming, Figures 5–4 through 5–6, pages 275–278. A relatively new concept of recording a family health history is by using the genogram, Figure 5–7. This method is a diagram of the family's medical history over several generations. Most genograms include at least three generations. This is most helpful to the physician in reviewing the patient's chances of developing particular hereditary diseases. The diagram makes it easy to check the family history at a glance to detect genetic tendencies. Because many diseases and conditions, such as heart attacks, strokes, cancer, and diabetes, "run in families" it makes good sense for a patient to know his or her family's medical history. This can provide the physician with valuable information in working out a personal individual health care plan for that patient. Knowledge of these family health facts can help a physician counsel patients in modifying their lifestyles toward better health practices. You may help with this aspect of promoting better health with the topics listed in this unit in patient education. Specialized printing companies can assist in designing a form for a particular practice. Forms may be color-coded for easy identification.

U N I T   3
Mensurations

The term **mensuration** simply means the measurement of things. In any medical facility many measurements of a patient are taken to establish a record for many reasons. A measurement can establish a baseline, a normal pattern, growth and development, or a change, whether it be a gain or loss. Keeping records accurately will be a primary daily responsibility for the medical assistant. Becoming swift and efficient in obtaining these measurements will come with experience. You should familiarize yourself sufficiently with the particular type of scales and measuring devices where you are employed so that you can confidently work directly with patients. You should also be readily able to convert inches to feet and inches accurately for patients when you measure their heights. They will ask how tall they are and will expect you to tell them without having to figure it out on paper. In order to do this you simply divide the number of inches by 12 (there are 12 inches in a foot). An example is: patient measures 64" tall. To find out how many feet and inches tall the patient is just divide 64 (what you got when you measured the patient) by 12. 64 divided by 12 = 5 feet with 4" left over. This means that the patient is 5' 4" tall. If you have trouble converting these mea-

FIGURE 5-4 General medical history form

Patient's Name_____ Date_____

Address:_____ Ins._____

Home Phone:_____ Business Phone:_____

Occupation:_____

Referred By_____ Age_____ B.D._____ Sex_____ S M W D

Family History: Father_____ Mother_____
Brothers_____ Sisters_____ Cancer_____
Tuberculosis_____ Mental Illness_____ Diabetes_____
Heart Disease_____ Hepatitis_____
Rheumatism_____ Gout_____ Goiter_____
Obesity_____ Nephritis_____ Epilepsy_____
Other_____

Past History: Diphtheria_____ Measles_____ Mumps_____
Chicken -Pox_____ Scarlet Fever_____ Smallpox_____ Thyroid_____
Infantile Paralysis_____ Malaria_____ Pneumonia_____
Dysentery_____ Jaundice_____ Boils_____ Rheumatic Fever_____
Tuberculosis_____ Asthma_____ Heart Disease_____
Hypertension_____ Diabetes_____ Infections_____
Gonorrhea_____ Syphillis_____ Tonsillitis_____
Nephritis_____ Operations_____

Menstrual: Onset_____ Frequency_____ Type_____
           Duration_____ Pain_____ L.M.P._____
Marital: Miscarriages_____ Abortions_____ Sterility_____
           Children_____
Habits: Alcohol_____ Tobacco_____ Drugs_____ Coffee_____
          Tea_____ Meals_____ Water_____ Sleep_____
          Bowel Movements_____ Exercise_____
          Amusements or Hobbies_____

Injuries:_____
_____

Allergies:_____
_____
_____

Present Illness:_____
_____
_____

PHYSICAL EXAMINATION: Ht._____ Wt._____ Temp._____ B.P._____
Pulse_____ Respirations_____ General Appearance_____
Skin_____ Mucous Membranes_____
Eyes: Vision: O.D._____ O.S._____ O.U._____
Ishihara_____ Near Vision_____

FIGURE 5–5   In-depth medical history form

Pupil _____ Fundus _____

Ears _____ Nose _____

Chest _____ Breasts _____

Heart _____

Lungs _____

Abdomen _____

Genitalia _____

Rectum _____

Vagina _____

Extremities _____

Lymph Nodes: Neck _____ Axilla _____ Inguinal _____

Abdominal _____ Reflexes _____

REMARKS: _____
_____
_____
_____

DIAGNOSIS: _____
_____
_____

TREATMENT: _____
_____
_____

FIGURE 5–5   Continued

surements you should practice until you are able to do it comfortably and quickly.

This unit deals with all of the measurements of the physical body. In Unit 4 you will learn about measuring vital signs.

OBJECTIVES ....

Upon completion of this unit, you will meet the following terminal performance objectives by verifying knowledge of the facts and principles presented through oral and written communication at a level deemed competent by the instructor or employer and will demonstrate the specific behaviors as identified in the terminal performance objectives of the procedures, observing all aseptic and safety precautions in accordance with health care standards.

1. Measure patients' height safely and accurately.
2. Weigh patients safely and accurately.
3. Record measurements of patients accurately.
4. Measure infant chest circumference accurately.
5. Measure infant head circumference accurately.
6. Record pediatric measurements on growth charts accurately.
7. Convert inches into feet and inches.
8. Spell and define, using the glossary at the back of the text, all the words to know in this unit.

WORDS TO KNOW ....

abnormalities	recumbent
horizontal	statistic
intersect	stature
mensuration	vertex
monitor	vertical
percentile	

MEDICAL HISTORY FORM

Date _____

Patient's name _____

Age	Date of birth	Sex

Address	City	State	Zip code

Phone ( ) _____

Insurance company	Policy number

Place of employment	Address

Phone ( )	Job responsibilities

Parent/Guardian if minor _____

Address	City	State	Zip code

Phone ( ) _____

Family History:

List family members: (mother, father, brothers, sisters, grandparents, etc.)—ages and health status (if deceased write their age at the time of their death and the cause). List allergies and/or any conditions or diseases they may have or have had, such as asthma, arthritis, tuberculosis, diabetes, cancer, heart disease, hypertension, kidney disease, mental illness, depression, or any other health problems that you know of in your family.

_____

_____

_____

Patient's Past History: Mark the boxes to the right either "yes" or "no" for the following questions:*

Do you ever have or have you ever had any of the following: **(yes) (no)**

SKIN

Rashes, hives, itching or other skin irritations ( ) ( )

EYES, EARS, NOSE, THROAT

Headaches, dizziness, fainting ( ) ( )
Blurred or impaired vision ( ) ( )
Hearing loss or ringing in the ears ( ) ( )
Discharge from eyes or ears ( ) ( )
Sinus trouble/colds/allergies ( ) ( )
Asthma or hay fever ( ) ( )
Sore throats/hoarseness ( ) ( )

CARDIOPULMONARY

Shortness of breath ( ) ( )
Persistent cough or coughing up blood or other secretions ( ) ( )
Chills and/or fever ( ) ( )
Night sweats ( ) ( )
Tuberculosis or exposed to TB ( ) ( )

Scarlet fever or rheumatic fever ( ) ( )
Chest pain ( ) ( )
Heart palpitations or rapid heartbeat or pulse ( ) ( )
High blood pressure ( ) ( )
Swelling of hands and/or feet ( ) ( )

GASTROINTESTINAL

Heartburn or indigestion ( ) ( )
Nausea and/or vomiting ( ) ( )
Loss of appetite ( ) ( )
Belching or gas ( ) ( )
Peptic ulcer, gallbladder or liver disease ( ) ( )
Yellow jaundice or hepatitis ( ) ( )
Diarrhea or constipation ( ) ( )
Dysentery ( ) ( )
Rectal bleeding, hemorrhoids (piles) ( ) ( )
Tarry or clay-colored stools ( ) ( )

GLANDS

Weight gain or loss ( ) ( )
Diabetes ( ) ( )

Thyroid or goiter ( ) ( )
Swollen glands ( ) ( )

GENITOURINARY

Kidney disease or stones, or Bright's disease ( ) ( )
Painful, frequent or urgent urination ( ) ( )
Blood or pus in urine ( ) ( )
Sexually transmitted disease (venereal disease) ( ) ( )
Been sexually active with anyone who has AIDS or HIV or hepatitis ( ) ( )

NEUROMUSCULAR

Problems with becoming tired and/or upset easily ( ) ( )
Nervous breakdown/depression ( ) ( )
Poliomyelitis (infantile paralysis) ( ) ( )
Convulsions ( ) ( )
Joint and/or muscular pain ( ) ( )
Back pain or injury/osteomyelitis/rheumatism ( ) ( )

Are you currently taking any medications? Yes ( ) No ( )
If yes, please list them _____
Have you ever had or been treated for cancer or any tumors? ( ) ( )
Are you anemic or have you ever had to take iron medication? ( ) ( )
Do you use tobacco? ( ) ( )
What type? _____
Do you use IV drugs or alcohol? ( ) ( )

WOMEN ONLY

Painful menstrual periods ( ) ( )
Pregnancy/abortion/miscarriage ( ) ( )
Vaginal infection or discharge/abnormal bleeding ( ) ( )

Last menstrual period _____
Birth control _____
List dates of all operations/surgeries, injuries, and illnesses that required hospitalization:

_____

Did you ever receive benefits from a medical insurance claim due to illness or injury? Yes ( ) No ( )
Were you ever rejected from the military or for employment? ( ) ( )
Were you absent from school/work in the past 10 years because of illness or injury? ( ) ( )
Did you ever file a Workers' Compensation claim? ( ) ( )
Did you ever seek psychological or psychiatric treatment? ( ) ( )

*Please use the back of this form to explain any "yes" answers. Thank you.

FIGURE 5–6 Medical history form

FIGURE 5–7   Example of a genogram

Height and Weight ....

The patient's height and weight must be recorded at the initial visit to serve as a reference point. Accuracy is important both in measuring and in recording this information. Infants and small children should have height and weight measured and recorded routinely for growth and development patterns to be established.

Using Figure 5–9A, page 282, as an example, you will see that the age of infant females ranges from birth (B) to 36 months across the top of the chart (it is also printed across the bottom). Each of the squares across the graph represents one month. After the measurements of the infant have been obtained at each check-up, they are plotted on this graph. The recumbent length of the child is recorded in either inches or centimeters, and the weight in pounds or kilograms. One must be consistent in measuring the child in the same manner to avoid discrepancies. To record these measurements, follow the age line (vertically) down to the child's length measurement on the left and follow the horizontal line to the point at where the two **inter-**

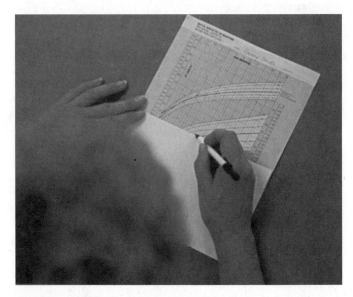

FIGURE 5–8   Medical assistant plotting a measurement on a growth graph

Patient education is a primary function of the medical assistant. Most patients are not trained health professionals and are somewhat confused by medical terminology, tests, procedures, and medications they encounter. Therefore, patient education becomes an important part of their medical care.

Whenever possible, the patient should be involved in making decisions about treatment or care. This will encourage the patient to participate more fully in the procedure. Patients will be more willing to cooperate if they understand the necessity for a particular procedure or treatment. Your careful and clear explanations of these procedures will encourage the patient to be more cooperative. If patients sense that you are truly concerned about their well-being, this will stimulate more cooperation. Always offer encouragement and praise where appropriate, even for the smallest accomplishment.

To instruct a patient properly, the medical assistant must know the material. Be prepared to answer any questions from the patient. If you cannot answer one of the patient's questions, tell the patient that you do not know the answer but will ask the physician. Never try to answer a question that you are not prepared to discuss. You could give incorrect information that could harm the patient's well-being. Never give information that is beyond your scope of practice.

In teaching a patient about health care and all that is involved in medical well-being, the primary goal of the medical assistant should be good communication. This means that each patient must be treated as an individual with particular needs. As the patient educator, you will have to meet these needs. You must communicate in the most efficient and effective manner for each individual. Listening is vital to this education. Patients may be shy or embarrassed by their problems or questions and may not ask direct questions. Therefore, you must listen carefully to the patient's comments and questions. Be familiar with information about the patient before proceeding with an explanation. This will help determine how to communicate best with each individual.

Never assume that a patient already knows the information you are conveying. Sometimes a patient will state that he understands something to keep from being embarrassed. If you sense that this is the situation you should briefly repeat the information and provide printed material for the patient to take home to read. Printed materials, such as one-page handouts, brochures, pamphlets, and booklets on various procedures and examinations, as well as diseases, conditions, and treatment plans, should be clear and concise in content. These informative materials should be appropriately distributed routinely to patients.

One very important aspect of patient teaching is your attitude toward the patient. The medical assistant must be open when approaching patients. This means that you must accept each patient as an individual who needs your help. There is no room in the medical office for prejudice. All patients should be treated with respect regardless of their financial status, race, religion, age, or station in life. Remember, your job is to provide assistance. If the patients sense any negative feelings on your part, then they will be less likely to pay attention to your instructions and suggestions.

Most patients are interested in getting better and staying healthy. Patient education involves not only instructing those who are sick, but helping healthy patients say well. By following current trends in wellness and prevention of medical problems, you can help patients help themselves to a healthier life.

The following are some general guidelines for patient education:

1. Become familiar with your office's or clinic's policy concerning patient care.
2. Thoroughly read all handout information given to patients to explain procedures, examinations, or treatment plans so that you can answer patients' questions intelligently.
3. Make yourself available to patients for answering questions. Always remember to ask patients if they have any questions about their treatment or diagnosis.
4. Always take the opportunity to explain procedures to patients and offer additional information, when appropriate, at the time of their visits. For example, be sure to explain warm-up and stretching exercises to the weekend athlete with a sprained ankle.
5. Attend continuing education programs to keep abreast of the latest medical information to pass on to patients.
6. Post charts, posters, and other information that will benefit the patient. Be sure that this information is kept current and is posted in areas where patients may spend time waiting.
7. Have current health-conscious magazines available in the reception area.
8. Post meeting times and information for patient support groups (weight control groups, stop-smoking groups, tough love meetings) and encourage their participation. Keep this information current.

sect and place a dot with your pen (or pencil); stay on the **vertical** (age) line and look to the right side of the chart for the weight of the child. Following the **horizontal** line from right to left, place a dot at the intersection of the weight and age line.

Record the head circumference in the same fashion by following the vertical age line down to the corresponding horizontal measurement (to the left of the chart) in inches or centimeters and place the dot with red ink or pencil where the two lines intersect. It is helpful to place a plain sheet of paper over the graph while finding the intersecting lines to avoid errors, Figure 5–8.

The dots are connected by drawing a straight line with a ruler from one point to another providing a neat and concise appearance.

The curved lines printed across the growth charts show the normal range of growth of infants and children in the United States. The numbers to the right of the chart in the boxes vertically between age 34 and 35 months show the **percentiles** of other children the same age. The National Center for Health Statistics (NCHS) growth charts become a permanent record of the child's development. Figures 5–9 A and B are examples. Additional growth graph charts for both boys and girls ages 2 to 18 years may be found in the appendix of the text. These give the physician a quick way to check the child's growth in relation to that of other children the same age. Growth charts aid in the diagnosis of growth **abnormalities** and nutritional disorders and diseases. Of course, hereditary factors also influence growth patterns, hence the importance of having the family history in the medical record.

In measuring **stature** (standing height), all patients over 3 years of age should be asked to stand tall and hold still until the measurement has been obtained. Children under 3 can be measured in either a standing or **recumbent** position. A child's length in the recumbent position will be nearly an inch greater than when standing, so it is necessary to be consistent in the method of measurement. Make a notation of which method is used when recording the measurement. It is recommended that a right-angle headboard be used to ensure accuracy in measuring children.

Since either the gaining or the losing of weight can change the course of a patient's diagnosis and treatment, proper balancing of the scales should be a routine practice.

Most physicians require that patients are weighed routinely at each visit. Measuring the height of patients should be done periodically after age 18 years of age because of certain degenerative conditions and anatomical changes of the body from aging. Patients are weight-conscious, so the remarks of the medical assistant should be positive ones, if any. A chart of desirable weight of men and women may be posted above the scale for patient education, Figure 5–10, page 285.

If there is no measuring device for use in obtaining the recumbent length of a baby, you may measure the length of the child by using a flexible measuring tape. Place the child on her back on the examination table and mark on the table paper with a pen the top (vertex) of the head and the bottom of the feet (the heel). Then measure the distance between the two marks with the tape measure to obtain the length of the child. Be sure that the baby was straight and still while marking the positions of head and heel for the measurement.

PROCEDURE

Weigh Patient on Upright Scale

PURPOSE: To obtain an accurate measure of the patient's weight.

EQUIPMENT: Upright balance scales, Figure 5–11, page 286, patient's chart, pen

TERMINAL PERFORMANCE OBJECTIVE: After the instructor has measured and recorded the weight of all students, each student will, in turn select five other students. Demonstrate on five other students each step in the weight measurement procedure to determine the accurate weight of each of the five students. The weight measurements obtained should agree with the weights for those five students as measured and recorded by the instructor ± ¼ lb.

1. Wash hands and balance scales.
2. Ask patient to remove shoes. *Some patients prefer to be weighed in a paper gown to give lowest weight.*
3. Place a paper towel on base of scale. **RATIONALE:**

Provides a clean surface for the shoeless foot.
4. Help patient onto scale.
5. Make sure patient is in center of platform. Ask patient to stand still while you adjust balance and read weight, Figure 5–12, page 286. If you are to obtain both the height and weight of a patient, it is best to have the patient remain on the scales. Raise the bar by pushing it up with one hand and holding the extension of the bar with the other hand protecting the patient from possible injury (the patient is still facing the measuring device). Refer to Step 4 of the procedure for measuring height to complete.
6. Help patient from scale and discard paper towel.
7. Record weight on patient's chart. Be sure to record whether patient was wearing street clothing or gown. *Note:* If patients are weighed with their clothes on, it is common to allow at least 3 pounds for women's clothing and 5 pounds for men's.
8. Return scale to balance at zero.

GIRLS: BIRTH TO 36 MONTHS
PHYSICAL GROWTH
NCHS PERCENTILES*

NAME _____ RECORD # _____

*Adapted from: Hamill PVV, Drizd TA, Johnson CL, Reed RB, Roche AF, Moore WM. Physical growth: National Center for Health Statistics percentiles. AM J CLIN NUTR 32:607-629, 1979. Data from the Fels Research Institute, Wright State University School of Medicine, Yellow Springs, Ohio.

© 1982 ROSS LABORATORIES

FIGURE 5–9A Growth chart for girls height and weight, from birth to age 36 months

NAME _____   RECORD # _____

MOTHER'S STATURE   GESTATIONAL
FATHER'S STATURE   AGE   WEEKS

DATE	AGE	LENGTH	WEIGHT	HEAD CIRC.	COMMENT
	BIRTH				

*Adapted from: Hamill PVV, Drizd TA, Johnson CL, Reed RB, Roche AF, Moore WM: Physical growth: National Center for Health Statistics percentiles. AM J CLIN NUTR 32:607-629, 1979. Data from the Fels Research Institute, Wright State University School of Medicine, Yellow Springs, Ohio.

c 1982 ROSS LABORATORIES

Ross
Growth &
Development
Program

B

FIGURE 5–9B Growth chart for boys height and weight, from birth to age 36 months

Weigh Infant

PURPOSE: To obtain an accurate weight measurement of an infant.

EQUIPMENT: Infant balance scales, towel, patient's chart, growth graph, parent's record booklet, pen

TERMINAL PERFORMANCE OBJECTIVE: Provided with at least three lifelike clinical or toy dolls (or an infant or small child under the close supervision of the parent, guardian, or the instructor) and an infant scales, demonstrate each step required in weighing infants and very small children by weighing each of the dolls; each weight must be within ± $\frac{1}{8}$ lb. of each weight as determined by the instructor beforehand.

1. Wash hands.
2. Ask parent to remove infant's clothing. **RATIONALE: Alleviates the infant's apprehension and conserves your time.**
3. Place a clean towel on scale cradle to avoid disease transmission and to decrease shock from the cold metal for infant. This will lessen chance that infant will move because of being uncomfortable or afraid. Keep diaper or towel over infant's genital area in case of an elimination.
4. Balance scale at zero with towel in place.
5. Place infant on scale holding one hand over infant

(almost touching) to give a sense of security. Talking in a quiet tone will also help keep infant still until reading has been taken. The age of the baby may determine how the child is placed on the scales. Small infants will be easier to weigh lying down; those who can sit up on their own will most likely be more cooperative sitting on the scales, Figures 5–13 and 5–14, page 286. In either case the safety of the baby is primary.

6. Slide weight easily until scale balances, which determines weight of infant. Read scale in pounds and ounces or kilograms.
7. Return infant to parent to dress.
8. Remove towel from scale, place it in proper receptacle, and balance scale at zero mark.
9. Record weight on growth chart, patient's chart, and parent's booklet. *Note*: If infant is unruly when weight is attempted, a notation should be made on chart that weight is approximate. Other attempts can be made at same visit. If weight is needed to determine nutritional needs or medication dosage you may have to weigh parent holding infant, then weigh parent, and subtract to get approximate weight of child.

Measure Recumbent Length of Infant

PURPOSE: To obtain an accurate measurement of recumbent length of an infant up to 36 months of age.

EQUIPMENT: Ruled measuring tape, yardstick, or meterstick; patient's chart; parent's record booklet; growth graph; pen

TERMINAL PERFORMANCE OBJECTIVE: Provided with at least three lifelike clinical or toy dolls (or an infant or small child under the close supervision of the parent, guardian, or the instructor) and a pediatric table or examining table along with a ruled measuring device, demonstrate each step required in measuring recumbent length of infants and small children and obtain a length measurement for each doll; each length measurement must be within ± $\frac{1}{8}$″ of each doll's actual length as determined by the instructor beforehand.

1. Wash hands and ask parent to remove infant's shoes and socks or booties.
2. Ask parent to place infant on examination table with the head against the table headboard at the zero mark of ruler. Gently straighten infant's back and legs to line up along ruler. Ask parent to hold infant's head against (end) headboard of table while you place infant's heels

against footboard. If there is no footboard (to place the infant's feet against) use your right hand as one, Figure 5–15, page 287. Place your left hand over the child's legs at the knees to secure the child in place and straighten the legs so you can read the recumbent length from the head **(vertex)** to the heel. **Placing your fingers behind the child's knees with your thumb over the kneecap applying gentle pressure will help to keep the legs straightened out for the procedure.**

3. Read length in inches or centimeters on ruler. *Note:* There may be discrepancies with measurement at birth or from another facility because of difficulty in getting an accurate reading. Infants are so used to fetal position that it is difficult to straighten the legs. The former reading may have been from measuring the infant's length from head to toe making the measurement of the recumbent length a few centimeters longer or more.
4. Return infant to parent.
5. Record measurement on growth chart, patient's chart, and parent's booklet of child's growth and development.

MEN			
Height	Small	Medium	Large
5' 2"	128–134	131–141	138–150
5' 3"	130–136	133–143	140–153
5' 4"	132–138	135–145	142–156
5' 5"	134–140	137–148	144–160
5' 6"	136–142	139–151	146–164
5' 7"	138–146	142–154	149–168
5' 8"	140–148	145–157	152–172
5' 9"	142–151	148–160	155–176
5'10"	144–154	151–163	158–180
5'11"	146–157	154–166	161–184
6' 0"	149–160	157–170	164–188
6' 1"	152–164	160–174	188–192
6' 2"	155–168	164–178	172–197
6' 3"	158–172	167–182	176–202
6' 4"	162–176	171–187	181–207

WOMEN			
Height	Small	Medium	Large
4'10"	102–111	109–121	118–131
4'11"	103–113	111–123	120–134
5' 0"	104–115	113–126	122–137
5' 1"	106–118	115–129	125–140
5' 2"	108–121	118–132	128–143
5' 3"	111–124	121–135	131–147
5' 4"	114–127	124–138	134–151
5' 5"	117–130	127–141	137–155
5' 6"	120–133	130–144	140–159
5' 7"	123–136	133–147	143–163
5' 8"	126–139	138–150	146–167
5' 9"	129–142	139–153	149–170
5'10"	132–146	142–156	152–173
5'11"	135–148	145–159	155–176
6' 0"	138–151	148–162	158–179

FIGURE 5–10 Chart of desirable weights for men and women

Head Circumference

Head circumference is a measurement that is routinely recorded on an infant's chart to alert the physician to any abnormal development. This procedure should be performed during routine visits until the child is 36 months old. Head circumference procedure requires a flexible measuring tape, Figure 5–17, page 288. Plotting the measurement on a growth chart is the most efficient way to keep records. Sample growth charts have a graph for plotting the head circumference measurements of children from birth to 36 months are shown in the Appendix.

Chest Measurement

Many physicians request the chest measurement of infants along with the height, weight, and head circumference at the regularly scheduled visits up to 12 months of age. This is per-

FIGURE 5-12 The weight of the patient may be read on either side of the scales.

FIGURE 5-11 The traditional beam balance scale with measuring bar

formed to **monitor** growth abnormalities. Patients of any age may require that this measurement be taken for a particular health history. Because of the extremely strenuous physical demands of some programs, additional body measurements are sometimes necessary to assess the condition of the person before they are accepted. Accuracy is vital in recording these and all measurements. Follow the procedure for obtaining chest measurement for infants and children and adapt for measuring adults. There is usually a request for measuring the chest while the patient inhales deeply, expanding the chest to full capacity.

Complete Chapter 5, Unit 3 in the workbook to help you meet the objectives at the beginning of this unit and therefore achieve competency of this subject matter.

U N I T   4
Vital Signs

OBJECTIVES ···

Upon completion of this unit, you will meet the following terminal performance objectives by verifying knowledge of the facts and principles presented through oral and written communication at a level deemed competent by the instructor or employer and will demonstrate the specific behaviors as identified in the terminal performance objectives of the procedures, observing all aseptic and safety precautions in accordance with health care standards.

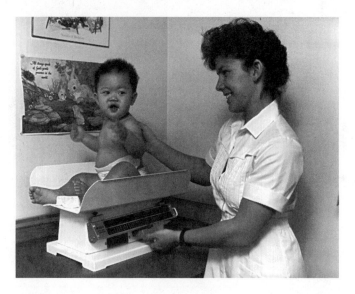

FIGURE 5–13 Weighing an infant sitting on scale

FIGURE 5–14 Weighing an infant lying on scale

1. Identify the four vital signs and the body functions they measure.
2. Explain how the body controls temperature.
3. Describe the different designs of glass clinical thermometers and their appropriate uses.
4. Demonstrate the cleaning and storing of mercury thermometers.

5. Accurately measure oral, rectal, and axillary temperature, identifying the normal temperature value and relative accuracy of each.

P R O C E D U R E

Measure Height

PURPOSE: To obtain an accurate measurement of a patient's height.

EQUIPMENT: Upright scale with extension measuring bar, patient's chart, pen (a measuring scale may be fixed to the wall)

TERMINAL PERFORMANCE OBJECTIVE: After the instructor has measured and recorded the height of all students, each student will, in turn, select five other students. Demonstrate on five other students each step in the height measurement procedure to determine the precise height of each of the other five students. The height measurements obtained should agree with the heights for those five students as measured and recorded by the instructor ± $\frac{1}{8}''$.

1. Raise measuring bar and extension higher than apparent height of patient. **RATIONALE: Avoids the possibility of striking the patient with the extension when it is raised.**
2. Ask patient to remove shoes. (Patients ready for physi-cal exams will not have on shoes.) Place a paper towel on platform of scale. **RATIONALE: Accurate measurement cannot be obtained if shoes are worn. The paper towel provides a clean surface for the shoe-less foot.**
3. Help patient onto scale facing you with his back to measuring device. Advise patient to stand erect, Figure 5–16.
4. Slide measuring bar down slowly and carefully to rest on top of patient's head, gently compressing hair. *Note:* Measurement of height is from the top of the head not the hair. This can cause a discrepancy in the reading.
5. Read measurement in inches or centimeters and tell patient what it is.
6. Help patient down from scale. Tell patient to put shoes back on unless ready for physical exam.
7. Place measuring extension bar back in place and dis-card paper towel.
8. Record height measurement on patient's chart.

PROCEDURE

Measure Head Circumference

PURPOSE: To obtain an accurate measurement of infants' and small children's head circumference in screening for head growth abnormalities.

EQUIPMENT: Flexible tape measure without elasticity, growth graph, patients's chart, pen

TERMINAL PERFORMANCE OBJECTIVE: Provided with at least three lifelike clinical or toy dolls and a flexible tape measure, demonstrate each step required in measuring the circumference of heads of infants and small children on each of the three dolls; each circumference measurement must be within ± ⅛″ (0.2 cm) of each doll's actual head circumference as determined by the instructor beforehand.

1. Wash hands.
2. Talk to infant to gain cooperation. Infant may be held by parent or lie on examination table for procedure. Older children of 2 or 3 years may stand or sit if they will remain still.
3. Use one thumb or finger to hold tape measure with zero mark against infant's forehead (above eyebrows). With other hand, bring tape around infant's head just above ears to meet in front. *Note:* Pull tape snugly to compress hair, Figure 5–17.
4. Read to nearest 0.1 cm or ½ inch.
5. Record on the measurement on the growth chart, parent's record booklet, and patient record.

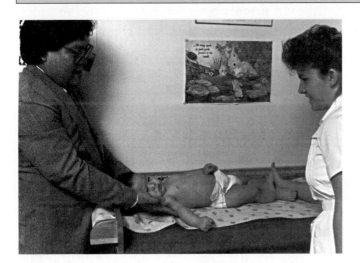

FIGURE 5–15 Measuring recumbent length of an infant

6. Explain situations when oral measurement is contraindicated.
7. Describe what causes pulse, why it can be felt, and name and locate five pulse points.
8. Identify normal pulse rates and describe five factors that affect the rate.
9. Measure radial and apical pulse and describe the quality characteristics to be observed.
10. Define pulse deficit, explaining its significance and how it is measured.
11. Measure respiration, identifying the normal rate and describing the quality characteristics to be observed.
12. Describe normal respiration and explain four abnormal breathing patterns.
13. List the five circulatory factors reflected by the measurement of blood pressure.

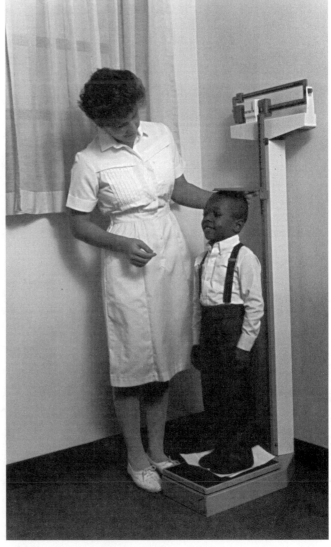

FIGURE 5–16 Measure the height of a child

Measure Infant's Chest

PURPOSE: To obtain an accurate measurement of infants' and small children's chests in screening for growth abnormalities.

EQUIPMENT: Flexible tape measure without elasticity, patient's chart, pen

TERMINAL PERFORMANCE OBJECTIVE: Provided with at least three lifelike clinical or toy dolls and a flexible tape measure, demonstrate each step required in obtaining the chest measurement of infants and small children on each of the three dolls; each chest measurement must be within ± ⅛″ (0.3 cm) of each doll's actual chest measurement as determined by the instructor beforehand.

1. Wash hands.
2. Talk to infant or child to gain cooperation. Infant or child may lie down on examination table or be held by parent or guardian for the procedure. Children of 2 or 3 years and older may sit or stand on their own if they will cooperate and remain still for the procedure. **RATIONALE: Accurate measurement cannot be achieved if the child is crying.**
3. Take the measurement of the chest just above the nipples with the tape fitting around the child's chest under the axillary region. Use one thumb to hold tape measure with zero mark against the infant's chest at the midsternal area. With the other hand, bring the tape around (under) the back to meet the zero mark of the tape in front. If you need assistance in holding the child still, ask the parent or another assistant. The measurement should be taken when the child is breathing normally, not with forced inspiration or expiration, Figure 5–18. **RATIONALE: Measurement would be inaccurate.**
4. Read measurement to the nearest 0.1 cm or ½ inch.
5. Record on patient's chart and in parent's record booklet.

Note: This procedure can be used for obtaining the chest measurement of patients of all ages.

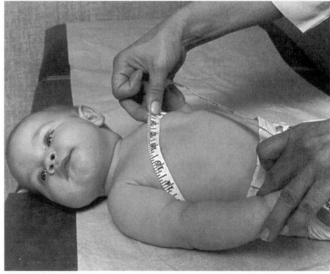

FIGURE 5–18 Measuring the chest of an infant

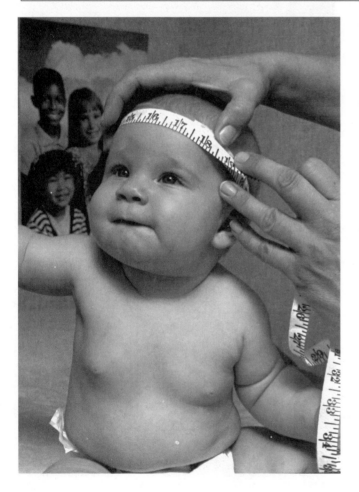

FIGURE 5–17 Measuring the head circumference of infant

14. Explain how the body maintains blood pressure.
15. Identify the phases of blood pressure, comparing them to the action of the heart.
16. Measure blood pressure by palpation and auscultation, explaining pulse pressure and normal findings.
17. Explain an auscultatory gap.
18. Spell and define, using the glossary at the back of the text, all the words to know in this unit.

WORDS TO KNOW ·····························

afebrile	hyperventilation
aneroid	idiopathic
antecubital	infrared
apex	inhale
apical	mercury
apnea	oral
arrhythmia	palpate
aural	pulse
auscultate	pulse deficit
axillary	pulse pressure
blood pressure	pyrogen
brachial	radial
cardinal signs	rales
carotid	rectal
Cheyne–Stokes	rhythm
dorsalis pedis	sphygmomanometer
dyspnea	stethoscope
essential	sublingual
exhale	temperature
fatal	thermometer
febrile	thready
femoral	vital
groin	volume

The term **cardinal signs,** or **vital** signs, is used by health care personnel to identify the measurement of body functions that are essential to life. The four vital indicators are **temperature, pulse,** respiration, and **blood pressure,** commonly referred to as TPR, and B/P. They indicate the body's ability to control heat; the rate, volume, and rhythm of the heart; the rate and quality of breathing; and the force of the heart and condition of the blood vessels. The vital signs give the physician an assessment of the status of the brain, the autonomic nervous system, the heart, and the lungs.

The correct measurement of vital signs is extremely important. Proper technique and attention to details are essential. Findings should be recorded immediately following measurement to avoid a memory error. Always repeat the procedure if you think you may have made a mistake in measuring or recording. Occasionally, you may have a problem measuring a vital sign because of a patient's unusual physical condition that makes measurement difficult. Inform the physician of your problem and follow the course of action advised. Avoid alarming the patient. *Never estimate* the measurement. The physician's choice of treatment and medication is often based on the findings; therefore, they must be accurate.

Temperature ·····························

The temperature of the body indicates the amount of heat produced by the activity of changing food into energy. The body loses heat through perspiration, breathing, and the elimination of body wastes. The balance between heat production and heat loss determines the body's temperature.

Conditions affecting body heat include metabolic rate, time of day, and amount of activity. Body temperature is usually lower in the morning following a period of rest. In the afternoon and evening, body temperature rises due to the heat produced by activity and the metabolism of food. These activities warm the blood that circulates though the body. "Normal" body temperature for an individual is that temperature at which his or her body systems function most effectively, Table 5-1. Not all people have the same normal oral temperature. An *average* normal temperature is 98.6°F (Fahrenheit) or 37°C (centigrade), Figure 5–19. Normal oral temperature of patients may vary from 97.6° to 99.6°F. A person with a temperature above normal is said to be **febrile** or to have a temperature elevation. A person with a temperature which is normal or subnormal is said to be **afebrile.**

Controlling Body Temperature   The temperature-regulating center in the body is located in the hypothalamus of the brain. The action of the hypothalamus can be compared to a thermostat that turns the furnace in your home off and on to keep the room temperature at the set number of degrees. As discussed previously, the brain, autonomic nervous system,

TABLE 5–1
Temperature Variations Considered "Normal"

	Oral	Axillary	Rectal
Average Temperature	98.6°F (37°C)	97.6°F (36.5°C)	99.6°F (37.5°C)
Range	97.6–99.6°F (36.5–37.5°C)	96.6–98.6°F (36–37°C)	98.6–100.6°F (37–38.1°C)

FIGURE 5–19   Normal body temperature on Fahrenheit and Celsius thermometers

blood vessels, and skin cooperate to regulate temperature. This is achieved through a feedback mechanism from temperature receptors. In the body, the hot and cold peripheral receptors in the skin send messages to the hypothalamus about the environment surrounding the body. Temperature receptors in the spinal cord, abdomen, and other internal structures send messages about the internal body temperature. One section of the hypothalamus also has many heat-sensitive neurons, which increase their output of impulses when temperature rises and decease their output when it drops. The signals from this section of the hypothalamus merge with those received in another section, along with the internal and skin receptors, to evaluate the situation and send signals to control heat loss or production. Therefore, this central center is referred to as the *hypothalamic thermostat.*

The hypothalamic thermostat is very effective. When receptors sense the body is too warm, they send a message to the brain, which in turn acts on the sweat glands of the skin to produce moisture. The moisture evaporates from the skin's surface and cools the body. At the same time, nerve impulses are sent to the surface blood vessels to dilate, which brings more blood in contact with the surface of the skin. The blood gives up heat, which cools the blood within the vessels and therefore cools the body.

When the body senses coolness, the opposite activities occur. Surface blood vessels constrict to keep the blood away from the surface of the skin and prevent the loss of heat. Impulses to the sweat glands are stopped when the temperature falls below normal. The small papillary muscles around the hair follicles contract causing gooseflesh. Heat is produced by the activity of the papillary muscles, thereby helping to warm the body. In addition, a portion of the hypothalamus becomes active when cold signals are received. Now hypothalamic messages are sent to skeletal muscles throughout the body, causing increased muscle tone that produces heat. When the muscle tone rises above a certain level, shivering results, and heat production is raised dramatically. The results are evident with an infectious process, such as influenza. Microorganisms cause the patient to experience chills and shivering until the temperature rises to warm the body and a fever develops.

During an infectious process, the presence of microorganisms cause **pyrogens** to be secreted, which raise the "set point" of the hypothalamic thermostat. Pyrogens are toxins from bacteria or a by-product of degenerating tissues. When the set point is higher than normal, the body's heat production and conservation processes are activated. Surface blood vessels constrict, causing the person to feel cold even though the temperature is above normal. No sweat is secreted. Increased white blood cell activity from fighting bacterial invasion also produces heat. Chills and shivering begin and continue until the temperature reaches the higher set point where the hypothalamus will continue to operate until the infectious process is reversed. Once this occurs, the hypothalamic thermostat is reset to a lower, or normal, value and the body's temperature reduction process results in profuse sweating and a hot, red skin from general vasodilation. After this onset reaction, the temperature will begin to fall.

The extent of the infection determines the amount of heat (fever) generated. A mild infection may cause the temperature to rise to 100°F. A moderate infection may elevate the temperature to 102°F. Fevers are categorized by the degree of body heat present as slight, moderate, severe, dangerous, or **fatal,** Table 5–2. Temperatures below normal are called subnormal. Collapse will occur at about 96.0°F, and death follows if temperature goes below 93.0°F except briefly. A fatality-associated elevated temperature also depends on the extent of time the fever is present. Fevers of short duration well above 106.0°F have not proved fatal, but immediate measures to reduce body temperature must be administered.

Thermometer Types and Designs   Body temperature is measured by means of a **thermometer** in the Fahrenheit scale or the metric system equivalent, Celsius. Thermometers are of the following main types: glass **mercury**, also called clinical; disposable, in the form of plastic strips; a self-contained digital, battery-operated electronic; and the most recent, a tympanic **infrared** thermometer. The mouth (**oral**), underarm (**axillary**), rectum (**rectal**), and ear (**aural**) may be used to measure body temperature. The large variety of thermometers, each with its own advantages and disadvantages, allow for personal preference in equipment selection for the physician's office. Table 5–3 briefly outlines the main features for each type.

Glass mercury thermometers are of three designs to measure the temperature by oral, rectal, and axillary method, Figure 5–20. An oral thermometer has a long slender bulb to fit under the tongue. A rectal thermometer has a fat rounded bulb that is stronger and safer to insert into the anus. An oral thermometer that is constructed with a rounded bulb is known as a stubby, or security, thermometer and is suitable for oral or axillary measurement. Many thermometers are further identifiable by a color-coded dot at the stem end. Blue indicates oral; red indicates rectal. Usually the word *oral* or *rectal* is inscribed on the stem.

It is extremely important that thermometers be used for their intended purpose. It is not safe to insert an oral thermometer into the rectum. The slender bulb may perforate (puncture) the tissues, and it is more easily broken. Be equally careful that a rectal thermometer is *never* used to measure an oral temperature.

TABLE 5–2
Classification of Fevers

	Fahrenheit	Celsius
Slight	99.6°–101.0°	37.5°–38.3°
Moderate	101.0°–102.0°	38.3°–38.8°
Severe	102.0°–104.0°	38.8°–40.0°
Dangerous	104.0°–105.0°	40.0°–40.5°
Fatal	over 106.0°	41.1°

TABLE 5–3

Comparison of Thermometer Types

	Advantage	Disadvantage
Glass mercury	Accurate, inexpensive, familiar	Slow, somewhat difficult to read, easily broken, requires cleaning and plastic cover
Plastic disposable	Single use avoids cross-contamination, no cleaning, relatively fast	Must protect from heat, somewhat unpleasant for patient; storage and inventory costs
Digital	Quick, signals when registered, easily read, self-contained	Moderate initial cost, platic cover and battery expenses
Electronic probe	Quick, signals when registered, easily read, self-contained	Fairly expensive, cumbersome cord, requires recharging, probe cover costs; may cause inaccurate readings if patient bites too hard on probe
Tympanic infrared	Instant results, easily read, core temperature, individualized probe cover, eliminates mucous membrane concerns	Expensive, probe cover costs, replacement battery costs

FIGURE 5–20 Types of mercury thermometers (Adapted from Caldwell & Hegner, *Nursing Assistant,* 5th ed. Copyright 1989, Delmar Publishers Inc. Used with permission.)

Reading a Mercury Thermometer and Recording Measurements

Clinical thermometers are slender glass rods with a hollow central cavity extending from a bulb reservoir of mercury. The stem of the Fahrenheit thermometer is calibrated in even tenths, [.2,.4,.6,.8] (Figure 5–21). The whole degrees are marked with long lines, but only the even-numbered degrees are printed on the thermometer. There is also a long line at 98.6° with an arrow, because this is the average normal body temperature when it is measured orally.

To view the numbers, lines, and column of mercury, hold the thermometer at eye level, between the thumb and index finger of the right hand, by the stem end only. Look directly at the edge of the glass triangle with the lines at the top and the numbers at the bottom. Rotate the stem slightly back and forth until you see the silver mercury column in the middle, Figure 5–22. The point where the mercury stops is read and recorded as the body temperature. **When the mercury is between tenth markings, it is read to the next highest two-tenths of a degree,** Figure 5–23. Many thermometers have markings printed in blue below the normal arrow and in red above to make temperature identification easier.

It is extremely important that you not only read the thermometer accurately but that you also record the findings accurately. Remember that every line on a Fahrenheit thermometer represents two-tenths of a degree. Note the difference between 100.2°F and 102.0°F. For example, Figure 5–24. When reporting verbally, 100.2° is referred to as "one hundred and two-tenths" or "one hundred point two." A temperature of 102.0° is reported as "one hundred two" or "one hundred two point zero." It is good practice to read the thermometer and record the temperature as soon as possible after measuring. After you have written it down, read the thermometer again and check what you wrote to be certain you are accurate. The implications of an error in reporting should be obvious.

FIGURE 5–21 Reading a thermometer. This thermometer reads 98.6°F (Adapted from Caldwell & Hegner, *Nursing Assistant,* 5th ed. Copyright 1989, Delmar Publishers Inc. Used with permission.)

FIGURE 5–22   Hold the thermometer at eye level to read (From Caldwell & Hegner, *Nursing Assistant*, 6th ed. Copyright 1992, Delmar Publishers, Inc.)

CAUTION: Taking temperatures requires contact with mucous membranes in the mouth or rectum. Discussion and procedure descriptions will reflect universal precautions. In any clinical setting, it is advisable to eliminate cross-contamination to prevent the spread of disease-producing organisms that cause hepatitis, AIDS, and many other transmittable diseases. Until a method of prevention or effective treatment is discovered, <u>EVERYONE</u> should be considered to be infected.

Care of Thermometers   Each time a temperature is taken, the thermometer must be cleaned and soaked in disinfectant. Even when covered with a plastic sheath, it is possible to accidentally contaminate the thermometer, depositing organisms on the bulb or stem. Glass mercury thermometers are extremely fragile, and care must be taken to prevent breakage.

When many thermometers are used daily, they will be processed in quantity. Each thermometer is cleaned and rinsed after use, then placed in a gauze-lined basin filled with disinfectant. Timing must begin after the last thermometer is added. All thermometers must be completely covered by the disinfectant. The thermometers are then removed from the solution, rinsed, and inspected. They may be stored in individual dry containers or placed in individual clean envelopes and stored in a drawer. Solution used in quantity disinfection is discarded after soaking time has elapsed.

FAHRENHEIT

99.4° F

FIGURE 5–23   A temperature reading of 99.4°F. **When the mercury is between the tenth markings it is read to the next higher tenth.** (From Caldwell & Hegner, *Health Care Assistant,* 5th ed. Copyright 1989. Delmar Publishers, Inc.)

THIS THERMOMETER READS 100.2° F

THIS THERMOMETER READS 102.0° F

FIGURE 5–24   It is important to read and record temperature accurately.

An individual container filled with disinfectant solution is not recommended. It is no longer considered safe to use an unsheathed thermometer even when it is cleaned after each use and returned to a solution-filled container. If such an individual storage method is used, wipe the solution from the thermometer with a cotton ball, from the bulb to the stem, and discard the cotton in a biohazardous waste container. Slip a sheath over the thermometer and continue as indicated in the procedure which follows. Stop and think, would **you** like to be your next patient? Remember your responsibility to others in stopping the threat of disease transmission. AIDS and hepatitis are very dangerous communicable diseases. Follow correct procedure each time you measure the temperature of any patient.

Slip-on Thermometer Sheaths   Clear plastic slip-on sheaths must be used when taking oral or rectal temperature with a glass thermometer. This narrow plastic cover slides over the thermometer like a loose skin. The covers come packaged in individualized narrow paper envelopes, Figure 5–25. The clean thermometer is inserted into the open end marked "insert." The opposite end is separated and peeled back revealing the plastic cover. Peel back the envelope to the stem end and snap off the tear tab. Check the cover to be certain it has remained intact before using. The thermometer is used exactly as if it were not covered. The covering is somewhat undesirable from the patient's viewpoint as it is a rather strange feeling to have a "minibaggie" under one's tongue.

When the temperature has been measured, the cover is simply held by the tear tab, pulled off, and discarded in the biohazardous waste container. The design is such that the sheath inverts itself, thereby reducing the chance of contamination of the thermometer. The temperature is then read and recorded and the thermometer cleaned, ready for use with the application of another sheath. A rectal thermometer *must* always be covered with a sheath and used only for rectal temperatures. It will require lubrication for ease of insertion.

Measuring Oral Temperature   Measuring temperature orally is the method of choice because it is relatively convenient, quick, and accurate. The oral clinical thermometer is placed in **sublingually** (under the tongue) and for a *minimum* of 3

FIGURE 5–25 Slip-on thermometer sheaths

minutes, Figure 5–26. (A study recently conducted indicated that 8 minutes was necessary to obtain the most accurate oral measurement.) Remember that a reading of 98.6°F or 37°C is considered normal.

Temperature readings will be inaccurate if the patient has smoked or had either a hot or cold drink within the previous 10 minutes. Always ask patients about this before placing the thermometer in their mouth. Tell them to keep the thermometer under their tongue with their lips closed around the stem. Readings will also be inaccurate if the patient breathes through the mouth. Caution the patient against biting down on the glass stem. It is possible to break the thermometer with the force of the teeth, cutting the tongue, gums, or inside of the mouth. The possible ingestion of glass fragments and poisonous mercury presents a real hazard.

Note: In temperature procedures, recording of findings is being delayed until after gloves have been removed and hands washed. This seems to be necessary to avoid contamination of pens, pencils, charts, and in turn yourself.

Contraindications to Oral Measurement Oral temperature measurement is not the method of choice in certain situations, such as with infants and children under 6; patients with respiratory complications that require mouth breathing or the use of oxygen; confused, disoriented, or emotionally unstable patients; patients with oral injuries, recent oral surgery, facial

---

 P R O C E D U R E

Clean and Store Mercury Thermometers

TERMINAL PERFORMANCE OBJECTIVE: Given soiled mercury thermometers, cotton balls, soap, water, gloves, and a prepared container, clean, inspect, disinfect, and store the thermometers aseptically, in accordance with procedure technique and observing aseptic and safety precautions. *Note:* Oral and rectal thermometers are cleaned and disinfected separately.

1. Wash hands and put on gloves. **CAUTION:** Remember, in order to comply with universal precautions guidelines, gloves must worn if there is any possibility of coming into contact with blood, body fluids, or wound drainage.
2. Take soiled thermometers to sink.
3. Apply soap to cotton ball and add water to make solution.
4. While holding thermometer by stem, rotate and wipe it from stem to bulb with soapy solution. **RATIONALE: Cleansing action forces soap into calibrations while working from clean to soiled area.**
5. Discard cotton ball in biohazardous waste container.
6. While holding by stem with bulb pointed downward, rinse thermometer in cool running water. **RATIONALE: Hot water will overexpand mercury and either damage or break thermometer.**
7. Inspect for cleanliness and condition. If still soiled, repeat steps 3 to 6. Discard a chipped or cracked ther-

mometer. **RATIONALE: A damaged thermometer is unsafe and may be inaccurate.**
8. Grasp stem firmly between thumb and index finger.
9. Shake mercury down to 95.0° or below. *Note:* Use a wrist-snapping action. Avoid striking faucet, sink, or counter. Remember, the mercury will not go down unless forced. **RATIONALE: Temperature will not be measured accurately if it is LESS than the previously measured temperature.**
10. Place thermometers in gauze-lined container filled with disinfectant. **RATIONALE: Gauze aids in preventing breakage.** *Note:* Thermometers must be completely covered and allowed to remain in solution for at least 20 minutes. If additional thermometers are added, timing must begin after last one is placed in the container.
11. Using correct procedure, remove and discard gloves.
12. Wash hands.
13. Set timer or note time.
14. Following adequate time for disinfection, wash hands. Rinse, inspect, and place clean thermometers in individual envelopes, individual dry holders, or storage container. Remember if stored in individual holders to place a cotton ball in the bottom to prevent breakage of the bulb.
15. Clean area and equipment. Return thermometers to appropriate locations.

paralysis, nasal obstruction, and so on. In such situations, temperature must be measured by either the rectal, axillary or aural (auditory canal) method.

Measuring Rectal Temperature   Rectal temperature is a very accurate measurement, simply because it is taken internally. Rectal measurement is always indicated with babies and with young children who have not yet learned how to keep an oral thermometer in place or who might break it by biting down. Often children complain bitterly about having a rectal temperature taken when they think they are "too big." The physician usually has a policy concerning the age limit for rectal temperatures, which you will follow.

When measuring the temperature, position infants as in Figure 5–27. If positioning on back, unfasten the diaper to expose the anus. Grasp the ankles securely with one hand, flexing the

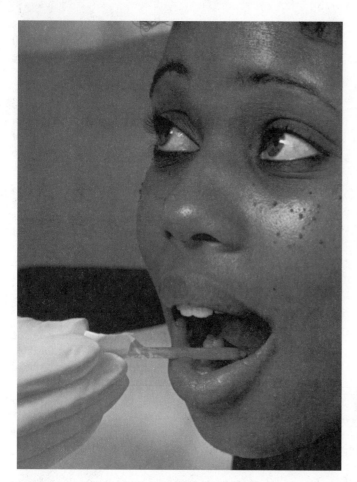

FIGURE 5–26   Place an oral thermometer siblingually in a heat pocket.

FIGURE 5–27   Positions (a and b) for measuring rectal temperature of infants

Measure Oral Temperature with Mercury Thermometer

TERMINAL PERFORMANCE OBJECTIVE: In a simulated or actual situation, given a patient, an oral mercury thermometer, latex gloves, thermometer sheath, watch, or timer, paper and pen or pencil, measure and record a patient's oral temperature. The procedure will be done with 100% accuracy, within 6-minutes, following correct procedural technique, and observing aseptic and safety precautions.

1. Wash hands, put on gloves. **CAUTION:** Remember, in order to comply with universal precautions guidelines, gloves must be worn if there is any possibility of coming into contact with blood, body fluids, or wound drainage.
2. Identify patient. **RATIONALE: Speaking to the patient by name and checking chart ensures that you are performing the procedure on the correct patient.**
3. Explain procedure.
4. Determine if patient has recently had a hot or cold drink or smoked. *Note:* If so, allow 10 minutes before measuring. **RATIONALE: Hot or cold substances in the mouth prevent accurate temperature measurement.**
5. Remove thermometer from holder or envelope. Avoid touching bulb end with fingers. **RATIONALE: Bulb must be untouched since it is inserted into the patient's mouth.**
6. Inspect thermometer. Discard a chipped or cracked thermometer. **RATIONALE: A damaged thermometer is unsafe and may be inaccurate.**
7. Read thermometer and shake down to 95° or below if

necessary. **RATIONALE: Temperature will not be measured accurately if it is LESS than the previously measured temperature.**
8. Put plastic sheath on thermometer. *Note:* Check that sheath is intact. **RATIONALE: Plastic sheaths protect against cross-contamination.**
9. Place bulb sublingually in patient's mouth. *Note:* **Take care not to probe. Sensitive sublingual tissues. RATIONALE: Heat pockets in the mouth are located sublingually (see Figure 5–29).**
10. Tell patient how to maintain proper position of thermometer: to keep lips closed, breathe through nose, and avoid biting.
11. Leave thermometer in position a minimum of 3 minutes. *Note:* Time by watch or timer.
12. Remove and read thermometer. *Note:* Reinsert for additional minute if reading is less than 97.0°.
13. Reread thermometer.
14. Holding by stem end, pull off plastic sheath and discard in biohazardous waste container.
15. Follow procedure for soiled thermometers.
16. Remove gloves and discard in biohazardous waste container.
17. Wash hands.
18. Record temperature.
19. Follow procedure to clean thermometer, returning to storage when completed. (*Note:* If greater accuracy is desired, adjust time and performance objective.)

knees to the abdomen. With the other hand insert the lubricated sheathed thermometer about 1 inch through the anal canal into the rectum. Hold the thermometer securely in place. Maintain your grasp on the ankles so the infant cannot turn over. Be prepared for the procedure to initiate urination or expelling of stool. It would be wise to cover the male infant's penis with a diaper to absorb the urine stream. When positioning the baby prone across a person's lap or on a table, be certain to maintain control of the infant or child's position to prevent turning over and causing injury to the rectum from the inserted thermometer. In either position, the thermometer position can be maintained by holding it securely between the index and middle finger with the palm of the hand against the buttocks.

Older children can be positioned either on their abdomen or side, whichever is preferred. Adults would be positioned on their side and draped with a sheet for privacy.

Temperatures measured rectally require a minimum of 3 minutes insertion time (5 minutes for greater accuracy). When recording a rectal measurement, place the letter R in parentheses following the reading, for example, 99.6°(R). Normal rectal

temperature is 99.6°F or 37.5°C, one full degree above normal oral temperature. Temperature must never be measured rectally if the patient has had recent rectal surgery. It is possible to damage the operative site or perforate newly sutured lines.

Measuring Axillary Temperature Temperature can also be measured by placing the thermometer in the axilla (armpit), Figure 5–28, page 297. This method is the least accurate and requires a full 10 minutes. Axillary measurement is appropriate only when oral measurement is contraindicated and rectal is inconvenient, undesirable, or contraindicated. An oral stubby or security design thermometer is best suited for axillary measurement. Normal axillary temperature is 97.6°F, or 36.4°C, one full degree *below* normal oral temperature. When recording axillary findings, place the letters Ax in parentheses following the reading; for example, 97.6°(Ax).

Disposable Thermometers Disposable plastic oral thermometers may be used in some offices, urgent care centers, and hospital emergency rooms. Since they are used

Measure Rectal Temperature with Mercury Thermometer

TERMINAL PERFORMANCE OBJECTIVE: In a simulated or actual situation, given a patient or manikin, a rectal mercury thermometer, tissue, lubricant, watch or timer, paper and pen or pencil, thermometer sheath, and latex gloves, measure and record a patient's rectal temperature. The procedure will be done with 100% accuracy, within 8 minutes, following correct procedural technique, and observing aseptic and safety precautions.

1. Wash hands and put on gloves. **CAUTION:** Remember, in order to comply with universal precautions guidelines, gloves must be worn if there is any possibility of coming into contact with blood, body fluids, or wound drainage.
2. Identify patient. **RATIONALE: Speaking to the patient by name and checking chart ensures that you are performing the procedure on the correct patient.**
3. Explain procedure and what you are going to do, to child and parent or to adult patient.
4. Place a small amount of lubricant on a tissue. *Note:* Lubricant should be water-soluble.
5. Remove thermometer from holder or envelope. *Note:* Hold by stem end only.
6. Inspect thermometer. Discard a chipped or cracked thermometer. **RATIONALE: A damaged thermometer is unsafe and may be inaccurate.**
7. Read thermometer and shake down to 95° or below if necessary. **RATIONALE: Temperature will not be measured accurately if it is LESS than the previously measured temperature.**
8. Place thermometer in plastic sheath. Check that sheath is intact. **RATIONALE: Plastic sheaths protect against cross-contamination.**
9. Rotate thermometer bulb in lubricant on tissue and place in convenient location. **RATIONALE: A lubricated thermometer inserts with less discomfort and reduces chance of injury.** *Note:* When performing this procedure on an adult patient, proceed with the following steps:
10. Instruct patient to remove appropriate clothing, assisting as needed. *Note:* Provide privacy.
11. Assist adult patient onto examining table and cover with drape. Avoid overexposure.
12. Position patient on side. Ensure patient's comfort and safety.
13. Arrange drape to expose buttocks.
14. With one hand raise upper buttock to expose anus.
15. With other hand, carefully insert lubricated thermometer into anal canal approximately 1½ inches.
    Note:
    a. Do not force thermometer. Rotating will often facilitate insertion.
    b. If opening is not apparent, request patient to bear down slightly; this will usually expose opening. When performing the procedure on infants or small children, ask the parent or accompanying adult to prepare the child while you prepare the thermometer.
16. Position as to parent's or physician's preference.
17. Ensure safety during procedure by maintaining control of the infant's or child's position. (A parent can be instructed to assist you, as in Figure 5–27(b), especially if it comforts the child.)
18. Expose anus.
19. Carefully insert well-lubricated thermometer 1 inch into anal canal. (See *Note* in Step 15 a.)
20. Hold thermometer in place for a minimum of 3 minutes (5 minutes for greater accuracy). *Note:* Time by watch.
21. Withdraw thermometer. Carefully remove plastic sheath and discard it in biohazardous waste container.
22. Read thermometer.
23. Reread to check temperature.
24. Place thermometer on tissue. **RATIONALE: A soiled thermometer must never be placed on an unprotected surface.**
25. Remove any excess lubricant from anal area with tissue. Wipe from front to back.
26. Ask parent or accompanying adult to dress infant or child.
27. Assist adult patient from examining table and instruct to redress. *Note:* Provide privacy as appropriate.
28. Follow procedure for soiled thermometer.
29. Remove and discard gloves in biohazardous waste container.
30. Record temperature, placing (R) after the finding.
31. Return thermometer to storage after cleaning.

only once and discarded, they are free from contamination, and no time or equipment is required for cleaning. One disadvantage is the cost factor. The patient's reaction may also be less than enthusiastic, however. The plastic is thin and almost sharp. Care must be taken to avoid touching the dot matrix portion, which is placed in the patient's mouth. The

dots can be placed up or down. The thermometer must be held under the tongue, as far back as possible in the heat pocket with the tongue pressed against the end and the mouth closed on the stem, Figure 5–29, page 297. Wait 60 seconds, then remove the thermometer. Allow 10 seconds for the dots to stabilize, then read and record the temperature. The heat in the

FIGURE 5–28 Measuring axillary temperature

mouth causes a reaction on the heat-sensitive dots printed on the surface of the plastic strip. Readings are calculated by counting the number of dots that change color within a degree grouping, Figure 5–30(b), page 298. The last changed dot on

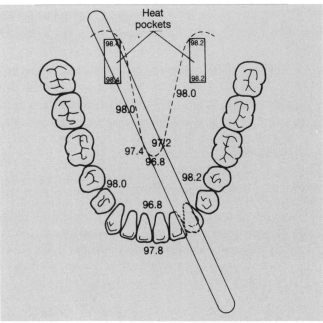

FIGURE 5–29 Dot matrix portion of disposable thermometer must be placed sublingually into a heat pocket. (Illustration courtesy of PhMaH Corporation, Sommerville, NJ.)

P R O C E D U R E

Measure Axillary Temperature with Mercury Thermometer

TERMINAL PERFORMANCE OBJECTIVE: In a simulated or actual situation, given a patient, a mercury oral security thermometer, tissues, watch or timer, paper and pen or pencil, measure and record axillary temperature with 100% accuracy, within 14 minutes, following correct procedural technique, and observing aseptic and safety precautions.

1. Wash hands.
2. Identify patient. **RATIONALE: Speaking to the patient by name and checking chart ensures that you are performing the procedure on the correct patient.**
3. Explain procedure and what you are going to do.
4. Remove thermometer from holder or envelope.
5. Inspect thermometer. Discard a chipped or cracked thermometer. **RATIONALE: A damaged thermometer is unsafe and may be inaccurate.**
6. Read thermometer and shake down to 95° or below if necessary. **RATIONALE: Temperature will not be measured accurately if it is LESS than the previously measured temperature.**
7. Place thermometer on tissue or in envelope in convenient location.
8. Assist patient, as necessary, to expose axilla. *Note:* Provide privacy.
9. Pat axillary space with tissue to remove perspiration. **RATIONALE: Perspiration prevents thermometer**

from coming into direct contact with skin. It also makes it more difficult to keep thermometer in place.

10. Place thermometer deep in the axillary space. Position so that the bulb is in direct contact with the top of the axillary space with the stem projecting anteriorly. *Note:* The thermometer may be placed with the stem extending posteriorly if desired.
11. Hold arm tightly against body. Have patient maintain position for a minimum of 10 minutes.
    Note:
    a. Time by watch or timer.
    b. Help weak or confused patient maintain position.
    c. Be certain thermometer remains deep in axillary space. Children will require close attention and assistance.
12. Remove thermometer and wipe with tissue from stem to bulb. **RATIONALE: Removes perspiration to facilitate reading. Action is from clean to soiled area.**
13. Read and record findings. *Note:* Place (Ax) after the reading.
14. Reread and check recording.
15. Help patient replace clothing.
16. Follow procedure for soiled thermometer.
17. Wash hands.
18. Return thermometer to storage after cleaning.

PROCEDURE

Measure Oral Temperature with Disposable Plastic Thermometer

TERMINAL PERFORMANCE OBJECTIVE: In a simulated or actual situation, given a patient, a disposable plastic thermometer, watch or timer, paper and pen or pencil, measure and record oral temperature with 100% accuracy in 4 minutes, following correct procedural technique and observing aseptic and safety precautions.

1. Wash hands.
2. Identify patient. **RATIONALE: Speaking to the patient by name and checking chart ensures that you are performing the procedure on the correct patient.**
3. Explain procedure and what you are going to do.
4. Determine if the patient has recently had a hot or cold drink or smoked. *Note:* If so, allow 10 minutes before measuring. **RATIONALE: Hot or cold substances in the mouth prevent accurate temperature measurement.**
5. Open package by peeling back top of wrapper to expose handle end of thermometer.

6. Grasp handle and remove from wrapper. *Note:* Do NOT touch dot matrix portion, which will be placed in the patient's mouth.
7. Insert thermometer into patient's mouth as far back as possible into one of the heat pockets (see Figure 5–29).
8. Instruct patient to press tongue down on thermometer and keep mouth closed. **RATIONALE: Firm direct contact is necessary for accurate measurement. Breathing through the mouth admits air which may affect accuracy.**
9. Maintain position for 60 seconds. *Note:* Time by watch or timer.
10. Remove thermometer and wait 10 seconds for dots to stabilize. *Note:* Take special care to avoid touching the portion that has been in the patient's mouth.
11. Read thermometer and discard in biohazardous waste container.
12. Wash hands.
13. Record temperature.

---

the matrix indicates the correct temperature. Then discard the thermometer in a biohazardous waste container. Plastic thermometers are not considered to be precisely accurate; however, for usual temperature determination, their single use and freedom from contamination may outweigh any minor disadvantages.

The disposable plastic thermometer can also be used to measure axillary temperature. The dot matrix portion is placed next to the body, deep in the axillary space, with the handle extending straight down the patient's side. The arm must be held tightly at the side. After 3 minutes, remove the thermometer, wait 10 seconds, then read and record the temperature.

A variation of the disposable thermometer is available for rectal use. It is packaged with a plastic sheath and is not recommended for infants or toddlers. The thermometer must be well lubricated and inserted until the dot matrix is completely covered. After 3 minutes, it is withdrawn and the sheath discarded.

FIGURE 5–30 (a) Disposable plastic thermometer. The matrix in (b) reads 101°F. (Adapted from Caldwell & Hegner, *Health Care Assistant*, 5th ed. Copyright 1989, Delmar Publishers Inc.)

A

Measure Oral Temperature Electronically

TERMINAL PERFORMANCE OBJECTIVE: In a simulated or actual situation, given a patient, an electronic thermometer unit, probe, sheath, paper and pen or pencil, measure the patient's temperature electronically. The temperature will be read and recorded at 100% accuracy in 2 minutes, following correct procedural technique, and observing aseptic and safety precautions.

1. Wash hands, assemble equipment.
2. Identify patient. **RATIONALE: Speaking to the patient by name and checking the chart ensures that you are performing the procedure on the correct patient.**
3. Explain procedure and what you are going to do.
4. Place probe connector in receptacle of unit base and check to make sure it is properly seated.
5. Holding it by the collar, remove appropriate probe from stored position.
6. Insert probe firmly into probe cover to ensure that it is properly seated.
7. Insert covered probe into mouth. *Note:* The probe and connecting cord is rather heavy and cumbersome. It

will be necessary to hold the thermometer steady in place.

8. Maintain covered probe in position until unit signals, approximately 10–15 seconds. **RATIONALE: Early removal results in inaccurate measurement.**
9. Remove probe from patient. Do not touch probe cover. **RATIONALE: Probe is contaminated with patient's saliva.**
10. Read and record temperature measurement. *Note:* Temperature is displayed digitally in window of unit.
11. Recheck your reading and recording.
12. Press the eject button to discard used probe cover into biohazardous waste container. **RATIONALE: All materials coming into contact with bodily secretions are deposited in biohazardous waste container.**
13. Return probe to stored position in unit. Thermometer display will read zero and shut off.
14. Store unit in charging stand. *Note:* A red light in the upper left hand area of the display indicates that the thermometer is charging. **RATIONALE: The unit should remain in the stand so it is is fully charged and ready for use.**

After 10 seconds, the temperature may be read and recorded. It would be necessary to wear gloves because the chances are great that you may contact secretions from rectal mucosa.

When exposed to high environmental temperatures the matrix dots on the thermometers will turn blue. If this should

occur, place them in a freezer for 1 hour for each box of 100 thermometers. Rectal thermometers will require 2 hours per 100 thermometers. Then let them stand at room temperature for a day. The thermometers will then be ready for use and their accuracy should not be affected.

Measure Core Body Temperature with an Aural Thermometer

TERMINAL PERFORMANCE OBJECTIVE: In a simulated or actual situation, given a patient, an aural thermometer, a probe cover, paper and pen or pencil, measure and record tympanic temperature with 100% accuracy within 3 minutes, following correct procedural technique and observing aseptic and safety precautions.

1. Wash hands.
2. Identify Patient: **RATIONALE: Speaking to the patient by name and checking the chart ensures that you are performing the procedure on the correct patient.**
3. Explain procedure and what you are going to do.
4. Remove aural thermometer from base. The display

should read "ready."

5. Attach a disposable probe cover to the ear piece.
6. Insert covered probe into ear canal, sealing opening.
7. Press the scan button to activate the thermometer.
8. Observe the display window, noting the temperature.
9. Withdraw the thermometer.
10. Press the release button on the thermometer to eject the probe cover into a waste basket.
11. Record the temperature using (T) or (Tc) to indicate tympanic or tympanic core temperature.
12. Return thermometer to base.

Note: Thermometers can be set to correlate with an oral or rectal reading. Usually, the oral mode is used and a reading of 98.6°F is considered "normal."

Electronic Thermometers The use of electronic thermometers is becoming more common. They are quick, sanitary, easily read, and do not require cleaning. A small, battery-powered unit with a digital read-out window is very accurate and capable of measuring a temperature within a few seconds, Figure 5–31. A metal probe, blue for oral, red for rectal, is used like a mercury thermometer. It is attached by a cord to the battery unit. A disposable cover slips over the probe to provide each patient with an individual thermometer. The covered probe is inserted in the patient's mouth like a mercury thermometer. It is usually held in place by the medical assistant since the time involved is short, and the probe, with its cord, is heavy and somewhat cumbersome. As soon as the temperature level has been reached, the unit will sound a signal and the final reading will appear in the window of the unit.

Electronic thermometers save time and are convenient, but they are somewhat expensive. Care must also be taken to adjust the unit frequently and correctly. It is critical that the dial be observed from a direct view at eye level while making adjustments. The unit must be returned to its charging stand after use to maintain the battery.

Electronic thermometers may also be used to measure axillary and rectal temperature. Use the rectal (red) probe to take a rectal temperature. Remove the rectal probe from its holder and attach a probe cover. The probe is inserted into the rectum $\frac{1}{2}''$ for adults and $\frac{1}{4}''$ for children. The use of lubricant is optional. The probe should be angled slightly to ensure contact with the rectal mucosa. After the reading is registered, remove the probe and discard the cover in a biohazardous waste container.

When taking axillary temperature, some manufacturers recommend using the rectal probe; others recommend the oral probe. Consult the instruction booklet with your equipment to determine which to use. Apply a probe cover and insert the tip well into the axillary space with the probe extending down and slightly forward along the patient's side. Press gently into the space to establish good tissue contact. Have patient lower arm over the probe. Hold the probe in position to maintain good contact. Remove and read after the unit signals completion. It should be noted that with an electronic thermometer a "normal" axillary temperature is 0.5°F (0.3°C) lower than an oral temperature.

Some units have built-in operator prompts to signal when technique or problems exist. If the phrase OPER ERR 9 (or something similar) shows on the readout window, it means the probe is not in contact with tissue. A readjustment of the thermometer will erase the message and allow the continued measurement of the temperature. A BAT LO (or similar) message indicates the unit's batteries do not have enough charge to take a temperature. The unit must be returned to the charger base for 6 to 8 hours to be fully charged or 45 minutes to permit a limited number of measurements. A PROB BAD (or similar) message indicates the probe is damaged and will not sense temperature properly. This can be corrected only by installing a new probe.

Another electronic thermometer is simple and self-contained. It is also a digital thermometer and is excellent for home use, Figure 5–32. The thermometer will register the temperature in about 60 seconds on an easy-to-read LCD panel that shows the temperature in tenths of degrees. The thermometer can be cleaned with soap and water and sanitized with a disinfectant. Probe covers are available for clinic or office use. It may be used for oral, axillary, or rectal measurement. Some models have a beeper that sounds when the maximum temperature is reached. This feature is especially appealing to children.

Tympanic Membrane Thermometers A totally new concept in temperature measurement is the instantaneous tympanic membrane (aural) thermometer. At the present time two manufacturers have models available. The Thermoscan Pro-1 is shown in Figure 5–33. The other, First Temp Genius

FIGURE 5–31 Electronic thermometer (From Caldwell & Hegner, *Health Care Assistant,* 6th ed. Copyright 1992, Delmar Publishers Inc.)

FIGURE 5–32 Electronic digital thermometer (Courtesy of Omron Marshall Products, Inc., Vernon Hills, IL.)

operates by the same principle. Both instruments measure the strength of the infrared heat waves generated by the tympanic membrane and will digitally display that temperature in less than 2 seconds. Because the tympanic membrane shares the same blood supply as the hypothalamus, it is believed the auditory canal is an ideal site for obtaining an accurate assessment of the body's core temperature. Studies conducted with temperature-sensing devices placed internally in a large blood vessel have shown strong correlation in results.

Although its greatest asset is the instant result, it has also become a real benefit to health care professionals in hospital emergency rooms, labor and delivery rooms, and pediatric units because it does not involve contact with mucous membranes and the site is so easily accessible. Another advantage is the readings are not affected by hot or cold liquids or smoking as are oral methods. In addition, the patient does not even need to be conscious.

The thermometer is extremely easy to use. You simply position the covered plastic tip inside the auditory canal, press the scan button, and an infrared beam measures the heat waves. The results are displayed digitally on the screen. A release button ejects the probe cover and in 10 seconds another temperature can be taken. The method is acceptable to patients and a real time saver to the health care worker. The units operate on three AAA alkaline batteries and will measure at least 10,000 temperatures before needing to be replaced. As the aural thermometer becomes more acceptable and less expensive, many clinics, urgent care centers, and group practices may use the new technology.

Celsius Thermometers The only difference between Celsius and Fahrenheit thermometers is the calibration. On a Celsius thermometer, each long line represents a degree. They are numbered consecutively, with the nine lines that are between each number representing one-tenth of a degree, Figure 5–34.

Temperature can be converted from one scale to another by a mathematical calculation. To convert Celsius to Fahrenheit, multiply the degrees by 9/5 and add 32. To change Fahrenheit to Celsius, subtract 32 and multiply by 5/9. Table 5–4 shows examples of temperature conversions and compares some common temperatures.

THIS TEMPERATURE READING IS 37.3° C

THIS TEMPERATURE READING IS 38.8° C

FIGURE 5–34 Reading a Celsius thermometer

FIGURE 5–33 Tympanic thermometer (Courtesy of Thermoscan Inc., San Diego, CA.)

TABLE 5–4
Temperature Conversion and Comparison
To convert Celsius to Fahrenheit:
$37°C \times \frac{9}{5} \left(\frac{333}{5}\right) = 66.6 + 32 = 98.6°F$
To convert Fahrenheit to Celsius:
$98.6°F - 32 = 66.6 \times \frac{5}{9} \left(\frac{333}{9}\right) = 37°C$

	Celsius (C)	Fahrenheit (F)
Freezing	0°	32°
Body Temperature	37°	96.6°
Pasteurization	63°	145°
Boiling	100°	212°
Sterilizing (Autoclave)	121°	250°

Pulse

Each time the heart beats, blood is forced into the aorta, temporarily expanding its walls and initiating a wavelike effect. This wave continues through all the body's arteries, causing the alternating expansion and recoil of the arterial walls, Figure 5–35. This effect can be **palpated** (felt) in the arteries that are close to the body surface and that lie over bone or firm structures. When the artery is pressed against the underlying structure, it is possible to feel the rhythmic pulsation, known as the pulse.

Pulse Points   The pulse can be felt in several locations on the body, Figure 5–36. The **radial** pulse point is on the thumb side of the inner surface of the wrist, lying over the radius bone. The radial pulse point is used most frequently when measuring pulse rate.

The **brachial** artery pulse point is on the inner medial surface of the elbow, at the **antecubital** space (crease of elbow). This point is used to palpate and **auscultate** (listen to) blood pressure.

The **carotid** pulse can be felt in the carotid artery of the neck when pressure is applied to the area at either side of the trachea. It is the carotid pulse that is palpated during the cardiopulmonary resuscitation (CPR) life-saving maneuver.

Two other points often palpated to evaluate circulation in the lower extremities are the **femoral,** located midway in the **groin** where the artery begins its descent down the femur, and the **dorsalis pedis,** on the instep of the foot.

Pulse Rate   The number of times the heart beats per minute is measured by counting the pulse in the radial artery. The average adult pulse rate is 72 beats per minute. The pulse rate is recorded as beats per minute preceded by a capital P; for example, P. 72.

The rate of the pulse is influenced by several factors. The most obvious is exercise or activity. With increased activity, the heartbeats per minute increase to meet the body's needs.

FIGURE 5–36   Pulse points of the upper and lower extremities and the neck

The rate should return to normal within 3 minutes after activity has stopped. Of course, the rate of increase will be in proportion to the level of activity.

Age is directly related to pulse rate. The younger the person, the faster the heartbeat. A sample of age-related average pulse rates is shown in Table 5–5.

Pulse rate is also related to the sex of the patient. A female's pulse is approximately 10 beats per minute more rapid than a male's of the same age. Pulse rate is also related to size; therefore the larger male will have a slower rate than a smaller male. The relationship of size is particularly evident in animals. The

FIGURE 5–35   Blood pumped from the heart causes a wavelike effect in the arteries.

TABLE 5–5
Pulse-Age Relationship

Age	Pulse Rate
Less than 1 year	100–170
2–6 years	90–115
6–10 years	80–110
11–16 years	70–95
Midlife adult	65–80
Aged adult	50–65

heart rate of a bird may be well over 200 beats per minute, whereas an elephant has a rate of about 30.

The physical condition of the body is another factor. Athletes, especially those who run or engage in strenuous sports, have a considerably slower pulse rate because of their more efficient circulatory system.

In general, the heart rate increases when the sympathetic nervous system is stimulated by such feelings as fear, anxiety, pain, or anger. The rate also increases with certain other conditions, such as thyroid disease, anemia, shock, or fever. A rate of over 100 beats per minute is known as *tachycardia.*

When the parasympathetic nervous system affects the heart, it causes the rate to be much slower. A rate below 60 beats per minute is known as *bradycardia.* This may also occur with the use of certain medications, heart disease, emotional depres-

sion, and drugs. A rate below 60 beats per minute is also normal for many athletes.

Pulse Characteristics   When measuring pulse rate, two other characteristics must also be observed and recorded. The force or strength of the pulse is referred to as its **volume.** Words used to describe this quality are: normal, full or bounding, weak, and **thready** (scarcely perceivable).

The quality of **rhythm** of the pulse refers to its regularity, the equal spacing of the beats. A pulse which lacks a regular rhythm is said to have **arrhythmia.** The pulse can be irregular (without a consistent pattern) or regularly irregular (unequally spaced but consistently the same beating pattern). A pulse can also be intermittent and occasionally skip or insert beats. Often caffeine or nicotine react on the heart to cause irregularity and increased rate.

Measuring Radial Pulse   The patient should be completely relaxed and sitting comfortably or lying down when the pulse is measured and evaluated. Ideally the arm should be well supported, with the wrist near the level of the heart. Place the tips of your first three fingers at the wrist area, about an inch above the base of the thumb, Figure 5–37. Never use your thumb to measure pulse rate; there is a chance you may feel and record your own heart rate in your thumb's artery.

An appropriate amount of pressure applied to the artery will

P R O C E D U R E

Measure Radial Pulse

TERMINAL PERFORMANCE OBJECTIVE: In a simulated or actual situation, given a patient, a watch with a sweep-second hand, paper and pen or pencil, within minutes, assess and record the quality, and measure and record the rate of a patient's radial pulse, within 2 beats per minute accuracy, following correct procedural technique.

1. Wash hands, assemble equipment.
2. Identify patient. **RATIONALE: Speaking to the patient by name and checking the chart ensures that you are performing the procedure on the correct patient.**
3. Explain procedure. Identify what you are going to do.
4. Determine patient's recent activity. **RATIONALE:** Exertion within past 3-5 minutes will cause temporary increase in pulse rate.
5. Have patient assume a comfortable position with arm supported, palm of hand down, wrist near level of heart or placed across upper abdomen if lying down.
6. Locate radial artery on thumb side of wrist. *Note:* Do not use your thumb. Place tips of fingers over the

artery; exert light pressure.
7. Observe quality of pulse before beginning to count. Determine if regular, strong, weak, or thready. **RATIONALE: Concentration on the quality prior to measurement assists in accurate evaluation.**
8. Check watch. Begin counting beats when second hand is at 3, 6, 9, or 12 (*Note:* Makes 30 seconds easier to observe.)
9. Count a *regular* pulse for 30 seconds and multiply results by 2. Note that this will always be an even number. If *irregular,* count for full minute, but do not multiply by 2. **RATIONALE: The pulse rate is recorded in beats per minute, you have already determined the total beats per minute.**
10. Record pulse in beats per minute. *Note:* Immediate recording helps eliminate errors.
11. Describe quality characteristics. **RATIONALE: In certain disease conditions the presence or absence of quality characteristics is a significant finding.**
12. Wash hands.

FIGURE 5–37 Measuring the radial pulse

permit the pulsations to be felt. Too much pressure will shut off the circulation and therefore eliminate the pulse beat. Too little pressure will not compress the artery sufficiently against the radius. With practice, applying the correct amount of pressure will become routine.

Measuring Apical Pulse In instances when measuring heart rate by the radial pulse is not appropriate, it is necessary to listen to the heart at its **apex** with a **stethoscope.** This is a very accurate method of measuring heartbeat. The contraction of the atria and the ventricles will be heard as two closely occurring sounds, known as the lubb dupp; however, both contraction phases are counted as only one beat. Whenever a pulse rate is measured at a point other than radial, that fact should be noted when recording the rate; for example, P. 97 (Ap). Note that an **apical** pulse is counted for a full minute, so it is possible to record an uneven number.

Locating the Apex. The bottom or lower edge of the heart is known as the apex. This is the point of maximum impulse of the heart against the chest wall. It can be palpated at the left fifth intercostal space in line with the middle of the left clavicle. This spot may be located by pressing the fingertips between the ribs and counting down five spaces on the left chest wall, Figure 5–38(a), page 305. Often the beat at the apex can be felt with the fingertips.

P R O C E D U R E

Measure Apical Pulse

TERMINAL PERFORMANCE OBJECTIVE: In a simulated or actual situation, given a patient, a watch with a sweep-second hand, stethoscope, alcohol wipe, paper, and pen or pencil, within 5 minutes, locate the apex of the heart, assess and record the quality and measure and record the rate of a patient's apical pulse. This procedure will be done with 100% accuracy, following correct technique, and observing aseptic precautions.

1. Wash hands.
2. Prepare stethoscope by wiping earpieces and chestpiece with germicidal solution to prevent transfer of organisms.
3. Identify patient. **RATIONALE: Speaking to the patient by name and checking the chart ensures that you are performing the procedure on the correct patient.**
4. Tell patient what you are going to do. If patient is an infant or small child, explain the procedure to parent.
5. Provide privacy and a gown or drape if indicated.
6. Uncover left side of chest. **RATIONALE:** Auscultation must be done directly against the skin surface.
7. Place earpieces in ears. Openings in tips should be forward, entering auditory canal.
8. Locate apex by palpating to left fifth intercostal space at midclavicular line. *Note:* If chestpiece does not have a chill ring, warm it in palm of one hand while locating apex. This also prevents accidental striking against

hard surface and resulting noise in ears.
9. Place chestpiece of stethoscope at apex.
10. Determine quality of heart sounds. *Note:* **Concentrate on rhythm and volume. RATIONALE: The quality of the beat is significant in evaluation of heart action.**
11. Concentrate on rate of beats. *Note:* Be certain of sounds and pattern.
12. Observe watch and begin counting rate when second hand is at 3, 6, 9, or 12. **RATIONALE: It is easier to measure 1 minute when beginning at one of these four numbers.**
13. Count beats for a full minute. *Note:* **Both pulse phases count as one beat. RATIONALE: Apical rates are indicated when quality or rhythm irregularities are present or possible; therefore, full-minute measurement is essential.**
14. Remove earpieces from ears.
15. Record rate and quality of heart sounds.
    Note:
    a. Immediate recording aids in eliminating errors.
    b. Indicate it is apical measurement.
16. Assist or instruct patient to dress unless physician also wishes to assess heart action. Determine this by asking physician prior to measurement of if your findings indicate the need.
17. Wipe earpieces and chestpiece of stethoscope with disinfectant. Return to storage.
18. Wash hands.

FIGURE 5–38   (a) Locating the apical pulse by counting intercostal spaces. (b) Alternative method for locating the apex of the heart

Another, quicker method for *estimating* the location of the apex is to place the outstretched left hand on the chest wall with the tip of the middle finger in the suprasternal notch and the thumb at a 45-degree angle, Figure 5–38(b). The end of the thumb will be approximately over the apex. This is only an approximate measurement since the size of the chest and the hand will vary. For a ready reference point, the apex should be just below the left breast. Again, this is a variable, particularly in the female, due to the size and placement of the breast.

Apical Indications.   Apical pulse measurement is indicated for infants and small children due to their normally rapid rate, which is easier to hear and count than to palpate. Patients with heart conditions, especially if being medicated with cardiac drugs, will require apical measurement for greater accuracy. Apical measurement is always indicated if you have difficulty feeling a radial pulse and believe you may be missing beats. Other indications are an excessively rapid or slow rate, a thready or irregular quality, or with an existing or suspected pulse deficit.

Measuring Apical-Radial Pulse   Certain heart conditions cause a symptom known as **pulse deficit.** A patient with a pulse deficit will have a higher apical than radial pulse rate. This difference indicates that some heart contractions are not strong enough to produce a palpable radial pulse. It is important to determine the extent of the deficit by measuring the apical and radial rate at the same time.

A procedure call *apical–radial pulse* requires one person to measure the pulse rate radially while another auscultates the apical rate with a stethoscope, Figure 5–39. The radial rate is then subtracted from the apical, the difference being the pulse deficit. Ideally, two people measure the rate at the same time.

If this is not possible, then the apical rate is measured and recorded, followed immediately by the radial. Apical–radial rates are always measured for a full minute.

Respiration

The third vital sign to be measured is respiration. One respiration is the combination of total inspiration (breathing in) and total expiration (breathing out). Other frequently used terms are **inhale** and **exhale.**

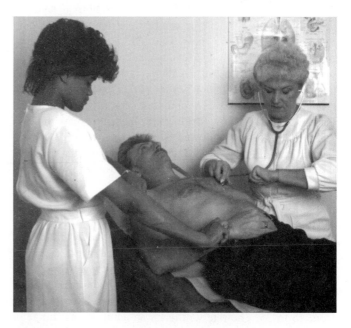

FIGURE 5–39   Measuring the apical–radial pulse

SHALLOW   DEEP   SHALLOW   APNEA

FIGURE 5-40 The Cheyne–Stokes breathing pattern

Respirations are usually measured as one part of total vital signs assessment. Since patients can voluntarily control the depth, rate, and regularity of their breathing to some extent, it is important that they not be aware the procedure is being done. To accomplish this, it is common practice to observe and measure respiration immediately after assessing the pulse, while maintaining your fingers at the radial pulse or auscultating the apex. Using this method, the patient assumes you are still measuring pulse rate.

Quality of Respiration Respirations should be quiet, effortless, and regularly spaced. Breathing should be through the nose with the mouth closed. Excessively fast and deep breathing, commonly associated with hysteria, is called **hyperventilation.** Difficult or labored breathing is called **dyspnea.** Frequently dyspnea is accompanied by discomfort and an anxious expression, due to fear of being unable to breathe. This patient will use the accessory respiratory muscles of the rib cage, neck, shoulders, and back to assist the breathing process.

The presence of **rales** (noisy breathing) usually indicates constricted bronchial passageways or the collection of fluid or exudate. Rales may be present with pneumonia, bronchitis, asthma, and other pulmonary diseases.

Respirations should be observed for the depth of inhalation. Three words are used to describe this quality: normal, shallow, or deep. Depth of inhalation can be determined by watching the rise and fall of the chest. The rhythm of the respirations must also be assessed. This quality can be described as regular or irregular. Absence of breathing is known as **apnea.** A breathing pattern called **Cheyne–Stokes** occurs with acute brain, heart, or lung damage or disease, and with intoxicants. It is characterized by slow, shallow breaths that increase in depth and frequency to be followed by a few shallow breaths, and then a period of apnea for 10 to 20 seconds, often more, Figure 5–40. This type of breathing pattern frequently precedes death.

Respiration Rate Normal respiration rate for adults is from 16 to 20 times per minute. The respiration rate in infants and children has a greater range and fluctuates more during illness, exercise, and emotion than adult rates do. In the newborn, the rate per minute may range from 30 to 80; in early childhood, from 20 to 40; and during late childhood from 15 to 25. The rate will reach an adult normal range of 16 to 20 by age 15. An abnormally slow rate of respiration is known as *bradypnea.* A faster than normal rate of respiration is known as *tachypnea.*

Counting Respirations It is necessary to observe the patient carefully while measuring respiration rate. If the patient is lying on the examination table, position the patient's arm across the upper abdominal area, placing your fingers over the radial pulse point. In this position you cannot only visualize respiration but feel it as well, Figure 5–41. With the patient in a sitting position, you will need to observe more carefully as

FIGURE 5-41 Measuring respirations

Measure Respirations

TERMINAL PERFORMANCE OBJECTIVE: In a simulated or actual situation, given a patient, a watch with a sweep-second hand, paper, and pen or pencil, assess and record the quality and rate of a patient's respirations with 100% accuracy, within 3 minutes, following the correct procedural technique.

1. Wash hands.
2. Identify patient. **RATIONALE: Speaking to the patient by name and checking the chart ensures that you are performing the procedure on the correct patient.**
3. In this procedure, it is preferable *not* to explain to the patient what you are about to do. If the patient knows that you will be counting respirations, control of breathing is possible, resulting in an inaccurate measurement.
4. Ask about recent activity level. **RATIONALE: Patient should have been relatively quiet for past 2–5 minutes to obtain accurate assessment.**
5. Place patient in comfortable position, either sitting or lying down.
6. Assume pulse measurement position. **RATIONALE: Respirations are more easily counted if patient's arm is across upper abdomen.**
7. Assess pulse quality. *Note:* Determine regularity, depth, quietness.
8. Count respirations for 30 seconds.
   Note:
   a. One rise and fall of the chest equals one respiration.
   b. Maintain radial pulse position. **RATIONALE: Patients must be unaware you are measuring respirations so that they do not unintentionally or purposely alter the rate or rhythm.**
   c. If respirations are irregular, count for a full minute; do not multiply results by 2. **RATIONALE: The rate per minute has already been determined.**
9. Multiply results by 2 and record.
10. Record quality characteristics. **RATIONALE: In certain disease conditions the presence or absence of quality characteristics is a significant finding.**
11. Wash hands.

you count the respirations. Remember, it is also necessary to keep your watch in view as you observe. With a little practice, you will be able to manage both at the same time.

When counting respirations as part of the TPR assessment, it is very important that you remember the number of heartbeats you have just counted. It may help you to use the following method:

1. Assume the pulse measuring position.
2. Observe, determine the characteristics, and describe to yourself the qualities of both the pulse and the respirations.
3. Count the number of heartbeats during the first 30 seconds.
4. Then repeat the pulse rate to yourself as you count the number of respirations during the second 30 seconds. (*Note:* You MUST use the word *and* between each respiration so you do not accidentally add counts to the pulse rate.)

For example, if your patient's pulse rate at 30 seconds is 40, repeat the rate as you count the respirations "40 and 1, 40 and 2, 40 and 3," an so on, until the second 30-second period is past. At the end of a minute, you will have both counts, which you will need to multiply by 2 and record.

Temperature–Pulse–Respiration Ratio

Respiration rate, like pulse, will increase with activity, excitement, fear, and other strong emotions, and certain disease con-

ditions. Respirations are, as is the pulse, in proportion to the degree of fever present. Table 5–6 demonstrates the relationship of the three vital signs.

Whenever a patient, either child or adult, has been upset and crying, a period of time must pass before an accurate measurement of either pulse or respirations can be made. Strong emotions elevate the vital signs and may make a true measurement impossible.

Blood Pressure

The fourth vital sign is blood pressure. Learning to assess blood pressure accurately requires attention to details, careful listening, and correct technique. The term *blood pressure* means the fluctuating pressure that the blood exerts against the arterial walls as the heart alternately contracts and relaxes. The blood pressure reflects the condition of the heart, the amount of blood forced from the heart at contraction, the condition of the arteries, and to some extent the volume and viscosity (stickiness) of the blood.

Blood pressure is measured in the brachial artery of the arm at the antecubital space, Figure 5–42. It should be measured in both arms, at least initially. There is normally a 5- to 10-mm difference. Subsequent readings should be made on the arm with the higher pressure.

Maintaining Blood Pressure Two main factors cooperate to maintain a fairly constant blood pressure. The first is the heart,

TABLE 5–6
Temperature—Pulse—Respiration Ratio

Respiration	Pulse	Temperature (F°)
18	80	99
19 (plus)	88	100
21	96	101
23	104	102
25 (minus)	112	103
27	120	104
28 (minus)	128	105
30	136	106

or pump, which exerts pressure on the blood. About 100,000 times a day the heart contracts, forcing blood into the aorta and throughout the blood vessels of the body. Without a strong, effective pump, the blood will not flow, and the pressure will drop.

The second factor is the brain, which controls, through the autonomic nervous system, the rate of the heart and the size of the opening or caliber of the arteries. When sensors in the arteries detect an increase in arterial pressure, a message is sent to the brain, which in turn directs the arteries to dilate slightly (reducing resistance to the flow of blood) and directs the heart to slow down (reducing the amount of blood being forced out). When the pressure drops too far, the message to the brain results in slightly increased heart action and constriction of the arteries, which cause the pressure to rise. Both actions are needed to maintain homeostasis.

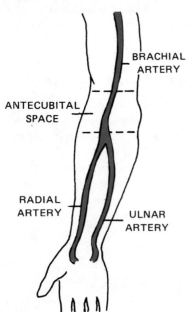

FIGURE 5–42 Blood pressure is measured in the brachial artery at the antecubital space.

Blood Pressure Phases   The phases of blood pressure are identical to those of the pulse. A contraction phase, known as *systole,* corresponds to the beat phase of the heart, and is the period of greatest pressure. The relaxation phase, known as *diastole,* corresponds to the resting or filling action of the heart, and is the period of least pressure.

Normal Blood Pressure   Blood pressure is measured in millimeters of mercury (mm Hg) using a stethoscope and a **sphygmomanometer,** which has either a calibrated column of mercury or an **aneroid** gauge. Figure 5–43. Blood pressure readings are measurements of systolic and diastolic pressure written as a fraction; for example, B/P 120/80, where 120 is systolic and 80 is diastolic pressure.

A normal adult will have a systolic pressure between 100 and 140 mm Hg, and a diastolic pressure between 60 and 90. Blood pressure readings persistently above 140/90 indicate *hypertension* (high blood pressure). Hypertension can result from conditions, such as stress, obesity, high salt intake, sedentary life-style, and aging. Physical conditions that cause hypertension are kidney disease, thyroid dysfunction, neurological disorders, and vascular conditions, such as atherosclerosis and arteriosclerosis, which make circulation more difficult, therefore requiring a greater pressure to circulate the blood. An elevated pressure without apparent cause is said to be **idiopathic,** or **essential,** hypertension. A blood pressure consistently below 90/60 indicates *hypotension* (low blood pressure), which may be normal for some persons. Hypotension will be present with heart failure, severe burns, dehydration, deep depression, hemorrhage, and shock.

Pulse Pressure   **Pulse pressure** refers to the difference between the systolic and diastolic reading and is an indicator of the tone of the arterial walls. For example, when the pressure is 120/80, the pulse pressure is 40, which is a normal finding. A pulse pressure over 50 or less than 30 mm Hg *may be* considered abnormal. A general rule is that the pulse pressure should be approximately a third of the systolic measurement. If less, the patient may have an auscultatory gap (absence of sound), and the pressure may have been incorrectly measured. This disorder will be described later.

Equipment Factors   It is important that sphygmomanometers be in proper working order and correctly calibrated. A mercury manometer that leaks mercury or has bubbles rising in the mercury column when used may not measure accurately. If correctly calibrated, the meniscus of the mercury is at 0 when viewed at eye level. The desktop manometer must always be placed on a flat, level surface. Wall-mounted units should be at a height permitting eye-level viewing. The medical assistant must either sit down or stoop to view a floor model manometer at eye level. Figure 5–44 shows various types of sphygmomanometers.

The aneroid dial should be calibrated occasionally by attaching it to a calibrated mercury manometer with a Y connector,

A

B

C

FIGURE 5–43 Blood Pressure measuring equipment. (a) Single- and dual head stethoscopes. (b) Aneroid sphygmomanometer gauge. (c) Mercury sphygmomanometer column

Figure 5–45, page 311. Elevate the manometers to 250 mm Hg together, then let the pressure fall, noting the reading at four different points. There should be no more than a 3-mm Hg difference according to the National Bureau of Standards. Mercury sphygmomanometers are much more accurate than aneroid models; however, they still need to be checked for faults every 6 to 12 months, depending on use. They should be serviced and calibrated to ensure accuracy in measurement. Aneroid models must be checked every 3 to 6 months over the entire pressure range against an accurate mercury manometer. Figure 5–45 illustrates how the manometers are connected together by a Y tube and measured simultaneously.

Studies have shown many sphygmomanometers used in family practice to be faulty. The primary areas of failure in both models are in the control valves of the cuffs, which result in leakage and in unsatisfactory condition of the mer-

cury columns either due to inadequate mercury in the reservoir or dirt from oxidation in the glass calibrated tube, which makes reading more difficult. The aneroid models showed a greater problem with accuracy due to dial errors because they are rarely calibrated.

It is important that sphygmomanometers be serviced regularly. Faults in aneroid models have to be corrected by service technicians or the manufacturer. A mercury manometer can be maintained by the owner if desired. The common sources of error—the mercury level, the glass tube, and the air vent—can be solved by topping off the mercury in the reservoir, cleaning the glass tube to permit better viewing and mercury flow, or replacing the chamois leather in the air vent. Because mercury is a harmful substance, it is probably best to use trained technicians to service the equipment.

The cuff is also critical in correct measurement. If the reading is to be accurate, the cuff must be the appropriate size, Figure 5–46. If it is too small for the upper arm, the reading will be falsely high; if too large, falsely low. To determine the proper size, compare the cuff width to the width of the upper arm. The cuff should be about 20% wider than the arm. When a cuff is too small and you do not have access to a wide adult cuff, measure to the width of the forearm. If the cuff is of adequate size, take the blood pressure reading in the forearm by placing the stethoscope over the radial artery.

Measuring Techniques   Because blood pressure readings are so critical to the determination of hypertension and consequently to the medication given for managing it, strict procedure techniques must be followed. Several factors affect the accuracy of results.

1. The cuff must be completely deflated when applied.
2. The patient must be comfortable, with the arm slightly flexed at the elbow and the brachial artery on a level with the heart. The arm must be bare and free of a constricting sleeve, Figure 5–47, page 313.
3. The center of the bladder in the cuff must be placed over the brachial artery. Fold the bladder area of the cuff in half to locate the center. Many cuffs have improper artery markings.
4. The manometer must be viewed directly from a distance of not more than 3 feet.
5. A palpatory reading should be taken first to determine proper inflation. Afterwards, deflate the cuff completely by compressing with the hands before reinflation.
6. A minimum of 15 seconds should elapse between inflations (30 is better) to allow blood pressure to normalize.
7. The cuff should be inflated rapidly to 30 mm Hg above the palpatory reading.

To obtain a baseline reading for new patients it may be desirable to measure the pressure twice in each arm, once while the patient is sitting and once while lying down.

Blood pressure has two phases, both of which must be determined. When the cuff is properly inflated, the valve must be opened carefully to allow deflation at a rate of 2-3 mm Hg per beat. Listen for the first sounds of heartbeat, and note the reading as the systolic pressure once you have heard at least two consecutive beats. Continue to listen and observe as the cuff is deflated until you hear a sudden change in sound to a softer, muffled tone. Note this reading as the diastolic pressure. Continue to observe the manometer until the sound disappears. Note this reading also, even if 0. To record, you would write, for example, B/P 140/90/70. You should ask the physician which

FIGURE 5–44   Types of sphygmomanometers (a) Aneroid (Courtesy of Omron Marshall Products Inc.) (b) Wall-mounted mercury (Courtesy of Tycos)

FIGURE 5–44   (continued) (c) Desk-type mercury (Courtesy of Omron Marshall Products, Inc.) (d) Standby mercury (Courtesy WA Baum Co., Inc.)

FIGURE 5–45   Testing an aneroid sphygmomanometer

Measure Blood Pressure

TERMINAL PERFORMANCE OBJECTIVE: In a simulated or actual situation, given a patient, stethoscope, mercury or aneroid manometer, alcohol wipe, paper and pen or pencil, measure palpatory and auscultatory blood pressure, recording findings, within 5 minutes, at 4 mm Hg accuracy, following correct procedural technique and observing safety and aseptic precautions.

1. Wash hands.
2. Assemble equipment
3. Clean earpieces and head of stethoscope with antiseptic. **RATIONALE: This prevents the transference of microorganisms.**
4. Identify patient. **RATIONALE: Speaking to the patient by name and checking the chart ensures that you are performing the procedure on the correct patient.**
5. Explain procedure. **RATIONALE: If it is new to a patient, especially if a child, explain that the cuff will squeeze but that they must not move.**
6. Place a mercury manometer on a flat, level surface near patient. Put aneroid type within easy reach.
7. Place patient in a relaxed and comfortable sitting or lying position.
8. Expose patient's upper arm well above elbow, extending arm with palm up. If sleeve is tight, remove garment. Arm must be bare for accuracy. *Note:* Arm must be relaxed, on a supporting surface, slightly flexed at elbow, with brachial artery approximately at level of heart.
9. With valve of inflation bulb open, squeeze all air from bladder, fold to identify center, placing bottom edge of cuff 1 to 2 inches above elbow. Wrap cuff smoothly and snugly around arm, with deflated bladder centered over brachial artery. If using mercury manometer, cuff and tubing may be disconnected for easier application. If using aneroid, be certain dial can be easily viewed and end of cuff does not interfere. (**CAUTION:** Be alert to patient's movements which could pull attached desk-type mercury manometer off table.)
10. Take position with mercury manometer or aneroid dial in a direct line at eye level.
11. With *one hand,* close valve on bulb, clockwise. *Note:* Do not overtighten or it will be hard to open.
12. Position other hand to palpate radial pulse.
13. Observing manometer, rapidly inflate cuff to 30 mm above level where radial pulse disappears.
14. Open valve, slowly releasing air until radial pulse is detected. (*Note:* Provides information for auscultatory measurement.)

15. Observe mercury or dial reading. *Note:* This is estimated for palpatory systolic pressure, which may be recorded, for example, as B/P 120 (P).
16. Deflate cuff rapidly and completely. Squeeze cuff with hands to empty. **RATIONALE: All the air must be expressed between inflations to obtain accurate results.** Adjust position if necessary.
17. Position earpieces of stethoscope in ears with openings entering ear canal.
18. Palpate brachial artery at medial antecubital space with fingertips.
19. Place head of stethoscope directly over palpated pulse. *Note:* Stethoscope head must not touch either cuff or clothing (creates static).
20. Close valve on bulb and rapidly inflate cuff to 30 mm above palpated systolic pressure. *Note:* A minimum of 15 seconds must have elapsed since the previous inflation. **RATIONALE: This is the minimum time required for the normalizing of blood flow through the artery.**
21. Open valve, slowly deflating cuff. *Note:* Pressure should drop 2–3 mm Hg per second.
22. With eyes at level of descending meniscus or directly in line or over dial, note reading at which you hear systolic pressure.
    Note:
    a. Must be at least two consecutive beats.
    b. Remember systolic measurement.
23. Allow pressure to lower steadily until you note a change in sound to a softer, more muffled sound. Note this as diastolic pressure (if so instructed).
24. Continue to release pressure until all sound disappears. Note point as diastolic pressure (if so instructed).
25. Release remaining air. Squeeze cuff between hands. **RATIONALE: This removes all the remaining air to make the patient more comfortable and ensures accurate results if reevaluation is necessary.**
26. Record systolic and whichever diastolic the physician prefers.
27. Reevaluate if indicated after a minimum of 15 seconds.
28. Remove stethoscope from ears.
29. Remove cuff from patient's arm.
30. Assist patient with clothing, if necessary.
31. Clean tips and head of stethoscope with alcohol to disinfect. Fold cuff properly and place with manometer and stethoscope in storage.
32. Wash hands.

FIGURE 5–46 Blood pressure cuffs in sizes to fit the arm of a small child to an adult thigh (From Caldwell & Hegner, *Nursing Assistant,* 6th ed. Copyright 1992, Delmar Publishers Inc.).

sound, the change or the absence, you are to record as the diastolic measurement. There are reasons to support either method.

Probably the mistake made most often in measuring blood pressure is reinflating the cuff after only partial deflation or too soon after complete deflation. Either error may cause a false reading and will also cause difficulty in hearing the sound changes because of venous congestion in the forearm.

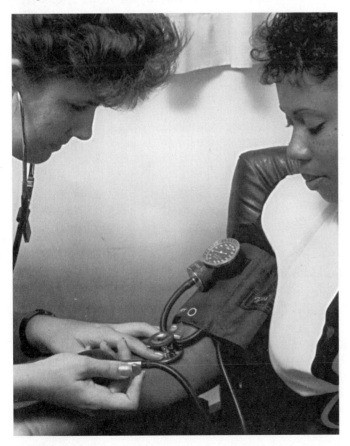

FIGURE 5–47 Measuring blood pressure

FIGURE 5–48 A technique to augment heart sounds in blood pressure measurement

Augmenting Sound. To augment heartbeat sounds when they are difficult to hear, use the following technique:

1. With the cuff properly applied and deflated have patient elevate arm above the shoulder and make and release a fist a few times to aid in emptying forearm veins, Figure 5–48.
2. With the patient's arm still raised, rapidly inflate the cuff to 30 mm Hg above palpated pulse.
3. Have patient lower arm.
4. Begin deflation, listening for initial beats. The sounds will be intensified because the blood spurting through the cuff tourniquet is striking against the walls of a near empty artery.

Auscultatory Gap. In some patients, usually those who are hypertensive, there is a silent interval between systolic and diastolic pressure, called an auscultatory gap, Figure 5–49, page 314. If this is not detected, it may lead to serious undermeasurement of the systolic pressure. For example, the patient's actual systolic pressure is 200, with a gap from 170 to 140, and a diastolic of 120/110. You inflate the cuff to 170

230
220
210
200
190
180
170
160
150
140
130
120
110
100
90
80
70
60
50
40
30
20
10
0

TRUE SYSTOLIC

AUSCULTATORY GAP

FALSE SYSTOLIC

MUFFLED DIASTOLIC
SILENT DIASTOLIC

FIGURE 5–49   Auscultatory gap

and hear nothing until the manometer reaches 140, which you presume is the systolic pressure. You would continue deflation and record 120/110 as the diastolic; therefore, you would have a pulse pressure of only 20 or 30 mm Hg. Keeping in mind the normal range for pulse pressure, however, you would view 20/30 as suspicious. Taking one-third of 140 would give you about 47. To be certain you had not missed a portion of the pressure, you would remeasure, palpating the systolic and then inflating the cuff 30 mm above. If sounds were still audible at that point you would reinflate it higher *after complete deflation* until you hear the first sounds of systolic pressure.

When recording a blood pressure with an auscultatory gap, list your complete findings; for example, B/P 200/120/110 with the auscultatory gap from 170 to 140.

Blood Pressure in Children   The blood pressure of infants and children is often omitted from the physical examination because it is so difficult to obtain. Variation in blood pressure due to anxiety and emotional upset make accurate readings very challenging. Basically, the procedure is the same as with adults. Often physicians prefer to do the measurement last after having established some rapport with the child.

The cuff size is important in measuring a child's pressure. It should be appropriate to the size of the arm. The inflatable bag must entirely encircle the extremity.

The level of systolic pressure gradually rises throughout childhood. Normal pressure for a 6-month-old is 70; at 1 year it is 95; and it rises to 100 at 6 years. By age 16, the systolic pressure will be 120, the adult average. The diastolic pressure reaches 65 by age 1 and does not change appreciably during childhood.

Complete Chapter 5, Unit 4 in the workbook to help you meet the objectives at the beginning of this unit and therefore achieve competency of this subject matter.

Ms. Right . . .

respects the privacy of each patient when obtaining information for medical records. She makes every effort to establish a good rapport with all patients by accepting each individual. She is ever mindful of the importance of confidentiality and obtains the proper authorization before release of information concerning patients. Ms. Right performs procedures and records results carefully and efficiently. She never guesses what a pulse or blood pressure reading is. If she is not sure of a result, she asks a supervisor or physician to check it. She also follows the statutes regarding the rights of minors in their medical treatment, reminding patients under age 18 that a parent or guardian must accompany them for their appointments.

Advancement potential: Excellent

Mr. Wrong . . .

disregards confidentiality, privacy, and respect regarding patients. He has a good rapport only with those patients he likes. He frequently forgets to obtain proper authorization to release information about a patient and often gives it over the telephone. He has told coworkers that sometimes if he cannot hear a blood pressure, he just records the reading from the patient's last visit. He pays little attention to the statutes concerning the rights of minors regarding medical treatment. He frequently has to be reminded by others to follow office policy.

Advancement potential: Poor (employment will most likely be terminated)

REFERENCES

The American Medical Association Family Medical Guide. New York: Random House, 1987.

Bates, Barbara A. *A Guide to Physical Examination.* Philadelphia: Lippincott, 1974.

Burch, George E., M.D., and Shewey, Lana, M.D. "Sphygmomanometer Cuff Size and Blood Pressure Recordings." *Journal of the American Medical Association.* 225:1215–1218, 1973.

Caldwell, Esther, and Hegner, Barbara. *Nursing Assistant: A Nursing Process Approach*, 6th ed. Albany: Delmar, 1992.

Diagnostic Tests, Nurse's Ready Reference. Springhouse, PA: Springhouse, 1991.

Fong, Elizabeth, Ferris, Elvira, and Skelley, Esther G. *Body Structures and Functions*, 8th ed. Albany: Delmar, 1993.

Mosby's Medical, Nursing, and Allied Health Dictionary, 3rd ed. St. Louis: C. V. Mosby, 1990.

Nurse's Reference Library, Assessment. Springhouse, PA: Springhouse, 1983.

Ohio's Health. Blood Pressure: Are You Reading it Right? Ohio Department of Health, Division of Chronic Disease, May 1984.

Perlman, Lawrence V., M.D., Chang, Benjamin N., M.D., and Keller, Jacob, MPH. "Accuracy of Sphygmomanometers in Hospital Practice." *Archives of Internal Medicine.* 125:1000–1003, 1970.

Reader's Digest Illustrated Encyclopedic Dictionary. Boston: Houghton Mifflin Lexical Databases, 1987.

Sarason and Sarason. *Abnormal Psychology: The Problem of Maladaptive Behavior*, 5th ed. Englewood Cliffs, NJ: Prentice-Hall, 1987.

Starr, Cecie, and Taggert, Ralph. Biology: *The Unity and Diversity of Life*, 5th ed. Belmont: Wadsworth, 1989.

Taber, Clarence W. *Taber's Cyclopedic Medical Dictionary*, 14th ed. Philadelphia: F.A. Davis, 1983.

U.S. Department of Health and Human Services, Public Health Service Centers for Disease Control. *Recommendations for Prevention of HIV Transmission in Health Care Settings.* Atlanta, 1987.

Zakus, Sharron. *Mosby's Fundamentals of Medical Assisting: Administrative and Clinical Theory and Technique*, 2nd ed. St. Louis: C. V. Mosby, 1990.

CHAPTER 6
Physical Examinations

UNIT 1
Head to Toe

UNIT 2
Positioning and Draping for Examinations

UNIT 3
Procedures of the Eye and Ear

UNIT 4
Specialty Examinations

The Medical Assistant is a significant **liaison** between the patient and the physician. You should be **discreet** and courteous at all times with all patients. You must listen carefully and observe them closely as they disclose their complaints and symptoms to you and while you are performing the many procedures dealing with their care. Some patients (themselves) may not even be aware of a condition or symptom that you could bring to their attention. Often a patient becomes so used to a problem that it may be overlooked, such as clearing the throat, a change in weight, or a skin discoloration. When changes like these happen gradually, sometimes the patient is really not aware of them. You can then alert the physician to initiate treatment for a problem that may have otherwise gone undetected.

In the pages that follow you will learn of many ways to be of assistance to both patient and physician. Pay special attention to the patient education sections for application to determine how they apply to the many procedures and examination preparations you provide for patients.

The overall preparation of patients for examinations performed by the physician is the responsibility of the medical assistant. To gain full cooperation of the patient for a particular examination the patient must understand completely what is expected. The medical assistant must keep in mind that these procedures and examinations, although routine to the medical staff, are not usually routine to patients.

In this chapter you will learn valuable skills to help you in getting patients ready for the doctor to see them. Patients will have appointments for a variety of reasons. The medical assistant's duty is to ascertain the reason the patient is visiting the physician (triage) and prepare the patient for the appropriate examination.

The patient will want to know: what the particular examination is (a brief definition); why it has to be done; how long it takes; if it hurts; when it must be done; and, of course, preliminary preparation if necessary. Even though the doctor tells the patient about all of these points concerning orders during the course of the visit, the patient may not ask questions (or even know what to ask). Often physicians leave these explanations up to the medical assistant who can review the information with the patient in a more relaxed setting. Usually this allows a few minutes for the patient to think about questions to ask before they leave the office.

Patient education is a primary function of the medical assistant. Most patients are not trained health professionals and are somewhat confused by medical terminology, tests, procedures, and medications they encounter. Therefore, patient education becomes an important part of their medical care.

Whenever possible, the patient should be involved in making decisions about treatment or care. This will encourage the participants to participate more fully in the procedure. Patients will be more willing to cooperate if they understand the necessity for a particular procedure or treatment. Your careful and clear explanations of these procedures will encourage the patient to be more cooperative. If patients sense that you are truly concerned about their well-being, this will stimulate more cooperation. Always offer encouragement and praise where appropriate, even for the smallest accomplishment.

To properly instruct a patient, the medical assistant must know the material. Be prepared to answer any questions from the patient. If you cannot answer one of the patient's questions, tell the patient that you do not know the answer but will ask the physician. Never try to answer a question that you are not prepared to discuss. You could give incorrect information that could harm the patient's well-being. Never give information that is beyond your scope of practice.

In teaching a patient about health care and all that is involved in medical well-being, the primary goal of the medical assistant should be good communication. This means that each patient must be treated as an individual with particular needs. As a patient educator, you will have to meet these needs. You must communicate in the most efficient and effective manner for each individual. Listening is vital to this education. Patients may be shy or embarrassed by their problems or questions and may not ask direct questions. Therefore, you must listen carefully to the patient's comments and questions. Be familiar with information about the patient before proceeding with an explanation. This will help determine how to communicate best with each individual.

Never assume that a patient already knows the information you are conveying. Sometimes a patient will state that he understands something to keep from being embarrassed. If you sense that this is the situation you should briefly repeat the information and provide printed material for the patient to take home to read. Printed materials, such as one-page handouts, brochures, pamphlets, and booklets on various procedures and examinations, as well as diseases, conditions, and treatment plans, should be clear and concise in content. These informative materials should be appropriately distributed routinely to patients.

One very important aspect of patient teaching is your attitude toward the patient. The medical assistant must be open when approaching patients. This means that you must accept each patient as an individual who needs your help. There is no room in the medical office for prejudice. All patients should be treated with respect regardless of their financial status, race, religion, age, or station in life. Remember, your job is to provide assistance. If patients sense any negative feelings on your part, then they will be less likely to pay attention to your instructions and suggestions.

Most patients are interested in getting better and staying healthy. Patient education involves not only instructing those who are sick, but helping healthy patients stay well. By following current trends in wellness and prevention of medical problems, you can help patients help themselves to a healthier life.

The following are some general guidelines for patient education:

1. Become familiar with your office's or clinic's policy concerning patient care.
2. Thoroughly read all handout information given to patients to explain procedures, examinations, or treatment plans so that you can intelligently answer patients' questions.
3. Make yourself available to patients for answering questions. Always remember to ask patients if they have any questions about their treatment or diagnosis.
4. Always take the opportunity to explain procedures to patients and offer additional information, when appropriate, at the time of their visits. For example, be sure to explain warm-up and stretching exercises to the weekend athlete with a sprained ankle.
5. Attend continuing education programs to keep abreast of the latest medical information to pass on to patients.
6. Post charts, posters, and other information that will benefit the patient. Be sure that this information is kept current and is posted in areas where patients may spend time waiting.
7. Have current health-conscious magazines available in the reception area.
8. Post meeting times and information for patient support groups (weight control groups, stop-smoking groups, tough love meetings) and encourage their participation. Keep this information current.

As you are getting patients ready for the physician's examination, it is an ideal time to provide them with **pertinent** information regarding the maintenance of their health.

The units that follow provide valuable information in preparing for and assisting with simple to complex preparations and examinations.

U N I T   1

Head to Toe

OBJECTIVES

Upon completion of the unit you will meet the following terminal performance objectives by verifying knowledge of the facts and principles presented through oral and written communication at a level deemed competent by the instructor or employer, and will demonstrate the specific behaviors as identified in the terminal performance objectives of the procedures, observing all aseptic and safety precautions in accordance with health care standards.

1. List the duties that involve the medical assistant in preparing for the complete physical examination (CPE) of a patient.
2. Name the instruments, equipment, and supplies used in the CPE, and state the function of each.
3. Identify each section of the CPE and describe how the physician conducts each part of the examination.
4. Explain the role of the medical assistant in the examination process.
5. List and discuss appropriate patient education for the various parts of the examination.
6. Identify the nine sections of the abdominal cavity and name the visceral organs therein.
7. Define the POMR and SOAP methods of charting patient information.
8. Establish reasons for progress reports.
9. Explain subjective and objective symptoms and give five examples of each.
10. Discuss the seven warning signs of cancer in adults and children.
11. Describe the physical examination schedules for adults and children.
12. Spell and define, using the glossary at the back of the text, all the words to know in this unit.

WORDS TO KNOW

acute	mensuration
alcohol-saturated gauze square	murmur
anxiety	nasal speculum
asymmetry	objective
audibility	occult
auscultation	otoscope
baseline	palpation
bimanual	penlight
bold	percussion
bruit	percussion hammer
caustic	pertinent
chronic	pitch
coordination	progress report
cytological	peripheral
detection	physical
dimpling	prolapse
douche	resonance
duration	R/O
enema	sphincter
evacuate	sphygmomanometer
explicit	steril gauze square
exudate	stethoscope
fasting	subjective
fistula	subsequent
gait	symmetry
glaucoma	tape measure
gooseneck lamp	tentative
guaiac test paper	tongue depressor
indigestion	tonometer
inguinal hernia	tuning fork
initial	vaginal speculum
inspection	visceral
L & A	void
laryngeal mirror	warrant
laxative	water-soluble lubricant
liaison	writer
manipulation	

Assisting with the complete physical examination (CPE), the general physical exam, H & P (history and physical), physical exam (PE), or just plain **physical,** as it is often termed, is not difficult, but complex in that it is a *set* of procedures. The

The patient needs to know why the physical examination must be performed accurately. Explain that the data collected form a database against which all future examinations and observations will be compared. The patient must understand what is taking place and why. It is very important for the patient to be relaxed while being examined. Some examinations can be embarrassing to a patient, but a clear explanation of each procedure can help relax the patient. You can assist the patient greatly by giving empathy and support. Never assume that a patient knows what clothing to remove or what position to assume simply because that patient has visited the office before. Be sure to answer all questions the patient has about the procedures to be performed.

responsibilities of the medical assistant are to prepare the room for the physician and patient, and then the patient for the physician to examine. You may also assist with the exam, or write the findings. In the following pages you will learn this process.

In many facilities, the medical assistant accompanies the physician in the examination room and records the findings while the physician dictates the information as the examination proceeds. The term **writer** is given to the medical assistant who writes what the physician dictates during the exam. One who performs this duty must have sound knowledge in medical terminology, anatomy, and physiology, and of course, good spelling and writing skills. Since the physician bases the diagnosis on these findings, accuracy is vital. Many physicians prefer to write their own findings on plain sheets of lined paper (a common practice is to use a rubber stamp that outlines a particular exam format), or on specially printed forms in the outlined order of their choice. Still other physicians prefer to dictate the findings of an examination into a recorder for transcription later by the medical assistant.

There is no absolute pattern of examination to follow as long as the examiner is consistent and forms a personal habit so as to be thorough and complete with each patient. The complete examination should include the whole body, from the head to the toes, and front to back, and inside and out. In your career as a medical assistant, you will work with many physicians who may be quite different in their systematic approach to patient care.

Physicians are skilled in a variety of techniques used in evaluating patients in the examination process. In assisting with the H & P, the medical assistant is expected to have a basic knowledge of these procedural terms.

The **initial** part of the exam is the **inspection,** in which the physician looks for any abnormalities of speech, skin condition, color, posture, **gait,** awareness, sensitivity, **anxiety,** grooming, or general appearance.

Whenever patients come in to the office or clinic for an appointment, whether it is for a check-up or a visit for an illness or injury, it is a perfect opportunity for you to motivate them to practice better health habits. The medical assistant usually has more time than the physician to talk with the patients because many procedures do take time to perform. While you are conducting these matters, you can suggest many different ideas to patients. Often for various reasons, the patient must wait for the physician. Making use of this time for patient education is wise. Sometimes a beginning medical assistant may be at a loss for words with patients and does not know what to talk about with them except for the weather. This may help you learn some appropriate topics to speak with patients about which may benefit them. Table 6–1 outlines the warning signs of cancer. A few other suggestions for topics to discuss with patients follow.

Palpation is a means of examination by touching with the fingers or hands. Digital (one-finger) palpation is used to examine the anus. **Bimanual** (two-handed) palpation is used in vaginal examinations. Palpation of the breasts is done with the fingertips of both hands.

Percussion is a means of producing sounds by tapping various parts of the body. The physician listens to the sounds to determine the size, density, and location of underlying **visceral** organs. **Pitch,** quality, **duration,** and **resonance** are terms

TABLE 6–1
The Seven Warning Signs of Cancer

Adults
1. Sore that does not heal
2. Annoying cough or hoarseness
3. Trouble with swallowing or frequent **indigestion**
4. Unusual bleeding or discharge
5. A thickened area or lump in breast or anywhere on the body
6. A change in a wart or a mole
7. Change in bowel or bladder habits

Children (same as for adults plus the following)
1. The over-all condition seems generally run-down
2. Unexplained stumbling
3. Infant or child cries continually for no apparent reason
4. Any bloody discharge; any spontaneous bleeding or failure to stop bleeding in usual time
5. Anywhere on the body: swelling, lumps, masses, or bumps
6. Change in size and looks of birth marks, moles, etc.
7. Nausea and vomiting for no obvious reason

used by physicians when referring to percussion. Direct percussion is termed *immediate* and is done by striking the finger against the patient's body. The type of percussion most often used is *indirect,* or *mediate.* With indirect percussion, the examiner's finger is placed on the area and struck with a finger of the other hand.

Auscultation is listening to sounds made by the patient's body. Indirect auscultation is done with the stethoscope to amplify sounds that arise from the lungs, heart, and visceral organs. Sounds heard by this method of examination include **bruits,** murmurs, and rhythms. Direct auscultation is done by placing the ear directly over the area.

Mensuration means measurement. In this part of the examination, the patient's chest and extremities are measured and recorded in centimeters. Usually a standard flexible tape measure is used.

Manipulation is the forceful, passive movement of a joint to determine the range of extension and flexion.

In documenting the physical examination, many physicians use the problem-oriented medical record (POMR) method. It is sometimes referred to as POS, or problem-oriented system. This system is used for a new patient workup and for patients with serious or **chronic** illnesses. It is also used to document specific multiple complaints of patients. For **acute** or single minor complaints, such as a sore throat or a splinter, this system may not be used, for the chief complaint would not **warrant** such detail. Using this system ensures that pertinent datais recorded in logical order on the patient's chart with each return visit to the physician. Data is recorded under the following headings:

S Subjective findings

O Objective findings

A Assessment of problems

P Plan for treatment

Under **subjective** findings are those symptoms which the patient feels but which cannot be seen by another. Nausea, joint pain, headache, and abdominal pain are examples of subjective findings. **Objective** findings are those symptoms that can be seen by another as well as by the patient, such as redness, rash, swelling, watery discharge, or bleeding. It can also include any information concerning the patient that a family member or friend has conveyed to either you or the doctor, and the patient's past health history. Assessment documents measurement of the symptoms. This includes laboratory reports, X rays, vital sign recordings, and other aids to diagnosis.

The **tentative** diagnosis is made in this section of the patient's chart. The final section of the system outlines the plan of treatment for the patient to follow. This includes referrals, medication, surgery, therapy, exercise, and any further orders to return the patient to better health. Patient education is obviously a great part of this systematic method of record keeping. All action taken in the course of the patient's treatment generates additional information that continually modifies the original data base. **Subsequent** visits of the patient are

A. To prevent injuries of the face and head:
 1. In working and recreational environments, wear protective head gear: hard hat at work (construction sites), helmet for sports (motorcycle riding, football).
    a. Wear protective face mask or goggles for sports, such as football, basketball, or wrestling to prevent possible eye injuries.
    b. Use ear plugs to protect the ears from exposure to loud noises that can lead to possible damage to auditory nerves, resulting in hearing loss (machinery, band concerts); water when swimming.
B. To protect the skin:
 1. Keep skin clean and soft by using mild soap and water for bathing and a moisturizing lotion as necessary.
    a. Discourage sun worship. Encourage keeping covered in the sun or the use of a sun block to prevent damage of ultraviolet rays if one must be in the sun for prolonged periods of time.
    b. Wash hands of (chemical) irritants immediately to prevent **caustic** burns.
C. To prevent diseases of the respiratory system and contagious diseases:
 1. Discourage eating, drinking, and so on after others to keep from transmitting viruses and other diseases to others.
 2. Wash hands after handling items in or from public places, which probably have been handled by multitudes of others (money, door knobs, etc.).
 3. Discourage smoking or tobacco use of any kind (post stop-smoking pamphlets or meetings for patients to read).
 4. Encourage *safe sex* by providing **explicit** information to teach patients about the dangers of sexually transmitted diseases and AIDS.
 5. Remind patients about immunizations and encourage their compliance.
D. To promote general good health and safety:
 1. Remind patients of the dangers of drug and alcohol use and abuse (display information about Alcoholics Anonymous meetings).
 2. Encourage exercise and physical fitness programs with the advice of the physician.
 3. Promote proper nutrition and weight control by reminding patients to eat well-balanced meals regularly and help them plan their diets.
 4. Discourage patients from using **laxatives** and **enemas** unless specifically ordered by the physician.
 5. Encourage patients to read labels for contents of the products they buy and use for their safety.
 6. Remind patients to use seat belts.
 7. Promote regular medical and dental checkups.

recorded in the same manner (SOAP) as was the initial visit on sheets termed *progress notes,* sometimes referred to as **progress reports** or chart notes. Following each entry on the patient's chart should be the signature or initials of the health care provider or the person who performed the procedure.

Preparation of the Examination Room ....

Getting the examination room ready consists of making sure that the temperature in the room is comfortable; that it is clean and tidy; that the examination table has a clean covering (either disposable table paper or a cloth sheet); and that all appropriate instruments, equipment, and supplies are arranged conveniently for use during the examination.

The medical assistant should routinely clean and restock the examination room. Carefully checking the room for necessary items will ensure efficient, expedient patient care. Make sure all equipment is in proper working order and that the room is cleaned following each patient.

These items are displayed and labeled in Figure 6–1 in the order in which they are commonly used for a complete physical examination. You should learn the name and function of each item.

Preparation of the Patient ....

It is a usual practice to schedule the CPE early in the morning because patients are normally required to fast (have nothing by mouth) from midnight on for blood chemistry tests, which are based on a **fasting** normal range. Other procedures within the examination process are more comfortable if the patient has not eaten before the physical.

1. stethoscope
2. penlight
3. guaiac/occult blood test developer
4. guaiac/occult blood test
5. flexible tape measure
6. urine specimen container
7. metal nasal speculum
8. tuning fork
9. percussion hammer
10. tongue depressr
11. ophthalmoscope (head)
12. okastic ear/nose speculum
13. otoscope head attached to base handle
14. sphygmomanometer
15. latex gloves

FIGURE 6–1 Instruments and supplies used in the physical examination

When these **preliminary** tasks have been completed, the medical assistant escorts the patient into the examination room and explains the proceedings, answers any questions, and may begin patient education where appropriate. Triage will have already determined what chief complaints the patient has. You may want to verify what the patient feels is the problem at this point. Make sure that you allow the patient time to use the restroom for comfort during the exam. You should ask the patient to urinate in a specimen cup if he or she did not bring a first morning specimen for you to test (complete instructions for specimen collection are in Chapter 7). Sometimes the physician must delay the examination of the abdominal area because the patient has to **void** or **evacuate** the bowel. Occasionally this is obviously unavoidable even if the patient has already made an elimination. Unnecessary interruptions are annoying besides hindering the patient flow schedule. The success of the physical examination is attributed largely to the preparation of the patient. Until you are sure of yourself in remembering details, it is helpful to keep a checklist in your uniform pocket for handy reference.

The next duty of the medical assistant is to ask the patient to disrobe and put on the examination gown. Explain how by showing the patient, for instance, whether the gown should be open in the front or the back. You should offer assistance with this and show the patient where to store belongings. Pull out the step at the end of the exam table (or provide a portable one) and help the patient up to the table. Cover the top of the patient's legs with a drape sheet, which provides both privacy and warmth.

General instructions about the physical may be offered at this point. You may want to tell the patient that some parts of the examination may be uncomfortable, but usually not painful. The patient should be urged to let the physician know of any pain or unusual discomfort during any part of the procedure, and to offer any complaint that has not previously been made known.

Physical Examination Format ....

In reviewing the medical history form in the previous chapter (see Figure 5–2), you will notice that the section immediately following, "present illness," has all of the areas outlined for recording the findings of the complete physical examination.

The format of the examination section of this form has been extracted and completed in the following text with an explanation of each of the body areas examined. Hopefully, this will help you become familiar with what the doctor does in each section of the physical examination. Even though H & P forms vary in appearance, the contents will be basically the same. In the spaces which say general appearance, skin, mucous membranes, and so on, a brief written description by the examiner is far more helpful for future reference than just writing "normal," or its equivalent N (negative or normal) or simply drawing a straight line which means, no comment.

Notice that the very first part of the physical includes measurement, vital signs, and vision screening, which the medical assistant normally completes. You may want to refer to appropriate units to review these procedures.

The instruments and equipment to be used in examining each area of the body are in bold print at the beginning of each section where necessary or appropriate. Certainly the patient's chart, pens (one with black ink, and one with red for alerting allergies), and any forms (laboratory request or others) necessary for completion should be at the disposal of the physician and the medical assistant to begin the examination.

(taken from the "in depth" medical history form)

Patient _____ Date _____

PHYSICAL EXAMINATION:

Ht.— recorded in: _____ cm (centimeters) or _____ "
(inches) or _____ ' (feet) and " (inches)

Wt.— recorded in _____ kg (kilograms) or _____ lbs
(pounds)

Temp.—recorded in degrees of _____ Fahrenheit or
_____ Centigrade

Pulse—recorded _____ per minute

Respirations— recorded _____ per minute

Blood Pressure—**stethoscope, sphygmomanometer**—Readings should be taken and recorded from both right and left arms and marked appropriately. It is generally advised that two or more readings be taken, preferably from two different positions (i.e., sitting and standing) and recorded as such.

General Appearance—This generally describes the patient and the state of health, such as "Mr. G. is a spirited, energetic, medium built, well-groomed 34-year-old Hispanic male who has a history of allergies. He has no speech or hearing defects."

Skin—Includes inspection of color (or discoloration), texture, temperature, and assessment of the condition of the hair and nails, as well as lesions, rashes, masses, or swollen areas, scars, wounds, warts, moles, bruises, or any other significant changes the patient reports.

Eyes—Vision: OD 20/30 OS 20/25 OU 20/30

Ishihara—Record plate numbers that are both seen and not seen by the patient for evaluation or physician may write that the patient's color vision is intact for red and green or normal or abnormal after interpreting the results of the test.

Near Vision—Record the number of the line that the patient can read most easily on the Jaeger card. Physician will determine if the patient's near distance acuity is normal or abnormal from test results.

Pupil—Fundus—**ophthalmoscope, tonometer**—The physician uses the ophthalmoscope to look deep into the center of the eye to check the condition of the tiny capillaries behind the retina; if there are no abnormalities there will be what is called a *red reflex,* or a red reflection that fills the pupil as the examiner views the eye. Then testing the pupils for reaction to light is done. During this part of the exam the overhead light is temporarily turned off (by the medical assistant) so that the doctor can watch for pupilary constriction, which if normal will happen right away. The patient is

FIGURE 6–2 Schioetz tonometer (Courtesy of J. Jamner Surgical Instruments Inc.)

instructed to keep looking straight ahead while this is done in both eyes. The examiner looks to see if the patient has eyelashes and brows (or not); checks ocular tension; if the patient exhibits a stare or any ocular protrusion; if the sclera is white; if there is any defect of the cornea or iris; if the pupils are round and equal in size, and if they react to light and accommodation (**L & A**). At some point during this part of the exam, the examiner will test the patient's **peripheral** vision and the horizontal and vertical fields. These tests are several hand or finger movements made by the doctor, which the patient is instructed to follow while the doctor observes. A test with the tonometer may be done next to detect **glaucoma**. There are several different types of tonometers; a picture of a commonly used one is shown in Figure 6–2. It measures the intraocular pressure by determining the resistance of the eyeball to an indentation made from an applied force. Assistance with this procedure consists of preparation (by instilling drops to anesthetize the eyes), instruction regarding the procedure, positioning the patient, and handing the instrument to the physician.

Ears—**otoscope, tuning fork**—The examiner inspects the ears for size and for any abnormalities, such as lesions or nodules, or diagonal creasing of the lobe. The otoscope is used to examine the inner ear. Refer to Figure 6–2 for use of the otoscope. The physician traditionally assesses the hearing during examination of the ear with the tuning fork.

Nose—**nasal speculum, penlight (otoscope), alcohol-saturated gauze square**—The physician checks for any outward signs of abnormalities, and then uses a nasal speculum to view the right and left nostril for any lesions, obstructions, **exudate,** tenderness or swelling. A test to check the sense of smell often is done at this point by having the patient close the eyes and identify a common substance such as alcohol.

Oral Mucous Membranes—**penlight, tongue depressor, sterile gauze square, laryngeal mirror, stethoscope**—The physician looks into the oral cavity with a penlight or by using the light of the otoscope (without the ear speculum attached), to check for any unusual condition of the teeth, tongue, throat,

FIGURE 6–3   The doctor performs auscultation of the neck to listen to the blood flow through the carotid artery.

FIGURE 6–4   Palpation of the patient's axillary region by the examiner

6–4. This allows the examiner to feel any nodules, lumps, swelling, or any other abnormal condition of the patient. Percussion is the next means of examination in which the doctor taps the fingers over several areas of the chest to evaluate the condition of the underlying structures. Figure 6–5 shows the examiner using blunt percussion to examine the kidney. The stethoscope is used finally in examining the chest to allow the physician to hear the sounds within the chest cavity, including

and so on. The patient is asked to tilt the head back, hold the mouth open, stick out the tongue, and say, "ahh," while the physician uses the tongue depressor, or a gauze square to hold the tongue to the side during the exam of the floor of the mouth. A laryngeal mirror may be used here to check areas difficult to view in the mouth, besides looking down the throat of the patient. It is a good opportunity to remind patients at this point to brush their teeth and use dental floss after eating and have regular dental checkups (especially if there is a noticeable need for dental care). The pharynx and neck are generally examined next by palpation. By auscultation the physician listens to the carotid artery bloodflow for any abnormal sounds. The sound made by the blockage of the carotid artery is referred to as bruit, Figure 6–3.

Chest—**stethoscope**—During this portion of the exam, the patient's gown must be removed to the waist so the physician can inspect the chest for visual signs of abnormality, such as lesions, tumors, swelling, skin disorders, and so forth, as well as observe the patient's breathing. The back is also checked in this manner. The chest is normally examined next by the physician palpating several areas, including the neck and axillary region by using the hands placed against the skin, Figure

FIGURE 6–5   The examiner uses blunt percussion to examine the kidney

breath sounds in the lungs and the heartbeat. The doctor will ask the patient to breathe through the mouth to make the sounds easier to hear while using the stethoscope.

Breasts—The inspection of the size, shape, **symmetry,** and position of the breasts and nipples is done first, then palpation while the patient is sitting and then lying down. The examiner looks for abnormalities, such as tenderness, discharge from the nipples, swelling or masses, lumps or nodules, **dimpling,** skin disorders, and any other signs of disease. Routinely, patient education should be done at this point in urging breast self-examination after her monthly menstrual period and in scheduling mammograms. An instruction booklet should be provided for the patient to take home, Figure 6–6. Men are also examined for abnormalities of the breasts.

Heart—**stethoscope**—Evidence of heart disease is indicated by many other areas of the body besides the findings from examination of the heart. The examiner visually inspects the chest and then palpates the chest wall to determine the cardiac border. The stethoscope is used to listen to the chambers of the heart to detect different characteristic heart sounds. The physician has the patient move into several positions to achieve maximum **audibility,** for instance, lying down, sitting up, leaning forward, while the doctor listens for any abnormal sounds, such as a heart **murmur.**

Lungs—See chest section.

Abdomen—**stethoscope**—Refer to Figure 6–7 for an out-lined description of the organs within the nine areas of the abdominal cavity. This will help you to understand the purpose of the various techniques used by the physician during the examination. For successful examination of the abdominal cavity, the patient should be lying in the supine position with the head supported by a pillow. The arms should be to the side or folded across the chest. The medical assistant should help the patient into position. You should place a drape sheet over the patient to provide privacy. The physician will inspect the skin (refer to discussion of skin previously), and proceed with the exam, usually in this order: inspection, auscultation, palpation, and percussion. The examiner looks for any abnormalities some of which may include hernias, masses, tenderness, or enlargement of organs.

Genitalia—**For both male and female patients, this is an ideal time to stress the importance of using latex condoms during sexual intercourse (vaginal and anal) each and every time.**

Males—**latex gloves, water-soluble lubricant**—(The physician wears latex gloves for this exam.) In general, the doctor inspects the external genitalia for gross **asymmetry,** comparing one side to the other, and checks for any deformities, lesions, swelling or masses, or varicosities, and if the patient has pubic hair or not. Skin temperature is also noted to determine circulation. The penis is examined for lesions, scars, masses, tumors, edema, and discharge. The scrotum is pal-

HOW TO DO BSE

1. Lie down and put a pillow under your right shoulder. Place your right arm behind your head.

2. Use the finger pads of the three middle fingers on your left hand to feel for lumps or thickening. Your finger pads are the top third of each finger.

3. Press hard enough to know how your breast feels. If you're not sure how hard to press, ask you health care provider. Or try to copy the way your health care provider uses the finger pads during a breast exam. Learn what your breast feels like most of the time. A firm ridge in the lower curve of each breast is normal.

4. Move around the breast in a set way. You can choose either the circle (A), the up and down (B), or the wedge (C). Do it the same way every time. It will help you to make sure that you've gone over the entire breast area, and to remember how your breast feels each month.

A   B   C

5. Now, examine your left breast using right hand finger pads.

You might want to check your breasts while standing in front of a mirror right after you do your BSE each month. You might also want to do an extra BSE while you're in the shower. Your soapy hands will glide over the wet skin making it easy to check how your breasts feel.

FIGURE 6–6   Breast self-examination (Courtesy of the American Cancer Society)

Right Hypochondriac	Epigastric	Left Hypochondriac

Right lobe of liver
Gallbladder
Part of duodenum
Hepatic flexure of
    colon
Part of right kidney
Suprarenal gland
	Pyloric end of
	    stomach
	Duodenum
	Pancreas
	Aorta
	Portion of liver
		Stomach
		Spleen
		    Tail of pancreas
		    Splenic flexure of
		    colon
		Upper pole of left
		    kidney

Right Lumbar	Umbilical	Left Lumbar

Ascending colon
Lower half of
    right kidney
Part of duodenum
    and jejunum
	Omentum
	Mesentery
	Transverse colon
	Lower part of
	    duodenum
	Jejunum and
	    ileum
		Descending colon
		Lower half of left
		    kidney
		Parts of jejunum
		    and ileum

Right Inguinal	Hypogastric	Left Inguinal

Cecum
Appendix
Lower end of ileum
Right ureter
Right spermatic
    cord in male
Right ovary in
    female
	Ileum
	Bladder
	Pregnant
	    uterus
		Sigmoid colon
		Left ureter
		Left spermatic
		    cord in male
		Left ovary in
		    female

FIGURE 6–7 The nine sections of the abdominal cavity with underlying visceral organs.

pated for content and then each side is pressed upward (palpated) while the patient holds his arms over his head and pushes downward with the abdominal muscles while the examiner observes for hernias (the patient is instructed to cough during the exam to detect any discomfort with abdominal straining). The physician places a gloved index finger (with water-soluble lubricant) into the rectum to examine the prostate gland and further check the patient internally for **inguinal hernia.** The patient usually stands for the exam; the examiner is seated. Patient education in testicular self-examination (TSE) to **detect** tumors of the testes is appropriate during this portion of the exam, Figure 6–8. Distributing pamphlets is recommended because of the increasing numbers of cases of testicular cancer being reported in young men aged 20 to 35. Early detection may save lives!

Female—**latex gloves, vaginal speculum, water-soluble lubricant, gooseneck lamp, tissues**—Refer to Unit 4 of this chapter for in-depth information regarding the gynecological (GYN) exam. At the time the patient schedules the CPE, she should receive instructions regarding this section of the exam. In general, female patients are advised not to **douche** or engage in sexual intercourse for 24 to 48 hours before the appointment. It is preferred that she make the appointment

either before or after the menstrual period (findings may be masked or misinterpreted during menses. Also remind her that routine vaginal douching should be done only by the direction of the physician). This part of the exam is often referred to as a pelvic exam. In general, you may help the patient lie down and then into the lithotomy position by placing your hand at the edge of the exam table and asking the patient to scoot down until she can feel your hand (the buttocks should be just at the edge of the table). Assist the patient in placing the feet in the stirrups and provide a drape for privacy. (The physician wears latex gloves for this exam.) The gooseneck lamp should be placed at the end of the examining table to aid in visual inspection. The physician first inspects the external genitalia for lesions or ulcers, reddening, scratches, edema, inflammation, tumors, cysts or masses, scarring, varicosities, bleeding, or discharge. During this exam, the patient should be instructed to try to relax and breathe slowly and deeply through the mouth. The vaginal speculum is warmed with water before being inserted into the vagina. This part of the exam is for internal inspection and to access vaginal and cervical scrapings, cultures, and **cytological** specimens. Using a water-soluble lubricant, a bimanual exam is performed to determine any abnormalities in the female reproductive organs. Offer tissues to the patient fol-

These symptoms may be evident with testicular cancer:
— a heavy feeling
— a dragging sensation
— the accumulation of fluid
— breast tenderness

The American Cancer Society recommends that men:
1. begin monthly TSE at 15 years of age;
2. perform careful 3 minute exam following a warm shower or bath when scrotal skin is relaxed;
3. observe for any changes in appearance;
4. manually examine each testis by gently rolling it between fingers and thumbs of both hands to check for any hard lumps or nodules.

FIGURE 6–8 Testicular self-examination. Men should be advised to be examined by a physician as soon as possible if there are any abnormal findings with TSE

lowing this procedure to remove excess lubricant. Help the patient out of the stirrups and to a sitting position. Your role in assisting is to hand items to the physician as needed and to offer the patient your support.

Rectum—Male—**latex gloves, water-soluble lubricant, guaiac test paper, tissues**—The patient stands with feet apart and bends over the examination table or is placed in the knee-to-chest position. The physician, wearing latex gloves and using a water-soluble lubricant, spreads the buttocks and inspects the patient for lesions, **fistulas,** external hemorrhoids, prolapse, or any other abnormalities. The internal exam determines **sphincter** control and any abnormalities and is performed as part of the examination of the genitalia (see above). It is followed by a guaiac test for **occult** blood by the placing of a small amount of stool from the gloved finger on the test paper.

Female—**latex gloves, water soluble lubricant, guaiac test paper, tissues**—The physician wears latex gloves for this exam. A water-soluble lubricant is used to insert the index finger into the rectum to palpate sphincter control, any fistulas, tumors, hemorrhoids, **prolapse,** or any other abnormalities. A guaiac test for occult blood is performed by placing a small amount of stool on the test paper from the gloved finger.

Vagina—see above, female genitalia.

Extremities—**tape measure**—This is a general overall examination of inspection that the physician does during the course of the examination. It begins with the head and neck, and includes evaluation of the patient's gait and posture, the appearance of the back, arms and legs. The examiner also looks for muscle strength, the condition of the patient's circulation, and the range of motion (ROM) of the joints. Sometimes measurements of the chest, arms, and legs are done at this point in the examination with a flexible tape measure and recorded in the patient's chart.

Reflexes—**percussion hammer**—The patient sits on the exam table with the legs dangling at the side. The patient must be relaxed during these procedures to elicit an involuntary reaction or response (as the absence of such response could mean neuropathy) as the physician strikes the tendon of each extremity. The examiner watches the response of the limb as contraction of the stretched muscle causes the sudden movement. The reflexes tested are biceps, triceps, patellar, Achilles, and plantar, Figure 6–9, page 328.

Lymph nodes—The physician palpates the lymph nodes of the neck, axilla, inguinal, and abdominal areas of the body during the course of the examination to determine if infection is present. Enlargement of these nodes may indicate infection; clustering of nodes may indicate pathology (see Figure 6–4).

In addition to the many examinations already discussed, the physician normally includes many others, such as:

1. *Romberg balance test*—Performed to detect any muscle abnormality. The patient stands with feet together and eyes open; if the balance seems all right, the examiner asks the patient to close the eyes. If there is any muscle abnormality, the patient possibly will fall. You should assist by standing close to help prevent this from happening.

2. Other tests involve checking for **coordination** and may include
   a. The patient sits up and spreads the arms out wide, and touches the fingertip to the nose, first the right and then the left quickly, with eyes open and then closed, Figure 6–10, page 329.
   b. The heel-to-shin test is performed by the patient while lying in the supine position; first the right heel traces the left leg down from the knee, and then the left heel down right leg; may also be done while patient stands.
   c. Alternating motion is a test that may involve tapping the foot or clapping.
   d. The heel-to-toe test of coordination requires having the patient touch the right heel to the left great toe, and then the left heel to the right great toe; it can be done while the patient is standing or lying down. The patient is observed and evaluated by the examiner.

Remarks—Physicians note additional observations of important information concerning the patient in this section of the form, such as, birth mark or scar, is noted.

Diagnosis (Diagnoses)—Here the physician makes a deci-

A Patient sitting

Patient lying down

B Patient sitting

Patient lying down

C Patient sitting

D Patient sitting

Patient lying down

Patient lying down

E

FIGURE 6–9 Percussion hammer is used by physician to test (a) biceps, (b) triceps, (c) patellar, (d) Achilles, (e) plantar reflexes

FIGURE 6–10 The physician observes the patient as the finger is touched to the nose to determine normal coordination

sion about the patient's condition based on the health history, symptoms, examination findings, and any other procedures and laboratory tests thought necessary to confirm the decision. The term, **R/O,** or *rule/out,* may be used to indicate that there is not yet conclusive evidence in the decision concerning a patient's condition or in confirming a diagnosis, such as, R/O gallbladder disease, (awaiting diagnostic X-ray studies).

Treatment—This section of the form is where all measures for management of the care of the patient are listed, including diet, exercise, physical therapy, medication, surgery, and any others.

Following the completion of the physical examination, the physician will usually leave the patient's chart in the chart holder on the door or in some other designated area for the medical assistant. You should then check the chart for orders to perform any additional procedures for the patient, such as ECG, lab tests, scheduling X rays, or an appointment with a specialist, and so on. After you have finished the procedures, you should write your initials after each one signifying that you completed the orders.

Always be sure to help the patient down from the examination table. Often after sitting there for some time, especially if the (elderly) patient has been lying down, he or she can become dizzy or lightheaded, and there is the possibility of a fall, which you could prevent. You may also offer the courtesy of assisting them in getting dressed when appropriate, again, with the elderly. Answer any questions they may have about the follow-up appointment or further studies. Always let the patient know how long to expect to wait for reports from lab, radiology, or other diagnostic procedures. Tell them when to call and with whom to speak when they phone for the report. It is a common practice to give the patient an appointment a week to 10 days after the physical for a report of the findings; others mail a report, Figure 6–11. Still others phone the patient or have the patient phone the office at a specific day and time. Whatever the policy where you are employed, you must realize that the patient is usually very concerned about what the physician will find and waiting makes the anxiety far worse. Letting patients know about their health status as soon as possible in a professional manner will be appreciated. Filing reports and phoning patients are also duties of the clinical medical assistant.

Patients may ask how often they need to have a physical or a checkup as they call it. You may use Table 6–2 as a guide in giving advice to adult patients about examination and specialty procedures routinely performed on patients. Some physicians recommend annual physicals for their patients, others every 2 to 3 years unless a specific or chronic medical problem exists. The age of the patient has some consideration in this matter. Pediatric patients should be examined more often than adults and monitored very closely since their growth and development, especially the first year, is so rapid. Initially infants are examined by the physician in the office or clinic at age 3 to 4 weeks. Diet and nutritional concerns are discussed and any laboratory tests or procedures are performed during each of these appointments besides the actual exam. At age 2 months the baby has a checkup and begins the immunization schedule (you will learn about this in detail in Chapter 10). At 4 and 6 months the baby has checkups and continues with the initial series of immunizations. Additional exams and immunizations are generally scheduled for the child at ages 9, 12, 15, and 18 months. Even though there are no immunizations needed again until between 4 and 6 years old, children should have annual examinations to detect any diseases or abnormal condition.

From the desk of Dr. H. N. Finklestein

(Today's date)

Dear Mr. G.:

We are pleased to inform you that the results of your physical examination, lab tests, EKG, and Chest x-ray were normal. Your next physical exam should be scheduled within the next 2 - 3 years unless you experience any medical problems. Please feel free to call if you have any further questions or concerns, or if we can be of service to you.

Sincerely,

H.N. Finklestein MD

H.N. Finklestein, M.D.

FIGURE 6–11 Example of report of physical exam

TABLE 6–2
Physical Examination Schedule

Procedure	Age
Electrocardiogram	PRN with **baseline** established at 40 if not before, thereafter as indicated
Eye exam	Tonometry and funduscopy at 40, then every 4 years
H & P	Every 3 years between ages 20–30 Annually after 40
Mammogram	Baseline at 35, then annually
PAP test pelvic	Begin age 20 (or whenever female becomes sexually active), annually thereafter
Pulmonary function tests	PRN for high-risk patients, chronic obstructive pulmonary disease and smokers
Sigmoidoscopy	two consecutive at 50, every 3–5 years thereafter
Rectal exam	Begin at 40, then annually
Stool for guaiac	Begin at 40, then annually
Thyroid screening	PRN; baseline at menopause; females every 2 years

This physical exam schedule is meant to serve as a guide. The medical needs of patients will vary as will physicians' recommendations.

You will, however, have to check with the physician who employs you, for office policies may vary.

The examinations discussed in this unit are by no means the only ones performed in medical offices and clinics. You will learn many others as you gain experience and knowledge in assisting. To learn other instruments used in medical offices or clinics, refer to the appendix of this text.

Complete Chapter 6, Unit 1 in the workbook to help you meet the objectives at the beginning of this unit and therefore achieve competency of this subject matter.

U N I T   2

Positioning and Draping for Examinations

OBJECTIVES ....

Upon completion of this unit, you will meet the following terminal performance objectives by verifying knowledge of the facts and principles presented through oral and written communication at a level deemed competent by the instructor or employer, and will demonstrate the specific behaviors as identified in the terminal performance objectives of the procedures,

observing all aseptic and safety precautions in accordance with health care standards.

1. Explain the purpose of each of the examination positions.
2. Demonstrate the proper method of positioning and draping patients for the various examinations.
3. Discuss safety precautions regarding both the medical assistant and patient in positioning for examinations.
4. Spell and define, using the glossary at the back of the text, all the words to know in this unit.

WORDS TO KNOW ....

anterior	horizontal recumbent
body mechanics	incompetent
dorsal	lithotomy
dowel	postpartum prolapsed
dyspneic	prone
fenestrated	shock
flexed	supine
genucubital	Trendelenburg
genupectoral	

Positioning and Draping Patient ....

Positioning the patient for examination is an important function of the medical assistant. There are a number of standard positions for specific examinations and treatments, which you should know. If a power table is used, you must learn how to operate it. The power table illustrated in Figure 6–12 is considered to be the most advanced power examination table in America. It is possible to program this table to the best height for the physicians who will use it and to the positions desired. The desired position is then achieved by the press of a button. This table has an optional plug-in foot control that could be used in the event of a failure in the computer circuit. This table also has two rolls of paper under the

> **PATIENT EDUCATION**
>
> Instruct the patient about the need for a specific position for the examination to be performed. This information should be included with the instructions on preparing for the examination. The patient must understand that the physician needs to examine certain parts of the body or perform certain procedures and tests, and the patient must be positioned in the most accessible manner.

A

B

FIGURE 6–12 (a). Midmark power table (b). Control panel
(Courtesy Midmark Corporation)

Assist Patient to Horizontal Recumbent Position

TERMINAL PERFORMANCE OBJECTIVE: In a simulated situation, using an appropriately prepared examining table and drape, assist the patient to assume the horizontal recumbent position while providing for safety and privacy according to standards identified in the procedure sheet.

1. Check examination room for cleanliness. *Note:* Always have clean paper on table and a clean pillow cover or clean towel over pillow. **RATIONALE: Every precaution must be maintained to prevent any possible cross-contamination of disease.**
2. Identify patient. **RATIONALE: Speaking to the patient by name and checking the chart ensures that you are performing the procedure on the correct patient.**
3. Give clear instructions to the patient regarding amount of clothing to be removed and where it is to be placed.
4. Instruct patient on use of gown. **RATIONALE: The procedure to be performed dictates whether the front or back should be open.**
5. Assist patient if help is needed. Otherwise respect privacy and modesty of patient by leaving room while patient changes.

6. Instruct patient to sit on side of table.
7. Instruct patient to lie flat on table with legs together.
8. Pull out end extension on table for leg support if needed.
9. Patient may rest head on small pillow if desired.
10. Instruct patient to cross arms on chest or put them at sides of body. To postion for dorsal recumbent, ask patient to put bottoms of both feet flat on table with knees flexed.
11. Drape sheet evenly over patient but leave loose on all sides. For vaginal or rectal examination, drape patient with one corner of sheet over chest, a corner wrapped around each leg, and fourth corner over pubic area. Physician will turn back sheet at pubic area.
12. Assist physician as necessary with examination.
13. Assist patient from table if help is needed when examination is completed. Patients may be dizzy from an abrupt change in position.
14. Clean room and replace supplies. *Note: Examination table surface and base must be thoroughly cleaned with disinfecting cleanser at regular intervals and following any contact with body fluids which may contain bloodborne pathogens.*

FIGURE 6–13 Examination positions: (a). Horizontal recumbent. (b). Dorsal recumbent. (c). Dorsal recumbent with diamond drape

frame at the head of the table so you should never run out of paper.

Most examination tables are vinyl-covered and easily cleaned with antiseptic soap and a sponge or cloth if any body fluids after being examined. The table needs to be cleaned regularly. The table is covered with a roll of paper, which needs to be the proper width to cover the table. The paper roll is usually inserted on a **dowel** under the head of the table and is secured at the bottom of the table with a strap. The strap is useful in

your practice of tearing off the paper when you pull down a clean paper for the next patient.

A female medical assistant should remain in the room when a female patient is being examined by a male physician. The patient should feel more relaxed and the physician is protected from lawsuits that could result from patients claiming the physician acted improperly during the examination. Patient gowns and drapes are made of cloth or disposable paper. The patient is instructed on the use of the gown to avoid unnecessary exposure. If the examination table is too high for the patient to sit on it comfortably, a foot stool should be provided. A very ill patient or a small child should never be left alone on a table; a member of the family may be asked to sit with them if you must leave the room.

Body mechanics are important. Never try to lift a patient who is obviously bigger than you can safely handle; have someone help you. If a patient needs help in moving on the table, reach under the arm at the shoulder and help the person move up. If it is necessary to help a patient out of a wheelchair, position the chair and lock the wheels before trying to help the patient move from the chair to the table. A procedure for this will be given later. The standing erect or anatomical position may be used especially for neurological examination, range of motion, and flexibility while the patient is being instructed by the physician in bending and walking. This position begins with the patient standing upright with arms at sides and palms facing forward. If the patient is well enough to sit on the edge or end of the table with feet hanging down and no back support this position may be used to begin the examination.

The **horizontal recumbent,** or **supine,** position is used for examination and treatment of the **anterior** surface of the body and for X rays, Figure 6–13. The term *dorsal recumbent* is used to indicate that the legs are **flexed.** This position allows for relaxation of the abdominal muscles and thus easier examination of the abdominal area. This position may also be used for vaginal or rectal examination and to test reflexes. The gown is open in the front and a drape sheet of cloth or paper is used to cover the patient. The **prone** position is used for examination of the back or spine, with the gown open in the back, Figure 6–14.

Sims' position is used in examination and treatment of the rectal area, for enemas, rectal temperature, and sigmoidoscopy, Figure 6–15. This position may also be used for pelvic examinations. This is also called the lateral position.

FIGURE 6–14 Prone position

FIGURE 6–15 Sims' position

P R O C E D U R E

Assist Patient to Prone Position

TERMINAL PERFORMANCE OBJECTIVE: In a simulated situation, using an appropriately prepared examining table and drape, assist the patient to assume the position while providing for safety and privacy according to standards identified in the procedure sheet.

1. Check examination room for cleanliness. *Note:* Always have clean paper on table and a clean cover or clean towel over pillow.
2. Identify patient. **RATIONALE: Speaking to the patient by name ensures that you are performing the procedure on the correct patient.**
3. Give clear instructions to patient regarding amount of clothing to remove and where it is to be placed.
4. Instruct patient on use of gown—to be open in back. Some offices furnish a modesty gown with a rectangular piece of material to be put on diaper fashion and tied on sides. If so, instruct in use.
5. Assist patient if necessary. Otherwise respect privacy of patient by leaving room while patient undresses.
6. Instruct patient to sit on side of table.
7. Instruct patient to lie flat on table with legs together.

8. Pull out end extension on table for leg support if needed.
9. Cover patient with drape sheet and instruct patient to turn toward you onto stomach, being careful to stay in center of table to avoid a fall. *Note:* Always instruct patient to turn toward your body to prevent a fall. You can grasp cover drape and keep it smoothly in place as patient turns over.
10. Instruct patient to turn head to side.
11. Instruct patient to flex arms at elbows with hands at side of head.
12. Drape sheet evenly and loosely on all sides.
13. Assist physician as necessary with examination.
14. Instruct patient to turn on back, being careful to stay in middle of table to avoid fall.
15. Instruct patient to sit up for a moment to regain balance before trying to leave table.
16. Clean room and replace supplies. *Note: The examination table surface and base must be thoroughly cleaned with disinfecting cleanser at regular intervals and following any contact with body fluids which may contain bloodborne pathogens.*

FIGURE 6–16 Knee-chest position

The knee-chest position is used for rectal examination and specifically for sigmoidoscopy examination, Figure 6–16. When properly done this position helps straighten out the sharp curve in the sigmoid colon and makes it safer and easier to pass the sigmoidoscope. This position is sometimes called the **genupectoral** and is used as therapy for a **postpartum prolapsed** uterus. The position is difficult to assume and to maintain for a long period of time. Special care must be taken to keep the patient from falling.

Fowler's position is used for patients with respiratory or cardiovascular problems, Figure 6–17. The patient who is dys-

FIGURE 6–17 Fowler's positions: (a). semi: (b). high

PROCEDURE

Assist Patient to Sims' Position

TERMINAL PERFORMANCE OBJECTIVE: In a simulated situation, using an appropriately prepared examining table and drape, assist the patient to assume the horizontal recumbent position while providing for safety and privacy according to standards identified in the procedure sheet.

1. Check examination room for cleanliness. *Note:* Always have clean paper on table and a clean cover or clean towel over pillow.
2. Identify patient. **RATIONALE: Speaking to the patient by name ensures that you are performing the procedure on the correct patient.**
3. Give clear instructions to patient regarding amount of clothing to remove and where it is to be placed.
4. Instruct patient on use of gown. **RATIONALE: The procedure to be performed dictates whether the front or back should be open.**
5. Assist patient if needed. Otherwise respect privacy and modesty of patient by leaving room while patient undresses.
6. Instruct patient to sit on side of table.
7. Instruct patient to lie on left side. A pillow may be placed under head.
8. Instruct patient to place left arm and shoulder behind body. This places weight of body on chest.
9. Instruct patient to flex right arm with hand toward head in front of body.
10. Instruct patient to flex left leg slightly with buttocks near edge of table, being sure patient does not fall.
11. Instruct patient to flex right leg sharply toward chest.
12. Cover patient with a **fenestrated** drape. If a regular sheet is used, hang drape free from under arms to below knees. Edge will be turned back for procedure.
13. Assist physician as necessary with examination.
14. Instruct patient to turn to back, sit up, and then move from table.
15. Clean and replace supplies. *Note: The examination table surface and base must be thoroughly cleaned with disinfecting cleanser at regular intervals and following any contact with body fluids which may contain bloodborne pathogens.*

PROCEDURE

Assist Patient to Knee-Chest Position

TERMINAL PERFORMANCE OBJECTIVE: In a simulated situation, using an appropriately prepared examining table and drape, assist the patient to assume the knee-chest position while providing for safety and privacy, according to standards identified in the procedure sheet.

1. Check examination room for cleanliness. *Note:* Always have clean paper on table and a clean pillow cover or clean towel over pillow.
2. Prepare examination equipment on tray with cover over instruments. Each office will have special equipment, which physician will want you to have ready. Check office procedure manual or make up your own card for each procedure.
3. Identify patient. **RATIONALE: Speaking to the patient by name ensures that you are performing the procedure on the correct patient.**
4. Give clear instructions to patient regarding which clothing to remove and where it is to be placed.
5. Instruct patient on use of gown. **RATIONALE: The procedure to be performed dictates whether the front or back should be open.**
6. Assist patient if needed. Otherwise respect privacy and modesty of patient by leaving room while patient undresses.
7. Instruct patient to sit on side of table.
8. Instruct patient to lie down on table.
9. Cover patient with drape.
10. Instruct patient to turn toward you onto stomach, being careful to stay in middle of table.
11. Instruct patient to get on hands and knees.
12. Instruct patient to flex arms and fold under head, bringing chest down to table. If this is too difficult, have patient rest on elbows (**genucubital** position).
13. Instruct patient to separate knees slightly and keep thighs at right angle to table.
14. A fenestrated drape is usually used, but two small sheets may be draped to meet at rectal area. Diamond drape may also be used.
15. Call physician immediately to complete examination.
16. Assist physician as necessary with examination.
17. Instruct patient to lie flat on stomach and then turn over on back (while lying in middle of table) and sit up before moving from table.
18. Clean room and replace supplies. *Note: The examination table surface and base must be thoroughly cleaned with disinfecting cleanser at regular intervals and following any contact with body fluids which may contain bloodborne pathogens.*

FIGURE 6–18   Lithotomy position

FIGURE 6–19   Trendelenburg position

pneic must be in a sitting or semisitting position to breathe comfortably. This position may be used to examine the trunk of the body (head, neck, and chest area). The position may be semi-Fowler's (partially sitting) or Fowler's (sitting upright). A female patient would be more comfortable in an examination gown opened in front if the sheet covers the chest area on down to the feet.

The **lithotomy** position is used for vaginal or rectal examination, Figure 6–18. This position can also be used for examination of the male genital area and for catheterization of a patient.

In the **Trendelenburg,** or **shock,** position the patient is supine with feet elevated slightly, Figure 6–19. This position may easily be accomplished with a power table. This position may be used for postural drainage with the patient turning into various positions. It can be used for a patient with low blood pressure and to displace organs for some abdominal surgical procedures. This position is also useful as a simple test for **incompetent** valves in persons with varicose veins. After being placed in this position the patient is asked to stand, and the physician observes whether the veins in the legs fill from above or below.

P R O C E D U R E

Assist Patient to Semi-Fowler's Position

TERMINAL PERFORMANCE OBJECTIVE: In a simulated situation, using an appropriately prepared examining table and drape, assist the patient to assume the semi-Fowler's position while providing for safety and privacy according to standards identified in the procedure sheet.

1. Check examination room for cleanliness. *Note: Always have clean paper on the table and a clean pillow cover or clean towel over the pillow.*
2. Identify patient. **RATIONALE: Speaking to the patient by name and checking the chart ensures that you are performing the procedure on the correct patient.**
3. Give clear instructions to patient if clothing is to be removed.
4. Instruct patient on use of gown. **RATIONALE: The procedure to be performed dictates whether the front or back should be open.**
5. Assist patient if needed or leave room while patient undresses.
6. Ask patient to sit at end of table.

7. Raise head of table to desired height for comfort of patient, usually 45-degree angle for semi-Fowler's and completely upright for Fowler's.
8. Ask patient to lean back on rest.
9. Support legs with extension rest at end of table.
10. Drape patient from underarms to below knees.
11. Assist patient as necessary.
12. Ask patient to sit up before lowering head of table. Be sure you understand how to lower head of table. **RATIONALE: Some tables have a release lever, and it is necessary to support head of table with one hand while releasing lever so that head of table will not fall with a crash.**
13. Assist patient from table.
14. Clean room and replace supplies. *Note: The examination table surface and base must be thoroughly cleaned with disinfecting cleanser at regular intervals and following any contact with body fluids which may contain bloodborne pathogens.*

Assist Patient to Lithotomy Position

TERMINAL PERFORMANCE OBJECTIVE: In a simulated situation, using an appropriately prepared examining table and drape, assist the patient to assume the lithotomy position while providing for safety and privacy according to standards identified in the procedure sheet.

1. Check examination room for cleanliness. *Note: Always have clean paper on the table and a clean pillow cover or clean towel over the pillow.*
2. Assemble necessary equipment.
3. Identify patient. **RATIONALE: Speaking to the patient by name and checking the chart ensures that you are performing the procedure on the correct patient.**
4. Give clear instructions to patient to remove clothing from waist down. If breast examination is also to be performed, ask patient to put on a gown.
5. Assist patient if needed or leave room while patient is undressing.
6. Ask patient to sit at end of table.
7. Instruct patient to lie back on table.
8. Support legs with extension on table. (If no extension, be sure patient moves back on table before lying down.) *Note: Newer examination tables allow patient to sit while table is tilted back, leg supports come up under legs, and end of table is lowered, all by use of a foot pedal.*
9. Position stirrups as far away from table as possible and adjust height if necessary. If heels are too close to table and buttocks, patient may get leg cramps.
10. Stabilize stirrups so they will remain in position during examination. *Note: Some tables are designed so that you must turn a knob at side of table. Some tables have several locking positions for stirrups as they swing outward.*
11. Ask patient to move toward end of table while you guide feet into stirrups. *Note: Place the back of your hand against the drape sheet at the end of the table. Request the patient to move until she touches your hand.*
12. Instruct patient to move down so that buttocks are at end of table.
13. Push in table extension, position stool for physician, and position light.
14. Assist physician with examination.
15. Ask patient to slide back up on table.
16. Instruct patient to sit up before moving from table.
17. Offer tissues to remove excess lubricant before dressing.
18. Clean room and replace supplies. *Note: The examination table surface and base must be thoroughly cleaned with disinfecting cleanser at regular intervals and following any contact with body fluids which may contain bloodborne pathogens.*

A special table would be needed for the jackknife position to be comfortable, Figure 6–20. The patient is in a semisitting position with the shoulders elevated and the thighs flexed at right angles to the abdomen. This position is especially useful for examination and instrumentation of the male urethra.

Complete Chapter 6, Unit 2 in the workbook to help you meet the objectives at the beginning of this unit and therefore achieve competency of this subject matter.

FIGURE 6–20 Jackknife position

U N I T 3

Procedures of the Eye and Ear

OBJECTIVES ....

Upon completion of this unit, you will meet the following terminal performance objectives by verifying knowledge of the facts and principles presented through oral and written communication at a level deemed competent by the instructor or employer and will demonstrate the specific behaviors as identified in the terminal performance objectives of the procedures, observing all aseptic and safety precautions in accordance with health care standards.

1. Discuss patient education concerning the eye and the ear.
2. Assist with examinations of the eye and the ear.
3. Administer screening tests of visual acuity.
4. List and describe screening tests of auditory acuity.
5. Demonstrate the procedure for eye irrigation.
6. Demonstrate the procedure for eyedrop instillation.
7. Demonstrate the procedure for eardrop instillation.
8. Demonstrate the procedure for ear irrigation.
9. Discuss the purpose of the Pelli–Robson and the Vectorvision visual screening chart.
10. Spell and define, using the glossary at the back of the text, all the words to know in this unit.

WORLDS TO KNOW ....

achromatic	lavage
acuity	liaison
anesthetize	occluder
audiometer	OD
auditory	ophthalmic
cerumen	OS
daltonism	otic
decibel	OU
discreet	pertinent
deuteranopia	protanopia
funduscopy	Snellen chart
instill	tonometry
irrigate	tritanopia
Ishihara	vertex
Jaeger	wick

Eye and Ear Examination ....

In assisting with eye and ear examinations, you will be expected to hand instruments to the physician as needed. Assembling the instruments in the order of their use will be most helpful. You will be responsible for making sure that the instruments are clean and in working order. Otoscopes and ophthalmoscopes should be checked to be sure that the light bulbs are providing a strong enough light.

These tiny light bulbs must be changed from time to time because they eventually burn out, as do any other kind of bulbs. If these instruments are the hand-held portable type, the batteries must also be changed periodically. The medical assistant is usually responsible for these minor but important tasks. More popularly used in most medical offices are the wall-mounted units with both otoscope and ophthalmoscope instruments, which have an electrically powered light source.

The ear speculum should be sterilized. Most physicians use the disposable plastic ear speculum, which eliminates the worry of disease transmission. The reusable ones must be washed after every use with a mild detergent and placed in a disinfectant solution for at least 20 minutes before they can safely be reused to examine another patient.

Proper lighting of the examination room is most important, because inspection is a large part of the examination of these sensory systems.

Some patients will need reassurance during the examination because of apprehension caused by an earlier experience or for other reasons. Usually a kind word and a reassuring smile will help them feel at ease, and their cooperation will follow. Remembering their comfort is vital.

Irrigate the Eye

PURPOSE: To irrigate the patient's eye(s) to soothe tissues, relieve inflammation, remove foreign objects, and aid the eye in draining.

EQUIPMENT: Latex gloves, small basin for irrigation solution, towel, emesis basin to catch the solution, bulb syringe or bottle of solution, patient's chart, pen

TERMINAL PERFORMANCE OBJECTIVE: Provided with a mannequin and all equipment required for the eye irrigation procedure, irrigate the eyes of the mannequin; each step of the procedure must be accurately demonstrated in proper order.

1. Wash hands and put on gloves. **CAUTION:** Remember, in order to comply with universal precautions guidelines, gloves must be worn if there is any possibility of coming into contact with blood or any body fluids.
2. Assemble items needed for procedure; prepare solution.
3. Identify patient. **RATIONALE: Speaking to the patient by name and checking the chart ensures that you are performing the procedure on the correct patient.**
4. Explain to patient reason for procedure and how it will be done.
5. Ask patient which position would be more comfortable, sitting or lying down, and assist in draping with towel to protect clothing.
6. Ask patient to tilt head back and to side. Place emesis basin against head for patient to hold to catch solution during irrigation. *Note: Placing a couple of tissues, gauze squares, or a towel between the face and the basin will help prevent the patient from getting wet during the procedure. You may have to hold the basin yourself, Figure 6–21, page 340.*
7. Wipe eye with gauze square from bridge of nose to outer corner to remove any particles before proceeding with irrigation.
8. Fill bulb syringe with ordered solution.
9. Hold affected eye open with thumb and index finger of one hand or with the little finger of the hand in which you are holding the bottle of solution and slowly release the solution over the eye gently and steadily. **RATIONALE: This must be done from inner canthus to outer canthus to prevent any solution from entering other eye, which may not be affected, and for comfort of patient in catching solution at side instead of near nose.**
10. When irrigation is completed, use sterile gauze squares or tissues to blot area dry and make patient comfortable.
11. Record procedure in patient's chart and initial. *Note: Be sure to record type of solution that was used, which eye was irrigated, results, and any other important information you may have observed while performing procedure.*
12. Wash items and return them to proper storage area.
13. Remove gloves and wash hands. *Note: Deposit gloves in an appropriate container based upon the conditions under which irrigation was performed.*

Patients with discharge of the ear or the eye will require **irrigation** (also known as **lavage**) to remove the irritant. The physician will then examine the ear or eye to ensure no damage was done by the discharge. A procedure for this will be given. You may also have the responsibility of **instilling** drops into a patient's eye or ear. This simply means dropping a solution into the patient's eye or ear to medicate the tissue or to soothe an irritation. Sterile technique should be used. Recording the amount of medication and the organ to which it is administered is a must.

Instillation of the ear is also performed to soften cerumen (ear wax). **Cerumen** is a protective secretion of the ear, produced to ward off invading microorganisms. Patients sometimes try to remove it by using a cotton-tipped swab, but often push it farther into the ear canal, where it becomes lodged and hardens. This buildup can be very uncomfortable and eventually impair hearing.

Procedures for eye and ear instillation follow. Sometimes it is necessary to instill medication into the ear to soften ear wax before an irrigation procedure can be performed. Irrigation of the eye and the ear may be ordered before a successful examination can be conducted by the physician.

Patients should have impacted cerumen removed by a member of the health care team to avoid further discomfort or possible injury to the ear. Many offices and clinics have adopted the water pic for this purpose because of the gentle flow it produces and its convenience for irrigation procedures. Some patients will need both irrigation and instillation procedures. A softening solution may be instilled into a severely impacted ear, followed by irrigation to remove the excess ear wax.

After having irrigation procedures performed, even with gentle care, many patients feel a little dizziness. You must be sure that patients are completely stable before permitting them to leave.

Irrigate the Ear

PURPOSE: To irrigate the ear canal to remove foreign objects, impacted cerumen, or to relieve inflammation and swelling.

EQUIPMENT: Latex gloves, small basin for ordered irrigation solution, towel, ear basin to catch solution, Pomeroy or bulb syringe, gauze squares, otoscope, ear speculum, and tissues.

TERMINAL PERFORMANCE OBJECTIVE: Provided with an anatomical model of the ear or a mannequin, and all equipment required for the ear irrigation procedure, first irrigate the anatomical ear, then the ears of the mannequin; in each process the steps of the procedure must be demonstrated in proper order.

1. Wash hands and put on gloves. **CAUTION:** Remember, in order to comply with universal precautions guidelines, gloves must be worn if there is any possibility of coming into contact with blood or any body fluids.
2. Prepare solution as ordered and assemble necessary items for procedure. *Note:* Solution is usually between 100°F and 105°F for patient comfort.
3. Identify patient. **RATIONALE: Speaking to the patient by name and checking the chart ensures that you are performing the procedure on the correct patient.**
4. Explain procedure.
5. View affected ear with otoscope to see where cerumen or foreign object is located so flow of solution can be directed properly. **RATIONALE: The flow should be directed upward and to one side (as you would rinse out a bucket with a hose).** To use the otoscope for viewing the ear canal, place one hand gently against the patient's head and grasp the auricle with your thumb and index finger pulling up and back for adults and down and back for babies up to 36 months. Hold the otoscope with the thumb, index, and great finger of your other hand to avoid using too much pressure as you insert the speculum into the ear canal, Figure 6–22.
6. Ask patient to turn head to side and back. Position ear basin under ear for patient to hold to catch solution as it returns during procedure. Place a towel over patient's shoulder to protect clothing, Figure 6–23. For pediatric patients, ask parent to hold the child on lap and assist you during procedure.
7. Use gauze square to wipe away any particles from outer ear before proceeding.
8. Fill syringe with ordered solution.
9. With one hand, gently pull auricle up and back for an adult (down and back for an infant or small child) **RATIONALE: To straighten ear canal.** With other hand place tip of syringe into canal and aim flow of solution upward so entire ear canal will be irrigated. DO NOT direct the flow of the solution straight into the ear or use force or the result will be quite painful for the patient and may damage the tympanic membrane.
10. Use gauze square to wipe excess solution from outside of patient's ear.
11. Give patient several gauze squares or tissues and have patient hold head tilted to side to allow drainage of excess solution from canal.
12. Inspect ear canal with otoscope to determine if desired results have been obtained. **RATIONALE: All material must be removed to adequately inspect the outer ear and tympanic membrane. Patients sometimes feel a little dizzy following this procedure. Allow the patient time to gain balance; assist patient from the examination table.**
13. Record procedure on patient's chart and initial. *Note:* which ear was irrigated, solution used, the results of the procedure, and any other important observations.
14. Wash equipment and return to proper storage area.
15. Remove gloves and wash hands.

A simple method of medicating the eye is by placing a small amount of ointment just inside the lower eyelid. The tip of the ointment tube must not touch the eyelid, where its contents would become contaminated by the secretions of the eye. Care must also be taken when instilling eyedrops so that the tip of the dropper does not come in contact with the eye.

Visual Acuity

Measuring visual **acuity** is a diagnostic screening procedure most often done by the medical assistant on the patient's initial visit prior to the physical examination. It should be done in a well-lighted room with no interruptions. Observation of the patient for any conditions or behaviors that may indicate visual disturbances is an essential part of the overall examination.

FIGURE 6–21 Irrigation of the eye is also referred to as lavage, which means to wash out.

FIGURE 6–22 The examiner is using the otoscope to view the ear canal. This instrument has a light source and a magnifying lens that assists with inspection.

acuity. This will help you determine whether or not the child is actually having trouble seeing, or if the child simply does not know what to call the letter or symbol you are pointing

The most common screening device for distance vision is a **Snellen chart,** which shows at what distance a patient can read. The regular chart has letters arranged in rows from largest to smallest.

Those who may have difficulty with reading, such as preschool children or non-English speakers, should be tested with the chart or cards of the letter *E* arranged in different directions. Figures 6–26, page 343 and 6–27, page 345, show the various Snellen vision screening charts, which are made to standard specifications. These charts are hung on the wall with a mark 20 feet away to show where the patient should stand or sit to read the chart. The chart should be at the patient's eye level. Charts are available on a lighted view box to increase the visibility of the letters.

Most preschoolers have a short attention span. You may need some assistance in screening them for visual acuity, either by having a parent or guardian help to interpret your instructions to them, or in the positioning and covering of their eyes during the screening process. It is best to familiarize the child with either chart (Big E or Kindergarten) at a short distance before you begin to screen them for visual

FIGURE 6–23 Drape the patient's shoulder and position the basin under the ear. Ask the patient to hold the basin as you position the syringe and straighten the ear canal.

to on the chart. You can make it fun for the child by taking your turn first to read the chart and then letting the child have a turn to read it to you. Remembering to praise the child will encourage good behavior. Usually it is not recommended to screen 3-year-olds below the 30-foot line. Make sure that you pay close attention to the patient (child or adult) during the procedure. The following are suggestions of what observations you should make while performing the test: tilting the head to the side or forward; blinking or watering of eyes; frowning or puckering of the face; closing of one eye when testing both eyes; or any other signs of straining to see.

P R O C E D U R E

Instill Eyedrops

PURPOSE: To instill medication (in the form of drops or ointment) into the eye(s) to relieve irritation; treat infection; dilate the pupil; or **anesthetize** the eye in preparation for an examination or for a surgical procedure.

EQUIPMENT: Latex gloves, ordered medication, sterile eyedropper, sterile gauze squares, tissues

TERMINAL PERFORMANCE OBJECTIVES: Provided with an anatomical model of the eye or a mannequin, and all equipment necessary to perform instillation of the eye, instill drops into the eyes of the anatomical model or of the mannequin; in each process the steps of the procedure must be demonstrated in proper order.

1. Verify medication ordered by physician in the patient's chart (check the expiration date) and assemble necessary items for procedure. **Ophthalmic** medications are often kept in the refrigerator after they have been opened, so it is necessary to bring them to room temperature by allowing the drops to sit out for a while or by running warm water over the bottle before using. This is for the comfort of the patient.

2. Wash hands and put on gloves. **CAUTION:** Remember, in order to comply with universal precautions guidelines, gloves must be worn if there is any possibility of coming into contact with blood or any body fluids.

3. Identify patient. **RATIONALE: Speaking to the patient by name and checking the chart ensures that you are performing the procedure on the correct patient.**

4. Explain procedure to patient.

5. **a.** Open the bottle of ophthalmic medication and draw into the dropper the ordered amount of drops for instillation. (Many prepared eye medications have their own dropper. It is vital that this dropper be used very carefully so as to keep it sterile. DO NOT touch the tip of the dropper to the eye!) **RATIONALE: If the dropper touches anything OTHER THAN the solution INSIDE the bottle it is considered contaminated.**

   b. If the medication ordered is an ointment, you should open the tube by removing the cap, being very careful not to touch the tip or it will become contaminated. Medication should be placed carefully and sparingly just inside the lower eye lid without touching the eye tissue. **RATIONALE: The tip can be contaminated if it is touched or touches any surface.**

6. Ask the patient to sit up straight and tilt the head back slightly (some patients may prefer to lie down). If the patient is very young or uncooperative, you may need to have another's help with holding the patient during the procedure.

7. Hand a couple of tissues to the patient before you begin. With one hand, use a sterile gauze square to touch the patient's skin just under the eye and gently pull down. This will expose a small pocket (a recessed area between the eye just inside the lower lid), Figure 6–24.

8. Hold the dropper steadily approximately $1/4$ inch from the area being careful NOT to touch the tissue. Tell the patient to look up while you gently drop the prescribed amount of drops into the pocket of the patient's eye. Ask the patient to blink to further distribute the medication. *Note: Advise the patient NOT to rub the eye and not to squeeze out the medications from the eyes. Remind the patient to use the tissues to gently blot excess medication from eyes and not to touch the eyes with bare hands.* (This is an ideal time to go over patient education material concerning the eyes.) Repeat for the other eye if ordered.

9. Close the bottle or tube of medication. Avoid touching the dropper to the outside of the bottle. *Note: If you have touched the patient's eye or anything else with the dropper, it must either be sterilized or replaced before any other doses of medication can be taken from the bottle, otherwise the contents will become contaminated.*

10. Remove gloves and wash hands.

11. Record procedure on patient's chart and initial. Be sure to note any complaints of the patient while performing the procedure, i.e., burning or other eye discomfort.

12. Return items to proper storage area.

Instill Eardrops

PURPOSE: To treat infections, relieve pain, and soften ear wax.

EQUIPMENT: Latex gloves, gauze squares, sterile cotton-tipped applicators and cotton balls, sterile dropper, ordered medication (may be in the form of drops or ointment), tissues.

TERMINAL PERFORMANCE OBJECTIVE: Provided with an anatomical model of the ear or a mannequin, and all equipment required to perform the ear installation procedure, first instill drops into the anatomical ear model, and then into the ears of the mannequin; in each process the steps of the procedure must be demonstrated in proper order.

1. Verify medication ordered by physician (and check expiration date) in the patient's chart and assemble necessary items for procedure. **Otic** medications are often kept in the refrigerator after they have been opened, so it is necessary to bring them to room temperature by running warm water over the bottle before using. This is for the comfort of the patient.
2. Wash hands and put on gloves. **CAUTION:** Remember, in order to comply with universal precautions guidelines, gloves must be worn if there is any possibility of coming into contact with blood or any body fluids.
3. Identify patient. **RATIONALE: Speaking to the patient by name and checking the chart ensures that you are performing the procedure on the correct patient.**
4. Explain procedure to patient.
5. **a.** Open the bottle of otic medication and draw into the dropper the ordered amount of drops for instillation. *Note: Many prepared ear medications have their own dropper. It is vital that this dropper be used very carefully so as to keep it sterile. DO NOT touch the tip of the dropper to the ear! It is a good practice to place the lid inside up or on side on a gauze square.* **RATIONALE: If the dropper touches anything OTHER THAN the solution INSIDE the bottle it is considered contaminated.**
   b. If the medication ordered is an ointment, you should open the tube by removing the cap, being very careful not to touch the tip. **RATIONALE: If the tip of the tube or inside of the cap is touched, they are con-**taminated. Medication should be instilled by placing a small amount on the tip of a sterile cotton applicator stick and applying it gently into the ear canal. Use extreme caution to avoid puncturing the tympanic membrane.

6. Ask the patient to sit up straight and tilt the head slightly to the left for instilling the right ear; and to the right for the left ear (some patients may prefer to lie down). If the patient is very young or uncooperative, you may need to have another's help with holding the patient during the procedure.
7. Hand a couple of tissues to the patient before you begin. Hold the auricle of the ear *gently* with one hand, while you hold the dropper in the other. To straighten the ear canal to allow the medication to enter, pull up and back for adults, and down and back for infants and children up to 36 months.
8. Position the dropper with the medication into (but not touching) the ear canal, Figure 6–25. Depress the bulb to release the prescribed amount of drops into the ear. *Note: Advise the patient to remain in this position for a minute or so to allow the medication to settle. Any excess may be wiped away with the tissues or gauze squares. (This is an ideal time to go over patient education material concerning the ears.) Repeat for the other ear if ordered.* Sometimes physicians will request that sterile cotton be inserted into the ear canal to hold the medication in. Simply place a small portion of the sterile cotton ball gently into the canal after instilling the medication; this is sometimes referred to as a **wick.** It is often saturated with the medication before being placed in the ear canal.
9. Close the bottle or tube of medication. Avoid touching the dropper to the outside of the bottle. *Note: If you have touched the patient's ear or anything else, the dropper must be either sterilized or replaced before any other doses of medication can be taken from the bottle.*
10. Remove gloves and wash hands.
11. Record procedure on patient's chart and initial. Be sure to note any complaints of the patient while performing the procedure, i.e., stinging or other discomfort.
12. Return items to proper storage area.

Often while you are preparing the child for this procedure, the parent may offer one or more reasons why the child was brought in for the examination. For instance, the child may hold story books too close to the face or rub the eyes frequently. You should record the symptoms on the patient's chart as well as the results of the visual screening. A list of common complaints that may indicate vision problems are in Table 6–3. These complaints pertain to both children and adults.

FIGURE 6–24 When instructing patients to use eyedrops at home, tell them to tilt the head back, look up (a), and gently pull the skin down just under the eye (b) to form a small pocket where the drops should be instilled

Patients should be screened with and without their corrective lenses and the results recorded as such on their charts. Note that if visual acuity does not exceed 20/200 in the better eye with corrective lenses, the patient is considered legally blind.

The **Jaeger** system is a most common method of screening for near vision acuity. The chart used for this procedure is very small compared with the wall-mounted charts for distance

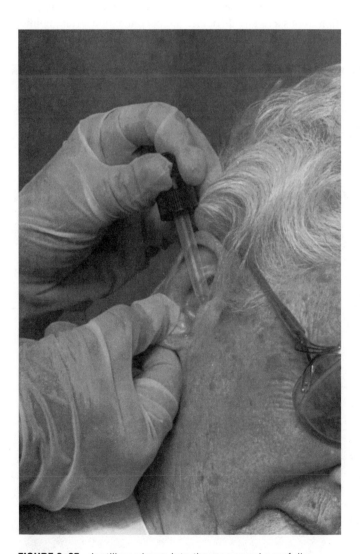

FIGURE 6–25 Instill eardrops into the ear canal carefully

FIGURE 6–26 Snellen visual acuity screening charts. On the left, letters appear in descending sizes; on the right, the letter E appears in various directions and in descending sizes

TABLE 6-3

Possible Indications of Visual Disturbance

During Activities That Require Reading Shows	Illness	Condition	Behaviors	Complaints
1. Difficulty with near or distant vision 2. Avoids reading, writing, and other related activities.	1. Childhood 2. Current infection/condition	1. Redness of the eye(s) or eyelid(s) 2. Crusting or swelling of eyelid(s) or styes 3. Poor eye coordination 4. Watering or discharge 5. Accident or injury to the eye	1. Looks cross-eyed 2. Rubbing eyes frequently 3. Confuses letters, i.e., *a* and *c*, *f* and *t*, *m* and *n* 4. Turns head or leans forward to see better 5. Blinks continually 6. Irritable at attempting close work	1. Blurriness of vision 2. Nausea 3. Headaches often 4. Dizziness 5. Eyes sensitive to light 6. Feels like something in the eye(s)

If a patient has a past history or a current complaint of any of the symptoms listed above, a visual disturbance is suggested.

visual acuity. The card is held by the patient between 14 and 16 inches from the eye. You should measure with a yardstick, meterstick, or a tape measure for accuracy. This is the distance at which one with normal vision is able to read printed material (a newspaper), or work on something that requires close attention (sewing). The Jaeger screening test consists of a series of reading material that has ascending sizes of type ranging from 0.37 mm to 2.5 mm, Figure 6–28, page 346. The test contains excerpts from a variety of paragraphs, none of which are the same. The medical assistant should pay careful attention to observe any difficulty the person exhibits (i.e., holding the chart right in front of the face, squinting, blinking, etc.)

P R O C E D U R E

Screen Visual Acuity with Snellen Chart

PURPOSE: To measure the visual acuity of a patient.

EQUIPMENT: Patient's chart, pen, Snellen chart Figures 6–26 and 6–27, pointer, occular eye **occluder,** card or paper cup.

TERMINAL PERFORMANCE OBJECTIVE: Provided with the necessary vision-screening equipment, measure the visual acuity of at least two other students or visitors by demonstrating each step of the vision-screening procedure; the results of each test will be accurately recorded on the individual patient's chart.

1. Identify patient. **RATIONALE: Speaking to the patient by name and checking the chart ensures that you are performing the procedure on the correct patient.**

2. Explain procedure to patient—that patient is to read each line from the chart as you point to it with pointer.

3. Ask the patient to read the chart with both eyes **(OU)** first, standing 20 feet from the chart.

4. Have patient cover left eye **(OS)** with a card or paper cup. If patient wears corrective lenses, procedure should be performed first wearing lenses and then without and recorded as such.
   Note:
   a. Chart should be at patient's eye level.

   b. Tell patient to keep both eyes open but to cover one eye. This prevents squinting and blurring.

   c. Record any observations of individual accommodations made to read chart, such as squinting, turning head, etc.

   d. Follow office policy in giving test. Asking patients to read only certain lines of chart is sometimes less time-consuming and less tiring for patient. Covering part of chart that is not being read keeps patients from "studying" for their eye test.

5. Record smallest line that patient can read without making a mistake.

6. Have patient cover right eye **(OD),** and test acuity of left, following same procedure.

7. Record the number of the lowest line that the patient can see. Distant visual acuity is written as a fraction, 20/20, which is average. The numerator is the number of feet, or the distance from the chart; the denominator is the numbered line the patient read. If one's distant visual acuity results are 20/100, it means that the person stood 20 feet from the chart and read the line that should be read at 100 feet. One who has 20/10 acuity can see at 20 feet what should be seen at a distance of 10 feet.

FIGURE 6-27 Kindergarten vision screening chart in descending sizes. Pictures must be reviewed with the child at a short distance before testing to be sure the child knows what you are pointing to during the test for accurate results.

while the patient reads this card (Figure 6–29, page 346). The medical assistant records the results on the chart. Record the line number that the patient can read easily. The screening procedure should be conducted in a well-lighted room without interruptions. The patient ought to be tested with and without wearing corrective lenses, and each eye should be tested separately for a complete assessment to be made by the physician.

Many devices for screening for visual acuity are available besides the methods already discussed in this unit. One compact instrument is the Titmus vision tester, Figure 6–30, page 348. In this system of screening, the patient looks into the instrument to view eight different specialized fields designed to detect all common vision problems. While administering this test, the medical assistant sits or stands next to the patient to operate the selection of visual fields. A vision occluder is within the device for testing each eye individually as the patient reads the various lines. Again, the medical assistant must be alert in observing and listening while the patient completes this test. All complaints or observations should be recorded on the patient's chart along with the results of the test. The instrument comes with forms for recording the results of the test.

Color vision acuity means that one can accurately recognize colors. Deficiency in this ability to perceive colors of the spectrum distinctly is commonly termed *color blindness*. This is due to changes that happen in the pigments of the cones in the retina of the eyes as they react to colored lights of red, green, and blue.

There are two primary types of color blindness: (1) **daltonism,** which is the most common, is a visual disorder in which the person cannot tell the difference between red and green. It is an hereditary disorder; and, (2) **achromatic** vision, which is total color blindness, and very rare, where the person cannot recognize any color at all. These people see everything in white, gray, and black. The probable cause for this condition is that the cones in the retina are defective or there may be none at all.

Several other conditions involve one's inability or weakness in distinguishing certain colors. In **deuteranopia,** the person has trouble in telling any difference between varying shades of green and also of bluish reds and neutral shades. **Protanopia** is partial color blindness. These people have trouble with the perception of reds, and sometimes yellows and greens are confused. This condition is often referred to as red blindness. **Tritanopia,** which is the rarest, means that the person cannot distinguish blue color.

A method for screening patients for defects in distinguishing color vision acuity is with the **Ishihara** color plates book. A sample of the series of multicolored charts in the test book is shown in Figure 6–31, page 348. Patients are asked to trace the patterns of color with their finger as you observe them. There are letters and numbers (and curved lines and shapes for nonreaders) that are one color within another. When administering this procedure, make sure that the room is well-lighted, preferably with natural daylight (not direct sunlight), so that the patient is able to follow your instructions without straining to see. Whatever method of color vision assessment is used where you are employed, it is vital that you are accurate in reporting the results. Medical assistants should first be tested to determine if they have normal color vision to administer the test to patients.

All patients with thyroid conditions should routinely be screened for color vision acuity during their scheduled visits.

No. 1.
.37M

In the second century of the Christian era, the empire of Rome comprehended the fairest part of the earth, and the most civilized portion of mankind. The frontiers of that extensive monarchy were guarded by ancient renown and disciplined valor. The gentle but powerful influence of laws and manners had gradually cemented the union of the provinces. Their peaceful inhabitants enjoyed and abused the advantages of wealth.

No. 2.
.50M

fourscore years, the public administration was conducted by the virtue and abilities of Nerva, Trajan, Hadrian, and the two Antonines. It is the design of this, and of the two succeeding chapters, to describe the prosperous condition of their empire; and afterwards, from the death of Marcus Antoninus, to deduce the most important circumstances of its decline and fall; a revolution which will ever be remembered, and is still felt by

No. 3.
.62M

the nations of the earth. The principal conquests of the Romans were achieved under the republic; and the emperors, for the most part, were satisfied with preserving those dominions which had been acquired by the policy of the senate, the active emulations of the consuls, and the martial enthusiasm of the people. The seven first centuries were filled with a rapid succession of triumphs; but it was

No. 4.
.75M

reserved for Augustus to relinquish the ambitious design of subduing the whole earth, and to introduce a spirit of moderation into the public councils. Inclined to peace by his temper and situation, it was very easy for him to discover that Rome, in her present exalted situation, had much less to hope than to fear from the chance of arms; and that, in the prosecution of

No. 5.
1.00M

the undertaking became every day more difficult, the event more doubtful, and the possession more precarious, and less beneficial. The experience of Augustus added weight to these salutary reflections, and effectually convinced him that, by the prudent vigor of

No. 6.
1.25M

his counsels. it would be easy to secure every concession which the safety or the dignity of Rome might require from the most formidable barbarians. Instead of exposing his person or his legions to the arrows of the Parthinians, he obtained, by an honor-

No. 7.
1.50M

able treaty, the restitution of the standards and prisoners which had been taken in the defeat of Crassus. His generals, in the early part of his reign, attempted the reduction of Ethiopia and Arabia Felix. They marched near a thou-

No. 8.
1.75M

sand miles to the south of the tropic; but the heat of the climate soon repelled the invaders, and protected the unwarlike natives of those sequestered regions

No. 9.
2.00M

The northern countries of Europe scarcely deserved the expense and labor of conquest. The forests and morasses of Germany were

No. 10.
2.25M

filled with a hardy race of barbarians who despised life when it was separated from freedom; and though, on the first

No. 11.
2.50M

attack, they seemed to yield to the weight of the Roman power, they soon, by a signal

FIGURE 6–28 The near distance visual acuity screening chart

The procedure should include testing with both eyes first, and then each eye separately to see if there is any difference in the perception of color in either eye. The eye not used should be covered and not held shut. Patients with Grave's disease especially need frequent assessment of their color vision acuity changes to detect possible damage to the optic nerve. In conditions such as this where swelling occurs behind the eye, pressure builds up, and hypertrophy of the tissues results. This interferes with the patient's ability to distinguish colors because the optic nerve is being compressed. The color vision test results may lead to earlier diagnosis and treatment of Grave's ophthalmopathy.

Pelli–Robson Contrast Sensitivity Chart ....

A recent advance in the measurement of visual acuity is the development of the Pelli–Robson contrast sensitivity chart, Figure 6–32, page 348. This chart measures contrast sensitivity by determining the faintest contrast that an observer can see. Recent clinical evidence shows that contrast sensitivity is affected by all of the major eye diseases—diabetic retinopathy, macular degeneration, glaucoma, and cataract. Therefore, mea-

suring contrast sensitivity provides a sensitive screening test for eye disease to provide earlier diagnosis and treatment.

Another contrast-sensitivity-screening method has been developed by Vectorvision. Even though all patients can be tested in this way, it is especially useful in screening small

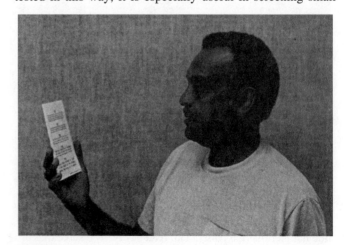

FIGURE 6–29 Patient holds near vision acuity screening card 14 to 16 inches from eyes to read.

Screen Visual Acuity with Jaeger System

PURPOSE: To determine near distance visual acuity of a patient using the Jaeger system.

EQUIPMENT: Jaeger near vision acuity chart, pen, patient's chart

TERMINAL PERFORMANCE OBJECTIVES: Using the Jaeger near vision acuity chart, in a well-lighted area, determine the near distance visual acuity of at least two other students or visitors by demonstrating each step of the visual acuity procedure; the results of each test will be accurately recorded on the individual patient's chart.

1. After identifying the patient, explain the procedure. **RATIONALE: Speaking to the patient by name and checking the chart ensures that you are performing the procedure on the correct patient.**
2. Have the patient sit up straight but comfortably in a well-lighted area.
3. Hand the Jaeger chart to the patient to hold, between

14 and 16 inches from the eyes. Figure 6–29 shows proper positioning of the card.

4. Instruct the patient to read (out loud to you) the various paragraphs of the card with both eyes open, first without wearing corrective lenses and then with. *Note: Each eye should be tested individually having the person cover the left eye first while reading the card and then the right. Observe carefully for any difficulty the patient has in reading any of the lines on the card. Listen also to any remarks made by the patient and note on chart.*
5. Record the results and problems, if any, on the patient's chart to assist the physician in determining the visual acuity of the patient. The smallest line of print that the patient can read should be recorded and initiated.
6. Thank the patient for cooperation and answer any questions.
7. Return Jaeger chart to proper storage.

children, foreigners, and illiterates. This test has a series of four groups of circles. In these rows of circles, some are solid gray colored and some have vertical lines within them. The patient is instructed to look at the first group and tell you which circles have lines within them. The last correctly identified circle in each group is charted on a graph. The results of this test are interpreted by the physician.

Auditory Acuity

The function of the ear is to enable sound to be perceived. If this process is impaired, hearing loss results. Diseases or conditions of the ear, if not treated, can cause damage to nerves and tissues, which may result in mild to complete deafness. Often patients try to hide a problem, such as hearing loss,

Determine Color Vision Acuity by Ishihara Method

PURPOSE: To determine color vision acuity of a patient using the Ishihara method.

EQUIPMENT: Ishihara book, pen, patient's chart

TERMINAL PERFORMANCE OBJECTIVE: Using the Ishihara book in a well-lighted area, determine the color vision acuity of at least two other students or visitors by demonstrating each step of the color vision screening procedure; the results of each test will be accurately recorded on the individual patient's chart.

1. Obtain chart from back of book. *Note:* Before administering this screening test, you should first be tested.
2. Explain procedure to patient.

3. Conduct the test by asking the patient first to read the plates with both eyes (if the patient wears corrective lenses, with them on). A common practice is to ask the patient to trace with the index finger the letters, numbers, or patterns of color printed in the various plates. Continue testing by having the patient cover the left eye to test the right eye, and then cover the right to test the left. Make sure to note any difficulty or complaint of the patient during the screening process.
4. Compare answers with those given on chart. Record frames patient misses and write down what patient reports so that degree of color impairment may be determined by physician.

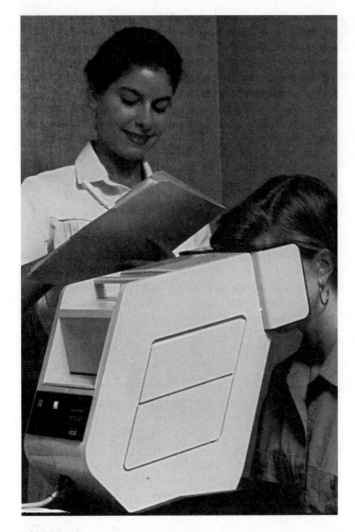

VRSKDR
NHCSOK
SCNOZV
CNHZOK
NODVHR
CDNZS
CSO

FIGURE 6–32 The Pelli–Robson contrast sensitivity chart. The faintest letters that can be read on this chart determine an individual's contrast sensitivity. The use of such a chart is an aid to earlier diagnosis of certain eye diseases.

FIGURE 6–30 The medical assistant records the visual acuity as the patient looks into the Titmus Vision Tester.

because it is an embarrassment to them. They are sometimes afraid they may have to wear a hearing aid or worry that they may need to have an operation. So that they can avoid making a decision, often the patient will try to compensate for the hearing loss by learning to read lips, always turning the best

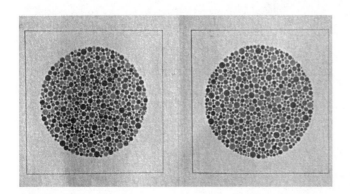

FIGURE 6–31 Sample color plate from Ishihara color acuity test

ear toward the sound source (or pretending that they heard), increasingly turning up the volume on audio equipment, standing very close during conversations, and sometimes by withdrawing from others. The family members of the patient may relate this information to you. You should advise the person to have the patient schedule a time to have the doctor examine the ears and have a hearing test. You should carefully note the information on the patient's chart and bring it to the physician's attention. The physician will discuss the problem with the patient during the scheduled appointment. Sometimes the problem may be as simple as the patient having impacted cerumen, and after an irrigation, the person's hearing usually returns to normal. Sometimes it is not that simple, and further measures are necessary. The medical assistant is in contact with the patient usually more than the physician. It is the assistant's responsibility to act in the best interest of the patient in conveying important information observed. You can watch for many behaviors as you are getting patients ready for their scheduled appointments or when you talk to them over the phone. One of your most important duties is relaying information to the physician about patients.

Common behaviors of patients that indicate they may have lost some hearing ability are: (1) being asked to repeat what you've said frequently during a conversation; (2) inappropri-

FIGURE 6–33 Noise levels associated with selected conditions, locations, and operations

ately loud voice when speaking to you; (3) no response at all when spoken to; (4) does not pronounce words well; and (5) responds only when you speak very loudly. Certain complaints may suggest hearing loss or **auditory** nerve damage. When patients disclose any of the following symptoms you should bring it to the attention of the physician for further assessment:(1) ringing in the ears; (2) decreased hearing in either ear (sometimes caused by impacted cerumen); (3) infection or injury to the ear(s); (4) bleeding or discharge from the ear(s); and (5) any unusual noise or feeling inside the ear(s). These signs, or any others, which patients tell you should be written on the chart during triage. Further examination by the physician is necessary to determine the extent of the problem and its treatment.

An **audiometer** is an instrument used to measure one's hearing. The audiometer determines the hearing thresholds of pure tones of frequencies that are normally audible by an individual. Some also measure bone and air conduction. The threshold of hearing is the point where a sound can barely be heard. A person with normal hearing should hear all frequencies up to 15 **decibels,** depending on the surrounding noise levels, Figure 6–33.

Audiometric devices are powered either by batteries or electricity. Whatever type is used in the facility where you are employed should be checked periodically for proper performance and accuracy. If the batteries need to be changed or if a wire is frayed, it should be taken care of before being used with patients, not only for their safety, but to make sure that it works efficiently. Several types of audiometers are available for use in determining hearing acuity. Many are still used requiring that the operator manually turn a dial to emit the var-

ious frequencies for the patient to hear during the test. Companies that manufacture audiometers offer in-service demonstrations to make sure their equipment is used properly. Operations manuals should be kept with the instrument for handy reference.

The procedure for every audiometer is basically the same. The patient is instructed to place the earphones (marked red for the right ear and blue for the left ear) over the ears. The medical assistant tells the patient in the soundproof booth how the earphones are to be placed and how to work the control signal, Figure 6–34. The printer on the table next to the booth records the results of the hearing test. The printout is called an audiogram, which is filed in the patient's chart after the physician reads the results of the test and makes an evaluation.

During the procedure in whichever ear that is not being tested, the sound is automatically blocked by the machine. In the ear which is being tested, the machine provides a series of tones. The patient listens and signals (either by raising a finger or by using a hand-held control) to the medical assistant as the various sounds are heard. The tones range in frequencies from very low to very high with a varied level of decibel intensity. After the right ear has been tested, the machine switches automatically to test the left ear. The medical assistant should report any complaints that the patient may have had before or during the hearing test and any unusual behavior to the physician. You should make a note of this information on the patient's chart along with the results of the test and place your initials indicating that you have completed the test.

Physicians use several audiometric assessment procedures to determine the cause of a patient's hearing loss, some of which are a part of the complete or routine physical examination.

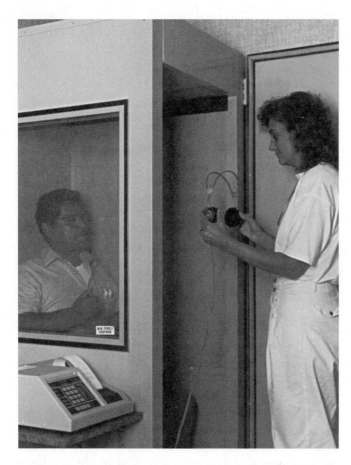

FIGURE 6–34 The patient presses the hand-held control button each time he hears a sound while in the soundproof booth. The signals are transmitted to the computer outside and printed as an audiogram.

FIGURE 6–35 The Weber test is normal if the patient can hear the sound in both ears equally well as the end of the tuning fork is placed against the skull.

PATIENT EDUCATION

1. Advise patients not to put anything into their ears to avoid damaging the tympanic membrane. The ear wax produced by the body has a purpose. It is to protect and moisten the membrane of the ear canal. Many people feel that they must completely remove this daily with a swab, which often results in packing it down into the ear canal where it hardens. This impacted ear wax (cerumen) must be removed by a qualified medical team member.

2. Instruct patients that eardrops and other ear medications should be used only with the advice of their physician. Earache, pain, or discharge should be reported to and examined by the physician as soon as possible.

3. Discuss the possibility of permanent hearing loss with patients who work around extremely loud noise or who have gotten into a habit of turning the volume way up when listening to audio systems, radios or TVs. Explain to these patients that protective ear coverings should be worn while on the job (it is a safety requirement) and advise those who listen to loud music to turn down the volume before their hearing is lost from damage to nerves.

4. Urge patients to have regular hearing tests to detect loss of hearing or other related problems. It is recommended that this be done annually unless otherwise instructed by the physician, or if there is a noticeable difference or problem with hearing. Patients who have a history of ear infections should have periodic hearing tests.

During the physical examination the physician will use a tuning fork to test the patient's hearing. A two-pronged metal tuning fork is used, its frequency varying with the size of the instrument. The common tests done are the Rinne and the Weber.

In the Rinne test, the examiner strikes the fork and then holds the shank (stem) against the patient's mastoid bone until the patient no longer hears the sound. The prongs of the tuning fork are then placed about 1 inch from the auditory meatus (opening to the ear) and then next to it. In a normal ear the sound is heard about twice as long by air conduction as by bone conduction. If hearing by bone conduction is greater, the result is spoken of as a negative Rinne.

In the Weber test the vibrating tuning fork is held against the vertex (crown of the head) or against the skull or forehead in the midline, Figure 6–35, page 350. The sound is heard best by the unaffected ear if deafness is due to disease of the auditory apparatus, by the affected ear if deafness is due to obstruction of the air passages.

A simple means of screening the hearing of infants and small children is to place a ticking watch behind their shoulder, without their seeing it, of course, and see how quickly they become aware of the noise.

A small amount of hearing loss may be temporary due to a patient's physical condition and a recheck in 1 or 2 weeks may be advisable.

Complete Chapter 6, Unit 3 in the workbook to help you meet the objectives at the beginning of this unit and therefore achieve competency of this subject matter.

U N I T 4
Specialty Examinations

OBJECTIVES

Upon completion of this unit, you will meet the following terminal performance objectives by verifying knowledge of the facts and principles presented through oral and written communication at a level deemed competent by the instructor or employer and will demonstrate the specific behaviors as identified in the terminal performance objectives of the procedures, observing all aseptic and safety precautions in accordance with health care standards.

1. Instruct a female patient for a Pap test appointment and explain why it is necessary.
2. List and describe the necessary instruments and supplies for a Pap test and pelvic exam.
3. Prepare a female patient for a Pap test and pelvic exam.
4. Demonstrate the proper way to assist with a Pap test and pelvic exam.
5. Prepare the Pap test specimen for laboratory analysis.
6. Explain breast self-examination.
7. Discuss patient education appropriate for females having a pelvic exam and Pap test.
8. Instruct a patient to prepare for a sigmoidoscopy and explain why it is necessary.
9. List and describe the necessary instruments and equipment for a sigmoidoscopy.
10. Explain how to assist with a sigmoidoscopy.
11. Discuss patient education appropriate for patients having a sigmoidoscopy.
12. Demonstrate how to administer an enema.
13. List the responsibilities of the medical assistant regarding obstetrics and pediatric patients.
14. Explain the appointment schedule for prenatal and obstetrics patients.
15. Discuss ways to gain compliance with pediatric patients.
16. Discuss topics that may be of concern to parents during office visits.
17. Explain how to make pediatric patients feel more at ease during their visits.
18. Spell and define, using the glossary at the back of the text, all the words to know in this unit.

WORDS TO KNOW

atypical cytology	intercede
cervical	Lamaze
constipation	lumen
diagnostic	maturation
disclose	mucosa
douche	obturator
endocervical	Papanicolaou
endoscope	pregnancy
enema	prenatal
evacuants	proctology
evacuate	risk
exfoliated	sigmoidoscopy
feces	stool
fetal monitor	suction
flatulence	tarry
flexible	trimester
formalin	tumor
gestation	ulceration
health check	vaginitis
heartburn	warranted
hormones	

Many special examinations are performed on patients in various medical practices. Specialties often require additional staff training in assisting with particular procedures.

It is important to stay within your boundaries until such time when you have been properly instructed and evaluated in specific areas.

In this unit, two very common procedures are discussed.

One is the Pap test and pelvic examination. In assisting with the CPE (Unit 1), the examination of the vagina and genitalia was described as a part of the total exam; the Pap test is not necessarily done at that time. Frequently, women schedule appointments with their general or family practitioners for the Pap test alone, definitely in the specialty of gynecology. One must make the distinction between a *physical* and a *Pap test*. The CPE is a review of systems (ROS) of the total body. The gynecological exam is that of the female reproductive organs only. As a rule, the specialists refer other symptoms or conditions of their patients back to the "family doctor" for treatment.

The sigmoidoscopy is another special diagnostic examination performed in most general or family practices, as well as in the specialty practice of internal medicine. Assisting with this procedure requires that you are familiar with the instruments and equipment used by the physician and that you have a sound understanding of the process in giving support to the patient.

With both of these exams it is essential that the patient receive proper preparation before the procedures can be successfully performed. Since the medical assistant is usually responsible for instructing patients, it is important that both verbal and written information is given. In consideration of the patient, the nature of both of these procedures can be embarrassing; having to go through the process only once will be appreciated.

The Pap Test and Hormonal Smears ....

The **Papanicolaou** technique, or Pap test, is a cytologic screening test to detect cancer of the cervix. This method of detection was developed by an American physician, George N. Papanicolaou, in 1883. This simple smear technique can also be used to screen tissue from other parts of the body for **atypical cytology** as the form in Figure 6–36 shows ("special cytology"). Female patients usually have the Pap test done routinely either as a part of the CPE with their family doctor or by their gynecologist. Patients who have complaints of severe menstrual pain or discomfort, unusual vaginal discharge, or lower abdominal pain (or any other problems) may have a Pap smear taken during the pelvic examination to rule out gynecological problems. Women should be especially conscientious in scheduling annual Pap tests if they have a family history of uterine or **cervical** cancer.

Some physicians recommend that females over age 35 have a Pap smear done every 6 months. Others feel that in healthy women one every 1 to 3 years is sufficient. The American Cancer Society recommends that females have a Pap test done at least every 3 years, beginning when they become sexually active, or at age 20 if there have been two initial negative Pap test results one year apart. You should check with your employer and advise patients accordingly.

Patients should not **douche** for 24 to 48 hours prior to the Pap test or the smear may be reported as negative because sloughed-off (**exfoliated**) cells would have been washed away.

The Pap test should not be done during the menstrual flow because red blood cells make the smear difficult to read. Patients should also be advised not to engage in sexual intercourse 24 to 48 hours before the scheduled appointment for the same reason.

Prior to bringing the patient into the examination room for the pelvic exam and Pap test, the medical assistant should make the necessary preparations. You should wash your hands before you begin. The exam table should have a clean protective covering, either table paper or a cloth sheet. Place a gown and drape sheet on the end of the table for the patient (either

C-4 REQUEST FORM

BILL
- [ ] ACCOUNT
- [ ] PATIENT SEE ①
- [ ] 3RD PARTY SEE ②

PLEASE LEAVE BLANK
AREA _____
DEPT. _____
BILL CD _____

INSTRUCTIONS: ① FOR PATIENT BILLING, COMPLETE BOX A.
② FOR 3RD PARTY BILLING, COMPLETE BOX A AND FILL IN DIAGNOSIS, THEN EITHER B, C, or D.

ABC LABORATORIES

PATIENT NAME (LAST) | (FIRST) | SPECIES | SEX | AGE YRS. MOS. | DATE COLLECTED MO. DAY YR. | TIME COLLECTED

PATIENT ADDRESS STREET | MISC. INFORMATION | DR. I.D. | MEDICARE: #

CITY STATE ZIP | DIAGNOSIS

PHYSICIAN | WELFARE: # | CASE NAME:

PROGRAM: | PATIENT 1ST NAME: | DATE OF BIRTH MO. DAY YR. ALL CLAIMS

INSURANCE GR. # | I.D. | SERVICE CODE:

SUBSCRIBER NAME: | RELATION: PHONE — —

CYTOLOGY | **INTERNAL USE ONLY**

DATE OF LAST MENSTRUAL PERIOD _____

Gravida _____ Para _____

Hormones (Type) _____

GYN Surgery _____ Date _____

Radiation Therapy _____ Date _____

Previous Cytology Number _____ Eval _____ Date _____

Pregnant ( ) Yes ( ) No
I.U.D. ( ) Yes ( ) No

PERTINENT CLINICAL HISTORY (Max. 35 Characters)

CYTOLOGY NUMBER

DATE RECEIVED

PAPANICOLAOU SMEARS AND MATURATION INDEX

Please mark source:

( ) Vaginal ( ) Cervical ( ) Endocervical

CHECK DESIRED TEST
8195 ( ) Pap Smear
8199 ( ) Pap and MI
8198 ( ) Maturation Index Only
8237 ( ) Pap added to Profile
8197 ( ) Pap included in Profile

SPECIAL CYTOLOGY
8202 ( ) Body Fluids, Misc Site _____
8203 ( ) Bronchial Washings, Brushings
8240 ( ) Cell Block
8200 ( ) Sputum
8201 ( ) Urine

8235 ( ) Endometrial Aspiration
8206 ( ) Eye (Ophthalmic)
8205 ( ) Fine Needle Aspirations
8204 ( ) Gastric Washings, Brushings

8232 ( ) Direct Smear
( ) Misc. Site _____
( ) Herpes Smear (Inclusion Bodies)
8233 ( ) Sex Chromatin (Barr Body)

SERIAL TESTS - Write in Number of Serial Samples Submitted Inside Parenthesis
8207 ( ) Serial Sputum ( ) Serial Urine

HISTOLOGY

9230 ( ) Surgical Pathology (Biopsy) preparation and pathologist interpretation)
8234 ( ) Bone Marrow Exam
9237 ( ) Stained Histology Slide (Without pathologist interpretation)
( ) Special Stain (Please Specify)
9251 ( ) Veterinary Pathology (Biopsy)

CLINICAL HISTORY

Source of Specimen _____
If Tumor, How Long Present _____
Post Operative Diagnosis _____
Previous History _____

UNLISTED TESTS
_____
_____
_____

FOLD THIS FORM IN HALF SO TEST(S) ORDERED IS CLEARLY VISIBLE

FIGURE 6–36 Cytology request form

cloth or disposable paper). On the Mayo tray near the end of the exam table you should place the instruments and supplies the physician will need to perform the pelvic exam and obtain the Pap smear. In Figure 6–37 the commonly used items for this GYN procedure are displayed. You must learn the names of the instruments and supplies, listed in the following procedure, to assist the physician efficiently. To aid in the inspection part of the pelvic exam, a gooseneck lamp should be placed within reach of the examiner's stool at the end of the table.

Escort the patient to the examination room. Before you continue further preparation of the patient, ask if she needs to empty her bladder and obtain a clean-catch midstream urine specimen if ordered by the physician. Pelvic examinations are uncomfortable for the patients if the bladder is full, besides making the examination difficult for the physician to perform. Examinations that have to be delayed while the patient goes to the rest room disrupt the schedule and are usually unnecessary. Certainly there are exceptions. Some patients may have trouble with bladder control or some other condition that could require frequent trips to the rest room. You should help these patients feel at ease for they will most likely feel embarrassed.

Complete the cytology request form (see Figure 6–36), by making sure that you ask the patient all necessary questions, including complaints she may have and the date of the last menstrual period (LMP, the first day of her last period). Instruct the patient about the procedure, letting her know what to expect, especially if it is the first time for her to have a pelvic exam. Never assume that a patient knows about a procedure whatever her age is. Unfortunately, some health care

FIGURE 6–37 A GYN/Pap tray setup

workers can often be remiss in giving important information to patients. Some patients are both afraid and embarrassed to ask questions because they figure they should already know about procedures. Try to make patients feel comfortable and at ease to help them relax for the exam. You should then instruct the patient to undress completely, where to put her belongings, and how to put on the exam gown (opened in front or back). You should politely offer your assistance. Ask her to leave the door unlocked, or slightly opened, when she is gowned. Allow the patient privacy to change for a couple of minutes. When the patient lets you know she is ready, pull out the foot step at the end of the exam table and help her step up to the exam table and sit at the end. Place the drape sheet over the top of her legs. This will give her privacy and warmth. You should remember to push the foot step back in after the patient has been seated to avoid injury to you or the physician.

Alert the physician that the patient is ready to be examined. (If the patient's appointment is for a Pap alone, or the physician has ordered a pelvic exam only, you should get everything ready, and then get the patient into the lithotomy position just before the doctor goes into the room, otherwise the patient will become uncomfortable and impatient staying in this position for any longer than necessary.) Most physicians prefer that the medical assistant (or nurse) accompany them into the exam room not only to assist with the procedure, but for legal reasons as well.

Because of the importance of early detection of breast cancer, physicians include the breast exam during the patient's annual appointment for the Pap and pelvic (patients should be urged to do breast self-examination each month following the menstrual period. Giving them a pamphlet of instructions to take with them for this procedure is recommended, Figure 6–38). Explain to the patient that the exam conducted by the physician with the annual Pap test is certainly noteworthy, but

insufficient in detecting abnormal breast tissue between visits to the physician. Most women discover a lump or mass in their breasts themselves and report it to the physician. This leads to early detection and treatment. The physician usually listens to the heart and lungs and does a brief general check of the patient first. Then the patient's gown is lowered to the waist while the patient is still sitting up for the inspection part of the breast exam and palpation for lumps and masses. You should then pull the table extension out to support the lower legs and feet and help the patient lie down in assisting the doctor in further palpation for any abnormalities of the breast tissue (often a towel is placed over the chest to provide a sense of privacy for the patient). The abdominal cavity is examined as the examiner palpates the pelvic area. Remind patients to breathe slowly through the mouth to help relax abdominal muscles during the exam.

Following this portion of the exam, you should help the patient into the lithotomy position. Assist her in getting her feet in the stirrups, adjusting them as necessary, and place the drape sheet over her knees. Ask her to scoot down to the end of the table until the buttocks are just at the edge (place your hand at the edge of the table and ask her to keep moving down until she feels the back of your hand). Be careful in assisting patients into positions as the exam tables are usually rather narrow and there *is* the possibility of a patient *falling off* the table. The gooseneck lamp should be adjusted at the end of the table and the stool placed comfortably into position for the physician. The medical assistant should put latex gloves on and hand the physician gloves. The vaginal speculum (after running warm water over it) should be handed to the doctor next for use in inspecting the cervix and in obtaining the smear, Figure 6–39, page 355. Hand the physician the spatula to obtain a sample of the vaginal secretions containing the exfoliated cells for analysis. The **endocervical** brush is used to obtain an endocervical tissue specimen. If the physician requests a Pap and **maturation** index (MI), it means that a **hormonal** evaluation is necessary in determining the patient's

FIGURE 6–38 Breast self-examination pamphlets and schedule

FIGURE 6–39 Lateral view of vaginal speculum in place for inspection and for obtaining specimens. (From Burke, *Human Anatomy & Physiology in Health and Disease,* 3d ed. Copyright 1992, Delmar Publishers Inc.)

condition. Hold the slides carefully at the frosted end and mark each slide accurately (in pencil) as the physician gives them to you: cervical–C, vaginal–V, endocervical–E. Immediately apply the commercial fixative spray to the slide(s) and put in the container, or place in the jar back to back with an alcohol–ether solution for transport to the lab. Make sure that you wrap the completed request form around the container and secure with a rubber band.

The bimanual exam is performed following the collection of specimens (Pap smear, cultures, etc.) so that the lubricant will not interfere in the lab analysis. The examiner inserts one finger (with a small amount of water-soluble lubricant) into the vagina, and palpates the pelvic area with the other hand, Figure 6–40. Normally the physician does a rectal examination next. You should hand the doctor another latex glove and lubricant. This is to prevent cross-contamination between the vaginal and rectal tissues. The medical assistant may be asked to write the findings of this examination while the physician conducts the exam alone. Whichever is your role, you will be a valuable assistant to both physician and patient.

When this exam has been completed, offer tissues to the patient to wipe away any residual lubricant. Discard the used tissues in an appropriate waste container, remove the gloves, and wash your hands. Push the stirrups and the extension of the table in and assist the patient in sitting up. After lying down for the exam the patient may either feel faint or dizzy; if she attempts to stand up too quickly she may fall. After she has let you know that she has regained her balance, help her down from the table and ask her to get dressed. Offer assistance to the patient.

Remember to advise her when to expect to receive the results of the Pap test and other reports in the mail, or when she should call to find out the report(s), Figure 6–41, page 357. Giving these instructions will decidedly reduce unnecessary phone calls to the office. If the physician requests a return appointment for the patient, politely assist her in scheduling it or direct her to the administrative area. As time permits, you may discuss patient education topics either before or after the exam as appropriate to the age and needs of the patient.

The medical assistant should return to the examination room to clean up the exam area. Wear gloves to protect yourself from disease transmission. Discard all disposables in biohazardous and appropriate containers, remove gloves, and wash your hands. Restock the supplies as necessary, making the room ready for another patient to be seen. Place the specimen(s) in the proper area for pick up by the lab representative.

Obstetrics Patients

The same principles apply in assisting with obstetrics patients as apply in assisting with the complete physical examination. You must be complete and efficient in documenting all information regarding patients. This enables the patient to provide quality care to patients.

Of primary concern with obstetrics patients is gaining their compliance with regular checkups. Some of your major responsibilities will be to provide patient education (both verbal and in printed form) and to give emotional support and encouragement. You should refer to Chapter 4, Unit 13 for review of the reproductive system and information regarding pregnancy, labor, and childbirth. You should be familiar with the terminology for explanation to the parents and for correct spellings.

Because such convenient home pregnancy tests are available to the public, many women in their childbearing years have already tested their urine at home. Often even after having performed the home test they still may not be certain of the results. When patients suspect that they are pregnant, their visit to the doctor is to confirm pregnancy. Usually the patient has missed one or two menstrual periods and suspects pregnancy. The diagnosis is made only after the patient has been given a complete evaluation. This is generally done by (1) interviewing the patient and obtaining a complete **prenatal** health assessment and history, (2) doing a complete physical examination, (3) ordering laboratory tests, such as urinalysis and pregnancy tests, blood tests, and cultures as **warranted,** and (4) performing any other diagnostic test indicated by the patient's condition.

The medical assistant's role in prenatal evaluation and care of patients is to instill the importance of keeping regular appointments, encourage patients to eat a sensible well-balanced diet, alert the doctor with any problems or concerns, and provide patient education materials with explanations. Follow the office policy regarding prenatal and childbirth classes and provide information about times and places of such programs as **Lamaze** classes.

Assist with a Gynecological Examination and Pap Test

PURPOSE: To assist in evaluation of the patient's gynecological condition.

EQUIPMENT: Two (or more) frosted-end glass slides, Mayo tray, cloth or paper towel, pen and pencil, fixative spray and container to hold slides (or jar with alcohol–ether solution), disposable latex gloves, water-soluble lubricant, vaginal speculum, endocervical brush, vaginal/cervical spatula (Ayer blade), sterile cotton-tipped applicators, tissues, lab request form, rubber band, (cultures and uterine dressing forceps as requested by physician) Figure 6–42.

TERMINAL PERFORMANCE OBJECTIVE: With all equipment and supplies provided, the instructor role-playing as the physician, and female students role-playing as patients, demonstrate (insofar as feasible) each of the steps required in assisting with the GYN examination and Pap test. The instructor will observe each step. Note that some steps will need to be simulated in the instructional setting.

1. Wash hands; place gown or drape sheet on exam table; cover Mayo tray with towel; assemble all necessary items on tray.
2. Take the patient into the examining room. Request her urine specimen if brought or ask the patient to go to bathroom to void if one is needed. Determine if the patient needs to empty her bladder before the examination is performed.
3. Obtain the necessary information and complete cytology request form, label slides.
4. Explain procedure, disrobing, and gowning to patient (assist if needed). Ask her to leave door unlocked when ready.
5. Assist patient onto the exam table and drape.
6. Accompany physician into exam room to assist both the doctor and the patient during the exam.
7. Assist patient into lithotomy position, helping her place her feet in the stirrups (adjust accordingly) and place drape sheet over the knees. *Note: Place the back of your hand against the drape sheet at the end of the table. Request the patient to move until she touches your hand.* Place a pillow under her head for comfort.
8. Physician will sit at the end of the exam table on exam

stool and adjust the lamp for inspection of vaginal and anal tissues. Hand gloves to the physician. You should also put on gloves. **CAUTION:** Remember, in order to comply with universal precautions guidelines, gloves must be worn if there is any possibility of coming into contact with blood or any body fluids. Run warm water over the vaginal speculum, and hand it and the vaginal spatula to the doctor to obtain Pap smear as you carefully hold the slide by the frosted end. The endocervical brush is used next to obtain a smear from the interior of the cervix. Slides for these specific areas must be marked appropriately: V–vaginal; E–endocervical; and C–cervical for proper analysis to be done at the lab.

9. Immediately apply fixative spray and place into container, or place in alcohol–ether solution, for transport to lab.
10. The physician performs the bimanual exam after smears have been taken. Assist by placing a small amount of lubricant on the doctor's gloved finger, and handing a fresh glove to the examiner for the rectal exam. Further assistance in obtaining cultures, a biopsy, or any other GYN procedures may be performed at this time. Refer to Figure 6–42 for other instruments that may be used in these procedures that you will assist in handing the physician.
11. Hand tissues to the patient for removal of any residual lubricant. Discard all disposables in biohazardous waste container. If metal speculum was used, place in cool water to soak until it can be properly washed, wrapped, and autoclaved, remove gloves, and wash hands.
12. Help patient sit up, push table extension and stirrups in, and help her down from table when her sense of balance has returned.
13. Instruct patient to dress (give assistance if needed).
14. Advise patient when results will be available and schedule follow-up appointment if indicated.
15. Place specimen(s) in lab pick-up area.
16. Clean and restock exam room to make ready for next patient.

Figure 6–43A&B shows an example of a medical history form used in assessing the health status of pregnant women. Subsequent findings during prenatal visits are recorded on progress notes. Careful attention should be given to sections regarding (1) medications, drugs, alcohol, and smoking (consumption and use); (2) preexisting **risk** factors; and (3) past menstrual and obstetrical health history.

Each time the patient comes in for an appointment you should

1. Ask her if she has been experiencing any problems and record symptoms.
2. Ask her to empty her bladder and obtain a urine specimen (preferred the first morning specimen).

FIGURE 6-40 Bimanual pelvic examination (From Burke, *Human Anatomy & Physiology in Health and Disease,* 3d ed. Copyright 1992, Delmar Publishers Inc.)

3. Weigh her and record the findings.
4. Take her vital signs and record.
5. Collect any reports from laboratory findings or other referrals and place them in the chart for the physician.
6. Assist the patient to the examination table and position and drape her appropriately.
7. Place flexible centimeter tape measure on the Mayo table, disposable latex gloves and lubricant and **fetal** (pulse) **monitor,** refer to Figure 6-44 (as appropriate for the visit—pregnancy is divided into three sections or **trimesters** of the 9-month (36 week) **gestation** period).
8. Assist with the examination.
9. Assist the patient from the examination table.

After the physician has completed the examination and talked with the patient, you should offer to answer any questions the patient may have. Encourage the patient to make her next appointment before leaving the facility. Give support and assistance by reminding her to call if there are any questions or problems.

To be of further assistance to both physician and patient, you may want to check all Medicare patients' charts to make sure that findings are documented in the SOAP method in a neat and

---

REPORT OF CYTOLOGICAL EXAMINATION PAPANICOLAOU TECHNIQUE

Laboratory I.D.   Patient Age   Date Received
Source of Material
Other Information

Patient Name   Physician Name

MATURATION INDEX

Estrogen (0-3+)	Trichomonas	% Superficial
Inflammation (0-3+)	Monilia	% Intermediate
Blood (0-3+)	Erosion Cells	% Parabasal

Class I Negative . . . . Absence of abnormal or atypical cytology.
Class II Doubtful . . . . Atypical cytology not suggestive of malignancy.
Class III Suspicious . . . . Cytology compatible with malignancy or other etiology.
Class IV Highly Suspicious . . . . Cytology strongly suggestive of malignancy.
Class V Positive . . . . Cytology practically conclusive of malignancy
Class C . . . . Insufficient for examination.

REMARKS & RECOMMENDATIONS

---

screened by

Cytologic
   Classifications for
   the Results of the
   Pap Smear

Class I: Negative, absence of abnormal cells.
Class II: Atypical cytology, but no evidence of malignancy. The atypical cells may be due to inflammation, which causes them to change in character.
Class III: Atypical cytology, suggestive of but not conclusive for malignancy.
Class IV: Abnormal cytology, strongly suggestive of malignancy.
Class V: Abnormal cytology, positive for malignancy

FIGURE 6-41 Cytology report form for Pap test

FIGURE 6–42 Additional gynecological instruments used in examinations and procedures: (a). Sims' uterine sound, graduated in inches: (b). Sims' uterine sound, graduated in centimeters: (c). Sims' uterine curette: (d). Randall uterine curette: (e). Toms-Gaylor uterine punch biopsy forceps: (f). Loufe uterine polyp (Courtesy of J. Jamner Surgical Instruments Inc.)

legible manner and signed by the physician. These records may be requested for on-the-spot checking at any time by Medicare to verify the diagnosis and coding. This will lead to more efficient and expedient payment.

Pediatric Examinations ....

When young patients come in to see the doctor, you must be especially pleasant and show genuine care and understanding. Your attitude may be the deciding factor in their cooperation during the visit. Greeting them with a smile and speaking to them on their developmental level will help to gain their trust and compliance. Often some youngsters have had traumatic experiences in emergency care centers due to serious illness or injury, which leaves them fearful of health care providers in general. If you take the time, showing consideration and patience, you can establish a rapport with the patients and

eliminate this potential problem. Patients of all ages are much more cooperative when they feel welcome.

Most medical facilities provide a play area for small children in the reception area or waiting room. This helps the children feel welcome and provides a comfortable environment. A variety of safe, durable, washable, educational toys is suggested. Toys that have many or tiny parts are not recommended because many small objects all over the floor would create an unsafe walkway and could cause others to fall and possibly be hurt. It could also be a potential problem for babies who put everything in their mouths. Keeping the toys clean and contained in one area will be one of your duties. Make it easy on yourself by recommending the purchase of large toys that have minimal accessory parts. Often a child will find an interesting toy while waiting to be called in to the examination room. Obviously the child's cooperation will be greater if the little patient is permitted to bring the toy in with him to keep occupied while awaiting the doctor. It will also help you in performing any necessary procedures for the child in preparation for the doctor's examination. You must make sure that when the child is finished with the toy that it is sanitized properly before returning it to the play area for other children. It should be noted that the play area should ideally be used for well children who are waiting for annual physical examinations or other well visits or for checkups, allergy injections, or immunizations. You should always bring in sick children to an examination room as soon as they arrive so you won't risk the transmission of their disease to others who are present. You

General Schedule for Prenatal or Obstetrical Appointments

FIRST TRIMESTER: Monthly into the second trimester or every 4 weeks through the 28th week.
THIRD TRIMESTER: Every 2 weeks in the 30th to 36th weeks. Every week in the 36th+ week up to delivery.

PLEASE USE BALL POINT PEN

NAME _____

ADDRESS _____

PHONE _____ RELIGION _____

AGE _____ GR _____ PARA _____ AB_____

BLOOD TYPE _____ RH _____SEROLOGY _____

HUSB. BL. TYPE _____ RH _____ GENOTYPE _____

_____

_____

_____

PAP SMEAR _____

SEND TOP (WHITE) COPY TO DEL. ROOM TERM_____

LMP_____ LIFE _____ EDC _____

NURSING _____ PEDIATRICIAN _____

ANESTHESIA _____

REFERRING M.D._____

PRENATAL PREPARATION _____

HUSBAND IN DELIVERY ROOM?_____

_____ RUBELLA TITER _____

MENSTRUAL CYCLE_____

G.C. CULTURE

P P A R S E T G.		DATE	WHERE CONFINED	WEEKS GESTATION	LENGTH OF LABOR	INFANT WT.	COMPLICATIONS
	1						
	2						
	3						
	4						

HISTORY AND PHYSICAL

CHILDHOOD _____

FAMILY _____

TRAUMATIC _____

ADULT_____

BLOOD TRANSFUSIONS _____

ALLERGIES _____

SURGERY _____

COMMENTS:_____

_____

MEDICATIONS _____

RH TITERS DATES: _____

HT. _____NORMAL WT. _____ NORMAL B.P._____

HEENT _____

HEART & LUNGS_____

BACK & BREASTS _____

ABDOMEN _____

SKIN & EXTREMITIES _____

PELVIC CAPACITY_____

PERIODIC VISITS		DATE	WEIGHT	BP	URINE	FHT	FUNDUS	PELVIC	COMMENTS
	1								
	2								
	3								
	4								
	5								
	6								
	7								
	8								
	9								
	10								
	11								
	12								
	13								
	14								

A

DELIVERY ROOM - TERM   SIGNATURE: M.D.

FIGURE 6–43A Example obstetrics/prenatal history form

must keep an open communication with the administrative medical assistant (receptionist) regarding the scheduling of these ill patients. Since you can never be sure of the health status of anyone, you must be vigilant in the practice of universal precautions. Sanitizing and disinfecting items and sufaces in the medical facility as needed is a vital part of your work day.

Even when you are frantically busy with an overbooked schedule, you must remember to follow universal precautions. It should become a habit that is second nature to you for your protection as well as for the protection of patients and other workers. A help in the effort to cut down on disease transmission is a commercial disinfectant spray. You can use this

PRENATAL RISK ASSESSMENT FORM

Please print or type:

Patient Name	Case Number	ADC Number	E.D.D.		
			month	day	year
Physician Name	Physician Telephone				

Please check all that apply:

AT RISK OF PRETERM BIRTH

ABSOLUTE FACTORS *(one factor puts patient at risk)*

OBSTETRICAL HISTORY
- ❑ 1. PRETERM DELIVERY
- ❑ 2. DES EXPOSURE
- ❑ 3. CONE BIOPSY
- ❑ 4. SECOND TRIMESTER ABORTION
- ❑ 5. 1st TRIMESTER SPONTANEOUS ABORTIONS, more than 2

CURRENT PREGNANCY
- ❑ 6. UTERINE ANOMALY OR FIBROIDS
- ❑ 7. MULTIPLE GESTATION
- ❑ 8. ABDOMINAL SURGERY

- ❑ 9. CERVIX DILATED, more than 1.5 cm before 29 weeks
- ❑ 10. CERVIX EFFACED, less than 1 cm before 29 weeks
- ❑ 11. IRRITABLE UTERUS, more than 6 contractions per hr. confirmed
- ❑ 12. POLYHYDRAMNIOS
- ❑ 13. BLEEDING, if significant after 12 weeks
- ❑ 14. PYELONEPHRITIS
- ❑ 15. PRETERM LABOR
- ❑ 16. SMOKING, more than 10 cigarettes per day
- ❑ 17. PROM, confirmed

❑ YES ❑ NO   At least ONE of the above conditions has been checked. Patient is at risk of preterm birth.

AT RISK OF POOR PREGNANCY OUTCOME

ABSOLUTE FACTORS *(one factor puts patient at risk)*

OBSTETRICAL HISTORY
- ❑ 18. INFANT DEATH, stillborn, neonatal, post neonatal
- ❑ 19. CONGENITAL ANOMALY, major
- ❑ 20. LOW BIRTH WEIGHT, less than 2500g.
- ❑ 21. ECLAMPSIA or severe preeclampsia
- ❑ 22. INCOMPETENT CERVIX

CURRENT PREGNANCY
- ❑ 23. HEART DESEASE, class III or IV
- ❑ 24. DIABETES, insulin dependent
- ❑ 25. SICKLE CELL ANEMIA or other hemoglobinopathy
- ❑ 26. MALIGNANCY or leukemia
- ❑ 27. THYROID DISEASE, confirmed
- ❑ 28. EPILEPSY or on anticonvulsant
- ❑ 29. HEPATITIS or chronic liver desease
- ❑ 30. ASTHMA, on medication
- ❑ 31. TUBERCULOSIS, active
- ❑ 32. PNEUMONIA

- ❑ 33. HYPERTENSION, on medication
- ❑ 34. DEEP VENOUS THROMBOSIS
- ❑ 35. PLACENTA PREVIA, 3rd trimester
- ❑ 36. OLIGOHYDRAMNIOS
- ❑ 37. ECLAMPSIA or preeclampsia
- ❑ 38. ALLOIMMUNIZATION associated with fetal disease
- ❑ 39. RUBELLA EXPOSURE with rising titer
- ❑ 40. POSITIVE SEROLOGY
- ❑ 41. ACTIVE HERPES or positive culture, 3rd trimester
- ❑ 42. PRIMIGRAVIDA, less than 17 years or more than 35 years
- ❑ 43. FAMILIAL GENETIC DISORDER, confirmed
- ❑ 44. PSYCHOSIS
- ❑ 45. MENTAL RETARDATION
- ❑ 46. DRUG OR ALCOHOL ABUSE
- ❑ 47. OTHER_____

❑ YES ❑ NO   At least ONE of the above conditions has been checked. Patient is at risk of poor pregnancy outcome.

RELATIVE FACTORS *(two factors put patient at risk)*

- ❑ 48. PRIOR C-SECTION
- ❑ 49. PRENATAL CARE NON-COMPLIANCE, most recent pregnancy
- ❑ 50. GRAND MULTIPARA, more than 5 of 20 weeks or more
- ❑ 51. RECENT DELIVERY, less than 1 yr.
- ❑ 52. LATE INITIAL VISIT, after 14 weeks of pregnancy
- ❑ 53. MISSED PRENATAL APPOINTMENTS, 2 consecutive
- ❑ 54. AGE, less than 17 years or more than 35 years
- ❑ 55. Height, less than 5 ft.
- ❑ 56. OBESITY, more than 20% weight for height
- ❑ 57. UNDERWEIGHT, more than 10% weight for height
- ❑ 58. WEIGHT LOSS, continuing after 14 weeks

- ❑ 59. ANEMIA, less than 10 Hgb. or less than 30% Hct.
- ❑ 60. GONORRHEA, positive culture
- ❑ 61. DIABETES, gestational, diet controlled
- ❑ 62. CHRONIC BRONCHITIS
- ❑ 63. TRAUMA, requiring hospitalization
- ❑ 64. ILLITERACY or language barrier
- ❑ 65. DOMESTIC VIOLENCE
- ❑ 66. OTHER_____

❑ YES ❑ NO   At least TWO of the above conditions have been checked. Patient is at risk of poor pregnancy outcome.

Physician's Signature	Date

B

FIGURE 6–43B Prenatal risk assessment form

quickly in between patients when you are hurried. The best way to eliminate a potential disease transmission is to remove the item when possible until it can be properly sanitized. Children (and patients of any age) becoming sick and vomiting is a concern you must be aware of in a medical facility. The administrative medical assistant should keep a disposable emesis basin near the window for this potential situation. You should also keep a commercial preparation accessible for use in cleaning up this type of waste material. Latex gloves, facial tissues, and biohazardous plastic waste bags should also be easily accessible. A covered waste receptacle lined with a bio-

hazardous plastic bag for disposal of contaminated items should be obtainable. There may be occasions where a parent or caregiver may bring a seriously ill or injured child into the facility unannounced. You must act quickly to provide immediate care to the patient and protect others who may be present from possible disease transmission in an emergency situation.

When you are assisting with the examination of a child, a very important responsibility you will have is relaying information to the doctor from the parent or caregiver, and from the doctor to the patient and parent or caretaker. Your careful observation of the child and the relationship between the par-

FIGURE 6–44 Fetal pulse monitor in use

ent or caregiver and the child may be critical to the physician in the course of the care and treatment of the patient. You are responsible for reporting any suspected cases of child abuse and neglect to the proper authorities (child protective agency) in your community. Make note of any unusual observations and advise the physician before the patient is seen.

Many caregivers or parents are unaware of developmental stages and what to expect from their children. Posting a chart for patient education regarding these growth and developmental stages of infants and children is most helpful for patient education. An example is shown in Figure 6–45. While you are preparing the child for the physician to come into the examination room is an ideal time to discuss such patient education topics with the caregiver as the child's eating habits, sleep and daily activities, immunizations schedules, toilet-training, and taking and recording a temperature. This is a great help to parents and caregivers in caring for their children. Printed booklets and pamphlets on a wide variety of topics should be offered to parents as appropriate to their childrens' ages.

Cooperation with youngsters is generally obtained by explaining, in a calm, simple manner appropriate to their stage of development, what you and the doctor are going to do and why. If you sense behavior that is not cooperative then you must ask the parent or caregiver to intercede. A child who is

unwilling to cooperate with a procedure that is necessary will have to be restrained safely by you and the parent, or another health care worker. Doing what has to be done as quickly as possible is the best way to handle a troublesome situation especially with a child.

Children are often amused with items that are not ordinary toys during an examination, such as a plastic drinking cup or tongue depressor (with supervision, of course). Giving children nonsharp instruments, such as a percussion hammer, stethoscope, or penlight, to examine may help them to overcome the fear of their use by the doctor during the exam. Be sure to clean these items properly when the child has finished with them.

Pediatric patients should be regarded as individuals and given the kindness and respect you should give to all patients you serve. You may want to make a "poncho" type covering for a little one made by folding a disposable drape sheet in fourths and cutting the point off to make an opening to go over the child's head. Young boys and girls are often embarrassed and chilled sitting on the examination table in their underwear awaiting the doctor. This is an easy way to help them feel more comfortable and keep warm. They like the special treatment.

Another common practice to help little ones feel special is to provide them with bandages in colorful prints or cartoon characters for their minor cuts and abrasions or for injection

FIGURE 6–45 Growth and developmental stages of infants and toddlers

sites following immunizations. Most health care providers in medical facilities that treat pediatric patients offer a small token reward, such as stickers, balloons, or trinkets, after their treatment or exam is completed. This gives the child positive reenforcement and helps to establish and keep a good rapport between the medical team and the child.

Chapter 5 contains the procedures that should be followed for preparing young patients for examinations. You will also be required to complete many types of forms requesting information derived from health checkups for various facilities, such as schools or day care centers. An example of a comprehensive health care program which requires careful documen-

It will most often be the medical assistant who tells the patient how to prepare for the **sigmoidoscopy** and explains how the test is performed. For successful examination, proper preparation is essential. In addition to having the patient restrict dairy products, raw fruits and vegetables, and grains and cereals from their diet, they should be encouraged to drink plenty of clear liquids and eat lightly the day before the scheduled appointment for the sigmoid colon exam. A plain commercially available **enema** (such as Fleet), should be self-administered at home approximately 2 hours before the exam. Physicians may vary the instructions according to the patient's condition. It is best to ask the examiner about the patient before proceeding with instructions. If patients are not completely informed about preparations and the exam is attempted with unsatisfactory results, it will have to be repeated, which is both costly and inconvenient. Satisfactory results are obtained by giving patients both oral and written instructions. This practice will also be helpful in reducing phone calls with **trivial** questions.

There are occasions, during an appointment for which the patient was "worked in" to the schedules, when the physician feels that the patient's condition warrants the examination of the sigmoid colon. In this case, the physician will order an enema to be given to the patient in the office. A procedure for both assisting with a sigmoidoscopy and administering an enema will follow in this unit.

Some exams, such as diagnostic sigmoidoscopy and X rays, require the use of **evacuants** by the patient the day before or the morning of the exam. This may present a problem in the patient's personal or employment schedule if instructions are not made clear before the appointment is scheduled. Most patients are fearful of what the diagnostic examination will **disclose.** Helping them choose a conve-nient appointment time and explaining the reasons for the preparations they must undergo will usually be appreciated.

When patients come in for rectal or sigmoidoscopy examinations here are a few informative topics that you may discuss with them.

1. Remind them that laxatives and enemas should only be used by direction of the physician.
2. **Constipation** may be avoided or relieved by including fresh fruits and vegetables, cereals, and grains in their diet, drinking plenty of liquids (water), and getting regular exercise.
3. Instruct them that if they have any of the following symptoms persistently it could mean that a disease or an abnormal condition is present and consulting the physician is strongly advised: **heartburn** or indigestion, nausea and/or vomiting, constipation or diarrhea, excessive gas or bloating, **stool** that is **tarry** (black) or other than a normal brown color.
4. Inform patients who are age 40 and over that they should routinely test their stool for **occult** blood every 2 years for detection of cancer of the colon, or more often if advised by the physician (if family history indicates). All patients over age 50 should test annually.
5. Advise patients to include high-fiber foods in their diets, avoid too much fat (and saturated fats) and cholesterol, and eat red meats very sparingly.
6. Urge patients to eat from a variety of foods (from the food pyramid in Chapter 2) and to eat four to six small meals rather than 1 or 2 large meals daily to promote better utilization of nutrients and more energy.
7. Suggest to patients that it is better to select snacks and beverages wisely, such as fruits, vegetables, and juices instead of coffee, tea, pop and high-calorie sweets or chips.

---

tation of examination findings is the federally mandated program called **Healthcheck.** This is for eligible Medicaid patients who are between the ages of birth and 21 years. This program requires regular routine health maintenance checkups to detect and treat medical problems. The parent or primary caregiver must accompany the child at each visit. The recommended schedule for examinations is as follows:

Age	Examinations per year
birth–12 months	6
1–2 years	2
2–21 years	1

The earlier a medical problem can be detected and treated, the better for the child. Health care officials have developed this program for periodic intervals of examinations so that potential problems can be caught before they become serious or beyond treatment stages. The screening procedures are simplified and relatively quick for determining abnormalities or illnesses. Whether a young patient requires further testing or other measures is determined from the results of these tests. This leads to earlier diagnosis and treatment of medical conditions. You should stress the importance of compliance with this program to the adult who is responsible for the child.

There are 13 areas that constitute the program:

1. health
2. developmental history from parent or primary caregiver
3. complete physical exam [unclothed] (including vital signs age 3–21 years) and height, weight, head and chest measurements
4. nutritional assessment—plot results on growth charts
5. vision (include color vision acuity)

6. hearing screening appropriate for the child's age
7. immunization needs using standard schedule
8. laboratory testing as indicated
9. anemia or sickle cell tests as indicated
10. urinalysis
11. lead poisoning absorption annually for ages 1 to 4 years and PRN

12. tuberculin test annually—Mantoux test on all individuals who have been or are suspected of having been exposed
13. dental assessment—refer to dentist

Any other laboratory tests, X rays, cultures, and so on should be performed as indicated from findings in the health history or during the examination. Your role is to be of assistance in gathering data, documenting information, performing the screening

---

P R O C E D U R E

Assist with Sigmoidoscopy

PURPOSE: To assist in examination of the sigmoid colon to determine its condition.

EQUIPMENT: Disposable latex gloves, water-soluble lubricant, gauze squares, sigmoidoscope, long cotton-tipped swabs, drape sheet (fenestrated–optional), suction machine (container with room temperature water), tissues, (if ordered by physician: biopsy forceps, specimen container for transport to lab, lab request form) pen, patient's chart

TERMINAL PERFORMANCE OBJECTIVE: With all equipment and supplies provided, the instructor role-playing the physician, and students role-playing patients, demonstrate (insofar as feasible) each of the steps required in assisting with the sigmoidoscopy procedure. The instructor will observe each step. *Note:* Some steps will need to be simulated in the instructional setting.

1. Explain procedure to identified patient. **RATIONALE: Speaking to the patient by name and checking the chart ensures that you are performing the procedure on the correct patient.** Ask patient to empty bladder and bowel.
2. Assemble all needed items on Mayo table near end of examination table. Plug in cord of light source to make sure it works properly, then unplug. **RATIONALE: If left on it will be uncomfortably warm for patient and may cause a burn. Note: If biopsy is scheduled complete lab request form and label specimen container.**
3. Instruct patient to disrobe from waist down and let you know when ready. Assist patient to sit at end of table and cover with drape sheet.
4. Both medical assistant and physician should wash hands and put on latex gloves. **CAUTION:** Remember, in order to comply with universal precautions guidelines, gloves must be worn if there is any possibility of coming into contact with blood or any body fluids.
5. Just before physician is ready to begin exam, assist patient into knee-chest or Sims' position, whichever physician prefers. *Note: Many physician's have an*

examining table which permits the patient to kneel on a pad and then be placed in a jacknife position to facilitate the procedure.

6. Assist physician by applying about 2 tablespoons of lubricant on gauze square for tip of obturator and tip of gloved fingers. *Note:* Physician makes digital examination of anus and rectum prior to insertion of endoscope.
7. As physician finishes digital exam, plug sigmoidoscope into light source. Secure air-inflation tubing and have it ready to hand to physician.
8. As physician inserts sigmoidoscope, be ready to hand items as needed. *Note:* Have suction machine plugged in and suction tip secured. **RATIONALE: Often fecal material or unexpelled enema fluid is present and must be removed before adequate viewing can be accomplished.**
9. If biopsy is indicated, hand biopsy forceps to physician and have specimen container open so physician can place tissue in it. a. Place cap on container securely and label properly. b. Complete lab request form and attach to specimen container with tape or rubber band.
10. Use tissues to clean lubricant and waste from patient's anal area and discard into biohazardous waste container. Assist patient to resting prone position.
11. Clean area and place used instruments in basin to soak in detergent solution. Remove gloves and wash hands.
12. Assist patient to a sitting position, allowing time for balance to return before helping down from table. Instruct patient to dress (unless patient has an appointment for additional examinations, such as X rays in the same office).
13. Disease transmission must be prevented. Wear gloves to clean the exam table and instruments. The metal scope and suction tip should be sanitized and prepared for sterilization (autoclaved). Restock the room and make ready for the next patient.
14. Record procedure on patient's chart and initial.

Following sigmoidoscopy, patients should drink plenty of clear liquids to help relieve the usual abdominal discomfort and **flatulence.** Patients may also find relief in lying in a prone position with a pillow across their midabdominal area to aid in the passage of gas.

FIGURE 6–46 Parts of the sigmoidoscope are labeled in this photo of the flexible sigmoidoscope setup with suction machine and necessary items for the exam.

tests as far as your skills and abilities, and being of assistance to both patient and physician as needed.

Accuracy in the documentation of each of these components is essential to quality care of these young patients. All screenings must be performed on site at a health care facility by qualified medical personnel. Use the time well with parents or caregivers and youngsters by providing patient education as indicated by the child's age and developmental stage and at the request of the adult.

Sigmoidoscopy ....

Sigmoidoscopy is a **diagnostic** examination of the interior of the sigmoid colon. It is a useful aid in the diagnosis of cancer of the colon, **ulcerations,** polyps, **tumors,** bleeding, and other lower intestinal disorders. The sigmoidoscope is a metal or plastic (disposable) instrument with a light source and a magnifying lens, which permits the mucous membrane of the sigmoid colon to be seen.

The metal and plastic types of scopes are still used to examine patients. Recently, another instrument has been gaining in popularity with physicians. A **flexible** sigmoidoscope is shown assembled with items necessary for the procedure to be performed in Figure 6–46. Since it is flexible, it can be inserted much farther into the colon. This instrument makes it possible to view more of the mucous membranes of the intestines.

An **obturator** is inserted into the sigmoidoscope. The tip of the obturator and scope are lubricated and carefully inserted into the rectum. Then the obturator is removed so that the S shape of the colon can be seen. Patients find this an unpleasant procedure.

As with any examination of the abdominal cavity, you should advise the patient to empty the bladder and **evacuate** the bowel before the procedure begins. This will make the exam easier for both patient and examiner. During the procedure the patient should be instructed to breathe through the mouth deeply and slowly to relax the abdominal muscles. Patients may feel the urge to defecate during any of these colon examinations because of the stretching of the intestinal wall by the instrument passing through and air being introduced with it. If patients use the breathing technique mentioned, this discomfort can be relieved. The procedure should last only a minute or two, especially if patients have followed preparation instructions.

Air is sometimes introduced into the colon (by the examiner's use of the inflation bulb attached to the scope with tubing) to distend the wall of the colon for easier placement of the **lumen** of the **endoscope.** Patients find this to be uncomfortable and sometimes painful. The physician may need to use a **suction** pump to remove mucus, blood, or **fecal** material that is obstructing the view of the colon.

Assistance in handling necessary items to the physician and giving support to the patient are your roles during these exams.

It is certainly not a common procedure to administer an enema to a patient in the medical office or clinic, but it is sometimes a necessity in the successful completion of a sigmoidoscopy, other rectal examination, or for other reasons. Even though a patient may have received proper instructions and carried them out before the scheduled appointment, there is no guarantee that the patient achieved success. In the event that the patient comes in for the appointment and is not sufficiently cleaned out for a sigmoidoscopy, the physician may order a cleansing enema so that the exam can be completed. It is generally best to proceed with the planned procedure, even with the delay of the enema. Usually this works out well for patient and staff, for rescheduling presents difficulties for everyone.

Often the patient did follow the list of instructions, but just did not retain the enema solution long enough for it to work. You will more likely be able to encourage the patient to hold the contents of the enema longer. You may want to explain that the longer the contents are held, the more successful the results will be. Otherwise, it may have to be repeated, or the exam rescheduled. Make sure that you use an examination room that is close to the rest room for the patient's convenience when you administer an enema. The enema is a quite simple procedure, one that patients can do at home when advised by the physician. Your patience and understanding are needed here, because most patients are embarrassed to have this done. The procedure that follows will provide the information you need to carry out this duty.

Administer Disposable Cleansing Enema

PURPOSE: To stimulate elimination of fecal matter from the lower intestinal tract (and in preparation for diagnostic examinations or tests).

EQUIPMENT: Prepackaged disposable enema (plain Fleet's), water-soluble lubricant, Mayo tray, towel, latex gloves, tissues, drape sheet, pen, patient's chart

TERMINAL PERFORMANCE OBJECTIVE: Provided with an anatomical model of the lower abdominopelvic cavity or a mannequin, and all equipment and supplies required to administer a cleansing enema, first administer the enema to the anatomical model, then the mannequin; in each process the steps of the procedure must be demonstrated in proper order.

1. Explain procedure to patient. **RATIONALE: Speaking to the patient by name and checking the chart ensures that you are performing the procedure on the correct patient.**
2. Instruct to disrobe from the waist down. Provide drape sheet and assist patient on to exam table.
3. Help patient into Sims' position, asking patient to lie on left side and to bring the right knee up to the waist. Adjust the drape sheet.
4. Wash hands and put on latex gloves. **CAUTION:** Remember, in order to comply with universal precautions guidelines, gloves must be worn if there is any possibility of coming into contact with blood or any body fluids.
5. Remove the protective covering from the tip of the enema container, and apply a small amount of lubricant if necessary (tip *is* prelubricated) to the tip.
6. With one hand separate the buttocks to expose the anus; with the other hold the enema bottle , and gently insert the tip into the rectum, making sure that the tip points in the direction of the patient's navel. Note: Advise the patient to breathe deeply and slowly through the mouth. **RATIONALE: This aids patient to relax and makes instillation easier.**
7. Express the entire contents from the bottle slowly (squeeze from bottom to top of bottle), asking the patient to retain the liquid for as long as possible. *Note: Five to ten minutes so that the solution will have time to work.*
8. Withdraw the enema tip slowly and provide patient with tissues. *Note: Tissues may be used to remove any lubricant or placed against the anus with pressure to aid in maintaining the enema. Discard in a biohazardous waste container if the tissues are left in the room.* Direct patient to rest room as necessary; ask patient to let you check results before flushing. Report to physician.
9. Clean room; discard disposables in appropriate waste containers.
10. Remove gloves and wash hands.
11. Initial chart (signifying that procedure has been completed).

Proper positioning of patients during the exam is important for both the physician's viewing of the rectum and sigmoid colon and the patient's comfort. **Proctology** tables are designed especially for this procedure. They provide support of the patient's chest and head with the arm resting against the headboard as the table is tilted to the knee-chest position. Those who cannot tolerate this position are assisted into Sims' position for the exam. Many physicians find this acceptable and it is certainly more comfortable for the patient. You should ask about the physician's preference in patient position since there are many variations.

The physician may wish to view the intestinal **mucosa** following a normal bowel movement. More often, the patient is instructed to eat a light diet containing plenty of clear liquids and avoiding dairy products for 24 hours before the exam, and to have a plain cleansing enema the morning of, or 2 hours before, the exam. Still other physicians may wish patients to use laxatives the day before and an enema the night before and also the morning of the exam. Patients have

FIGURE 6–47 Rectal examination setup

usually eaten little within the past few days because of their abdominal distress.

In the diagnosis of hemorrhoids, fissures, and ulcerations, the physician usually begins investigative procedures by examining the anus and the interior of the rectum with a proctoscope, Figure 6–47. During the sigmoidoscopy, the physician may want to take a biopsy of questionable tissue from the sigmoid colon to aid in confirming the diagnosis. It is a good rule to have all possible necessary items available. When the patient has been prepared and the examiner is ready to begin the exam, the medical assistant hands the necessary instruments and supplies to the physician as needed. Remember to advise patients to report any problems, such as bleeding, discharge, swelling, or any other unusual discomfort following any procedure. A biopsy lab request form must be completed and accompany the tissue to the lab. Containers for biopsy specimens have a **formalin** solution to preserve the tissue until the analysis is done.

There are many other proctological procedures that may need to be performed by the physician for patients in the office setting. Some of the instruments used in these procedures are shown in Figure 6–48. All instruments and items that come in contact with a body cavity must be sterile. One of the duties that the medical assistant is generally responsible for is to make certain that this is so. Autoclaving, which is a method for sterilization of instruments, is discussed in Chapter 9.

Complete Chapter 6, Unit 4 in the workbook to help you meet the objectives at the beginning of this unit and therefore achieve competency of this subject matter.

FIGURE 6–48 Additional instruments used in rectal examinations: (a). Brinkerhoff rectal speculum: (b). Turrell rotating shaft rectal biopsy forceps: (c). Norwood rectal snare (Courtesy of J. Jamner Surgical Instruments Inc.)

MEDICAL–LEGAL
ETHICAL HIGHLIGHTS

Mrs. Right . . .

obtains a written contract for third-party payment and the written authorization for release of medical information from patients. She respects each patient and keeps information disclosed confidential. She reports suspicious injuries to the proper authorities and sexually transmitted diseases to the health department. She practices safety, assists patients when necessary, and respects their choice of treatment.

Employment outlook: Excellent

Miss Wrong . . .

forgets frequently to obtain written authorization to release information. She is careless about keeping information confidential. She won't take the time to report suspicious injuries or sexually transmitted diseases because it is too much trouble. She is often careless about safety practices, and shows little respect to patients.

Employment outlook: Poor

REFERENCES

A Guide for Eye Inspection and Testing Visual Acuity. National Society for the Prevention of Blindness, Inc., 1991.

Kunz, Jeffrey R. M. and Finkel, Asher J., Eds. *The American Medical Association Family Medical Guide.* New York: Random House, 1987.

Morbidity and Mortality Weekly Report (MMWR) 32, no. 1, (January 14, 1983): 1–17.

MMWR Supplement, 36, no. 25 (August 21, 1987).

Mosby's Medical, Nursing, & Allied Health Dictionary, 3d ed. St. Louis: C.V. Mosby Company, 1990.

Ohio Department of Health, 246 N. High St., Columbus, OH 43215; and Columbus Health Department, 181 S. Washington Blvd., Columbus, OH 43215. "Child Daycare Center Communicable Disease Chart." Columbus, February 1986.

Reader's Digest Illustrated Encyclopedic Dictionary. Pleasantville, NY: Reader's Digest Association, Inc., 1987.

Schneidman, Rose; Lambert, Susan; and Wander, Barbara. *Being a Nursing Assistant,* 3d ed. Robert J. Brady, 1982.

Sherman, Jacques L. Jr. and Fields, Sylvia K. *Guide to Patient Evaluation History Taking, Physical Examination, and the Nursing Process,* 5th ed. New York: Medical Examination Publishing Company, Elsevier Science Publishing Co., Inc., 1988.

Simmers, Louise. *Diversified Health Occupations,* 3rd ed. Albany: Delmar, 1993.

_____. Nurses Reference Library, Assessment. Springhouse, PA: Springhouse, 1983.

Taber, Clarence W. *Taber's Cyclopedic Medical Dictionary,* 14th ed. Philadelphia: F. A. Davis Co., 1983.

Titmus Optical, Inc. Petersburg, VA, 1985.

U.S. Department of Health and Human Services, Public Health Service Center for Disease Control, Atlanta, GA 30333. "Recommendations for Prevention of HIV Transmission in Health Care Settings." Atlanta, 1987.

Webster's *New World Dictionary, The 100,000 Entry Edition.* New York: Penguin, 1971.

C H A P T E R   7

Specimen Collection and Laboratory Procedures

UNIT 1
The Microscope

UNIT 2
Capillary Blood Tests

UNIT 3
Venous Blood Tests

UNIT 4
Urine, Sputum, and
Stool Specimens

UNIT 5
Bacterial Smears and Cultures

The medical assistant will be responsible for a number of laboratory testing procedures when assisting the physician in the medical office. To be effective in this role, you must know the normal range of various laboratory tests and the proper preparation and procedure for each. An office policy manual for laboratory procedures, as well as one from the laboratory where specimens are sent for analysis, should be kept in a handy place for reference. The knowledgeable medical assistant can make patients feel more at ease about these procedures and elicit more cooperation.

You must follow laboratory instructions exactly in obtaining, preparing, labeling, and sending all specimens for analysis. Accurate typing or printing of all the necessary information on the lab request forms will help to expedite testing and reporting from the laboratory and eliminate unnecessary phone calls. As reports of tests are returned, it will be your responsibility to alert the physician to any abnormal results. This is usually done by circling or underlining the abnormal finding in red ink. As ordered by the physician, you may contact the patient concerning the reports and follow-up procedures.

All lab reports should be filed in the patient's chart as soon as possible after the physician has read them. A special marking, stamp, or the physician's initials on the lab reports will indicate that they are ready to be filed.

Almost every medical practice is equipped with a standard microscope, which is used to examine objects that cannot be seen with the naked eye. The microscope is most helpful in identifying microorganisms in urine and other body fluids and tissues. It is also used in determining blood cell counts. You must develop basic skill in operation and care of the microscope.

Public health officials at the Centers for Disease Control in Atlanta, Georgia, recommend that **all health professionals follow universal precautions.** These "universal blood and body-fluid precautions," or "universal precautions," are required as a means of infection control and should be used consistently for all patients, especially when the health status of the patient is unknown (such as in an emergency situation). Making these universal precautions a *habit* is *vital* for your future health. The precautions recommend:

1. Routine use of appropriate barriers and **PPE (Personal Protective Equipment)** to prevent contact with mucous membranes, blood, or any other body fluid of a patient
2. Routine, proper, thorough handwashing
3. Immediate placing of used sharps and needles in biohazard puncture-proof containers
4. Use of disposables in resuscitation procedures
5. Refraining from direct patient care if you have an exudative skin condition (or other contagious disease)
6. Especially strict adherence to precautions during pregnancy.

Many serious diseases can be spread by careless acts. The two most feared are hepatitis B (HBV) and human immunodeficiency virus (HIV), which is the cause of acquired immunodeficiency syndrome (AIDS). Research continues in an effort to find vaccines for AIDS and HIV. There is a vaccine for the prevention of HBV, which all health care providers should have administered at no cost to employees if they will be exposed to **bloodborne** pathogens or other hazardous body fluids or infectious waste in the course of their duties. If all health care workers follow these precautions to help in the control of contagious diseases, it will set a good example for the public (remember, actions speak louder than words).

Guidelines for Lab Safety ....

1. Proper handwashing before and after any and every procedure, before and after gloving, must become a habit for all health workers for self-protection from disease transmission. (Immediately washing **any** skin surface thoroughly that has been contaminated with any blood or body fluids is vital.)
2. Gloving is always a must when handling *any* blood or body fluid specimens.
3. Cover all scratches, paper cuts, or any breaks in the skin with a bandage after handwashing and before gloving for self-protection against possible contamination.
4. Never eat, drink, chew gum, smoke, or place hands or fingers to your mouth or face or place any item, such as a pen or pencil, in your mouth while working.
5. A completely separate storage area, including refrigerator and freezer, must be provided for all food and drink for employees and for all blood and other specimens awaiting analysis. It is federally mandated that employers follow OSHA standards of December 1991.
6. Wear protective gloves, mask, gown (or apron), and goggles when splashing of any blood or body fluids is possible while you are working, Figure 7–1.
7. Always recap or close bottles, jars, tubes, and other containers immediately after desired amounts are obtained to avoid spills, waste, and accidents.

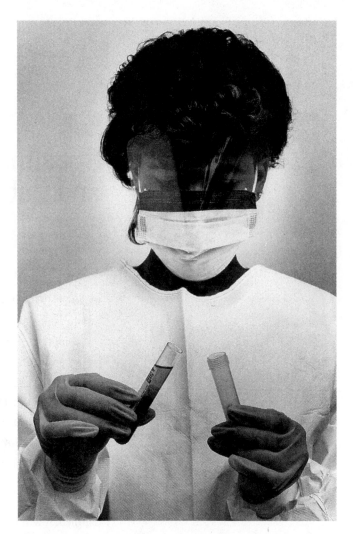

FIGURE 7–1 This medical assistant is wearing protective barriers—latex gloves, gown, face shield and mask—as she prepares to pour serum from a centrifuged blood tube to the transfer for laboratory analysis.

8. Clean up spills immediately to avoid accidents, Figure 7–2. Spilled blood or any body fluids should be flooded with a liquid germicide or bleach solution (a 1:10 ratio) before cleaning up with paper towels (wear latex gloves). Commercial preparations may also be used to solidify liquids, which makes cleanup easier.
9. Record lab test results immediately on charts or in logs to ensure accuracy.
10. Work in a well-lighted, properly ventilated, uncluttered, quiet area for better concentration.
11. Discard all disposable sharp instruments, lancets, syringes and needles (intact) in proper biohazard puncture-proof containers, Figure 7–3 (**never** break needles off, handle after use, or reuse). Place reusable metal instruments in a disinfectant solution after rinsing in cold water in preparation for proper cleaning and sterilization.
12. Discard *all* hazardous waste in proper containers, Figure 7–4.

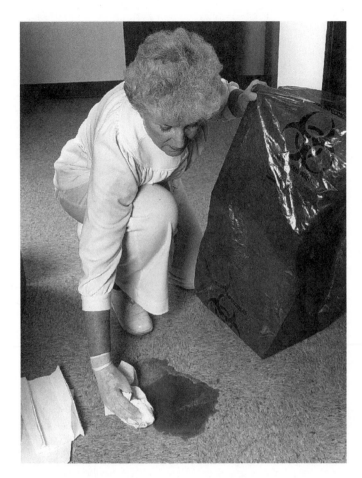

FIGURE 7–2 This medical assistant is wearing latex gloves to clean up a specimen spill. The biohazardous waste bag is used to dispose of the contaminated materials.

FIGURE 7–3 A few of the various sizes of biohazard puncture-proof containers are displayed (they are a bright red or yellow to alert caution). Biohazardous waste containers should be autoclaved when full and returned to the biohazard agency for proper disposal.

FIGURE 7–4 This medical assistant is placing a sturdy disposable plastic bag marked with the biohazardous waste symbol into a durable cardboard box marked the same for collection of infective waste material. When full, these boxes are picked up by an agency for incineration or for autoclaving before disposal in a public landfill.

13. Make periodic checks of all electrical appliances and equipment for frayed wires or faulty operation and tag for repair if needed.
14. Make sure that your hands are dry before using any electrical appliances or equipment.
15. Report all accidents to your supervisor or instructor immediately.
16. Clearly post emergency phone numbers near the telephone in the lab (i.e., local fire, police, emergency medical unit, and poison control center), Figure 7–5, page 372.
17. Have available (nearby or in the lab) first aid items (i.e., sterile gauze, bandages, tape, etc.) for emergency use.
18. Clearly post the sign over the functional emergency eye wash station in the lab, Figure 7–6.
19. Do not wear loose-fitting or bulky clothing or jewelry that could contribute to accidents while working with machines or equipment in the lab or any area in the office or clinic.

20. Use gas or air valves and Bunsen burners with caution. Keep flammable chemicals away from them.
21. Use only disposable paper cups for drinking.
22. Designate a "dirty" and a "clean" area in your lab, and enforce this policy.
23. Package broken glass or any sharp usable item in a sturdy cardboard box or puncture-proof container marked "caution—broken glass" to discard in the proper waste receptacle. (This will protect unsuspecting custodial personnel from injury.)
24. Never lean into work area when working with flame or chemicals (pour at arm's length) to avoid self-injury or accident.

U N I T 1
The Microscope

OBJECTIVES ....

Upon completion of this unit, you will meet the following terminal performance objectives by verifying knowledge of the facts and principles presented through oral and written communication at a level deemed competent by the instructor or employer, and will demonstrate the specific behaviors as identified in the terminal performance objectives of the procedures, observing all aseptic and safety precautions in accordance with health care standards.

1. Identify the parts of the microscope and the purpose of each.
2. Adjust and focus the objectives and state their magnification power.

EMERGENCY PHONE NUMBERS		
EMS		911
Police		555-1111
Emergency Squad		555-1010
Fire Dept.		555-0000
Rescue Squad		555-5050
Hospital:		555-7171
	ICU	ext. 210
	CCU	ext. 250
	ER	ext. 265
	Admitting	ext. 200
Ambulance		555-1818
Poison Control Center		555-6101
Coroner		555-9914
Taxi		555-2222

FIGURE 7–5 Example of recommended phone numbers to post near each phone for emergency assistance.

Many patients may be frightened or confused about some of the laboratory procedures requested by the physician to aid in diagnosis. You may perform some of these in the office or clinic setting or send the patient to the lab for tests. If you send patients elsewhere, make sure you give accurate directions on how to get there.

Each test or procedure must be explained clearly and concisely to relieve patients' anxiety. Use language that patients will understand. Most people have little or no knowledge of medical terminology.

Certain lab tests require preparation by patients prior to arrival (i.e., fasting, taking or omitting certain medications, etc.). Be sure to instruct patients in these preparations and have clear, concise, written instructions available. Do not presume that patients know all about a procedure even if they have had the test before. Often new techniques require additional or different instructions for preparation. Medical technology is constantly changing. It is important for health care providers (including medical assistants) to keep abreast of new developments in medicine. Inform patients that some procedures can cause temporary discomfort and how it may be relieved.

Give patients enough time to look over the printed instruction sheet or pamphlet and make certain you answer all of their questions thoroughly before they leave.

FIGURE 7–6 The emergency eye wash fountain connects to existing plumbing. The two streams of water wash both eyes continuously and simultaneously.

Use Microscope

PURPOSE: To gain skill in the use of the microscope.

EQUIPMENT: Microscope, electrical outlet for light source of microscope, specimen on glass slide with frosted end, cover glass (used usually for wet specimens only), lens cleaning tissues, latex gloves

TERMINAL PERFORMANCE OBJECTIVE: Provided with all necessary equipment and supplies, demonstrate the use of the microscope following the steps in the procedure with the instructor observing each step.

1. Wash hands and put on latex gloves. **CAUTION:** Remember, in order to comply with universal precautions guidelines, gloves must be worn if there is any possibility of coming into contact with blood or any body fluids.
2. Assemble necessary equipment.
3. Clean ocular lens with lens cleaning tissues. **RATIONALE: Removal of makeup, oil, and eye secretions is necessary to ensure clear viewing and eliminate transmission of disease among office personnel.** *Note: Use only lens tissue paper to prevent damaging the surface of the lens.*
4. Plug microscope light source into electrical outlet and turn on light switch at front base of microscope.
5. Place specimen slide on stage with frosted end up, between clips, and secure over opening of stage.

Note: Frosted end is used for labeling the specimen in pencil.

6. Watch carefully as you raise substage so that it does not come into direct contact with slide.
7. Turn revolving nosepiece to low-power objective (10X) and begin to focus coarse-adjustment dial until a wide shaft can be seen.
8. When outline of specimen is in view, turn fine-adjustment dial until specimen can be seen in detail.
9. Adjust substage diaphragm lever or adjust mirror to obtain proper lighting.
10. If sharper detail is needed, carefully turn revolving nosepiece to intermediate-power objective and adjust fine-focus dial.
11. When using oil-immersion lens objective or hpf, oil should be used very sparingly. *Note: A cover slide should be used and lens must be cleaned after each use. Adjustment must be made for amount of light needed by adjusting diaphragm lever under stage.*
12. When specimen has been identified turn off light and return all items to proper storage area. *Note: Microscope stage should be cleaned as well as any slides that are not disposable.*
13. Remove gloves and wash hands.
14. Results of examination should be recorded or reported to physician as directed.

---

3. Adjust the light and mirror for proper viewing.
4. Demonstrate how to clean the microscope (lens, stage, mirror).
5. Explain the general purpose of the microscope in the medical office.
6. Demonstrate the proper way to carry a microscope.
7. Spell and define, using the glossary at the back of the text, all the words to know in this unit.

WORDS TO KNOW ....

binocular	monocular
bloodborne	objective
compensate	PPE (personal protective
condenser	equipment)
hpf (high-power field)	proficient
lpf (low-power field)	specimen
magnify	technical
minute	

The microscope is an essential piece of equipment in the laboratory of almost every medical practice. It is used to examine and identify **minute** objects that cannot be seen with the naked eye. Microscopes are fine and expensive **technical** instruments that must be handled with great respect. The operation and care manual should be kept handy for reference, because each microscope is slightly different. The amount of routine maintenance required will vary with the amount of use.

The part of the microscope that supports the eyepiece is called the arm. Figure 7–7, page 375, shows the labeled parts of a **binocular** microscope. The proper way to carry the microscope is to grasp the arm with one hand and place the other hand under the base, holding it at waist level. The electrical cord for the light source should be loosely wrapped and secured with a twist tie or a rubber band. Wrapping the cord too tightly may cause the enclosed wires to break and lead to a short that could cause an electrical fire. The cord of the microscope should be kept loosely wrapped and out of the work area when not in use. It should always be unplugged by grasping the plug, never by pulling the cord. As with any electrical appliance, all surrounding surfaces and hands should be dry. Wet hands, floors, and so on, can lead to electric shock.

A binocular microscope has two eyepieces. The **monocular** microscope has only one eyepiece, or ocular lens. The eyepiece is in the upper part of the tube of the microscope and contains a lens to **magnify** what is being seen.

The body tube leads to the revolving nosepiece. Attached to the revolving nosepiece are three (sometimes four) small lenses called **objectives**, each of which has a different magnifying power. The shortest has the lowest power. It is called the **low-power field**, or **lpf**. On most microscopes, it will magnify the object to be viewed 10 times, or make it 10X larger than when viewed by the naked eye. The low-power field is the lens used to scan the field of interest and to focus in on the specimen. To position each objective, you simply rotate the nosepiece until you hear a click.

For greater detail in viewing the specimen, turn the nosepiece to the next longer objective, the high-power (hpf, high-power field) lens. It will magnify the object approximately 40 times, or 40X. The longest objective is the oil-immersion objective. This high-power lens magnifies objects about 100 times, or 100X. Using the fine-focus dial will bring the specimen into good definition.

The stage of the microscope has two clips which hold the **specimen** slide to be viewed. Just underneath the stage is a substage where a **condenser** is held that regulates the amount of light directed on the magnified specimen. It has a shutter or diaphragm to control the amount of light desired. The substage may be raised or lowered in focusing on the specimen.

A supply of lens tissue paper should be kept nearby to clean the lenses after each use. Makeup, oil, secretions from the eyes, and dust can make it difficult to see through the lens, besides being a possible means of transmitting disease among office personnel. Eyeglasses are not necessary when performing microscopic work, because the microscope may be focused to **compensate** for all visual defects except astigmatism.

It will take time and patience to learn how to operate the microscope. The supervision of an experienced operator is essential to becoming **proficient** in its use and care.

Complete Chapter 7, Unit 1 in the workbook to help you meet the objectives at the beginning of this unit and therefore achieve competency of this subject matter.

U N I T   2

Capillary Blood Tests

OBJECTIVES ....

Upon completion of this unit, you will meet the following terminal performance objectives by verifying knowledge of the facts and principles presented through oral and written communication at a level deemed competent by the instructor or employer, and will demonstrate the specific behaviors as identified in the terminal performance objectives of the procedures, observing all aseptic and safety precautions in accordance with health care standards.

1. State the purpose of wearing latex gloves when performing laboratory procedures.
2. List and discuss the regulatory bodies that govern the POL.
3. List and discuss the laboratory practices that yield quality assurance in the POL.
4. Explain the reasons for performing capillary blood tests in the medical office.
5. Perform skin puncture procedures to obtain capillary blood specimens.
6. Complete a health department request form for the PKU test and obtain the blood specimen for it.
7. Obtain hemoglobin and hematocrit levels.
8. Operate a microhematocrit centrifuge.
9. Operate a hemoglobinometer.
10. Perform a blood glucose screening test with glucometer (or color chart on bottle) from reagent strip.
11. Explain the purpose of the GTT (glucose tolerance test).
12. Give instructions and patient education for the preparation of a patient for a GTT.
13. Make calculations of blood cells using the hemocytometer.
14. Perform a red and white blood cell count.
15. Prepare a blood smear for a differential count.
16. List each type of white blood cell and state the function of each.
17. Spell and define, using the glossary at the back of the text, all the words to know in this unit.

WORDS TO KNOW ....

allosteric	metabolism
carbohydrates	neonate
centrifuge	OSHA (Occupational Safety and Health Administration)
CLIA (Clinical Laboratory Improvement Amendments)	pallor
differential	percentage
diffuse	phagocytosis
erythropoiesis	phenylalanine
glucose	PKU (phenylketonuria)
HCFA	POL (physician's office laboratory)
hematocrit	
HHS (U.S. Department of Health and Human Services)	polycythemia
	puncture
implement	regulatory
insignificant	reticuloendothelial
insulin	stat
laboratory	sterile
lancet	tolerance
meniscus	waiver

Laboratory Classification and Regulation ....

The physician's office **laboratory (POL)** falls under many **regulatory** bodies. The complexity of the laboratory tests performed will determine which classification the POL is and

TABLE 7-1
Laboratory Classifications

Proposed Certificate of Waiver Tests (Exempt)

Urinalysis by reagent strip or tablet
Microscopic urine sediment
Urine pregnancy tests
Occult blood in stool
Microscopic examination of:
    Pinworm preparation
    Vaginal wet mount preparation
    KOH (Potassium hydroxide) preparation of cutaneous
       scrapings
    Semen analysis
    Gram stain (of discharge and exudate)
Screen-slide card agglutination test for
    ASO (antistreptolysin O)
    CRP (C-reactive protein)
    Infectious mononucleosis screening
    Rheumatoid factor screening
    Sickle cell screening (nonelectrophoresis method)
Ovulation tests (visual color test for human luteinizing
       hormone)
Whole-blood-clotting time
Glucose reagent strip screening
Spun microhematocrit
Erythrocyte sedimentation rate

Proposed Level I Tests

Cholesterol screen (qualitative and semiqualitative determinations)
Urine cultures for colony counts (excluding identification and
    susceptibility)
Red and white blood cell counts
Hematocrit
BUN (blood urea nitrogen) uric acid
Glucose
    Creatinine
Direct strep-antigen test

Proposed Level II Tests

All other remaining tests under CPT 80000 series, including
Automated multichannel chemical profiles
Radioimmunoassay procedures
Drug and toxicology procedures
Coagulation studies

These classifications are based on the complexity of the tests and the risks involved in the reporting of an error in the results.

FIGURE 7-7 Parts of the microscope (From Caldwell & Hegner, *Nursing Assistant,* 6th ed. Copyright 1992, Delmar Publishers Inc. Photo courtesy of Bausch & Lomb Inc.)

under which body it is regulated. Table 7–1 outlines the three laboratory classifications under **CLIA**-88 (Clinical Laboratory Improvement Amendments, 1988).

A certificate of **Waiver** allows *only* those tests to be performed in a POL that are on the final list of waivered tests. Waivered tests are those that basically have an **insignificant** risk to the patient if an error is made in the test results. This means that there would be no significant risk or harm done to the patient. Application for this certificate is obtained from **HHS** (U.S. Department of Health and Human Services). Laboratory tests on the certificate of waiver list may be billed to Medicare and Medicaid. This certificate must be renewed every 2 years for a moderate fee. Tests performed in the POL must be restricted to this list.

Level I laboratory tests must be performed under more strict regulations. Any abnormal test results that apply to a previously undiagnosed condition of a patient must be referred to a level II lab to be verified.

Regulatory bodies periodically inspect laboratories and medical offices to ensure quality assurance and quality control. Quality assurance in the health care field refers to all evaluative services and the results compared with accepted standards. Quality control implies that operational procedures are used to **implement** the quality assurance program. To determine these standards many aspects of care are taken into account. First, the cost, place, accessibility, treatment, and benefits of health care are evaluated. The next step is comparing the findings with standard results. Finally, the appropriate recommendations for improving health care are noted.

Both level I and II laboratories are required to follow quality assurance programs. The purposes of quality assurance programs are to evaluate the quality and effectiveness of health care

Puncture Skin with Sterile Lancet

PURPOSE: To obtain a few drops of capillary blood for screening tests.

EQUIPMENT: Latex gloves, sterile **lancet,** Figure 7–9, page 379, alcohol, cotton balls, gauze squares, Mayo table.

TERMINAL PERFORMANCE OBJECTIVE: Provided with all necessary equipment and supplies, and using other students as patients, demonstrate the skin puncture procedure following all steps to obtain capillary blood for test(s) specified by the physician or instructor. The instructor will observe each step.

1. Identify patient. **RATIONALE: Speaking to the patient by name and checking chart ensures that you are performing the procedure on the correct patient.**
2. Explain the procedure to the patient.
3. Inspect patient's fingers (or other puncture sites) and select most desirable site.
   Note:
   a. *Main sites are ring or great finger, earlobe, infant's lateral areas of heel.*
   b. *Some patients have a preference for a particular site.*
   c. *Earlobe is less sensitive to pain than fingers.*
   d. *Do not use areas that are bruised, calloused, or injured.*
4. Wash hands, put on latex gloves, and assemble needed items on Mayo table. **CAUTION:** Remember, in order to comply with universal precautions guidelines, gloves must be worn if there is any possibility of coming into contact with blood or any body fluids.
5. Wipe desired site with an alcohol-saturated cotton ball

and let dry. Do not blow the skin to expedite drying; **RATIONALE: You may contaminate the area with microorganisms in the exhaled air**
6. Take **sterile** lancet out of package without contaminating point. *Note: Another must be used if point is touched*
7. Hold patient's finger (or other site) securely between your thumb and great finger. In your other hand hold lancet, pointed downward, with thumb and index or great finger. Puncture site quickly with a firm, steady down-and-up motion to approximately a 2-mm depth. *Note: Control entry and exit of lancet in same path to avoid ripping skin. To obtain a better blood sample, puncture across fingerprints not parallel to them.*
8. Discard first drop of blood by blotting away with dry gauze square. **RATIONALE: First drop may contain traces of alcohol or tissue fluid that would dilute sample and make test inaccurate**
9. Keep applying gentle pressure on either side of puncture site until necessary amount of blood has been obtained. *Note: Too much pressure will cause tissue fluid to mix with blood resulting in diluted sample and incorrect test results.*
10. Wipe site with alcohol-saturated cotton ball and ask patient to hold dry gauze square over it for a minute or two. *Note: Check site to be sure bleeding has stopped. Determine if patient is allergic to adhesive before applying bandage to puncture site (use guaze square and hypoallergenic tape if allergic).*
11. Remove gloves, wash hands, and discard used items in proper receptacle.

---

according to accepted standards and to ensure accuracy and validity in testing procedures. These levels of POLs must also participate in proficiency-testing programs for the test procedures that they perform and keep strict records of quality control.

Other federal bodies that provide regulation inspections of a POL are **HCFA** (Health Care Financing Administration) and **OSHA** (Occupational Safety and Health Administration). Private agencies also issue accreditations or state licensing for approved operation of the POL. The laboratory may be operated under a provisional certificate, which is issued until the HHS inspects the facility. Certificates must be renewed every 2 years. Inspections may be made, unannounced, anytime. If OSHA, an inspecting body separate from CLIA, finds a POL in noncompliance of regulations during a visit (scheduled or not), a $10,000 fine per item, per employee (per visit) applies.

In the POL, no matter what classification, the following practices should be followed to ensure reliable and accurate data, and to ensure quality health care to patients; quality assurance involves *proper*

1. Patient identification
2. Patient preparation and specimen collection
3. Specimen processing and transportation
4. Instrumental and technical performance
5. Safety
6. In-service training and education of all health care personnel

All state and federal health and safety regulations and laws apply to the POL according to the three lab classifications. It is important to stay abreast of the current regulations that apply to the facility where you are employed.

Skin Puncture

Capillary blood tests are frequently performed in the medical office or clinic because of the small amount of blood required, usually one to a few drops. Because most patients are extremely apprehensive, you must develop skill not only in performing the

PROCEDURE

Puncture Skin with Autolet

PURPOSE: To obtain a few drops of capillary blood for tests.

EQUIPMENT: Autolet, disposable platform (yellow—standard puncture depth of approximately 2 mm, orange—super-puncture depth of approximately 3 mm), sterile lancet, alcohol, cotton balls, gauze squares, latex gloves, Mayo table.

TERMINAL PERFORMANCE OBJECTIVE: Provided with all necessary equipment and supplies, and using other students as patients, demonstrate the steps in the procedure for obtaining capillary blood using the Autolet. The instructor will observe each step.

1. Identify patient. **RATIONALE: Speaking to the patient by name and checking chart ensures that you are performing the procedure on the correct patient.** *Note: When providing patient education be certain you are instructing the person who will be performing the procedure.*
2. Explain procedure to patient.
3. Inspect patient's fingers (or other puncture sites) and select most desirable site.
4. Wash hands, put on latex gloves. **CAUTION:** Remember, in order to comply with universal precautions guidelines, gloves must be worn if there is any possibility of coming into contact with blood or any body fluids. Assemble all necessary items on Mayo stand. *Note: Explain that gloves are not necessary when doing self-testing; however, washing hands is essential to prevent infection. Discuss home arrangement of equipment.*

5. Pull arm of Autolet back to activating button. It holds in place when click is heard.
6. Place sterile lancet securely into socket. Next, place appropriate platform, recessed surface down, into platform slot at base of Autolet.
7. Wipe puncture site with alcohol-saturated cotton ball and let dry.
8. Twist protective covering from tip of sterile lancet and press recessed surface against site firmly so that skin enters opening of platform, Figure 7–10.
9. Hold patient's finger steady with one hand and with other hand press activating button to pucnture site with lancet. Rest Autolet on Mayo stand and proceed.
10. Apply gentle pressure to both sides of puncture site with your thumb and great finger. Blot first drop of blood from puncture site with dry gauze square. **RATIONALE: The first drop of blood may contain traces of alcohol or tissue fluid that would dilute sample and make test inaccurate**
11. After a sufficient amount of blood has been obtained for desired test, wipe puncture site with alcohol-saturated cotton ball and ask patient to apply gentle pressure to site with dry gauze square for a minute or two. *Note: Check site to be sure bleeding has stopped. Determine if patient is allergic to adhesive before applying bandage to puncture site (use gauze square and hypoallergenic tape if allergic).*
12. Remove gloves, wash hands and discard used items in proper receptable.

---

procedures but in conveying reassurance to the patient. When skin **puncture** procedures are done correctly, the patient should feel minimal discomfort. Displaying confidence in carrying out the procedures competently will ensure patient safety and comfort.

Capillaries are minute blood vessels which convey blood from the arterioles to the venules. At this level, blood and oxygen **diffuse** to the tissues, and products of metabolic activity enter the bloodstream. For this reason, capillary blood is an ideal sample for the screening of **hematocrit**, hemoglobin, blood glucose, and PKU levels and other screening tests that require a very small amount of blood.

Capillary blood is just under the surface of the skin. The most practical sites to use are the ring and great finger, the earlobe, and in infants the heel or great toe, Figure 7–8(a) and (b).

The Autolet is widely used by diabetics (and other) patients in their homes for simple blood tests that require capillary blood, Figure 7–10(a), and (b). Patients may perform their own cholesterol tests at home using a drop of capillary blood with

the FDA approved (3/93) ChemTrak, Inc. Cholesterol Test Kit. This product gives results in 15 minutes by matching a color chart for the reading of the test strip. Patients should be instructed to sanitize the skin puncture device as necessary. You may be given the duty of instructing patients in use of the Autolet. Patients who use this technique daily at home should simply wash the puncture site thoroughly with soap and water. Alcohol tends to toughen the skin if used for extended periods.

With strict regulations regarding quality control and quality assurance, it is advisable to keep a log book to record all specimens and the results of the tests performed. The log should include

1. The date
2. Patient's name
3. Test performed
4. Results of the test
5. Your initials

Most patients, especially youngsters, are apprehensive about having blood taken. The medical assistant must calmly explain to each patient that screening tests, such as a hemoglobin or a blood glucose, are performed with a small amount of blood taken from the finger, earlobe, or infant's heel. Let the patient know ahead of time what you are going to do to gain cooperation. You should tell the patient that there will be a little pain or discomfort during the initial skin puncture, but it will not last long. Reassure the patient that this procedure is short-lived and necessary for the physician to make a diagnosis or evaluate the condition. Remember to advise the patient to keep the puncture site clean and dry for 24 hours with a fresh bandage as necessary.

PKU Test ....

A screening test done with capillary blood from an infant's heel or great toe is the **PKU (phenylketonuria)**. Phenylketonuria is a congenital disease due to a defect in the **metabolism** of the amino acid, **phenylalanine**. This unmetabolized protein, phenylalanine, accumulates in the bloodstream and can prevent the brain from developing normally. If this condition goes undetected and untreated, the result is mental retardation. This screening is required by law in most states and all Canadian provinces, either by blood test or urinalysis. The blood test requires that a few drops of the infant's blood be soaked through the outlined circles (from the back) of the treated paper attached to the health department form, Figure 7–11. This duplicated form must be completed accurately. Parents usually bring the form with them on the infant's first office visit unless the procedure was performed at the hospital nursery. After completion of the instructions, the form (intact with all copies) should be mailed to the health department. A report of the results of the screening test will be mailed back to

P R O C E D U R E

Obtain Blood for PKU Test

PURPOSE: To obtain a blood specimen for determination of PKU (phenylketonuria) level in blood.

EQUIPMENT: PKU helath department form, Autolet or sterile lancet, latex gloves, cotton balls, alcohol, gauze squares, round adhesive bandage, patient's chart, pen, stamped envelope addressed to health department.

TERMINAL PERFORMANCE OBJECTIVE: Provided with all necessary equipment and supplies, and using other students as patients, demonstrate the steps of the procedure for obtaining a blood speciment for determination of phenylketonuria level in the blood. The instructor will observe each step.

Note: This procedure may be simulated by using a clinical lifelike doll and milk colored with red food coloring for practice.

1. Wash hands, put on latex gloves, and assemble needed items on Mayo table. **CAUTION:** Remember, in order to comply with universal precautions guidelines, gloves must be worn if there is any possibility of coming into contact with blood or any body fluids.
2. Identify patient. Ask parent to name patient and check chart to avoid error.
3. Explain procedure to parent and ask for necessary information to complete form. Be sure to write the exact birth weight of the infant on the form and the date and time the test was performed. **RATIONALE: Accurate**

results depend on the ratio of findings to birthweight. Ask for their assistance in holding infant still during procedure.

4. Wipe desired site with alcohol-saturated cotton ball and let dry.
5. Take sterile lancet out of the package without containinating point.
6. Secure infant's great toe or lateral heel with your great finger and thumb and gently apply pressure to produce a large drop of blood. Carefully blot onto one of outlined circles on end of form soaking the test paper from the back of the form. *Note: Repeat until each circle has been entirely saturated*
7. Wipe puncture site with alcohol-saturated cotton ball and apply dry gauze square. Ask parent to hold against puncture site. Then place small round bandage over area.
8. Place completed test form into protective envelope and then into an envelope addressed to health department with physician's return address.
9. Record procedure on patient's chart and initial.
10. Remove gloves, wash hands, discard used items in proper receptacle, and return items to proper storage area.
11. File report in patient's chart when received in return mail after physician has checked the results.

Infant's heel/great toe · Earlobe · Ring/great finger

B.

FIGURE 7–8 (a) These skin puncture sites are recommended because of abundant capillary blood flow for obtaining a specimen. They are also desirable sites for convenience of the patient. (b) Skin punctures should be made across the fingerprints, not parallel to them.

the physician to be filed in the infant's chart. This test is limited to newborns (**neonates**) and their biological parents.

Symptoms of PKU are severe mental retardation, hyperactivity, convulsions, and a musty sweat and urine odor.

In addition to the PKU test, public health officials recommend that infants are screened for the following genetic and endocrine diseases and disorders that cause mental retardation

FIGURE 7–10(a) Autolet components: (a) platform, (b) platform slot, (c) spring-loaded arm, (d) activating button, (e) lancet, (f) lancet socket

YELLOW
2.4 mm

ORANGE
3.0 mm

FIGURE 7–9 A variety of sterile lances and devices to use for obtaining capillary blood samples

and other problems if not detected and treated shortly after birth. *Galactosemia* is the body's inability to digest galactose, a milk sugar. A buildup of galactose in the blood interferes with the body's use of sugars and starches. This can cause damage to the brain, liver, and eyes, and if not detected and treated may lead rapidly to death. A well-balanced milk-free diet is the treatment.

Homocystinuria is an inability to utilize methionine (an amino acid, which is found in proteins) because of the absence of a liver enzyme that is necessary for growth. If this is not treated, the results are not detected until it is too late. The abnormalities caused by this disease are mental retardation, bone and blood vessel deformities, blood clots, and eye com-

FIGURE 7–10(b) Press the recessed surface against the site so that the skin enters the opening of the platform.

FIGURE 7–11 (a) PKU blood test form (b) Instructions

INSTRUCTIONS FOR NEWBORN SCREENING SPECIMENS

1. Cleanse infant's heel with alcohol swab.
2. Puncture heel in fleshy lateral or medial posterior portion with sterile disposable lancet. Wipe puncture site with dry sterile swab.
3. Allow large blood droplet to form. Touch blood droplet to center of circle on ONE SIDE of filter paper card ONLY. Observe reverse side of card and insure that blood has soaked completely through before removing card from infant's heel.
4. Repeat step 3 to fill ALL FIVE CIRCLES. DO NOT squeeze heel excessively to obtain blood.
5. Allow card to AIR DRY 2 hours at room temperature on a non-absorbent surface. DO NOT stack cards together while drying.
6. After blood spots are completely dry, place card in ODH self-addressed laboratory mailing envelope. MAIL within 48 HOURS.

CORRECT   INCORRECT

B

plications. This is also treated with well-balanced diet and vitamin therapy. Regular checkups and monitoring of methionine levels are recommended.

Hypothyroidism, which is a lack of thyroid hormone, results in slow mental and physical development. Lifelong thyroid hormone replacement therapy is necessary for normal growth and development.

Hemoglobin and Hematocrit

Hemoglobin and hematocrit screening tests also require a few drops of capillary blood. Usually the ring or great finger is used in children and adults because these fingers are not as sensitive as the index finger. The thumb is usually too tough-skinned, and the little finger is generally too small and would not yield an adequate amount. The patient's age or preference will help you decide which site to choose.

Hematocrit is a screening test to determine anemia. *Anemia* is a condition in which there is a lack of circulating red blood cells. Erythrocytes transport oxygen to the entire body. When there are not enough of them to supply all of the cells, symptoms of paleness, fatigue, drowsiness, among others, become apparent in patients. **Polycythemia,** a condition of having an excessive number of erythrocytes, may be indicated by an abnormally high reading. Some of the symptoms are similar to anemia—weakness and fatigue. Redness of the skin (opposite of anemia) and pain of the extremities, often with black-and-blue spots, is observed in some patients with polycythemia. You should become familiar with all of the symptoms of the diseases for which you perform screening tests so that you may alert the physician to any changes that patients may tell you. Often patients disclose important information to you and then do not say anything to the doctor because they think you have already reported it.

To perform a microhematocrit screening test, you begin by cleansing the skin site with alcohol using a gauze square or

FIGURE 7–12 Skin puncture is made with a sterile lancet across the fingerprints.

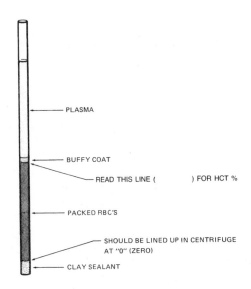

FIGURE 7–14 A labeled hematocrit tube after centrifugation

Labels on figure:
- PLASMA
- BUFFY COAT
- READ THIS LINE (   ) FOR HCT %
- PACKED RBC'S
- SHOULD BE LINED UP IN CENTRIFUGE AT "0" (ZERO)
- CLAY SEALANT

cotton ball. A sterile lancet is used to puncture the skin, Figure 7–12. Very small glass tubes, called microhematocrit tubes, are used to collect the blood sample, Figure 7–13. Many of them are marked with a fill line at about the three-quarter point. The tube fills very quickly by capillary action if the puncture site is deep enough, usually about 2 mm. A small amount of clay sealant is carefully placed in one end of the microhematocrit tube to seal the opening so that blood will not leak out. Make sure that there is no trace of red visible around the end of the tube with clay (even a minute hairline path of red will cause *all* of the blood in the tube to spin out during centrifugation).

The tube is then placed in a microhematocrit **centrifuge** where spinning for approximately 3 minutes separates the blood components by centrifugal action. The tube after cen-

FIGURE 7–13 Microhematocrit tubes

trifugation has three layers: plasma, a thin yellowish layer called the buffy coat, and packed red blood cells, Figure 7–14. Contained in the buffy coat are the white blood cells and the platelets.

The hematocrit is expressed as the **percentage** of the total blood volume made up of red blood cells (erythrocytes) or as the volume in cubic centimeters (cc) of erythrocytes packed by centrifugation in 100 cc of blood. The normal hematocrit range for adult males is 40 to 54% and for adult females 37 to 47%.

Figure 7–17, page 386, shows a centrifugal hematology system that analyzes finger-puncture or venous blood samples to provide the following values:

- hematocrit
- platelet count
- total white blood cell count
- total granulocyte count
- percentage granulocytes
- total lymphocyte and monocyte count
- percentage lymphocytes to monocytes

Figure 17–18, page 387, shows the steps in preparing the blood tubes for use in centrifugal hematology system.

In determining the hemoglobin (Hb) level of the blood, a conversion chart may be used when the hematocrit percentage (Hct %) is known; it may also be used to check the red blood cell count when hemoglobin and hematocrit (H & H) are known, Table 17–2. Hemoglobin is an **allosteric** protein found in erythrocytes, which transports molecular oxygen in the blood. A most reliable and simple way to determine hemoglobin level is with the hemoglobinometer, Figure 17–19, page 388. The normal range of hemoglobin for males is 14 to 18 grams per 100 mL of blood, and for females 12 to 16. Physicians may order an H & H to get a more definite idea of the patient's red cell volume.

TABLE 17–2

Approximate Relationship Between Hematocrit, Red Cell Count, and Hemoglobin in Adults

For Red Cells of Normal Size—To Be Used for Checking Purposes Only*		
Hematocrit (%)	Red Cell Count (x 1 million per cubic millimeter of blood)	Hemoglobin (in grams per 100 cc)
30	3.4	9.8
31	3.6	10.4
32	3.7	10.7
33	3.8	11.0
34	3.9	11.3
35	4.0	11.6
36	4.1	11.9
37	4.3	12.4
38	4.4	12.8
39	4.5	13.1
40	4.6	13.3
41	4.7	13.6
42	4.8	13.9
43	4.9	14.2
44	5.1	14.8
45	5.2	15.1
46	5.3	15.4
47	5.4	15.7
48	5.5	16.0
49	5.6	16.2
50	5.7	16.5
51	5.9	17.1
52	6.0	17.4
53	6.1	17.7
54	6.2	18.0
55	6.3	18.3
56	6.4	18.6
57	6.6	19.1
58	6.7	19.4
59	6.8	19.7
60	6.9	20.1
61	7.0	20.3
Normal Hematocrits	Normal Red Cell Counts	Normal Hemoglobins
Men: Range 40–54%	Men: Range 4,600,000–6,200,000	Men: Range 14.0–18.0 g
Aver. 47%	Aver. 5,400,000	Aver. 15.8 g
Women: Range 37–47%	Women: Range 4,200,000–5,400,000	Women: Range 11.5–16.0 g
Aver. 42%	Aver. 4,800,000	Aver. 13.9 g

*The relationship shown between hematocrit and red cell count is based on normal cells (which have an average mean corpuscular volume of 0.87). The relationship between hemoglobin and red cell count is based on normal cells (with a mean corpuscular hemoglobin of 29). These relationships do not hold true in cases of microcytic or macrocytic anemias, which probably will not be more than 5 to 10% of blood examined by clinical laboratories and blood banks.

Determine Hematocrit (Hct) Using Microhematocrit Centrifuge

PURPOSE: To determine the volume of packed erythrocytes in whole blood.

EQUIPMENT: Autolet or sterile lancet, microhematocrit tube(s), sealing clay, microhematocrit centrifuge, latex gloves, cotton balls, alcohol, patient's chart, pen (if hemoglobin is done by this procedure, conversion chart will also be needed to determine Hb), Table 7–2.

TERMINAL PERFORMANCE OBJECTIVE: Provided with all necessary equipment and supplies, and using other students as patients, demonstrate the steps in the procedure for determining hematocrit (Hct) readings using the microhematocrit centrifuge. The instructor will observe each step.

1. Assemble needed items on Mayo table. Check to see that centrifuge is plugged into the elctrical outlet.
2. Identify patient and explain procedure. **RATIONALE: Speaking to the patient by name and checking chart ensures that you are performing the procedure on the corrent patient.**
3. Put on latex gloves. **CAUTION:** Remember, in order to comply with universal precautions guidelines, gloves must be worn if there is any possibility of coming into contact with blood or any body fluids.
4. Follow desired skin puncture procedure.
5. Hold microhematocrit tube as you would hold a pencil or pen, horizontally with opening next to drop of blood that appears at puncture site. **RATIONALE: Holding tube horizontally slightly tilted downward assists the flow of blood to enter the tube by capillary action until it reaches the fill line or three-quarter point. See Figure 7–15(a), page 384. Hold tip of gloved finger over Hct tube to keep blood from flowing out. Obtain as many tubes as ordered, usually one or two.**
6. Wipe outside end of glass tube with gauze square, while still holding it horizontally, Carefully seal *only one end* of the tube by placing it into the clay and turning it until the entire end is solid clay, *Note: Do not*

apply too much pressure or the glass tube will break, Figure 7–15(b). Only a very small amount of clay is needed. You may leave the tube standing up in the tray until you are finished tending to the needs of the patient.
7. Have patient hold dry gauze square on puncture site. *Note: Check to make sure bleeding has stopped.*
8. Secure sealed end of tube against rubber padding in centrifuge (clay end of tube is always toward you). Balance centrifuge with another tube opposite it. *Note: If two or more patients' tubes are placed in centrifuge at same time, make sure that you note numbers of spaces to avoid a mix-up* Figures 7–16(a) and (b), page 385. **RATIONALE: Accurate identification is essential to assigning results to proper patient.**
9. Close inside cover carefully over tubes and lock into place by turning dial clockwise. Then close and lock outside cover. Listen for it to click into place.
10. Turn timer switch to 3–5 minutes. (Most timing switches indicate that you turn past desired time and then back to time you want set.) It will automatically turn off.
11. Wait until centrifuge has completely stopped spinning and unlock covers. (Opening a centrifuge before it stops spinning is most dangerous—centrifugal force pulls objects, such as hair, jewelry, loose sleeves of lab coats into it.
12. Read results by placing bottom line of packed RBCs (up to buffy coat but not including it) against calibrated chart in centrifuge where tube is resting, Figure 7–16(c)(d). (There is usually a magnifying glass attached to centrifuge to assit in reading Hct accurately.) Keep cover of centrifuge closed when not in use.
13. Discard used items in proper waste receptacles, remove gloves, and wash hands.
14. Record reading on patient's chart as a percentage, for example, Hct 47% and your initials.
15. Return items to proper storage areas.

Blood Glucose Screening ....

Another capillary blood test performed in most medical practices today is the blood **glucose** screening. It is done with a drop of blood obtained from a skin puncture. A drop of blood is applied directly to a chemically treated reagent strip. After timing (as directed by the manufacturer), the strip is blotted and read by comparing the color of the reagent strip with the color chart on the bottle. A more accurate reading may be obtained by reading the reacted reagent strip in a glucometer,

Figure 7–21, page 388. There are several types, some of which may take a few moments to warm up before they can be used for reliable testing. Unless the machine has an automatic calibration mechanism incorporated within it, you should calibrate the glucose meter and follow directions for use according to the manufacturer's specifications. The operation manual and directions should be kept near the instrument for reference.

The normal fasting blood glucose range is from 80 to 120 mg/100 mL blood. The term *fasting* means that the patient has had nothing to eat or drink for a specific period of time,

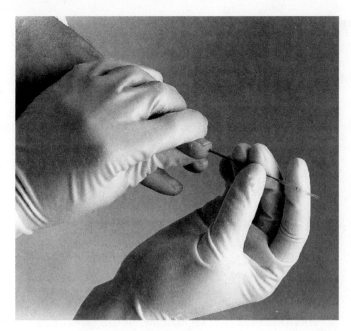

FIGURE 7–15(a) To fill the microhematocrit tube, hold the tip just to the drop of blood.

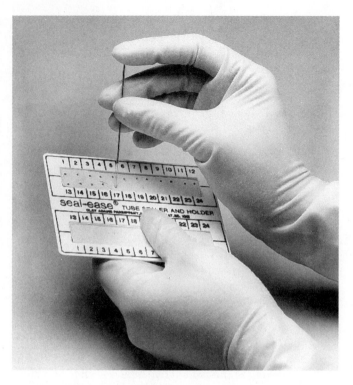

FIGURE 7–15(b) Carefully push the glass tube into the clay to seal one end before centrifugation.

usually for 8 to 12 hours prior to the test. Fasting means that the patient should not even chew gum, eat mints, smoke, or drink water. Any stimulation of the digestive system may alter the results of the scheduled laboratory test.

GTT–Glucose Tolerance Test ....

The standard glucose **tolerance** test (GTT) determines a patient's ability to metabolize **carbohydrates**. This test is used primarily to aid in the diagnosis of diabetes mellitus and hypoglycemia. Usually, the patient is advised to eat a high-carbohydrate diet for 3 days before the scheduled GTT. The night before the procedure, the patient is required to have nothing to eat or drink from midnight on, or to fast for 8 to 12 hours before the test begins.

Fasting samples of blood and urine are obtained from the patient to begin this procedure. Then the patient is given 100 g of glucose (commercial preparation) orally. A half hour after the patient has consumed the glucose drink, samples of blood and urine are taken. Every hour thereafter, both blood and urine samples are taken for up to 6 hours, or for whatever time period the physician has ordered. Since accuracy is critically important in this test, timing and precise readings of the tests are vital in assessing glucose metabolism.

With today's highly skilled **laboratory** technicians, you will probably do few blood tests in the medical office. Some offices have their own labs in which laboratory technicians are employed to carry out tests that the medical assistant is not trained to do or is not licensed to do by law. The blood screening tests already mentioned are simple and require a minimal amount of instruction to perform. Proficiency in performing these minor tests will come with practice.

Blood Cell Count ....

Be sure to determine if it is lawful and within laboratory governing regulations before performing *any* diagnostic laboratory tests. Many of these tests must be performed by only licensed clinical laboratory technicians. These regulations have been made for quality assurance purposes. On occasion the physician wants to know a patient's red or white blood cell count immediately rather than waiting for lab results, to aid in diagnosis. Performing the test right in the office offers convenience to the physician and the patient as well. There are also times when the laboratory service may not be available, such as evenings and weekends when the physician is on call. For these reasons, especially in rural settings where a clinical laboratory may not be readily available, the medical assistant may be asked to perform a red or white blood cell count. Medical offices or clinics may have mechanical devices specifically designed to perform these types of blood counts for which in-service training should be provided by your employer, Figure 7–25, page 390.

To do these procedures, you must become proficient in the use of a method of obtaining the blood sample and mixing it with a diluting solution to prepare the blood cells for counting on the hemocytometer. Mouth pipetting is an obsolete procedure on the advice of public health officials because of the danger of disease transmission. Mechanical devices are now used to draw solutions into a pipette as necessary. Figure 7–26, pages 392-393, presents a commonly used method for determining

FIGURE 7–16(c) This medical assistant is obtaining a hematocrit reading by looking down onto the tube against the values chart within the centrifuge.

FIGURE 7–16(a) There are grooved slots for up to six microhematocrit tubes to be centrifuged at once. Be sure to note the space number for each patient's hematocrit tube and write it down to avoid a mixup. The clay sealant tray also has numbers along its side to help you keep track of several patients' specimens.

You may want to use the same number on the tray as in the centrifuge for each patient when there are two or more.

FIGURE 7–16(d) After centrifugation the hematocrit reading is obtained by placing the sealed end of the tube against the padding, making sure that the line between the packed red cells and the clay is at 0 (zero). Read the hematocrit at the bottom of the meniscus (the curved line where the red cells and the buffy coat meet). The reading in this photo is 35%.

FIGURE 7–16(b) Carefully place the sealed end of the tube (toward you) against the rubber padding in the microhematocrit centrifuge.

red and white blood cell counts. It is important to make certain which diluting fluid is used for either red or white blood cell counts. The reservoirs are marked, as are the containers they come in, as to which should be used. Practice in performing the procedures for erythrocyte and leukocyte counts is necessary for you to gain expertise in this skill.

Red Blood Cells. A red blood cell (erythrocyte) count is performed when symptoms indicate possible anemia. A decrease in the number of RBCs constitutes a form of anemia. The normal RBC count range for males is 4 to 6 million per cubic millimeter of blood and for females 4 to 5 million.

The function of the RBC is to transport oxygen to and carry carbon dioxide from the cells. It also contributes to the acid–base balance of the blood. If there is an insufficient number of RBCs in the bloodstream, the patient's symptoms will be lack of energy, fatigue, and, in severe cases, shortness of breath (SOB), pounding of the heart, rapid pulse, and **pallor**.

The iron-carrying protein, hemoglobin, gives the RBC its color. Erythrocytes have a biconcave disk shape and no nucleus when mature. They are formed in the red bone marrow of

FIGURE 7–17 The QBCII, a centrifugal hematology system (Courtesy of Becton Dickinson and Company.)

P R O C E D U R E

Hemoglobin (Hb) Determination Using the Hemoglobinmeter

PURPOSE: Estimating the amount of Hb (iron-carrying protein) in the blood.

EQUIPMENT: Hemoglobinometer, glass chamber slide, hemolysis applicator (plastic or wooden), Autolet or sterile lancet, cotton balls, alcohol, latex gloves, gauze squares, Mayo table, batteries and light bulbs (as needed), patient's chart, pen

TERMINAL PERFORMANCE OBJECTIVE: With all necessary equipment and supplies provided, and using other students as patients, demonstrate the steps required to perform a hemoglobin determination using the hemoglobinometer. The instructor will observe each step.

1. Assemble all needed items on Mayo table, check patteries and light bulb in hemoglobinometer and change if needed.
2. Explain procedure to identified patient. **RATIONALE: Speaking to the patient by name and checking chart ensures that you are performing the procedure on the correct patient**.
3. Wash hands and put on latex gloves. **CAUTION:** Remember, in order to comply with universal precautions guidelines, gloves must be worn if there is any possibility of coming into contact with blood or any body fluid. Follow the desired skin puncture technique (procedure in this unit).
4. Pull the glass chamber out of the side of the hemoglobinometer and fix the lower part of the slide so that it is slightly offset.
5. Place a large drop of blood directly onto the offset glass chamber surface from the patient's finger (or other puncture site), Figure 7–20(a), page 388 Wipe the patient's finger

with an alcohol-saturated cotton ball and give patient a dry gauze square to hold over the puncture site. *Note: Check to be sure bleeding has stopped.*

6. Mix the blood on the slide with the hemolysis applicator to break down the cell membranes to release the hemoglobin. *Note: This is seen when the appearance of the blood becomes clear from cloudy and will take up to 45 seconds.* Figure 7–20(b).
7. Push the chamber into the clip and place into the slot on the left side of the hemoglobinometer, Figure 7–20(c).
8. Hold the hemoglobinometer in your left hand at eye level, while using your left thumb to turn on the light by depressing the button on the bottom of the instrument. Look into the instrument to see a split green field.
9. Slide the button on the right side of the meter with your right thumb and index finger while still looking into the meter until a matching solid green field occurs. Leave the sliding scale on the calibrated line where the solid green field appeared.
10. Read the hemoglobin level at the top calibration scale for it is most frequently used (there are 4 on the scale). It is read in grams of hemoglobin per 100 mL of blood.
11. Wash chamber (and hemolysis applicator if reusable) with a detergent solution, rinse, dry and return to the hemoglobinometer for the next use. Discard disposable items in proper receptacle, return items to proper storage area.
12. Remove gloves and wash hands. Place gloves in the proper receptacle.
13. Record the reading in the patient's chart, i.e., 14.5 g/100mL, initial.

Blood-Tube Preparation Sequence

Centrifugal Hematology System

Capillary Tube Preparation
Specimen: Finger-puncture blood

Venous Tube Preparation
Specimen: EDTA-anticoagulated venous blood, well mixed and at room temperature.

1

From end *nearest* two black lines, fill tube to level between the lines. Roll tube between fingers to mix blood with tube coating. Wipe blood from tube with lint-free cloth.

Insert end of tube nearest red lines into Pipetter. Aspirate blood specimen. Wipe blood from tube with lint-free cloth.

2

Invert slightly and allow blood to flow to other end. Roll tube between fingers AT LEAST 10 TIMES OR FOR AT LEAST 5 SECONDS to mix blood with orange coating.

Press distal end of tube into closure. Remove tube from Pipetter. Twist closure to form a leak-tight seal.

3

Press distal end of tube into closure. Twist closure to form a leak-tight seal.

Roll tube between fingers AT LEAST 10 TIMES OR FOR AT LEAST 5 SECONDS to mix blood with tube coatings.

4

Slide tube over float. Gently push until float is inside tube as far as possible. Carefully lift closure end of tube until float is free of tray slot.

Slide tube over float. Gently push until float is inside tube as far as possible. Carefully lift closure end of tube until float is free of tray slot.

5

Insert open end of tube under flange of rotor nut, then lower tube into rotor slot of centrifuge. Slide closure against outer rim. Balance rotor if necessary, but retain tube identification. Install rotor cover and close lid. Centrifuge for 5 minutes.

Insert open end of tube under flange of rotor nut, then lower tube into rotor slot of centrifuge. Slide closure against outer rim. Balance rotor if necessary, but retain tube identification. Install rotor cover and close lid. Centrifuge for 5 minutes.

6

Press the "CAP" mode key of the Reader. Insert the QBC Capillary-Blood Tube. Read the 7 interfaces according to instructions on reverse side of this card.

Press the "VEN" mode key of the Reader. Insert the QBC Venous-Blood Tube. Read the 6 interfaces according to instructions on reverse side of this card.

BECTON DICKINSON

Becton Dickinson
Primary Care Diagnostics
One Becton Drive
Franklin Lakes, NJ 07417-1882

© 1988 Becton Dickinson and Company.
QBC is a trademark of Becton Dickinson and Company.
Printed in U.S.A.

QBC-7538H 6/88

4270-000-025 Rev A (7/88)

The QBC System is protected by U.S. Patent Numbers: 4,027,660; 4,082,085; 4,077,396; 4,159,896; 4,156,570; 4,091,659; 4,141,654; 4,137,755; 4,181,609; 4,209,226; 4,259,012; 4,190,328; as well as many foreign patents. Other patents pending.

FIGURE 7–18 Blood tube preparation sequence. After preparing the blood tubes, insert them into the QBCII for reading. (Courtesy of Becton Dickinson and Company.)

FIGURE 7–20 (a) Place the capillary blood on the glass chamber. (b) Mix the (hemolyze) blood with a hemolysis applicator (wooden stick). (c) Push the chamber into the clip and place it in the slot in the side of the hemoglobinometer.

FIGURE 7–19 The hand-held hemoglobinometer

FIGURE 7–21 The Glucometer III for blood glucose screening tests. (Courtesy of Banyan International Corporation.)

adults (**erythropoiesis**) and in the liver, spleen, and bone marrow of the fetus. The average life span of the RBC is about 120 days. The **reticuloendothelial** system, mostly the liver, bone marrow, and spleen, removes the worn-out red blood cells from the circulatory system.

White Blood Cells A white blood cell (leukocyte) count is done when symptoms indicate possible infection in the body. An increase in WBCs signifies that the process of **phagocytosis** (WBCs combating infection by engulfing microorganisms or other foreign particles or cells and forming pus) is taking place. The normal leukocyte count for males and females is from 5 to 10 thousand per cubic millimeter of blood. Leukocytes are formed in the bone marrow, lymph nodes, spleen, and the lining of various visceral organs. The chief function of the WBCs is to aid in the body's defense against disease.

Differential Count One of the most vital tests generally performed with the complete blood count (CBC) is the **differential** count. This count determines the number and percentage of each of the five different types of white blood

PROCEDURE

Screen Blood Sugar (Glucose) Level

PURPOSE: To determine the sugar (glucose) level of the blood.

EQUIPMENT: Autolet or sterile lancet, reagent strips, bottle (for color chart) glucometer, latex gloves, cotton balls, alcohol, gauze squares, watch or clock, facial tissue

TERMINAL PERFORMANCE OBJECTIVE: Provided with all necessary equipment and supplies, and using other students as patients, demonstrate the steps required in the procedure for determining blood glucose levels. The instructor will observe each step.

1. Assemble all needed items on Mayo table. *Note: If glucometer is to be used, make sure it has been turned on required time and has been calibrated for accuracy (follow manual of instruction).*
2. Identify patient and explain procedure. **RATIONALE: Speaking to the patient by name and checking chart ensures that you are performing the procedure on the correct patient.** *Note: If test is to be for a fasting blood sugar level, be certain patient has not had anything by mouth for past 8 to 12 hours.*
3. Wash hands and put on latex gloves. **CAUTION:** Remember, in order to comply with universal precautions guidelines, gloves must be worn if there is any possibility of coming into contact with blood or any body fluids.

4. Follow desired skin puncture procedure.
5. Open reagent strip bottle and take one of plastic strips out without touching chemically treated pads. **RATIONALE: Heat and moisture from skin may alter results.** Reclose bottle.
6. From patient's finger apply large drop of blood so pad is completely covered.
7. Begin timing *immediately* (**stat**) for *exactly* the amount of time specified by the manufacturer. Give patient dry gauze square to hold over puncture site after wiping it with alcohol-saturated cotton ball.
8. After the specified time, immediately blot pad firmly and quickly. *Note: Follow manufactuer's instruction prcisely for timing and blotting.*
9. Immediately place the reagent strip into glucometer and close the door. *Note: Color begins to fade after a few seconds. Delay may cause inaccurate reading of results.* The number displayed is the blood glucose level, Figure 7–24, page 390, OR Hold pad next to color chart on reagent strip bottle to compare color. The closest color match will indicate approximate glucose (sugar) level in blood.
10. Discard all used items in proper receptacle, remove gloves, and wash hands.
11. Record in patient's chart; for example, 98 mg/100 mL of blood. Initial.

ORAL GLUCOSE METABOLISM

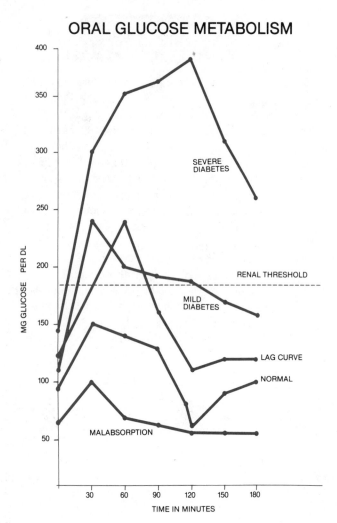

FIGURE 7-22 Graph of 3-hour glucose metabolism

DATE	PATIENCE		ADDRESS	
☐ GLUCOSE TOLERANCE TEST			_____ HOURS	
TIME	BLOOD SUGAR	URINE SUGAR	ACETONE	PATIENT'S CONDITION (SYMPTOMS)
FASTING	mg/100m			
1/2 HR	mg/100m			
1 HR	mg/100m			
2 HR	mg/100m			
3 HR	mg/100m			
4 HR	mg/100m			
5 HR	mg/100m			
6 HR	mg/100m			
PHYSICIAN	PHONE		TECHNOLOGIST	

FIGURE 7-23 Laboratory report form for glucose tolerance test

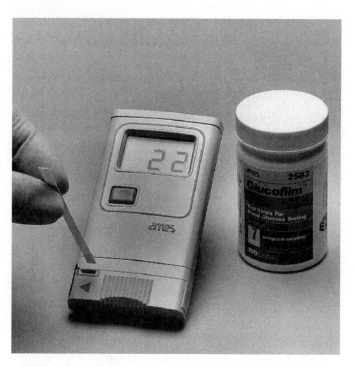

FIGURE 7-24 Insert a reagent strip into the glucometer after hearing the beep at 22 seconds and read the glucose level .

FIGURE 7-25 The Coulter JT3 hematology system was designed to meet the needs of the moderate-volume health care facility.

cells (leukocytes). Each has a specific function as outlined in Table 7–3, page 395. Preferably the differential count is made from a fresh whole-blood specimen. This blood smear is usually sent to a clinical or hospital laboratory where it is stained by a skilled certified laboratory technician who also determines the platelet count. The morphology of the erythrocytes is also noted during this microscopic examination. Figure 7–28, page 395, is a drawing of normal blood cells.

Some laboratories provide an apparatus for slide preparation of blood smears, which will be demonstrated at your request. A blood smear can be obtained from capillary or venous blood by placing a moderate drop of blood on a glass slide (frosted side up) and labeling it with pencil. A second glass slide is used to distribute the blood cells evenly over three-fourths of the slide, ending in a feathered tip. Practice is necessary in developing skill and proficiency in making good blood smears.

Count Erythrocytes (RBCs) Manually

PURPOSE: To estimate the number of RBCs in a blood sample.

EQUIPMENT: Disposable self-filling diluting pipette with a plastic reservoir prefilled with exact amount of diluting solution, hemocytometer with cover glass slide, microscope, hand tally counter, pad and pen, patient's chart, detergent solution, gauze squares, latex gloves, paper towels, Mayo table

TERMINAL PERFORMANCE OBJECTIVE: Provided with all necessary equipment and supplies, demonstrate each of the steps required to perform a manual RBC count. The instructor will observe and check each step.

1. Wash hands and put on latex gloves. Assemble needed items on Mayo table near patient. **CAUTION:** Remember, in order to comply with universal precautions guidelines, gloves must be worn if there is any possibility of coming into contact with blood or any body fluids.
2. Explain procedure to identified patient and perform skin puncture to obtain capillary blood sample.
3. Refer to Figure 7–25, and follow directions for filling the Unopette® pipette and reservoir.
4. Wait for 2–3 minutes after charing hemocytometer with solution. **RATIONALE: Waiting allows time for cells to stop movement to ensure accurate counting.**
5. Carefully place slide on stage of microscope, turn light source on, and move nosepiece to select low-power objective. Scan square in ruled area fro even distribution of cells. Check other side of slide in the same manner.

6. When an equal distribution of cells has been determined, turn nosepiece to high-power objective and focus on top left square in red counting area, Figure 7–27(a), page 395 *Note: Ruling is much smaller than in white blood cell field. Adjust light and fine focus as necessary.*
   a. Count only cells with a concave, disklike appearance that are on the top and left lines and within squares.
   b. Count in a pattern to avoid recounting cells, Figure 7–27.
   c. Count cells in all five squares in order from A to E. There are 16 smaller squares in each larger square.
   d. Write the number of cells counted in each larger square.
   e. Count both sides to be certain of equal distribution of cells.
7. Add total number of cells counted in all five squares (of one side of hemacytometer) and multiply by 10,000. **RATIONALE: This method provides the number of RBCs in a cubic millimeter of blood.**
8. Record RBC count on patient's chart and initial.
9. Wash hemocytometer with detergent solution, rinse, and dry with paper towels. Return items to proper storage area, discard used disposable items in proper receptacle, remove gloves, and wash hands.

Count Leukocytes (WBCs) Manually

PURPOSE: To estimate the number of WBCs in a blood sample.

EQUIPMENT: Disposable self-filling diluting pipette with a plastic reservoir prefilled with exact amount of diluting solution, hemocytometer with cover glass slide, microscope, hand tally counter, pad and pen, patient's chart, detergent solution, gauze squares, latex gloves, paper towels, Mayo table

TERMINAL PERFORMANCE OBJECTIVE: Provided with all necessary equipment and supplies, demonstrate each of the steps required to perform a manual WBC count. The instructor will observe and check each step.

1–5. Same as for RBC counts.
6. When an equal distribution of cells has been determined, leave nosepiece on low-power objective and focus on top left square in the WBC counting area, Figure 7-27(a), page 395.

a. Count the cells in each of the 16 small squares, counting those on the top and left lines and all cells within the squares.
b. Adjust the fine focus as needed. White blood cells will look like solid dark dots, like periods on this page.
c. Follow the pattern for counting cells as in Figure 7–27(b), page 395. Use the hand tally counter to record the number of cells you see.
d. Count cells in all four large outer squares in order from 1–4.
e. Write the number of cells counted in each of the four large squares.
7. Add total number of cells in all four squares and multiply by 50. **RATIONALE: This method provides the number of WBCs in a cubic millimeter of blood.**
8–9. Same as for RBC counts.

1. Puncture diaphragm

Using the protective shield on the capillary pipette, puncture the diaphragm of the reservoir as follows:
a. Place reservoir on a flat surface. Grasping reservoir in one hand, take pipette assembly in other hand. Push tip of pipette shield firmly through diaphragm in neck of reservoir, then remove.

b. Remove shield from pipette assembly with a twist.

2. Add sample

Fill capillary with sample and transfer to reservoir as follows:
a. Holding pipette *almost* horizontally, touch tip of pipette to sample. (See alternate methods in illustrations above.) Pipette will fill by capillary action. Filling is complete and will stop automatically when sample reaches end of capillary bore in neck of pipette.

b. Wipe excess sample from outside of capillary pipette, making certain that no sample is removed from capillary bore.

c. Squeeze reservoir slightly to force out some air. Do not expel any liquid. Maintain pressure on reservoir.

d. Cover opening of overflow chamber with index finger and seat pipette *securely* in reservoir neck.

e. Release pressure on reservoir. Then remove finger from pipette opening. Negative pressure will draw blood into diluent.

f. Squeeze reservoir *gently* two or three times to rinse capillary bore, forcing diluent into, *but not out of,* overflow chamber, releasing pressure each time to return mixture to reservoir.

CAUTION: If reservoir is squeezed too hard, some of the specimen may be expelled through the top of the overflow chamber.

g. Place index finger over upper opening and gently invert several times to thoroughly mix sample with diluent.

3. Count cells (option 1)

Mix diluted blood thoroughly by inverting reservoir (see 2g) to resuspend cells immediately prior to actual count.

a. Convert to dropper assembly by withdrawing pipette from reservoir and reseating securely in reverse position.

b. Invert reservoir, gently squeeze sides and discard first three or four drops.

c. Carefully charge hemacytometer with diluted blood by gently squeezing sides of reservoir to expel contents until chamber is properly filled.

OR

3. Transfer contents (option 2)

Transfer thoroughly mixed contents of each reservoir to appropriately labeled test tubes or corresponding cuvettes as follows:

a. Convert reservoir to dropper assembly by withdrawing pipette and reseating securely in reverse position as shown above.

b. Place capillary tip into appropriately labeled test tube or cuvette which will accommodate 5.0 ml of reagent and squeeze reservoir to expel entire contents.

OR

3. Store diluted specimen (option 3)

Cover overflow chamber with capillary shield or remove capillary and insert tip of shield firmly into reservoir opening. (Note time for which diluted specimen remains stable for each test.)

FIGURE 7–26 Procedure for using the Unopette system to collect and prepare blood specimens for hematology and chemistry studies. Each unit of the system consists of a disposable diluting pipette and a plastic reservoir containing a premeasured volume of reagent for diluting. (Courtesy of Becton Dickinson Vacutainer Systems.)

The procedure for making a blood smear for the purpose of a differential count includes directions regarding various methods of obtaining blood specimens.

Complete Chapter 7, Unit 2 in the workbook to help you meet the objectives at the beginning of this unit and therefore achieve competency of this subject matter.

PROCEDURE

Making a Blood Smear

PURPOSE: To make an adequate blood smear for a *differential* white blood cell count.

EQUIPMENT: Latex gloves, sterile lancet (or skin puncture device with sterile lancet) or CBC (lavender-stoppered) blood collection tube with needle adapter attached, or needle and syring (for venipuncture procedure), alcohol, cotton balls or gauze squares, fresh clean glass slides with frosted ends, pencil, pen, laboratory request form, patient's chart

TERMINAL PERFORMANCE OBJECTIVE: Provided with all necessary equipment and supplies, demonstrate the steps required to make an adequate blood smear for a differential white blood cell count. The instructor will observe and check each step.

1. Explain procedure to identified patient. Complete laboratory request form. Print patient's name and date on the frosted end of the glass slide with the pencil. This appropriately identifies slide in case multiple slides are in the laboratory area.

2. Assemble all needed items on Mayo table near patient.

3. Wash hands and put on latex gloves. **CAUTION:** Remember, in order to comply with universal precautions guidelines, gloves must be worn if there is any possibility of coming into contact with blood or any body fluids.

4. Perform desired method for obtaining blood specimen (either capillary or venous blood may be used).

5. Place a small drop of blood approximately a quarter inch from the frosted end of the glass slide (the drop of blood should be approximately one-eighth of an inch in diameter), Figure 7–29, page 396.
   Note:
   a. *If blood is obtained from the patient's finger, touch the drop of blood carefully to the slide (do not press the blood onto the slide or smudging will occur).*
   b. *If the blood is obtained by needle and syringe, depress plunger to allow a drop of blood to fall onto the end of the glass slide.*
   c. *If the blood is obtained from the needle and adapter, press in on the CBC blood tube attached*

(within the adapter) to allow a drop of blood to fall onto the glass slide.

6. a. Hold the corners of the frosted end of the glass slide down on a flat surface with the thumb and index finger of one hand, and with the other hand hold the second glass slide with the thumb and index (or great) finger at a 45 degree angle. *Note: If smear is too thick, the angle of spreading should be decreased; too thin, increased).*
   b. Rest the spreader slide against the first one and move it back carefully into the drop of blood. The blood will follow the edge of the slide evenly across the glass.
   c. Move the angled slide toward the frosted end quickly and gently (pressure will hemolyze blood cells). (The second glass slide is used to evenly spread the blood over the first slide, thereby distributing the blood cells for the differential white blood cell count.) *Note: The smear should have a feather-edge.* This is the area of the blood smear where the technician examines the cells. If the slide has been prepared properly, the red cells will be in an even monolayer and the white blood cells will be evenly distributed. It should not be too thick or cells are overly crowded, making counting difficult; if too thin it results in an inadequate number of cells to count.

7. Allow the blood smear to air dry, or *carefully* fan it in the air to expedite drying. **RATIONALE: Quicky drying helps cells maintain their shape and size.** *Note: Avoid blowing on the smear to dry. It may disturb the cells.*

8. Place blood smear into appropriate container (attach completed lab request form) for transport to laboratory. Generally the slide will accompany a CBC request with a lavender-stoppered blood-filled tube.

9. Remove latex gloves and wash hands. Discard all waste in appropriate containers.

10. Initial procedure on patient's chart.

TABLE 7-3

Categories of White Blood Cells and Their Functions

White Cell Type	Percent in Normal WBC	Function
Granulocytes		
Neutrophils		Phagocytosis and killing of bacteria; release of pyrogen that produces fever
Segmented	56.0	
Band	3.0	
Eosinophils	2.7	Phagocytosis of antigen–antibody complexes; killing of parasites
Basophils	0.3	Release of chemical mediators of immediate hypersensitivity
Lymphocytes	34.0	
B lymphocytes		Humoral immunity; production of specific antibodies against viruses, bacteria, and other proteins
T lymphocytes		Cell-mediated immunity, including delayed hypersensitivity and graft rejection; regulation of immune response
Monocytes	4.0	Phagocytosis of microorganisms and cell debris; cooperation in immune response

FIGURE 7–27 Counting blood cells. (a) The ruled counting area on the surface of the counting chamber (hemocytometer). White blood cells are counted in the four large outside corner squares (labeled 1, 2, 3, and 4), and red blood cells are counted in the five smaller squares (labeled A, B, C, D, and E) contained in the middle square. (b) Pattern for counting cell

PATIENT EDUCATION

Explaining the procedure and making the patient comfortable will be of great importance. If the patient shows any signs of apprehension, ask the patient to lie down and try to relax. This eliminates the possibility of a patient falling as the result of fainting during the procedure. Some patients experience a queasy (nauseated) feeling, so it is a good idea to keep an emesis basin nearby. Displaying competency and efficiency in carrying out the procedure will gain the patient's confidence and cooperation.

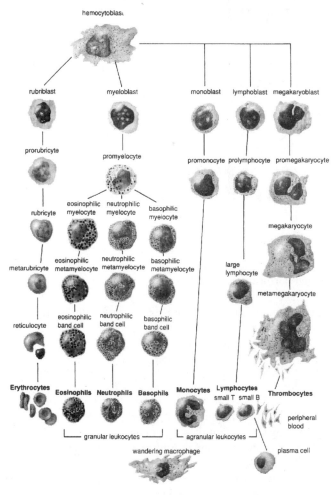

FIGURE 7–28 Blood cells and platelets

FIGURE 7–29 Making a blood smear for a differential white blood cell count

U N I T   3
Venous Blood Tests

Upon completion of this unit, you will meet the following terminal performance objectives by verifying knowledge of the facts and principles presented through oral and written communication at a level deemed competent by the instructor or employer and will demonstrate the specific behaviors as identified in the terminal performance objectives of the procedures, observing all aseptic and safety precautions in accordance with health care standards.

1. Prepare blood specimens to be sent to an outside laboratory.
2. Perform a venipuncture by either the sterile needle and syringe method or the vacuum method.
3. Explain how to obtain serum from whole blood.
4. Determine an erythrocyte sedimentation rate (ESR).
5. List the different colors used to code blood specimen tubes and what they stand for.
6. Spell and define, using the glossary at the back of the text, all the words to know in this unit.

WORDS TO KNOW ....

elasticity	oxygenate
gauge	prothrombin
hematoma	sedimentation
hemolysis	tourniquet
heparin	venipuncture
legible	venous
meniscus	

Venous means pertaining to the veins. As veins return blood to the heart and lungs to be **oxygenated** and recirculated, they carry the waste products of the body. Venous blood tests permit measurement of the kind and amount of those waste products.

Venipuncture ....

When more than a few drops of blood are required to perform tests, a venipuncture is performed. **Venipuncture** is the surgical puncture of a vein.

Usually the patient is seated in a chair with the arm supported for the venipuncture procedure. In the event that a patient does faint from this position, the needle must be withdrawn, the **tourniquet** removed, and a bandage held over the puncture site first. Then the patient must be helped carefully to the floor. Spirits of ammonia may be used to help revive the patient. The physician should check the patient before you proceed further. Patients who say they feel faint should put their head down between their knees. Usually this will help within a few minutes, and the procedure can be accomplished with no further interruptions. Often following a complete physical examination, the patient may still be lying on the examination table. This makes an ideal work area for the medical assistant and the position for the patient is most comfortable. In case the patient feels faint there is no worry of accidental falling when the patient is lying down. The law regarding venipuncture varies from state to state. Usually the physician is aware of it and will not ask you to perform the procedure unless it is lawful.

The area of choice for venipuncture is most often the inner arm at the bend of the elbow, Figure 7–30. The veins in this area are the median basilic and the median cephalic (commonly referred to as antecubital veins). A tourniquet is a means of promoting better palpation and sometimes visual position of the veins. Tourniquets are available in many materials. Soft, flat vinyl or rubber tubing is probably most popular. It is also economical. It comes in widths of 1 to 2 inches and can be cut into any length desired, usually from 12 to 16 inches. Thinner vinyl or rubber tubing is also popular, but it tends to pinch the skin. Tubing is easily washed with a detergent solution and quickly cleaned with alcohol and a cotton ball. Velcro tourniquets are cloth strips, approximately 1½ to

FIGURE 7–30 The veins of the arm. The median cephalic vein is most often used for venipuncture.

2 inches wide. They are not so easily cleaned and are not elasticized, so they cannot be used on patients with larger than average arms.

The tourniquet is placed on the patient's upper arm, about 2 inches above the elbow. Before applying the tourniquet it is a good idea to check both arms of the patient or simply ask which arm is better for this procedure. Many patients have had the procedure performed and know that one arm is better. Some patients will have a preferred arm because of their work or planned activities. Some patients are extremely difficult to obtain blood from. It may be necessary in these cases to draw the sample from a vein on the back of the hand using the sterile needle and syringe method. These veins are small and the procedure is painful. The tourniquet should be

applied just above the wrist in this case. Venipuncture must always be done carefully to avoid causing a **hematoma** (collection of blood just under the skin). Gentle pressure applied immediately on withdrawing the needle will help avoid this problem.

Use a cotton ball saturated with alcohol to swab the entire area. The alcohol will help make the skin more sensitive to your touch. Slowly move your fingertip across the patient's arm at the bend of the elbow. Veins have **elasticity** and will give somewhat when depressed. Feeling the subtle spring-back movement will help you find a suitable vein for the procedure. Having the patient clench the fist will help make the veins stand out to the touch if not to the sight.

There are two methods of performing this procedure: (1) the syringe and sterile needle method, and (2) the vacuum tube and sterile needle method. Sterile technique must be used because a foreign object is introduced directly into the vein.

A 20 or 21-**gauge** needle is usually used. The gauge must be large enough to allow blood to flow through the needle without causing **hemolysis** (breakdown of blood cells).

The needle and syringe method is always used when very small veins are involved because it is less damaging to the tissues than the vacuum method, Figure 7–31. The size of the syringe will vary according to the amount of blood needed. Usually a 20 to 30-cc syringe is used when drawing several tubes, each 5 to 15 ml.

The vacuum method is probably the most popular because it is so convenient. Blood specimens enter directly into the tubes for the desired tests rather than having to be transferred. It is vital that the correct tubes be used, however.

FIGURE 7–31 Collecting a venous blood specimen by needle and syringe method

Specimen test tubes are color-coded for the various hematology departments in the lab, Figure 7–32. Red-stoppered tubes come in sizes ranging from 3 to 15 mL. They are used to collect whole blood that is allowed to clot so that the serum can be obtained by centrifugation. The serum can be drawn out by a disposable pipette and deposited into a transfer tube, which is labeled for the particular test to be done. There are other methods to transfer serum easily from the centrifuged tube. The most efficient way is to use the red-gray stoppered tube, which has a gel in the bottom. During centrifugation, the gel liquifies and travels to the center of the tube, separating the red cells from the serum. You can then carefully pour the serum into a transfer tube and label for analysis. Another method is to place a slender rubber-tipped tube down carefully into the centrifuged tube (pushing the tube down forcefully will result in hemolysis) just to the **meniscus** of the packed red cells. The screened filtered opening at the rubber end of the inner tube allows the serum to fill the tube leaving the red cells at the bottom. You pour off the serum into a transfer tube and label for analysis. Lavender-stopped tubes, or CBC tubes, are usually 5 to 10 mL. They are also used to collect whole-blood specimens, but they contain an anticoagulant so that tests which require whole blood may be performed. Gray-stoppered tubes are used in blood glucose tests and are usually 5 ml. They contain a different anticoagulant from the CBC tubes. Blue-

stoppered tubes (sometimes green) are most often 5 ml and are used to collect specimens for testing **prothrombin** time,

FIGURE 7–32 Blood connection tubes (from left to right): red/gray for whole blood with gel for serum separation; red for whole or clotted blood specimens; blue for whole blood for coagulation tests (contains anticoagulant); gray for whole blood for glucose tests (contains anticoagulant); lavender for whole blood tests (contains anticoagulant)

USA
LABORATORIES

NAME: KREBS, HERBERT E

ACCT: #987654321

Requested by:
Physician _____
Address _____
Phone _____

Age: 74Y

SEX: M

T35474 COLL: 12/22/92 10:00   REC: 12/22/92 10:02 PHYS: PULTZ, ANDREW J.
  LIPID PROFILE
    GLUCOSE FASTING   94   [72–128]   mg/dL
    CHOLESTEROL   218   [160–330]   mg/dL
    TRIGLYCERIDE   75   [10–190]   mg/dL
    HDL   51   [30–65]   mg/dL
    LDL   PENDING
    VLDL CHOLESTEROL   PENDING
    CHOLESTEROL/HDL   4.27
                                    ½   AVERAGE   3.43
                                        AVERAGE   4.97
                                    2x AVERAGE   9.55
                                    3x AVERAGE   23.99
  LPE INTERPRETATION   PENDING

FIGURE 7–33A Lab report of normal lipid profile

blood gases, and pH. The anticoagulant is different from the glucose tube or the CBC tube and is called **heparin**. Tests drawn in the blue tubes should be performed within 2 hours for accurate results. Blood should be drawn into the tubes in the order that they have been discussed if tubes for various tests have been ordered.

Blood in specimen tubes that contain an anticoagulant must be mixed immediately in a figure-eight motion 8 to 10 times. Gentle mixing will prevent hemolysis. The tubes with the red stoppers must be allowed to stand vertically and undisturbed for at least 20 to 30 minutes to allow clotting to occur. The tube(s) must then be properly balanced in a centrifuge and spun for 20 to 30 minutes. The serum, which is a clear, light yellow liquid, is then carefully drawn off with a pipette (usually disposable ones provided by the laboratory) or by using one of the methods discussed earlier. Refer back to Figure 7–1, page 370, to see the serum separated from the centrifuged red blood in the tube the medical assistant is holding and preparing to pour into the transfer tube.

Blood collection tubes and supplies must be checked for the expiration date, and if out of date, not used. This is in compliance with quality control and quality assurance regulations. A log book must be kept of all specimens collected and sent for analysis. The log book must contain the following legible information:

1. Date collected

2. Patient's full name, address, and phone number
3. Date sent to lab
4. Test requested
5. Date results received
6. Test results

Be sure to tell patients who to ask for and when to call in for the results of their lab tests. Figure 7–33(a) is an example of a normal lipid profile lab report.

Often specimens are sent by mail or shipped to out of town or out of state to laboratories for analysis, Figure 7–33(b), page 400. The federal government requires that specimens are shipped and transported in securely closed, watertight containers. Blood tubes should be enclosed in a second durable watertight container. Then specimens should be wrapped in layers of paper towels to absorb any possible breakage or leakage during transportation. The doubly secured specimens are then placed in a shipping container of fiberboard, wood, or heavy cardboard with a label stating it is biohazardous. It is then ready for safe transport to the reference laboratory. A second label should read: In case of breakage send to this address: Centers for Disease Control, Attention: Biohazards Control Office, 1600 Clifton Road, Altanta, GA 30333.

Figure 7–34, page 404, shows instructions for use of the Saf-T Clik shielded blood needle adapter. It was designed to protect the phlebotomist from accidental needle injury, thereby reducing possible disease transmission. This adapter may be

STANDARD PROFILES				SINGLE TESTS			
2987 ( )	Diagnostic (Multi-Chem) Profile	8350 ( )	Immunologic Evaluation*	5165 ( )	ABO and Rho (B) (S)	6526 ( )	Neonatal T₄ (S)
2804 ( )	Health Survey (SMA-12)	2814 ( )	Lipid Profile A	6555 ( )	Alpha-Fetoprotein RIA (S)	6525 ( )	Neonatal TSH (S)
2824 ( )	Executive Profile A	2817 ( )	Lipid Profile B	3015 ( )	Alk. Phosphatase (S)	7941 ( )	Neonatal T₄, Blood Spot
2825 ( )	Executive Profile B	2003 ( )	Lipid Profile C	3041 ( )	Amylase (S)	3019 ( )	Phosphorus (S)
2826 ( )	Executive Profile C	2805 ( )	Liver Profile A	5163 ( )	Antibody Screen ( ) If pos. ID & Titer (S) (B)	4132 ( )	Platelet Count (B) (S)
2858 ( )	Amenorrhea Profile	2867 ( )	Liver Profile B	5166 ( )	Antibody ID (B&S)	3026 ( )	Potassium (S)
7330 ( )	Anticonvulsant Group	2868 ( )	MMR Immunity Panel	5164 ( )	Antibody Titer (B&S)		Pregnancy Test. (S or U)
2927 ( )	Autoimmune Profile	2869 ( )	Myocardial Infarction Profile		(Previous Pat.# _____)	5187 ( )	Premarital RPR (S)
2801 ( )	Calcium Metabolism Profile	2585 ( )	Parathyroid Panel A (Mid-Molecule)	5208 ( )	ANA, Fluorescent (S)	6505 ( )	Prostatic Acid Phospha-
2859 ( )	Diabetes Management Profile	2586 ( )	Parathyroid Panel B (Dialysis)	5169 ( )	ASO Titer (S)		tase (RIA) (S)*
7701 ( )	Drug Abuse Screen	2587 ( )	Parathyroid Panel C (Adenoma)	3147 ( )	Bilirubin, Direct (S)	2992 ( )	Protein Electrophoresis (S)
( )	Drug Analysis Comprehensive	2818 ( )	Prenatal Profile A	3010 ( )	BUN (S)		IEP if Abnormal ( ) 9085
	(S & U or G)	2819 ( )	Prenatal Profile B	3018 ( )	Calcium (S)	4149 ( )	Prothrombin Time (P)*
( )	Drug Analysis, Qual. (U/G)	2820 ( )	Prenatal Profile C	6472 ( )	CEA (RIA) (Plasma Only)	4144 ( )	Reticulocyte Count (B)
7340 ( )	Drug Analysis, Quant. (S)	2877 ( )	Prenatal Profile D	2995 ( )	CBC with Automated Diff.	5207 ( )	RA Latex Fixation (S)
2022 ( )	Electrolyte Profile	( )	Respiratory Infection Profile A		(Abnormal Follow-Up Studies) (B) (SL)	5194 ( )	RPR
( )	Exanthem Group	( )	Respiratory Infection Profile B	2996 ( )	CBC less Diff. (B)	5195 ( )	Rubella H.I. (S)
( )	Glucose/Insulin Response	( )	Respiratory Infection Profile C	3022 ( )	Cholesterol (S)	3016 ( )	SGOT (S)
2871 ( )	Hepatitis Profile I	( )	Respiratory Infection Profile D	3042 ( )	CPK (S)	3045 ( )	SGPT (S)
2872 ( )	Hepatitis Profile II	2821 ( )	Rheumatoid Profile A	6500 ( )	Digoxin (S)	3031 ( )	T-3 Uptake (S)
2873 ( )	Hepatitis Profile III	2878 ( )	Rheumatoid Profile B	6501 ( )	Digitoxin (S)	3032 ( )	T-4 (S)
2874 ( )	Hepatitis Profile IV	2882 ( )	T & B Lymphocyte Differential	3606 ( )	GGT (S)	2832 ( )	Thyroxine Index Free (T₇) (S)
2875 ( )	Hepatitis Profile V		Panel	3006 ( )	Glucose (S) Fasting	3036 ( )	Triglycerides (S)
2876 ( )	Hepatitis Profile VI	2883 ( )	Testicular Function Profile	3009 ( )	Glucose (P) Fasting	4111 ( )	Urinalysis (U)
2879 ( )	Hepatitis Profile VII	2832 ( )	Thyroid Panel A	3023 ( )	Glucose P.P. (P)	5277 ( )	Urogenital GC Assay
2864 ( )	Hirsutism Profile	2032 ( )	Thyroid Panel B		Hrs. _____		UNLISTED TESTS OR PROFILES
2865 ( )	Hypertension Screen	2833 ( )	Thyroid Panel C	3650 ( )	HDL Cholesterol (S)		
				5180 ( )	Heterophile Screen (Mono) (S)		
				5179 ( )	Heterophile Absorption (S)		
				3342 ( )	Hemoglobin A₁c (B)		
				6416 ( )	IgE (S)		
				3078 ( )	Iron and T.I.B.C. (S)		

*FROZEN • (B) BLOOD • (P) PLASMA • (U) URINE • (S) SERUM • (SL) SLIDES

(Rev. 1-84)

FOLD THIS FORM IN HALF SO TEST(S) ORDERED IS CLEARLY VISIBLE

FIGURE 7–33B Laboratory request form for hematology

used with all standard blood collection needles and does not change the procedure for venipuncture. After its use, the phlebotomist simply slides the protective sheath forward until the "click" is heard, and the needle is safely covered and locked so that there is no danger of injury to the phlebotomist or patient. Figure 7–35 (page 404) is an actual photo of Saf-T Click shielded blood needle adapter covered and locked after use. It is completely disposable and must be discarded in the biohazardous waste receptacle.

Erythrocyte Sedimentation Rate ....

The erythrocyte **sedimentation** rate is also known as the ESR, the sed rate, and the SR. It is the rate at which red blood cells settle in a particular calibrated tube within a given amount of time, usually 1 hour. Some physicians are interested in 15-minute readings in addition to the standard 1-hour reading. The purpose of the test is to determine the degree of inflammation in the body. When inflammation is present, red cells become heavier than normal. The ESR may be performed in the medical office or clinic. Whole blood is required, and the usual procedure is to draw blood into a lavender-stoppered tube that contains an anticoagulant. The test should be performed within 2 hours of being drawn for accurate results. The erythrocyte sedimentation rate is useful in the diagnosis and evaluation of diseases of the respiratory tract, and in cancer, arthritic, and patients with collagen disease. It may also be used in determining

P R O C E D U R E

Obtain Venous Blood with Sterile Needle and Syringe

PURPOSE: To obtain venous blood specimens when the amount needed is more than a few drops.

EQUIPMENT: Sterile needle (20–21 G, 1–1½ in. length), adequate size syringe for specimen tubes, pen, patient's chart, alcohol, latex gloves, cotton balls, tourniquet, lab request form, rubber band, gauze squares, adhesive bandage, spirits of ammonia, emesis basin, and biohazardous waste container should be within reach

Note: A utility bucket is a convenient way to carry all necessary items for venipuncture procedures. It should be stocked with lab request forms, specimen tubes, cotton balls, alcohol dispenser, syringes, sterile needles, sharps container, latex gloves, tourniquet, frosted-end slides, adapter for vacuum tube method, pen and pencil, rubber bands, gauze squares, spirits of ammonia, and bandages. This handy carrier may be set next to the patient. It should be restocked daily during routine checking of supplies.

TERMINAL PERFORMANCE OBJECTIVE: Provided with all necessary equipment and supplies, and using a training arm model, demonstrate the steps necessary for obtaining venous blood using the sterile needle and syringe method. The instructor will observe each step. *Note:* The instructor will determine the student's skill in the performance of this procedure on other students as patients. Use the picture guide in Figure 7–31, page 397, to help you with this procedure.

1. Wash hands, put on latex gloves, and assemble all needed items on Mayo table next to patient. **CAUTION:** Remember, in order to comply with universal precautions guidelines, gloves must be worn if there is any possibility of coming into contact with blood or any body fluids. *Note: Label all required specimen tubes and complete lab request form.*

2. Identify patient. **RATIONALE: Speaking to the patient by name and checking chart ensures that you are performing the procedure on the correct patient.**

3. Explain procedure to patient and ask if there is a preferred venipuncture site. If patient has no preference, visually check both arms and select a vein which can be palpated (felt) easily with your fingertip after application of alcohol. *Note: Ask patient to lie down if there is any sign of apprehension. Most often patient will be sitting down with arm extended and supported on arm rest of chair or on a table. Providing a comfortable position will relax the patient and elicit better cooperation.*

4. Secure needle onto syringe by holding needle guard in one hand and turning syringe barrel clockwise. Push in plunger of syringe all the way to release any air from barrel.

5. Apply tourniquet to patient's upper arm, about 3 in.

above bend in elbow. **RATIONALE: The tourniquet slows down blood flow increasing volume within the vein, thereby aiding palpation and visualization of the blood vessel.**

   a. Bring ends of tourniquet up evenly and cross them.

   b. Switch, so that you are holding an end in each hand comfortably.

   c. Stretch end in your right hand to apply gentle pressure over area of arm while you hold other end against patient's arm.

   d. Tuck any excess of stretched end under section which is held against arm so that there is nothing in way of puncture site. *Note: Proceed quickly, as tourniquet should not be left on longer than 1 minute. If tourniquet is applied too tightly it will prevent blood flow and patient will be most uncomfortable.*

6. Clean site lightly with alcohol-saturated cotton ball and let it air dry. **RATIONALE: Blowing on site to dry it will contaminate tissue.** Ask patient to make a fist and hold it until you say to release it. **RATIONALE: This will assist further in making vein stand up.** Take off needle guard and, with the bevel of needle up, insert needle tip into vein with a quick and steady motion, following path of vein at approximately 15-degree angle. *Note: Holding skin at site to stretch it slightly will help keep vein from moving as puncture takes place. Needle should be inserted no more than ¼–½ inch, or it may pass through the vein.* **RATIONALE: This helps maintain position of vein.**

7. Hold barrel of syringe in one hand and with other hand pull plunger back slowly and steadily until barrel is filled with amount of blood needed to fill specimen tubes.

8. Ask patient to release clenched fist. Release tourniquet by quickly pulling up on end of portion which is tucked in. Pull needle out in same path as it was inserted and place gauze square over site as needle is withdrawn. *Note: Have patient apply gentle pressure and slightly elevate arm.*

9. Quickly fill required specimen tubes by inserting needle into rubber-stoppered end. Gently push plunger of syringe to fill. **RATIONALE: Forcing blood into tubes will cause hemolysis. Vacuum tubes fill easily because vacuum draws in blood.** *Note: Specimen tubes must be filled quickly, for clotting will begin within minutes in the syringe and needle.* Fill tubes with blood from syringe into blood culture tubes first, red then blue, green, gray, and last. lavender. **RATIONALE: Blood in syringe contains no anticoagulant.** Blood smears should be made at this time if needed.

10. Stand red-stoppered tubes vertically to clot so that serum can be drawn after centrifugation. *Note: Do not shake blood or hemolysis will occur.* In tubes that contain an anticoagulant, use a figure-eight motion to gently mix the blood.

11. Deposit needle and syringe intact in sharps biohazardous waste container. Wrap labeled specimen tubes together with lab request form and secure with rubber band. *Note: Keep near centrifuge so that serum-only transfer tube(s) may be added when completed.*

12. Attend to patient's needs; apply bandage over puncture site.

13. Discard disposables in proper receptacle and return items to proper storage area. Remove gloves and wash hands.

14. Record procedure in log book on patient's chart and initial.

P R O C E D U R E

Obtain Venous Blood with Vacuum Tube

PURPOSE: To obtain venous blood specimens when the amount needed is more than a few drops.

EQUIPMENT: Multiple sample sterile needles (20–21 G, 1–1½ inch length), plastic adapter (the Saf-T Click shielded blood needle adapter is recommended for safety), labeled specimen tubes (vacuum), alcohol, latex gloves, sharps container, cotton balls, gauze squares, tourniquet, lab request forms, rubber bands, pen, patient's chart, bandages, biohazardous waste container.

TERMINAL PERFORMANCE OBJECTIVE: Provided with all necessary equipment and supplies, and using a training arm model, demonstrate the steps necessary for obtaining venous blood using the vacuum tube method. The instructor will observe each step. *Note: The instructor will determine the student's skill in the performance of this procedure on other students as patients.*

1–2. Same as for needle and syringe procedure.

3. Secure needle onto adapter by screwing grooved end of needle into grooved tip of adapter, holding needle guard and turning adapter in clockwise motion. Set aside.

4. Same as for needle and syringe procedure.

5. Clean site with lightly alcohol-saturated cotton ball and let air dry. (Blowing on site to dry it will contaminate skin.)
   a. Push rubber-stoppered end of vacuum tube into adapter until needle is inserted just into rubber to hold tube in place, Figure 7–36.
   b. Ask patient to make a fist and hold it. This will assist further in making vein stand up.
   c. Take off needle guard and, with bevel of needle up, insert tip of needle into vein with a quick and steady motion, following path of vein at approximately a 15-degree angle.
   Note: Holding skin at site to stretch it slightly will help keep vein from moving as puncture takes place. Needle should be inserted no more than ¼ to

½ inch or it may pass through vein.

6. Hold adapter with one hand and with other hand place your index and great fingers on either side of protruding edges of adapter. Push vacuum tube completely into adapter with your thumb, allowing needle to puncture rubber stopper. Blood will flow into tube by vacuum force if other end of needle is in vein properly. When tube is filled, pull it out of adapter by holding it between your thumb and great finger and pushing against adapter with your index finger. *Note: Fill required number of tubes for tests ordered by physician.* Begin with blood culture tubes first, then red, blue, green, gray, lavendar, in that order. **RATIONALE: This order will prevent any possible traces of anticoagulant from entering the "serum-only" specimen tube.** Remember to mix blood with anticoagulant gently using a figure-eight motion.

7. Ask patient to release clenched fist. Release tourniquet by quickly pulling up on and of portion which is tucked in. Pull needle out of vein in path of insertion and place gauze square over site as needle is withdrawn. Ask patient to elevate arm slightly to help stop bleeding and apply gentle pressure. *Note: If a blood smear is needed for a differential, turn CBC (lavender) tube (still attached to adapter) upside down and gently press tube down to release drop of blood onto glass slide.* Make blood smear, or as many as have been ordered, label frosted end with pencil, air dry quickly, and send with other specimens.

8. Set red tubes vertically to clot so that serum can be obtained by centrifugation for serum-only tests.

9. Same as steps 10–14 for needle and syringe procedure except for disposing of needle from plastic adapter carefully into biohazardous waste or sharps container. If Saf-T Click is used, dispose of the entire locked unit in the biohazardous waste or sharps container. Table 7–4 lists laboratory normal value ranges of commonly performed venous blood test results.

Complete an ESR Using the Wintrobe Method

PURPOSE: To determine the rate at which the red blood cells (erythrocytes) fall in a given amount of time (usually 1 hour). Sometimes, additionally, physicians request recorded readings at 15-minute intervals up to 1 hour.

EQUIPMENT: (Disposable) calibrated glass ESR tube-Wintrobe method, rubber bulb, plastic disposable pipette, tube holder with level, fresh blood specimen from CBC tube, timer or timepiece, latex gloves, pen, patient's chart, paper towels. Figure 7–37, page 405, shows the medical assistant adjusting the dials on either side of the tube rack to make it stand level.

TERMINAL PERFORMANCE OBJECTIVE: Provided with all necessary equipment and supplies, demonstrate all required steps to complete the procedure for an ESR. The instructor will observe each step.

1. Assemble needed items on level counter space. Wash hands and put on latex gloves. **CAUTION:** Remember, in order to comply with universal precautions guidelines, gloves must be worn if there is any possibility of coming into contact with blood or any body fluids.

2. Carefully set tube in leveled stand. **RATIONALE: The instrument must be level to obtain accurate readings at meniscus at eye-level.** *Note: If more than one ESR is being done, record slot number next to*

patient's name on a notepad near stand and time it was set.

3. Carefully fit rubber bulb onto large end of pipette. Depress bulb end of pipette and place tip of pipette into bottom of blood-filled specimen tube. Slowly fill the pipette with blood by letting up on depressed bulb. Place tip of blood-filled pipette to the very bottom of calibrated sed rate tube carefully without touching sides.

4. Slowly press bulb and fill Wintrobe tube to precisely the 0 line, keeping tip of pipette below meniscus, Figure 7–38.

5. Immediately set time for 1 hour, or write down exact time that you set tube in stand and check reading in exactly 1 hour.

6. Discard disposables, wash and return other items to proper storage area, remove gloves, and wash hands.

7. Read Wintrobe tube at calibrated line where red cells and plasma separate, Figure 7–39. If meniscus of plasma is above 0 line (2 lines are allowed) add 1 or 2 to reading, depending on line that meniscus is closest to when time is up. *Note: Normal range for ESR, Wintrobe method is males, 0 to 6.5, females 0 to 15 mm/h.*

8. Record on patient's chart; for example, ESR 29 mm/h. (Wintrobe) and initial.

---

the extent of dehydration in burn victims. Sed rates are performed with several different types of calibrated cylindrical tubes. The most common methods and their normal ranges are:

	Males	Females
Culter	0–8	0–10 mm/h
Wintrobe	0–6.5	0–15 mm/h
Westergren	0–15	0–20 mm/h

The normal rate at which red blood cells fall is 1 mm every 5 minutes. Since the readings vary according to which method is used, it is essential that the method be recorded with the results on the patient's chart. Females tend to have higher readings than males, especially during menstruation and in pregnancy.

Complete Chapter 7, Unit 3 in the workbook to help you meet the objectives at the beginning of this unit and therefore achieve competency of this subject matter.

UNIT 4

Urine, Sputum, and Stool Specimens

OBJECTIVES ....

Upon completion of this unit, you will meet the following terminal performance objectives by verifying knowledge of the facts and principles presented through oral and written communication at a level deemed competent by the instructor or employer, and will demonstrate the specific behaviors as identified in the terminal performance objectives of the procedures, observing all aseptic and safety precautions in accordance with health care standards.

1. Explain the methods of urine collection: clean-catch midstream, catheterization, infant collection, random.

Saf-T Clik Shielded Blood Needle Adapter

Instructions For Use
PREPARATION

1. Before attaching needle, push ends of Saf-T Click® together to insure outer sleeve is seated.

2. Open needle cartridge. Twist to break the tamperproof seal. Remove cartridge cap to expose rear needle with threaded hub. Do not remove front needle cover. Use up to 1½" blood collection needle.

3. Attach needle to Safety Adapter. Screw needle into Safety Adapter until firmly seated.

AFTER VENIPUNCTURE

4. When sampling is complete, grasp the Safety Adapter's outer sheath sliding it forward over the exposed contaminated needle until a distinctive "CLICK" is heard. "LOCKED, LOCKED" is visible when Adapter is locked. The contaminated needle is now safely covered.

Two Handed Technique   One Handed Technique

5. Discard the Safety Adapter/Contaminated Needle Assembly according to hospital procedures. Do not reuse needle/Safety Adapter.

FIGURE 7–34 Instructions for using the Saf-T Clik shielded blood needle adapter (Courtesy Ryan Medical, Inc.)

FIGURE 7–35 The Saf-T Clik adapter locked after use (Courtesy of Ryan Medical, Inc.)

2. Perform routine urinalysis: physical, chemical, and microscopic examination.
3. Instruct patients in collection of urine, sputum, and stool for analysis.
4. Obtain a catheterization urine specimen from a female patient.
5. Determine specific gravity of urine using a urinometer.
6. Describe the reagent strips used in chemical urinalysis.
7. Describe the proper storage of urine specimens until analysis can be performed and the reasons for it.
8. Complete a lab request form.
9. Record the results of a urinalysis on the patient's chart.
10. Discuss patient education regarding respiratory, digestive, and urinary systems.
11. Discuss the collection process of specimens sent for drug or alcohol analysis.
12. Spell and define, using the glossary at the back of the text, all the words to know in this unit.

amber

cancer

chemical

clarity

crenated

dextrose

last menstrual period (LMP)

physical

quantity not sufficient (QNS)

random

renal threshold

supernatant

turbidity

urinalysis

urinary tract infection (UTI)

urination

In addition to obtaining blood specimens and preparing them for laboratory tests, the medical assistant will probably be responsible for collecting specimens of other body fluids from patients or instructing the patients to do so. The specimens that you must obtain and prepare for analysis most

TABLE 7–4

Normal Values of Commonly Performed Laboratory Tests

Chemistry	
Total cholesterol	130–200 mg/dL
HDL cholesterol	45–65 mg/dL
LDL cholesterol	90–130 mg/dL
Glucose	80–120 mg/dL
Triglyceride	40–150 mg/dL
Creatinine	0.7–1.4 mg/dL
Uric acid	3.5–7.5 mg/dL
BUN	8–20 mg/dL
Sodium	132–142 mEq/L
Potassium	4–5 mEq/L
Chloride	98–106 mEq/L
CO_2	25–32 mEq/L

Hematology	
White blood cell count	5.000–10,000/mm^3
Red blood cell count	3.5–5.5 x 10/mm^3
Hemoglobin	12–16 g/dL
Hematocrit	35.5–49%
Sedimentation rate	0–10 mm/h
Platelet count	150,000–350,000/mm^3
Coagulation	
Prothrombin time	11–13 s

FIGURE 7–36 The Vacutainer system for venous blood collection

— Sterile blood collection needle

— Needle holder/Adapter

— Color coded rubber stoppered cap

— Pre-measured vacuum glass specimen tube

often are urine, sputum, and stool. The same standard information (the patient's name, age, sex, etc.) should accompany each specimen on the appropriate laboratory request form. In addition, specimens must be obtained and sent to the lab in the

FIGURE 7–37 The sedimentation tube rack must be level for accurate reading of the ESR tube.

PROCEDURE

Catheterize Urinary Bladder

PURPOSE: To obtain a sterile urine specimen from the urinary bladder for laboratory analysis.

EQUIPMENT: Sterile tray covered with sterile towel, sterile gloves, sterile towels, sterile specimen container with lid, sterile basin to catch excess urine, sterile catheter (French type, sizes 12–16), sterile cotton balls, sterile medicine cup, sterile 4 3 4 inch gauze squares, sterile forceps, sterile plastic sheet, antiseptic solution, sterile lubricant, sterile gloves, gooseneck lamp, Mayo table

TERMINAL PERFORMANCE OBJECTIVE: With all equipment and supplies provided, and using a female training model or mannequin in lieu of a patient, demonstrate the steps required to perform a urinary bladder catheterization. The instructor will observe each step. *Note: To prevent injury, disease transmission, or embarrassment, this procedure should not be practiced before other students. Simulation should be made by the instructor if models are not available.*

1. Place catheter kit on Mayo table next to examination table and explain procedure to identified female patient. Adjust position of lamp and turn on.

2. *Note: Normally patient to be catheterized has already been examined and gowned or is covered below the waist with a drape sheet.* Assist her into dorsal recumbent position with her feet in stirrups. Drape patient with sheet and expose external genitalia.

3. Pull out the footrest. Place sterile kit on footrest and open outer wrapping. Touching only corners, place sterile plastic sheet under patient's buttocks. Ask patient to keep her knees apart.

4. Wash and dry hands and put on sterile gloves, being careful not to contaminate your gloved hands. Pour antiseptic solution over cotton balls in medicine cup. Open urine specimen container and keep on sterile field. Apply sterile lubricant to one of gauze squares.

5. With left hand spread labia and wipe genitalia once with each of three antiseptic-soaked cotton balls (front-to-back motion) and discard onto Mayo table, using

right hand. Keep left hand in place and do not touch sterile items with it as it is now contaminated. Place tip of catheter in lubricant and other end of catheter tube into basin.

6. Holding catheter tube about 4 inches from lubricated tip with your right thumb and index finger, insert tip gently into urinary meatus (located below clitoris and above the vaginal opening) about 2 to 3 inches. Figure 7–43, page 409. Patient should be instructed to breathe slowly and deeply to relax abdominal muscles and tissues so that procedure is not painful. Tell patient that uncomfortable feeling will last only a few minutes until tube is withdrawn. Procedure should not be painful to the patient. Any unusual complaints should be brought to physician's attention immediately.

7. After inserting tip of catheter, urine should begin to flow immediately into basin. Flow may be stopped by closing metal clamp attached to tubing. Position other end of tube into specimen container and release clamp to collect urine specimen. Allow remainder of urine from bladder to flow into basin.

8. Withdraw catheter tube gently once specimen is obtained and dry area with sterile gauze squares or cotton balls. Secure lid onto urine specimen container and set aside. Turn lamp off and return it to usual position. Remove all items from footrest.

9. Assist patient to sitting position then from table to dress.

10. Place any reusable items in basin of cold water to soak until you have time to wash and sterilize them. (*Note: Remember to wear gloves later when handling any items that have come into contact with blood or any body fluids.*) Clean off examining table. Discard gloves and disposable items in biohazardous waste bag.

11. Wash hands. Label specimen for analysis and complete request form if sending it to outside lab.

12. Record procedure on patient's chart and initial. Include information about physical properties of urine, rate of flow, and any abnormal or significant observations.

---

proper containers to avoid misunderstanding by lab personnel.

Most specimens should be refrigerated if there is a delay in transporting them to the laboratory. Many specimen containers already have a preservative added to prevent deterioration so that refrigeration is not necessary. A laboratory procedure manual should be kept at hand for reference on how to prepare specimens.

Urine Specimens ....

Urinalysis is probably the most frequently performed test in the medical office. Examination of urine consists of three major areas of testing: **physical, chemical**, and microscopic, Figure 7–40.

Specimens for urinalysis are usually collected in plastic disposable containers, Figure 7–41. The time that the urine speci-

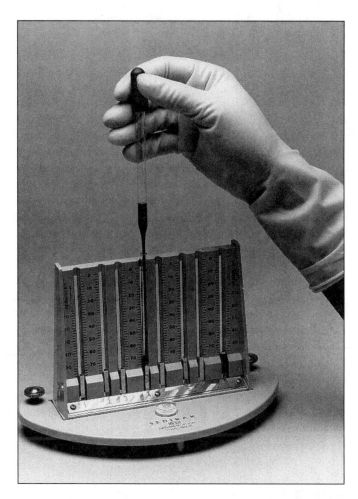

FIGURE 7–38 Fill the calibrated tube from the solid blood-filled pipette, keeping the tip just below the meniscus to precisely the 0 (zero) line.

FIGURE 7–39 Reading a Wintrobe tube: The tube on the left reads 16 mm/h, on the right 29 mm/h.

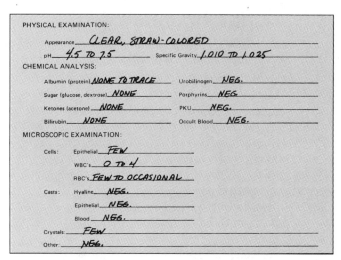

PHYSICAL EXAMINATION:

Appearance _CLEAR, STRAW-COLORED_

pH _4.5 TO 7.5_   Specific Gravity _1.010 TO 1.025_

CHEMICAL ANALYSIS:

Albumin (protein) _NONE TO TRACE_   Urobilinogen _NEG._

Sugar (glucose, dextrose) _NONE_   Porphyrins _NEG._

Ketones (acetone) _NONE_   PKU _NEG._

Bilirubin _NONE_   Occult Blood _NEG._

MICROSCOPIC EXAMINATION:

Cells: Epithelial _FEW_

WBC's _0 TO 4_

RBC's _FEW TO OCCASIONAL_

Casts: Hyaline _NEG._

Epithelial _NEG._

Blood _NEG._

Crystals: _FEW_

Other: _NEG._

FIGURE 7–40 The lab report shows normal values for a routine urinalysis.

men was obtained should be noted on the container with the patient's name, the date, and the test to be performed on the specimen. Ideally, urinalysis should be performed within 2 hours of collection to avoid bacterial growth and the decomposition of cells. If there is a delay, the specimen should be refrigerated.

The first morning **urination** is the most concentrated and therefore most often the choice for accurate test results. In addition, patients usually have little difficulty in obtaining **random** urine specimens upon request in the medical office. *Random* means nonscheduled or that no preparation is required. Most physicians prefer that the specimen be a midstream sample. Partial voiding before catching the specimen

FIGURE 7–41 Urine specimen cup with identification label (From Caldwell & Hegner, *Health Care Assistant,* 5th ed. Copyright 1989, Delmar Publishers Inc.)

During the patient's office visit you may have an opportunity to discuss a few of the following areas which may help the patient better understand proper health habits in regard to urinary problems.

1. Remind female patients to avoid using perfumed toilet articles (i.e., tissue, tampons, soaps, etc.) that are irritating to delicate vaginal tissues.
2. Advise patients to void when they feel the urge because delay can cause bladder stress and irritation.
3. Instruct female patients to practice Kegel exercises to increase the sphincter control of the bladder to improve urine retention. This exercise is done by pushing down with the lower pelvic muscles (as in forcing urination), counting to 10, and then squeezing back counting down to 1. Repeating this routine several times a day helps to strengthen muscle control.
4. Remind patients that they should drink plenty of fluids, avoiding caffeine drinks.
5. Remind patients (especially females) that taking a shower instead of a tub bath reduces the possibility of infection. (Bubble baths should be taken rarely because they irritate delicate vaginal tissues.)
6. Advise female patients that wearing pants that are too tight, as well as nylon underwear, may be irritating to delicate vaginal tissues. Cotton is recommended because it allows heat and moisture to escape.

will clear the urethra of any sloughed off cells, bacteria, mucus, or other debris that could interfere with accurate test results. Patients should be instructed to wash the genital area with soap and water, rinse well, wipe the genitals with several antiseptic-soaked cotton balls (usually zephrin chloride is used), begin to void into the toilet, and after a few seconds catch about 3 ounces in the urine container.

The 24-Hour Urine Specimen On occasion, a 24-hour urine specimen will be called for. Usually a written laboratory order will be given to the patient, and instruction will be given by the laboratory technician, but you may be given this responsibility. Printed instruction sheets are most helpful in this procedure. The patient is given a large container with a preservative already added. This container will hold all of the urine the patient voids in a 24-hour period and must be refrigerated throughout this time. The patient must keep a

record of the date and exact time that the collection begins, which should be at the second urination of the day. Then every time the patient voids, day and night, for the next 24 hours, the patient should urinate into a clean smaller container and add the urine to the larger container. The last specimen included in the test period is the first urination of the next morning. When completed, the specimen should be taken to the laboratory as soon as possible, and kept cool during transporting with ice in a portable cooler. Again, it is necessary to check the lab manual for directions in preparing specimens because some 24-hour urine samples should not have the preservative added.

Pediatric urine collection bags fit over the genital area of either sex and are secured with adhesive, Figure 7–42. The infant's skin should be washed and dried thoroughly before application if the bag is to stay in place. You may have to instruct the parent in the procedure so that it can be done at home. It may be necessary to transfer the urine into a regular specimen container for transporting. You should advise the parent to label the specimen with the baby's name and the date and time of the urine collection.

The lab report will be given to the physician within a few days depending on the type of tests performed. As with any lab test, the patient will be anxious to know the results and should be notified as soon as possible.

FIGURE 7–42 Pediatric urine collection unit in place: (a) Female (b) male

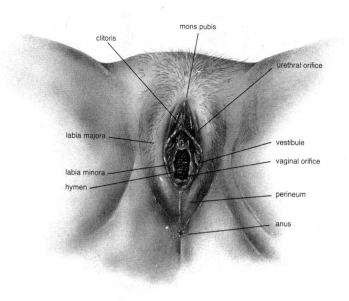

FIGURE 7–43 External female genetalia (From Caldwell & Hegner, *Nursing Assistant,* 6th ed. Copyright 1992, Delmar Publishers Inc.)

Catheterization. You may be asked to either perform or assist with the procedure of urinary bladder catheterization, the introduction of a catheter (tube) through the urethra into the bladder for withdrawal of urine.

There are basically three reasons for catheterizing patients:

1. To obtain a sterile urine specimen for analysis
2. For relief of urinary retention
3. To instill medication into the bladder, after the bladder is emptied

This procedure is not performed routinely. In most cases, it is done by a urologist, a physician who specializes in diseases of the urinary system. However, some physicians in obstetrics–gynecology and general and family practice may delegate this duty to the medical assistant to aid in the diagnosis of the patient. Generally, the physician will order a culture and sensitivity analysis of the urine obtained from catheterization. This is done to determine what microorganism is present and what medication will be effective in treatment. You must be authorized by the physician to perform the procedure. The physician generally will have you observe several catheterizations to become familiar with the procedure. After you have demonstrated the skill under the direct supervision of the physician, you will be released to perform catheterizations alone. If any doubt or problem occurs during the catheterization procedure, the physician should be notified immediately.

Generally, physicians will catheterize male patients for it is a more difficult procedure and sometimes painful. Assistance in assembling the necessary items and helping the physician during the procedure may be the medical assistant's role.

Sterile technique must be maintained throughout the procedure. Contamination of any of the items during the procedure is possible, and these should be discarded and another

sterile item used to continue the procedure. Carelessness may result in severe bladder infection or injury to the patient. You should follow the procedure for putting on sterile gloves given later in the text.

French catheters are used in performing simple catheterizations. The Foley catheter is used when the catheter will remain in the urinary bladder. Sterile, disposable catheterization kits are available that contain all the necessary items to perform the procedure. Some have only the catheter tube, which attaches to the sterile specimen container directly. This is convenient for obtaining a sterile urine specimen. Other items must be assembled to properly carry out the procedure.

Physical Urinalysis Physical properties of urine include the appearance (color), specific gravity, and **turbidity (clarity)**. Standard color descriptors are light straw, dark straw, light **amber**, amber, and dark amber. Clarity is described as clear, slightly cloudy, cloudy, and very cloudy. Specific gravity indicates the concentration of urine. It is measured with a glass urinometer and calibrated float, Figure 7–44. The weight of substances contained in urine is assessed by comparing the specific gravity of urine with that of distilled water, which is 1.000. The specific gravity of urine is normally from 1.010 to 1.025. Lighter colored urine usually has a lower specific gravity, and darker urine a higher one.

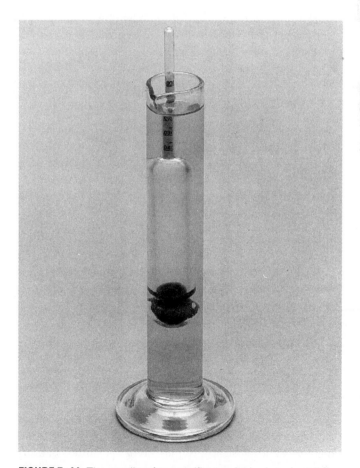

FIGURE 7–44 The reading for specific gravity is done immediately at the meniscus when the spinning stops.

P R O C E D U R E

Determine Specific Gravity Using Urinometer

PURPOSE: To determine the specific gravity of urine.

EQUIPMENT: Clean dry glass urinometer and float, fresh urine specimen, tongue depressor, and disposable gloves

TERMINAL PERFORMANCE OBJECTIVE: Provided with the necessary equipment and supplies, demonstrate the steps of the procedure for determining specific gravity of urine. The instructor will observe each step.

1. Wash hands, put on gloves, and assemble all needed items on level counter. **CAUTION:** Remember, in order to comply with universal precautions guidelines, gloves must be worn if there is any possibility of coming into contact with blood or any body fluids.
2. Mix urine well with tongue depressor and fill glass container about three-fourths full. **RATIONALE: Urine must be well mixed to distribute solutes evenly throughout the specimen.** *Note: If there is not enough*

urine to complete the specific gravity test write QNS (quantity not sufficient).

3. Hold the slender, clear end of the float between your thumb and index finger and place the larger end into the glass container holding the urine.
4. Roll the tip of the float quickly between your thumb and index finger.
5. Watch the spinning action at eye level and read the measurement at the meniscus immediately when it stops. **RATIONALE: If measurement is not read immediately, float tilts, resulting in an inaccurate reading.**
6. Record the reading on the patient's chart.
7. Discard urine and tongue depressor. Wash, rinse, and dry urinometer and float. Remove gloves and wash hands. **RATIONALE: The float should be kept dry and handled carefully because the bottom may be easily cracked.**

The color of urine can be affected by disease, some medications, and food. Urine with a strong ammonia-like odor may be alkaline from a high concentration of bacteria. Urine with a high glucose level (glycosuria) may have a fruity sweet odor. Glycosuria is caused by a high glucose level in the blood, which spills into the urine when the **renal threshold** is reached.

Blood in the urine (*hematuria*) may give the specimen a red or rusty color. However, foods with strong color, such as beets, also produce redness in the urine and stool. Patients should be advised that this is only temporary and told not to worry. If medication is known to cause urinary discoloration, the patient should be told in advance to avoid undue stress.

Chemical Urinalysis Any urine specimen that has been refrigerated should be returned to room temperature before testing.

Reagent strips are convenient and relatively inexpensive diagnostic tests which reveal the presence of abnormal substances in the urine. The reagent strips provide both qualitative and quantitative assessment. Qualitatively, they reveal the presence of an abnormal substance; quantitatively, they determine how much of the substance is present. The substances include sugar (glucose), protein (albumin), ketone (acetone), bilirubin, urobilinogen, blood, nitrite, pH, leukocytes, and specific gravity. The treated end of the reagent strip reacts chemically with the urine, and if a sufficient amount of a substance is present in the urine, the strip changes color. The strip is then compared with the color chart on the bottle.

Fresh urine specimens should be used, and exact timing of the tests is vital. Adequate lighting is also important to view the colors of the reagent strips and the changes that may occur. If there is no reaction (no change in color), the results are recorded as negative.

Care must be taken to protect the reagent strips from exposure to light, heat, and moisture. Reagent strip bottles must be capped immediately after use and stored in a dry, cool area (but not refrigerated). The strips are bottled in light-resistant glass with a moisture-absorbent agent included. They must not be used after the expiration date on the bottle.

Many companies manufacture urine tests. One test that is commonly used because of its wide range is the Multistix 10 SG reagent strip test (Ames Co.), Figure 7–45. Each reagent strip bottle has a package insert with instructions, which should be precisely followed.

The Multistix 10 SG is also used in the Clinitek 100 urine chemistry analyzer, Figure 7–46. This instrument provides standardized readings of reflectance photometry on a screen (with abnormal results highlighted) as well as a printed record for the patient's file.

The pH range for normal urine is from 5.0 to 7.0, Figure 7–47. Above 7.0 is considered alkaline, and below 5.0 is acid. If a urine specimen has a pH over 7, it probably contains a great number of bacteria, which make the urine alkaline. This will destroy the urinary casts that are formed in the kidney. Urinary casts are important in the diagnosis of a patient's condition.

Diseases of the kidney and **urinary tract infections (UTI)** produce protein (albumin) in the urine that is not normally present. A patient with a trace or a reading of 1+ or more of pro-

Test Urine with Multistix 10 SG

PURPOSE: To detect pH, protein, glucose, ketones, blood, bilirubin, urobilinogen, leukocytes, and specific gravity in urine.

EQUIPMENT: Multistix 10 SG reagent strips, fresh urine specimen, disposable gloves, watch or other timepiece, tongue depressor, patient's chart, pen, adequate lighting to read color chart on reagent bottle (for accurate test results, use before expiration date on the bottle)

TERMINAL PERFORMANCE OBJECTIVE: Provided with all necessary equipment and supplies, demonstrate the steps required to perform the procedure for using Multistix 10 SG. The instructor will observe each step.

1. Wash hands, put on gloves, and assemble all needed items on cleared counter. **CAUTION:** Remember, in order to comply with universal precautions guidelines, gloves must be worn if there is any possibility of coming into contact with blood or any body fluids.

2. Stir urine with tongue depressor to evenly distribute solates throughout specimen.

3. Remove cap from bottle and take out one reagent strip without touching test paper end. Place cap securely back on bottle. *Note: Study times given on bottle for reading each test section.*

4. Dip test paper end of reagent strip into urine specimen. With reagent side of strip down, pull across inside of specimen container opening to remove excess urine. **RATIONALE: If strip is too saturated, treated test paper chemicals will run together and make results inaccurate.**

5. **a.** Place reagent strip next to color chart on bottle by holding bottom of bottle in left hand and strip by right thumb and index finger.
   b. Read results by comparing color of reacted reagent strips with color chart on bottle.
   c. Place bottle on its side and hold it at bottom with left hand.
   d. Hold reagent strip in right hand with thumb and index finger and line up with color chart on bottle.
   e. Read test results from bottom to top in order of shorter to longer timings. Proper timing is essential for accurate results.

6. Begin timing tests immediately. *Note: The scale below is in the same order as reagents on strip and on color chart on bottle when properly aligned and observed from left to right.*
   2 minutes—leukocytes
   60 seconds—nitrite
   60 seconds—urobilinogen
   60 seconds—protein (albumin)
   60 seconds—pH
   50 seconds—blood
   45 seconds—specific gravity
   40 seconds—ketone
   30 seconds—bilirubin
   30 seconds—glucose (quantitative)
   10 seconds—glucose (qualitative)

7. Discard used reagent strip, gloves, and other disposables into proper receptacle. Wash hands. Return Multistix 10 SG to proper storage area.

8. Record results as indicated for each section on patient's chart along with name of test. Initial.

---

tein on a random specimen will probably be asked to have a first morning sample checked to see if the protein is in the concentrated urine.

Ketone (acetone) bodies are not normally present in the urine. They are the result of fat metabolized in the digestive tract. Their presence could indicate severe diabetes mellitus, starvation, a high-fat diet, or body wasting. A highly concentrated amount of ketones is called *ketonuria*. Many patients who have been fasting before coming in to the medical office for blood and urine tests may show a high ketone urine level, which is usually insignificant.

Bilirubin (bile) is an orange or yellowish pigment which is a product of degenerated RBCs that release hemoglobin in the liver. This waste product is normally excreted through the intestines. In patients who have liver damage or disease,

bilirubin will appear in the urine, often before they develop symptoms and appear jaundiced.

Urobilinogen is bilirubin that has been converted in the intestines by coliform bacteria. This chemical reaction gives feces its brown color. Urobilinogen is excreted through the intestines normally. Large amounts are produced when the heart, spleen, and liver are diseased or dysfunctioning.

Blood in the urine is termed hematuria. The presence of blood in the urine indicates damage of the kidney from injury or from disorders and diseases of the urinary tract. Blood is found normally in the urine specimens of menstruating females. If the specimen is necessary immediately for a diagnosis, a catheterized specimen may be required.

Nitrite is present in urine that contains microorganisms. The action of the invading bacteria converts nitrates in the nor-

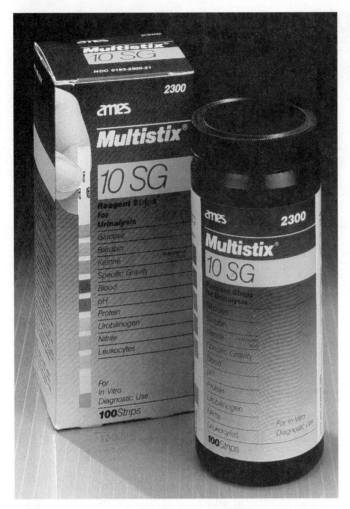

FIGURE 7–45 Multistix® reagent strips for urinalysis (Courtesy of Miles Inc. Diagnostic Division.)

FIGURE 7–46 This urine chemistry analyzer provides quick and accurate test results. (Courtesy of Miles Inc. Diagnostic Division.)

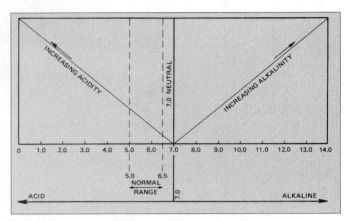

FIGURE 7–47 Scale of pH for urine

mally sterile urine to nitrate. Urine which has been left unrefrigerated may contain nitrite due to the action of bacteria present in an alkaline urine. This is why urinalysis should be done as soon as possible after collection.

Phenistix is a reagent strip that detects the presence of phenylketonuria (PKU) in infants. This test may be done like the others by dipping the reagent strip into a fresh urine specimen and timing the reaction.

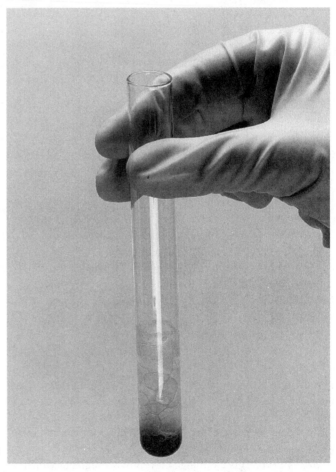

FIGURE 7–48 Carefully hold the test tube at the top to avoid possible burns from boiling caused by the chemical reaction of the Clinitest tablet with the solution.

P R O C E D U R E

Determine Glucose Content of Urine with Clinitest Tablet

PURPOSE: To determine the glucose content of urine.

EQUIPMENT: Clinitest tablets with color chart for test result (must be used before expiration date to ensure accurate results), disposable glass test tubes, eyedropper, fresh urine specimen, disposable latex gloves, small container of water, test tube rack, tongue depressor, watch or time-piece, proper lighting

TERMINAL PERFORMANCE OBJECTIVE: Provided with all necessary equipment and supplies, demonstrate the steps in the procedure for using Clinitest tablets. The instructor will observe each step.

1. Wash hands, put on gloves, and assemble needed items on adequate counter space. **CAUTION:** Remember, in order to comply with universal precautions guidelines, gloves must be worn if there is any possibility of coming into contact with blood or any body fluids.
2. Stir urine with tongue depressor and fill dropper halfway with urine. **RATIONALE: Stirring mixes liquid and solutes in urine for more accurate testing.**
3. Hold test tube near top between thumb and index fin-

ger and with other hand release 5 drops of urine into test tube.
4. Rinse dropper and fill halfway with water. Release 10 drops of water into test tube. Shake gently to mix.
5. Set test tube in rack and open Clinitest bottle. Without touching tablets, shake one tablet directly into Clinitest bottle cap. **RATIONALE: Moisture on hands may cause a chemical reaction with the tablet, causing a burn. Recap the bottle.**
6. Watch reaction, Figure 7–48. As soon as boiling stops, allow exactly 15 seconds before carefully grasping test tube at top, gently tilting it back and forth and swirling contents, and then comparing color of mixture in bottom of test tube with closest color on chart, Figure 7–49. Results are determined in percentage of miligrams per deciliter.
7. Return items to proper storage. Discard disposable items. Remove disposable gloves and discard in proper receptacle. Wash hands.
8. Record reading on patient's chart and initial.

Glucose (sugar, **dextrose**) is not normally present in the urine, but it may spill out from the kidney when the blood-stream is saturated. Female patients may have a high glucose level during pregnancy and postpartum. Further tests should then be performed to determine the cause. Glucose in the urine may indicate the presence of the disease diabetes mellitus. Some patients have a low renal threshold, which may explain the presence of glucose in the urine. Patients with a high glucose level are usually asked for several specimens from different times of the day, with blood tests. The results are evaluated by the physician with other findings from the patient's history before a final diagnosis is made.

Another reliable way to determine the amount of glucose in the urine is with the Clinitest tablet. Instructions for use are enclosed with each kit and may be used by diabetic patients in daily monitoring of their glucose level at home. Bottles which contain Clinitest tablets are light-resistant and should be kept in a dry, cool storage area to ensure accurate test results. As with all medications and chemical preparations, Clinitest should be kept out of the hands of children. These tablets should not come in contact with skin, or a **caustic** reaction with the skin's moisture will result in a burn. Patients who use Clinitest, or other home test kits, keep a record of the results and either phone the medical office or bring the report in to be filed in their chart.

Pregnancy tests are often performed with urine specimens.

Female patients usually bring a urine specimen into the medical office in their own containers. They should be instructed to wash, rinse, and dry these carefully before collecting the specimen.

The ideal urine specimen for pregnancy testing is obtained from the first morning urination, which contains the greatest concentration of chorionic gonadotropin, the hormone on which most pregnancy tests are based. For certain biological pregnancy tests, animals are used. If this type of test is to be performed, the patient should be instructed to discontinue medications or the test results may be inaccurate.

If pregnancy tests are performed in the medical office, the package insert instructions should be followed exactly. Most are simple and easy to complete. Pregnancy tests performed in the medical office take only a few minutes, and patients may want to wait for the results. If the test is positive (meaning that pregnancy is evident), the patient may have several questions and may wish to consult further with the physician. Routine scheduling of an appointment is advised.

Patients are usually advised to bring a urine specimen for a pregnancy test no earlier than 10 days after the first missed menstrual period. Refrigeration is necessary if the specimen cannot be taken directly to the laboratory. The laboratory request form and patient's chart should contain the age of the patient and the date of the **last menstrual period (LMP)** along with the standard information requested.

P R O C E D U R E

Obtain Urine Sediment for Microscopic Examination

PURPOSE: To obtain urine sediment to determine microscopic contents of urine.

EQUIPMENT: Fresh urine specimen, disposable latex gloves, two glass test tubes, centrifuge, frosted-end glass slides with cover glass, tapered pipette, patient's chart, pen, pencil, tongue depressor, microscope with light source, urine sediment chart, timer or timepiece

TERMINAL PERFORMANCE OBJECTIVE: Provided with all necessary equipment and supplies, demonstrate all steps required in the procedure for obtaining urine sediment. The instructor will observe each step.

1. Wash hands, put on gloves, and assemble all needed items on cleared counter surface near centrifuge. **CAUTION:** Remember, in order to comply with universal precautions guidelines, gloves must be worn if there is any possibility of coming into contact with blood or any body fluids.
2. Stir urine specimen with tongue depressor and pour equal amounts (approximately 10 cc) into each of two test tubes or use plain water in one of test tubes. *Note: Remember that equal weight is required for proper operation of centrifuge.*
3. To balance centrifuge, place test tubes on opposite sides. Urine should be spun at 1500 revolutions per minute for 3 to 5 minutes. *Note: Set timer or write down time.*
4. When centrifuge has completely stopped, lift out tube containing urine specimen and carefully pour off urine (**supernatant**).
5. There will still be a few drops of urine in the bottom of test tube with sediment. Gently tap bottom of tube on counter or against your palm to mix urine and sediment together.
6. Obtain a drop or two of urine sediment with a tapered pipette and place it on a clean frosted-end glass slide.
7. Place a cover slip over specimen, allow it to settle, and place on microscope stage.

Unless you are highly experienced in this area, the physician will conduct the examination from this point on. Consult with your employer about the office policy in this matter before proceeding with the examination.

8. View slide under low-power objective first. Scan for casts and epithelial cells, Figure 7–50. *Note: Use dim light.* **RATIONALE: Dim light enhances visualization; bright light causes glare, interfering with vision.**
9. Change to high-powered objective to view structures, such as blood, bacteria, and crystal cells. At least 10 different fields should be viewed. Turn light off when finished. **RATIONALE: Heat from light will dry out slide and destroy specimen.**
10. Record microscopic observations on patient's chart. Casts and epithelial cells are counted as few, moderate, or many; for example:

    blood casts—few/lpf
    epithelial cells—many/lpf

    Red and white blood cells and bacteria are counted by number seen under microscope using high-power objective or by terms *occasional* or *loaded* (to describe too many to count); for example:

    WBCs—loaded/hpf
    bacteria—occ/hpf

    Red blood cells which are shrunken, or **crenated** will appear smaller than average and will have a jagged surface.
11. Rinse glass items, wash in detergent solution if not disposable, rinse well, and dry on paper towels. Test tubes may be placed bottom-up to drain on paper towels. Return items to proper storage area. Remove disposable gloves and discard in the proper receptacle. Wash hands.

Collection of Specimens for Substance Analysis You may be given the responsibility of collecting specimens for drug (chemical) and alcohol analysis. You must be sure to explain the procedure thoroughly before you have the patient complete and sign the consent-release form for the blood or urine test (or both). The form will state that the purpose of the test is to screen for the presence of drugs, alcohol, and chemical substances. The signature of the patient on this form gives authorization for you to collect the specimen(s) for this purpose, prepare it for transport to the laboratory for analysis, and release the results to the agency (employer) where it was requested. Generally this information is an employment requirement. It can also be required for legal reasons. These specimens should be collected very carefully. The consent form and the test request form must accompany the specimens to the laboratory. Information regarding the samples includes:

1. Purpose of the test
2. Number of specimens
3. Comments about: (urine) color, temperature, pH and specific gravity
4. Collector's name
5. Site of collection, date, and time

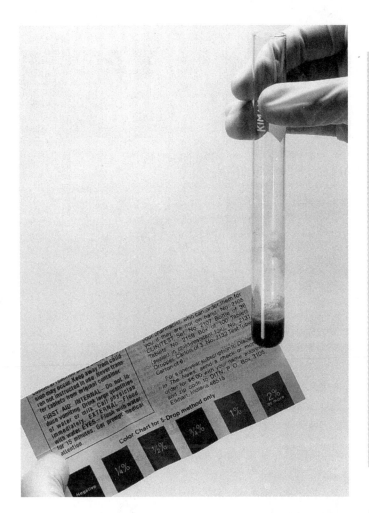

FIGURE 7–49 Compare the reaction color with the chart 15 seconds after boiling stops after gently swirling to mix the solution.

The signature of the collector then verifies that the sealed specimen sent is the same one that was received from the patient (at the site) whose name is on the request and consent forms. This multiple-(five) copy form is color-coded for routing purposes. Copies are given to

1. Medical review officer
2. Laboratory
3. Patient
4. Collector
5. Employer

An example of a *chain of custody* multicopy request form for substance analysis is shown in the Appendix.

Patients should be informed that all medications, drugs, and alcohol which have been consumed within the last 30 days prior to the test will be revealed by the testing process. OTC (over-the-counter) medications are included. Explain that concealing information is certainly not advised because it would only make a possible problem situation worse for them. A section on the form allows the patient to list all substances consumed in the last month. Patients should be

advised to be specific and state what was taken and how much. Ask patients to think about this before completing the form so that they can remember exactly to complete the form accurately.

Because of the odor caused by the bacterial growth, discarding specimens may present a problem. Urine specimens should be flushed down the toilet carefully.

Sputum Specimens ....

Sputum specimens are sent to the laboratory for analysis of the secretions from the patient's lower respiratory tract. The patient is instructed to obtain the specimen by deeply coughing up the secretions from the bronchial tubes, the trachea, and the lungs into a sterile specimen container. Saliva and mucus from the mouth and nasal passages are not the desired secretions for the sputum analysis and interfere with the test results. The physician may wish to induce coughing in some patients to obtain the specimen in the medical office. Otherwise the patient should be instructed to collect the secretions at home. The patient must understand that the most productive cough will probably occur in the morning soon after waking. This specimen will be the most concentrated. Explain why it is important to follow directions in obtaining a sputum specimen, and that the physician

CRYSTALS FOUND IN ACID URINE

URIC ACID (BRIGHTFIELD) URIC ACID (POLARIZED) TYROSINE (BRIGHTFIELD) LEUCINE (BRIGHTFIELD) CYSTINE (BRIGHTFIELD) CYSTINE (POLARIZED)

CRYSTALS FOUND IN ALKALINE URINE

TRIPLE PHOSPHATE (BRIGHTFIELD) AMMONIUM URATES (BRIGHTFIELD)

CRYSTALS FOUND IN ACID, NEUTRAL, AND ALKALINE URINE

HIPPURIC ACID (BRIGHTFIELD) CALCIUM OXALATE (BRIGHTFIELD)

CELLS FOUND IN URINE

RBCs WBCs RENAL TUBULAR & WBC (SEDI-STAIN) RENAL TUBULAR TRANSITIONAL SQUAMOUS

CASTS AND ARTIFACTS FOUND IN URINE

GRANULAR HYALINE WBC CASTS RBC CASTS

BACTERIA, FUNGI, PARASITES FOUND IN URINE

BACTERIA YEAST TRICHOMONAS VAGINALIS

FIGURE 7–50 Crystals, cells, and casts found in urine sediment (Courtesy of Miles Inc. Diagnostic Division.)

needs accurate information to make a diagnosis. Instruct the patient that this procedure will help identify certain organisms that might not be diagnosed otherwise. Be sure to answer all questions about the process of obtaining the specimen.

The sterile specimen cup (usually a disposable cardboard or plastic container) should be prelabeled with the patient's name and other standard information. The patient should be instructed to fill in the time and date of the specimen and transport it to the medical office as soon as possible. The container should be no more than half full and securely sealed. If

it will be more than an hour until the specimen is received by the lab, it should be refrigerated.

Some sputum specimens require collection of secretions of the patient's productive coughing episodes over a period of 24 hours or up to 72 hours. In this case, the secretions will be placed in a larger container and must be refrigerated and appropriately labeled. The appropriate laboratory request form, Figure 7–51, page 417, must be completed with important information regarding the specimen and the patient and accompany the specimen to the lab for proper analysis.

C-5 REQUEST FORM

BILL
- [ ] ACCOUNT
- [ ] PATIENT SEE (1)
- [ ] 3RD PARTY SEE (2)

PLEASE LEAVE BLANK
AREA _____
DEPT. _____
BILL CD _____

INSTRUCTIONS: (1) FOR PATIENT BILLING, COMPLETE BOX A
(2) FOR 3RD PARTY BILLING, COMPLETE BOX A AND FILL IN DIAGNOSIS, THEN EITHER B, C, or D.

ROCHE BIOMEDICAL LABORATORIES, INC.
P.O. BOX 2289
COLUMBUS, OHIO 43216
614 889-1061

PATIENT NAME (LAST) (FIRST) SPECIES SEX AGE YRS MOS DATE COLLECTED MO DAY YR TIME COLLECTED

PATIENT ADDRESS STREET MISC INFORMATION DR ID MEDICARE #

CITY STATE ZIP DIAGNOSIS

PHYSICIAN WELFARE # CASE NAME

PROGRAM PATIENT 1ST NAME: DATE OF BIRTH MO DAY YR. ALL CLAIMS

INSURANCE GR # I.D. SERVICE CODE:

SUBSCRIBER NAME: RELATION: PHONE

VIROLOGY

VIRUS ISOLATION

9325	( )	GENERAL VIRUS
9326	( )	INFLUENZA VIRUS
9327	( )	HERPES SIMPLEX VIRUS
9328	( )	CYTOMEGALOVIRUS
9329	( )	CHLAMYDIA CULTURE
9330	( )	ROTAVIRUS ANTIGEN SCREEN
9332	( )	C DIFFICILE TOXIN SCREEN

CLINICAL INFORMATION

VIRUS SUSPECTED

SOURCE OF SPECIMEN _____

DATE COLLECTED _____

IS PATIENT PREGNANT YES ___ NO ___

PATIENT SYMPTOMS _____

EPIDEMIOLOGIC FACTORS
SIMILAR ILLNESS IN FAMILY _____
LOCAL EPIDEMICS _____
RECENT TRAVEL _____
ANIMAL CONTACT _____

IMMUNIZATION (SPECIFY TYPE AND DATE OF LAST DOSE)

POLIO _____ INFLUENZA _____ OTHER _____
MISCELLANEOUS INFORMATION

MICROBIOLOGY

SOURCE OF SPECIMEN _____

9219	( )	ACID FAST CULTURE & SMEAR
9220	( )	ACID FAST SMEAR ONLY
9245	( )	ANAEROBIC CULTURE
9209	( )	BETA STREP (A) FA
9214	( )	BLOOD CULTURE
9226	( )	FECES, FAT & MUSCLE FIBER
9225	( )	FECES, OCCULT BLOOD
9309	( )	FECES, OVA & PARASITES
9221	( )	FUNGUS CULTURE
9204	( )	FUNGUS ID, COMPLETE
9222	( )	FUNGUS, KOH PREP
9232	( )	GENERAL CULTURE
9215	( )	GONOCOCCUS CULTURE
9218	( )	GRAM STAIN ONLY
9207	( )	LEGIONELLA CULTURE
9228	( )	PINWORM EXAM
9241	( )	POST VASECTOMY EXAM

9233	( )	SALMONELLA & SHIGELLA SCREEN
9203	( )	SPUTUM CULTURE
9227	( )	STOOL, COMPREHENSIVE
9206	( )	STREP SCREEN, THROAT
9202	( )	UPPER RESPIRATORY TRACT CULTURE
9212	( )	URINE, COMPREHENSIVE CULTURE
9213	( )	URINE, SCREEN CULTURE
9234	( )	UROGENITAL CULTURE

UNLISTED TESTS

ADDITIONAL CLINICAL INFORMATION:

SENSITIVITIES ARE PERFORMED AS PART OF THE ROUTINE CULTURE AT NO ADDITIONAL CHARGE WHERE ORGANISMS ARE CONSIDERED PATHOGENIC SENSITIVITIES ARE NOT PERFORMED ON NORMAL FLORA, ALPHA STREPTOCOCCUS, PNEUMOCOCCUS OR BETA STREPTOCOCCUS ROUTINELY

(Rev 1-84)

FOLD THIS FORM IN HALF SO TEST(S) ORDERED IS CLEARLY VISIBLE

FIGURE 7–51 Laboratory request form for identification of microorganisms.

The sputum specimen is analyzed for fungal infections, tuberculosis, and pneumonia. **Cancer** is detected from sputum by the Papanicolaou stain. This test requires a special request form identifying the source of the specimen, Figure 7–52, page 419. This specimen should be sent in the appropriate container with a 95% alcohol solution.

Stool Specimens

Stool specimens (**feces**) are probably the most difficult to instruct patients to obtain. There is a certain amount of embarrassment for both the patient and the medical assistant in regard to this procedure. Nevertheless, it is an extremely important specimen. Microbial organisms, ova, and **occult** (otherwise invisible or hidden) blood may be determined from careful examination of the fecal material.

Patients are instructed to obtain the stool specimen at home, usually within a few days of the request. For the patient who has a daily bowel movement, this will be no problem. For patients who have difficulty with daily elimination, it may take a few days. Patients should use **laxatives** only by order of the physician. Straining during a bowel movement may cause hemorrhoids and is never recommended. You may suggest that the patient drink plenty of fluids to help avoid constipation.

A very small amount of stool is required for laboratory tests. The patient is usually advised to use a tongue depressor or similar stick that can be disposed of to get a sample of stool (the size of a half dollar) from the toilet after a bowel movement. Female patients should be careful not to contaminate the

PROCEDURE

Instruct Patient to Collect Sputum Specimen

PURPOSE: To instruct patients in collection of an adequate sputum specimen for laboratory analysis.

EQUIPMENT: Sputum specimen container and lid, label, pen, patient's chart, lab request form, note pad, rubber band, printed instruction sheet (optional)

TERMINAL PERFORMANCE OBJECTIVE: Provided with all necessary equipment and supplies, and using other students as patients, demonstrate the steps of the procedure for instructing a patient in the collection of a sputum specimen for analysis. The instructor will observe each step.

1. Assemble items next to patient.
2. Write patient's name on specimen cup label and complete lab request form.
3. Explain physician's orders to identified patient. Give printed instructions or write out if you feel patient has a difficult time understanding you.
4. Instruct patient to remove lid from sterile specimen container and to expel secretions from a first morning coughing episode into the center of cup, being careful

not to touch inside of cup. Container should not be more than half full.

5. Instruct patient not to allow tears, sweat, mucus from nose or mouth, or any other substance to enter cup. *Note: Secretions must be coughed up (expectorated) from lower respiratory tract (lungs, bronchial tubes, and trachea) or test will not be acceptable.*
6. When secretions have been obtained and cup sealed with its cover, patient should write time and date that it was obtained on label and lab request form and bring it to lab or medical office as soon as possible. *Note: If patient cannot bring specimen in within 2 hours after collection, it should be refrigerated.*
7. Secure completed lab request form to specimen container with a rubber band or tape. Send to lab. *Note: If patient prepares specimen at home, show patient how to do this.*
8. Record that instruction was given to patient in sputum collecting and initial.

PROCEDURE

Instruct Patient to Collect Stool Specimen

PURPOSE: To instruct patients to obtain an adequate stool specimen for laboratory analysis.

EQUIPMENT: Specimen container with lid, lab request form, pen, patient's chart, label, rubber band, printed instructions (optional), tongue depressors, note pad

TERMINAL PERFORMANCE OBJECTIVE: With all necessary equipment and supplies, and using other students as patients, demonstrate the steps of the procedure for instructing a patient in collecting an adequate stool specimen for laboratory analysis. The instructor will observe each step.

1. Assemble items next to patient.
2. Write identifying information on request form and label (usually cover) and affix to specimen cup.
3. Identify patient and explain physician's orders. **RATIONALE: Speaking to the patient by name and checking chart ensures that you are performing the**

procedure on the correct patient. Give printed instructions or write out if necessary.

4. Instruct patient to obtain a small amount of stool (about a tablespoon) from next bowel movement, within next few days. Explain that nothing else should be placed in cup besides stool (no tissue paper, urine, etc.). Patients may defecate onto a paper plate and obtain a small specimen from plate, which is then discarded. Or they may use a tongue depressor to obtain specimen from toilet bowl.
5. Instruct patient to place specimen in cup, secure cover tightly and write date and time specimen was obtained on cover of cup; then bring specimen to lab or medical office with request form as soon as possible. *Note: To prevent bacterial growth, specimen should be refrigerated if it cannot be received by lab within 2 hours.*

CYTOLOGY-PAP
TECHNIQUE

PLEASE PRINT

Patient's Name

☐ PAP ONLY
☐ PAP & M.I.
☐

THIS SPACE FOR INFORMATION
DESIRED ON REPORT

Physician's Name
Address
City

PLEASE DO NOT WRITE IN THIS SPACE

Date

Address Line Should Only Be Filled In
When Address Is Desired On Report

Separate Address Forms Required For Bill Patients

PLEASE PENCIL PATIENT'S NAME
ON FROSTED END OF SLIDE.

State   Zip

DIAGNOSTIC INFORMATION
(Please complete this section)

Patient's Age _____ Sex ____
Source of Material _____
Last Menstrual Period (First Day) _____
Vag. Bleeding ☐   Vag. Discharge ☐
No. of Pregnancies _____
Menopause _____
Hormone Therapy _____
Irradiation _____
Chief Complaint _____
Clinical Diagnosis _____

☐ Additional information or instructions to laboratory
on reverse side of form.

FIGURE 7–52 Cytology request form

specimen with urine or blood. The stool should be placed in a container which has been labeled with the date and time of collection, Figure 7–53. If the specimen cannot be taken directly to the lab or brought to the medical office, it must be refrigerated to prevent bacterial growth.

Complete Chapter 7, Unit 4 in the workbook to help you meet the objectives at the beginning of this unit and therefore achieve competency of this subject matter.

FIGURE 7–53 Laboratory stool specimen container with identification lid (From Caldwell & Hegner, *Health Care Assistant,* 5th ed. Copyright 1989, Delmar Publishers Inc.)

U N I T   5

Bacterial Smears and Cultures

OBJECTIVES ....

Upon completion of this unit, you will meet the following terminal performance objectives by verifying knowledge of the facts and principles presented through oral and written communication at a level deemed competent by the instructor or employer, and will demonstrate the specific behaviors as identified in the terminal performance objectives of the procedures, observing all aseptic and safety precautions in accordance with health care standards.

1. Obtain a smear for bacteriological examination.
2. Heat-fix a smear for staining.
3. Explain the reason for heat-fixing specimens.
4. Complete a Gram stain.
5. List common diseases caused by gram-positive and gram-negative bacteria.
6. Obtain a throat culture and streak an agar plate.
7. Describe growth media for cultures.
8. Label specimens for analysis.
9. Record information concerning specimens on the patient's chart.
10. Spell and define, using the glossary at the back of the text, all the words to know in this unit.

P A T I E N T E D U C A T I O N

Instructing patients in the collection of stool specimens is a good opportunity to give helpful advice in regard to bowel problems. The following is a list of suggestions for discussion with patients.

1. Advise patients to drink plenty of fluids to help reduce the incidence of constipation.
2. Urge patients to refrain from using laxatives, enemas, or suppositories unless specifically ordered by the physician.
3. Instruct the patients regarding straining during a bowel movement, which could cause hemorrhoids (and other problems). Sitting or standing for prolonged periods can also be a factor in the development of hemorrhoids.
4. Remind patients that a change in bowel habits should be reported to the physician.
5. Advise patients that a proper well-balanced diet (from the food guide pyramid), consistent meal times, and exercise is the best way toward regularity regarding bowel habits.
6. Remind patients to wash their hands with soap and water before *and* after using the bathroom each time to avoid spreading germs.

The possibility of disease transmission is extremely high in handling any type of specimen, especially those of patients suspected of having infections. Proper hand-washing and sterile technique must be used at all times to break the cycle of the infection. Eating, drinking, chewing gum, smoking, and any hand-to-mouth gesture should be avoided to prevent possible self-contamination. Any items used must be carefully washed or properly disposed of to prevent others from becoming infected. Disposable items are almost exclusively used in medical practice today for this reason.

Bacteriological Smear

Identification of microorganisms that cause disease is accomplished by obtaining a smear or a culture from the area of the body that appears to be infected. To make a smear, a sample of the **exudate** (drainage) is taken from the throat, mouth, ear, eye, nose, vagina, anus, the surface of the skin or from within a wound by introducing a sterile cotton swab into the area, Figure 7–54. The swab is then rolled over two-thirds of a frosted-end slide, Figure 7–55. The smear is air dried at room temperature and then *heat-fixed,* or passed through a flame, Figure 7–56. This seals the specimen to the glass so that it won't wash off during the staining process.

After preparation of a bacteriological smear, determination of the microorganism causing the infection must be made by the physician. Your role is that of obtaining and preparing the smear.

FIGURE 7–55 Rolling the specimen onto the glass slide from left to right covering two-thirds of the area

Culturing

Culturing is a means of isolating a disease-causing microorganism for identification. It takes far longer than a bacteriological smear but is still a relatively simple procedure. A specimen is obtained and placed in a culture medium, which contains nutrients comparable to human tissue to encourage growth of microorganisms. The medium is **agar**, a gelatin-like substance, mixed with sheep's blood.

Explain to the patient that a throat culture is necessary to identify certain organisms. Be sure to tell the patient that there

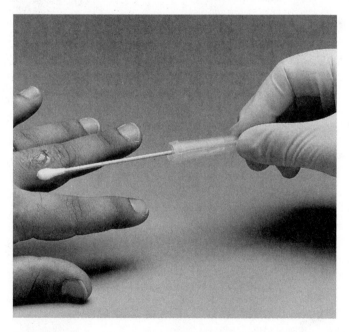

FIGURE 7–54 Use a sterile swab to obtain a specimen from a wound.

FIGURE 7–56 Heat-fixing the specimen onto the glass slide

FIGURE 7–57 Pattern for smearing a plate (From Simmers, *Diversified Health Occupations,* Copyright 1988, Delmar Publishers Inc.)

might be some momentary discomfort in obtaining the specimen, and answer all questions about the process of obtaining the specimen. The specimen is taken directly from the affected area of the patient with a sterile swab and distributed over the agar in a Petri dish of clear plastic using the pattern shown in Figure 7–57. Many cultures are streaked with a fine wire loop (pictured in the foreground of Figure 7–56, page 420), which is sterilized by flame to prevent cross-contamination when distributing the specimen. The culture plate is then placed in an incubator for 24 to 48 hours to provide the proper temperature for bacterial growth. Many physicians in pediatrics, general, and family practice obtain, incubate, and read their own cultures, not only for the patient's convenience, but for their own.

The Petri dish must be properly labeled for identification purposes, including the patient's name, the date and time the specimen was taken, and the source of the specimen. This information should be written on the bottom of the Petri dish with a wax crayon or label.

Petri plates and other types of transport media for culturing specimens should be prepared according to the outside laboratory's directions. The culture media are disposable and should be discarded in securely tied biohazardous plastic bags in the proper receptacle.

Gram Staining ....

The purpose of Gram staining is to make heat-fixed bacteria visible for **microscopic** identification, Figure 7–61. The two most common divisions of bacteria are **gram-positive** and **gram-negative**. The infectious diseases most commonly caused by these bacteria are

PROCEDURE

Prepare Bacteriological Smear

PURPOSE: To adhere a specimen to a glass slide for examination under the microscope.

EQUIPMENT: Specimen (on labeled cotton swab), disposable gloves, clean frosted-end glass slide, forceps, Bunsen burner, matches, slide staining rack, pencil, pen, patient's chart (if sent to outside lab: slide holder, lab request form, rubber band or tape)

TERMINAL PERFORMANCE OBJECTIVE: With all necessary equipment and supplies provided, demonstrate the steps of the procedure for preparing a bacteriological smear for microscopic analysis. The instructor will observe each step.

1. Wash hands and put on latex gloves. Assemble all needed items on counter space. **CAUTION:** Remember, in order to comply with universal precautions guidelines, gloves must be worn if there is any possibility of coming into contact with blood or any body fluids. Pencil patient's name on frosted end of glass slide. Complete lab request form, including source of specimen.
2. Prepare as many smears of specimen as ordered by physician by rolling cotton swab evenly over two-thirds of glass slide, holding slide with thumb and great finger.
3. Light Bunsen burner or other source for flame and adjust to a blue flame. **RATIONALE: Blue flame is hottest.**
4. Hold frosted part of slide with your thumb and index finger or with forceps and pass specimen portion of slide through blue part of flame, smear side up, slowly (taking about 2 seconds) two or three times. **RATIONALE: The yellow portion must be avoided as it leaves carbon deposits on slide, obscuring visualization.** *Note: Excessive heating will destroy specimen.* Turn Bunsen burner or other source off.
5. Place heat-fixed smear on staining rack to cool for staining procedure or place on microscope stage for observation by physician.
6. Discard used disposables and return other items to proper storage area. Remove disposable gloves and discard in the proper receptacle. Wash hands.
7. Record procedure on patient's chart and initial.

Obtain a Throat Culture

PURPOSE: To isolate a disease-causing organism to determine effective treatment of the patient.

EQUIPMENT: Culture plate (Petri dish), sterile cotton swabs, sterile tongue depressor, disposable gloves, pen, patient's chart, penlight (optional), wax crayon or label for culture plate (if sent to outside lab, request form and label for culture plate, clear tape, tissues)

TERMINAL PERFORMANCE OBJECTIVE: Provided with all necessary equipment and supplies, and using a lifelike clinical doll infant or small child under close supervision, or other students as patients, demonstrate the steps required to perform the procedure for obtaining a throat culture. The instructor will observe each step.

1. Assemble needed items near identified patient. Label culture plate and complete request form if required. Wash hands and put on gloves. **CAUTION:** Remember, in order to comply with universal precautions guidelines, gloves must be worn if there is any possibility of coming into contact with blood or any body fluids.
2. Identify patient. **RATIONALE: Speaking to the patient by name and checking chart ensures that you are performing the procedure on the correct patient.**
3. Explain procedure to patient and assist patient to comfortable position. Sitting is usual position for adults. It may be easier to work with children if they are lying down. Assistance may be necessary.
   Note: If you must obtain a throat culture from a small child or infant without assistance, it may prove easier if you sit with child on your lap. Place child's right arm under your left arm. Hold child's left wrist with your left hand and cradle head between your left wrist and left shoulder. This will free your right hand to obtain specimen. Gently touch child's throat with back of your left thumb to encourage mouth to open. With your right hand, hold swab securely, quickly insert it and swab back of throat with a rolling motion. (Insert swab at corner of mouth behind teeth to prevent child

from biting it.) Use flexible swabs (wooden stick swabs may break if bitten, and splintering is a danger when working with small children or infants). Touch only back of throat.

4. Open sterile swab and ask patient to open mouth as wide as possible. Quickly examine with light source.
5. Depress tongue with sterile tongue depressor held in one hand. Hold sterile swab in other. Ask patient to say "ah" to assist depression of tongue (this also prevents patient from feeling gag reflex by diverting attention). Quickly insert swab into back of throat and roll over at least two areas, touching areas with obvious exudate.
6. Remove swab and depressor from patient's mouth. *Note: Some physicians order a nasopharyngeal culture (NPC) in which a specimen is obtained from the nasal passages and throat. This is accomplished by inserting a sterile swab into nasal cavities (one for each nostril) and applying each to culture plate, or into a transport media if sent to a lab, Figure 7–58.* Attend to patient, offer tissues. Tearing may result from procedure.
7. Immediately apply specimen to agar in Petri dish, smearing it as shown in Figure 7–59 or place swab into container for transportation to lab. Tape request form securely.
8. Place identification label on bottom of Petri dish or write patient's name, date, time, and source on bottom with wax crayon. Secure cover with clear tape.
9. Discard all disposable items in proper receptacle. Remove gloves and dispose of them in the proper receptacle. Wash hands. Place culture in incubator agar side up. **RATIONALE: The growth of microorganisms releases moisture which collects on cover and will drip onto agar, drowning microorganisms if agar is on bottom, Figure 7–60.**
10. Remove gloves and wash hands.
11. Record procedure on patient's chart and initial.

- *Gram-positive bacteria:* botulism, diphtheria, lobar pneumonia, rheumatic fever, streptococcal sore throat, tetanus
- *Gram-negative bacteria*: bacillary dysentery, cholera, gonorrhea, meningitis, pertussis, plague, typhoid fever

Bacteria have certain characteristic formations and are identified by their size and shape. Cocci appear in clusters. Staphylococci form grapelike clusters. Bacteria that form

pairs are called diplococci. Those that form chains are streptococci. Bacteria with capsule-like coverings are called spore-forming.

Gram-positive bacteria take a violet (purple) color from the Gram stain procedure. Gram-negative bacteria take a red or pink color from the counterstain. Without the staining process the bacteria are colorless. In preparing the slide, you should avoid getting the crystal (or gentian) violet dye on your hands,

FIGURE 7–58 Place the swab with the specimen into the transport container with a culture media for laboratory analysis.

clothing, or counter as it is difficult (sometimes impossible) to remove. Alcohol and acetone are helpful in removing the dye in some cases.

Refer to Table 7–5, page 426, for examples of how different bacteria stain the particular color of purple (positive) or pink (negative).

Complete Chapter 7, Unit 5 in the workbook to help you meet the objectives at the beginning of this unit and therefore achieve competency of this subject matter.

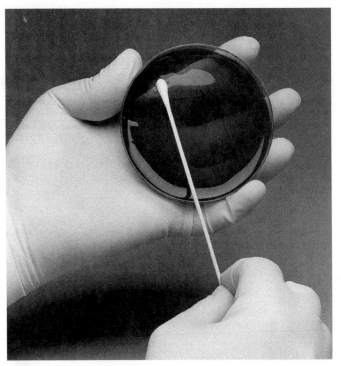

FIGURE 7–59 Smear the culture plate with the specimen from the swab.

FIGURE 7–60 Place the culture plate in the incubator agar side up.

As you obtain throat cultures from patients you may want to give them some helpful advice concerning their condition. Generally when a person has a sore throat it is associated with other respiratory symptoms as well. The following suggestions may provide some relief from discomfort and help them toward better health.

1. Advise patients to drink plenty of liquids (fruit juices) and to eat sensibly from the basic food groups.
2. Urge patients to get extra rest and dress comfortably (according to the weather and temperature outside).
3. Suggest the use of gargles or throat lozenges (or both) to relieve painful sore throat.
4. Remind them to avoid tobacco and smoking.
5. Instruct them to cough and sneeze into tissue and discard them into proper waste containers to prevent the spread of germs.
6. Remind them not to eat or drink after others and to use disposables at home when there is illness.

BACILLI WITH CENTRAL AND TERMINAL SPORES

FIGURE 7–61 Shapes of bacteria

| 1. Crystal violet | 60 sec. | 2. Wash | 2 sec. | 3. Gram's iodine | 60 sec. | 4. Decolorize with alcohol | 10-20 sec. |

| 5. Wash | 2 sec. | 6. Safranin | 20 sec. | 7. Wash | 2 sec. | 8. Blot dry |

FIGURE 7–62 The Gram-staining procedure

P R O C E D U R E

Prepare Gram Stain

PURPOSE: To stain a heat-fixed bacteriological smear for microscopic identification.

EQUIPMENT: Heat-fixed slide (frosted end labeled), slide rack and tray, crystal (or gentian) violet dye, water wash bottle, forceps, Gram's iodine, alcohol (or acetone), safranine solution (or dilute fuchsin), timer or timepiece, immersion oil, microscope with light source, pen, patient's chart, pencil, cover glass slides, eyedroppers, paper towels; disposable latex gloves and plastic apron (optional)

TERMINAL PERFORMANCE OBJECTIVE: Provided with all necessary equipment and supplies, demonstrate the steps in the procedure for preparing a Gram stain. The instructor will observe each step.

1. Assemble all needed items on counter and wash hands. *Note: Apron and disposable gloves are to be used; put them on now.* **CAUTION:** Remember, in order to comply with universal precautions guidelines, gloves must be worn if there is any possibility of coming into contact with blood or any body fluids.

2. Place heat-fixed slide on staining rack, specimen side up, over tray. *Note: Recap all solutions immediately after each use to avoid accidents.*

3. Open crystal violet (gentian) dye and fill dropper. Apply over entire specimen area of the slide and time for 60 seconds, Figure 7–62.

4. Hold frosted end of slide with forceps or thumb and index finger and tip slide to allow stain to run off into tray. Wash slide with water, letting flow begin at top and run down.

5. Place slide flat on rack. Fill dropper with Gram's iodine and apply over entire specimen. Leave on for 60 seconds. Tilt slide to allow iodine to run off into tray.

6. Wash slide with water, tilting to direct runoff into tray, and replace flat on rack.

7. Apply alcohol (or acetone) with dropper for a few seconds until purple color in excess runoff is gone.

8. Tilt slide and wash with water immediately. Return flat to rack.

9. Apply safranine solution with dropper to counterstain specimen and wash off with water immediately.

10. Hold slide by frosted end and wipe excess solutions from back. Tap side of slide onto paper towel to help remove excess liquid. Allow slide to air dry. *Note: Slide may be blotted between paper towels, but be careful not to rub slide or specimen may be destroyed.*

11. Apply small drop of immersion oil to specimen and place on microscope stage to view under oil-immersion objective. Turn light on to view and turn off when finished. A slide cover may be used to help preserve specimen for future viewing.

12. Discard disposables, wash used items, and return items to proper storage. Wash hands.

13. Record procedure and results on patient's chart and initial.

M E D I C A L - L E G A L
E T H I C A L   H I G H L I G H T S

Ms. Right . . .
enters laboratory specimens in the log book as they are received. She efficiently follows up by reporting the results as soon as possible. She is ever mindful of universal precautions and respects the privacy of patients keeping all records confidential.

Promotion outlook: Excellent

Miss Wrong . . .
is careless in recording laboratory specimens in the log book. She is also negligent in following universal precautions. Results are not reported in a timely fashion because she misplaces them, thereby jeopardizing confidentiality and privacy of patient information.

Promotion outlook: Poor

TABLE 7–5

Some Important Pathogenic Bacteria and Their Reaction to the Gram Stain

Gram-Positive Reaction (+) (Reaction of Purple Stain)		Gram-Negative Reaction (−) (Loss of Purple Stain)		Gram-Variable Reaction (+/−)	
Bacterium	Disease It Causes	Bacterium	Disease It Causes	Bacterium	Disease It Causes
Bacillus anthracis	Anthrax	Bordetella pertussis	Whooping cough	Mycobacterium leprae	Leprosy
Clostridium botulinum	Botulism (food poisoning)	Brucella abortus (bovine strain)	Infectious abortion in cattle and undulant fever in man	Mycobacterium tuberculosis	Tuberculosis
Clostridum perfringens	Gas gangrene, wound infection	Brucella melitensis, (goat strain)			
Clostridium tetani	Tetanus (lockjaw)	Brudella suis (porcine strain)			
Corynebacterium diphtheriae	Diphtheria	Esherichia coli	Urinary infections		
Staphylococcus aureus	Carbuncles, furunculosis (boils), pneumonia, septicemia	Haemophilus influenzae	Meningitis, pneumonia		
Streptococcus pyrogenes	Erysipelas, rheumatic fever, scarlet fever, septicemia, strep throat, tonsillitis	Neisseria gonorrhoeae	Gonorrhea		
		Neisseria meningitidis	Nasopharyngitis, meningitis		
Streptococcus pneumoniae	Pneumonia	Pseudomonas aeruginosa	Respiratory and uro-genital infections		
		Rickettsia rickettsii	Rocky mountain spotted fever		
		Salmonella paratyphi	Food poisoning, paratyphoid fever		
		Salmonella typhi	Typhoid fever		
		Shigella dysenteriae	Dysentery		
		Treponema pallidum	Syphilis		
		Vibrio cholerae	Cholera		
		Yersinia pestis	Plague		

(From Fong and Ferris, *Microbiology for Health Careers*, 4th ed. Albany: Delmar, 1987.)

Fong, Elizabeth, and Ferris, Elvira. *Microbiology for Health Careers,* 4th Ed. Albany: Delmar, 1987.

Garza, Diana, and Becan-McBride, Kathleen. *Phlebotomy Handbook,* 3rd ed. East Norwalk, CT: Appleton and Lange, 1993.

Miller, Benjamin F., and Keane, Claire Brackman. *Encyclopedia and Dictionary of Medicine and Allied Health,* 3d ed. Philadelphia: W.B. Saunders Co., 1983.

Mosby's Medical & Nursing Dictionary, 3d ed. St. Louis: C.V. Mosby, 1990.

Nurse's Ready Reference Diagnostic Tests. Springhouse, PA: Springhouse, 1991.

Ohio Department of Health, Division of Maternal and Child Health, Genetics Project. 1992, Columbus, Ohio

OSHA Bloodborne Pathogens Final Standard: Summary of Key Provisions. Washington, D.C.: Government Printing Office, 1993.

Raphael, Stanley S. *Lynch's Medical Laboratory Technology,* 3d ed. Windsor, Ontario: W.B. Saunders Co., 1976.

Taber, Clarence W. *Taber's Cyclopedic Medical Dictionary,* 14th ed. Philadelphia: F.A. Davis, 1983.

Ware, Barbara E. *CLIA '88 Physician's Office Laboratory, Are You Ready?* June 1991.

C H A P T E R   8

Diagnostic Tests, X Rays, and Procedures

UNIT 1
Diagnostic Tests

UNIT 2
Cardiology Procedures

UNIT 3
Diagnostic Procedures

UNIT 4
Diagnostic X-ray Examinations

D iagnostic tests, X rays, and procedures will be discussed in this chapter. The medical assistant has a multiple role in these diagnostic aids. You will be responsible for instructing and preparing patients for procedures, tests, and X rays. In some cases, you will either carry out the test(s) or procedure(s), or assist the physician. After completion, you will alert the physician of the results, and from the order of the doctor notify the patient, and then file the report of the results in the patient's chart.

Often as a part of the CPE the physician may order certain tests or other procedures, such as chest X ray, mammography, intravenous pyelegram, and so on. If these diagnostic tests are performed on site, the results may often be determined while the patient is still present. If referrals must be made for diagnostic tests, patients may be asked to return within a week to 10 days for a final report of the findings. This gives the medical assistant and the physician time to gather reports in the patient's chart for review and evaluation. You may want to advise patients to bring a list of their concerns with them so they won't forget to ask necessary questions. This practice may reduce the number of phone consultations required.

U N I T   1

Diagnostic Tests

OBJECTIVES ··

Upon completion of this unit, you will meet the following terminal performance objectives by verifying knowledge of the facts and principles presented through oral and written communication at a level deemed competent by the instructor or employer and will demonstrate the specific behaviors as identified in the terminal performance objectives of the procedures, observing all aseptic and safety precautions in accordance with health care standards.

1. Describe scratch, patch, and intradermal skin tests, state their purpose; and perform each test under supervision.
2. Describe the schedule and instructions for administering allergy injections.
3. Discuss patient education concerning allergies and treatment.
4. Spell and define, using the glossary at the back of the text, all the words to know in this unit.

adrenalin   extract

adverse   histamine

anaphylactic   hypersensitive

antibody   immune

antigen   interpret

contact dermatitis   obsolete

desensitizing   systemic

eosinophil   venom

epinephrine   wheal

Skin Tests ....

Three procedures are commonly used to determine allergic reactions in patients. They are the scratch, intradermal, and patch tests. The physician determines the diagnosis by evaluating the results of the tests along with the patient's medical history, physical exam, and other laboratory tests. The medical assistant may assist the physician in performing these tests or may perform them by order of the physician. Tests should always be performed under the direct supervision of the physician.

These tests involve introducing an **antigen** directly into the patient's skin to induce a reaction. If the reaction is negative (normal) there will be no change in the appearance of the skin following testing. A normal **immune** reaction occurs in the body when an antigen and **antibody** unite and the foreign substance is excreted by the body.

A positive allergic reaction to a test is shown by a raised area on the skin, much like a mosquito bite, called a **wheal,** see Figure 8–6, (hive). This is due to interaction of the antigen and antibody, which releases **histamine** and is termed a **hypersensitive** reaction. Histamine is naturally produced by the body to attach itself to certain cells to cause dilation of blood vessels and contraction of smooth muscles. Most cells release histamine during allergic reactions. As a part of the normal inflammatory response of the body, histamine protects tissue against injury (the scratch test) and it is the reason that redness and a wheal are produced. The inflammatory response of the body is specific in that it is the whole body's defense against infection, chemicals, or other physical factors.

Besides histamine, researchers are still finding that other chemicals are released during the allergic response. Millions of people have allergies to a variety of substances, including certain foods, pollens, dust, drugs (medications), chemicals, **venom** of stinging insects, animal dander, molds, pollutants, and other allergens. Reaction to these substances ranges from slight to severe. Severe reactions can be life-threatening. A life-threatening reaction must be counteracted with an injection of **adrenalin** immediately to prevent **anaphylactic** shock. Symptoms of anaphylactic shock initially include intense anxiety, weakness, sweating, and shortness of breath. Symptoms may continue and include hypotension, shock, arrhythmia, respiratory congestion, laryngeal edema, nausea, and diarrhea.

PATIENT EDUCATION

Certain diagnostic tests, X rays, and procedures may be frightening and sometimes even painful to patients. Careful explanation of the reasons for performing such procedures will help relieve some of the patient's tension. Some tests might require advanced preparation on the part of the patient. Be sure that the patient not only understands what the procedure entails, but also how to prepare for the examination. Give clear verbal and written instructions to the patient including time frames to be followed. Make sure there are no unanswered questions. Remember, if the patient is not adequately prepared for certain tests and examinations, then the tests must be rescheduled. Letting the patient know when the results will be available will also help reduce some anxiety.

Those who have known allergies to the venom of stinging insects, for example, or to certain foods that produce intense life-threatening allergic reactions are instructed to carry an anaphylactic shock kit with them at all times. The kit contains a self-injecting dose of adrenalin for emergency use.

Treatment for many allergy patients consists of an allergy immunotherapy program. Over a considerable time, this therapy gradually provides immunization against the substance that the person is allergic to. Increasing amounts of the allergen are injected as long as the patient can tolerate each dose. Treatment generally takes a few years. It is usually effective in reducing symptoms of most allergies. Often patients bring their serum from the allergy specialist to the family doctor's office or clinic for administration. All allergy serum should be refrigerated unless otherwise specified. These **desensitizing** injections of allergy serum (which patients refer to as "allergy shots") should always be administered under the direct supervision of a physician because anaphylactic shock can occur within seconds even in unsuspecting individuals. Following any injection, the patient must be observed for 20 minutes for possible reaction. Any reaction or unusual symptom must be reported to the physician and noted on the patient's chart, as well as on the schedule sheet accompanying the allergy serum. An example of this schedule is shown in Figure 8–1.

Since patients generally continue this therapy once a week (or even more frequently) over a few years, it is wise to change the injection sites frequently. A practical method of keeping a record of where the allergy serum is injected each time is by alternating arms and numbering the injection sites. This pattern allows up to 18 injection sites and then it can be repeated. This may help in preventing tissue damage from recurring frequent injections of the same area. Keep track of the pattern on the schedule that comes with the allergy serum, or in the patient's chart by recording which arm, the number of the injection site, and of course, the date and your initials.

Figure 8–2, page 430, shows an illustration of (a) a suggested clockwise pattern and (b) charting method. Refer to

Company's Name
(maker of serum)

Physician's Name/Allergist
Address and Phone Number

Patient's Name   Lot Number of Serum
Account Number   Expiration Date

INSTRUCTIONS FOR ADMINISTRATION

—Preparations should always be made for physician to treat anaphylaxis should it occur.

—Patients who are being treated with beta-blocker medications should not be given allergy serum.

—Use 27G 1/2" needle.

—Administer 3/8" to 1/2" into subcutaneous tissue between deltoid and biceps muscle (but not into the muscle).

—Aspirate plunger of syringe to ensure needle is not in a blood vessel.

—Reschedule patient for injection if s/he is feverish or is wheezing.

—Observe patient for possible reaction for 20 minutes following injection.

—Administer cold packs on site if local redness, itching, or wheal develops—alert physician for administration of antihistamine PRN.

—If a systemic or general reaction occurs, such as hives, sneezing or wheezing, alert physician for dosage and administration of epinephrine (subcutaneous).

—**Contact allergist for rescheduling instructions if systemic reaction occurs.**

SCHEDULE

Administer allergy serum injections every _____ days. If no adverse reaction occurs, resume scheduled dose. If adverse local reaction occurs, resume schedule with the last well-tolerated dose. Proceed with the following schedule until maximum dose is reached and well-tolerated. Then repeat maximum dose tolerated until vial is empty.

Dose	Date Administered	Adverse Reaction
0.10 cc	month/day/year	type of reaction
0.15 cc	initials of one who	if any (note the
0.20 cc	administered the	severity and
0.30 cc	injection	symptoms of
0.40 cc	and which arm	the patient)
0.50 cc	was injected	
*0.50 cc	Rt or L	

*Reorder before last dose is administered. Allow 2 weeks for delivery.

FIGURE 8–1   Example of a schedule and instructions for allergy serum injections

Chapter 10 for the procedure for administering injections.

The size of the wheal is **interpreted** by the physician after a timed 20- to 30-minute period. Wheals are measured in centimeters by using a tape measure or by comparison, Figure 8–3, page 430. A trained skin tester may observe the reaction and make an interpretation by inspection alone.

Extracts of substances that are commonly the cause of allergy in patients are manufactured in applicator bottles. These should be refrigerated and the expiration date noted for accurate test results. Many of the skin-testing extracts vary in strength from one company to another. Since specific allergens may also differ geographically, skin tests are sometimes unreliable. Stan-

dardization would be helpful, but new methods are being researched, and skin testing may one day become an **obsolete** procedure.

Scratch Test   Desirable sites for the scratch test are the arms and the back, depending on the number of tests to be performed and, in some cases, the preference of the patient. Small children are easier to restrain if they are lying face down while the test is being administered. The area to be tested should be comfortably accessible to both patient and physician or assistant. The patient must stay in the same position for at least 20 minutes, so comfort is essential for compliance.

The tests should be numbered in a pattern with washable ink on the surface of the skin. Explain to the patient that there will be some discomfort when administering either the scratch test or the intradermal test, but it will not last long. Instruct the patient to inform you of any itching or swelling at the site of injection. Advise the patient to avoid scratching the area for accurate interpretation following the prescribed timing of the test(s). Several extracts may be applied to the patient's skin in rows from evenly spaced applicators that have been dipped into various bottles of allergen substances. The applicator provides a small drop of the substance on the skin in preparation for the scratch test. Figure 8–4 shows a medical assistant applying seven different extracts on the patient's skin. Usually the skin is prepared with alcohol and allowed to air dry. Alcohol may also be used to remove the ink after the test is completed. A sterile needle or lancet is used to tear the surface of the skin in a scratch of about ⅛ inch or less to allow a drop of the antigen to enter the epidermis, Figure 8–5. Some test materials are packaged in sealed glass capillary tubes, the contents of which are shaken onto the skin after the tube is snapped. Only a small drop should be used. Otherwise, antigens may run together, and test results will be inaccurate. The scratches should be from 1½ to 2 inches apart, allowing possible reactions to spread without interfering with each other. A control is used for comparison in interpreting the results. This is a nonallergy-producing plain base fluid.

Reactions usually occur within the first 20 minutes (Itching at the test site may be relieved by application of cold or ice packs), Figure 8–6, page 432. Many physicians wish to recheck the test sites in 24 hours for delayed reactions. If the physician's interpretation of the skin tests is consistent with the patient's history and physical examination findings, more advanced studies will not be necessary. It is not advisable to perform intradermal tests on patients who have had positive scratch tests.

Intradermal Test   The intradermal test, thought to be more accurate than the scratch test, is often performed if the scratch test is negative or unclear. Although the solutions used for intradermal tests are about 100 times more dilute than those used for scratch tests, they are still potentially dangerous. Severe reactions may occur, however, with either method.

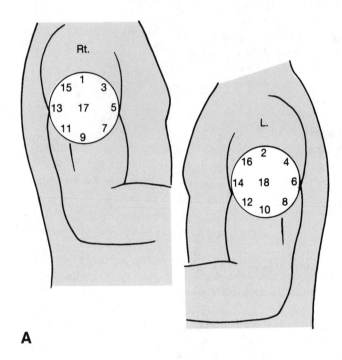

A

FIGURE 8–2 (a)   This alternating pattern of injection allows 18 sites to help prevent possible tissue damage. Repeat as needed.

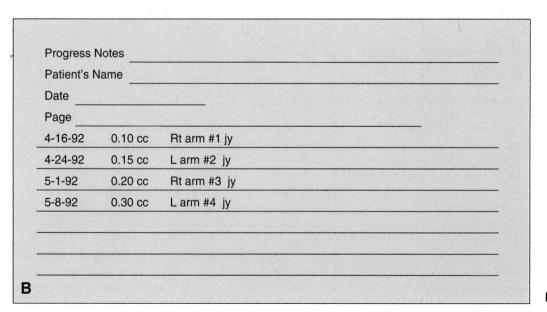

B

FIGURE 8–2 (b)   Example of charting allergy serum injections on a patient's chart

Progress Notes		
Patient's Name		
Date		
Page		
4-16-92	0.10 cc	Rt arm #1 jy
4-24-92	0.15 cc	L arm #2 jy
5-1-92	0.20 cc	Rt arm #3 jy
5-8-92	0.30 cc	L arm #4 jy

+1

+2

+3

+4

FIGURE 8–3   Sizes (+1 to +4) of wheals in reactions to skin tests

FIGURE 8–4 Placing allergy extract solutions on the skin with the multiple applicator

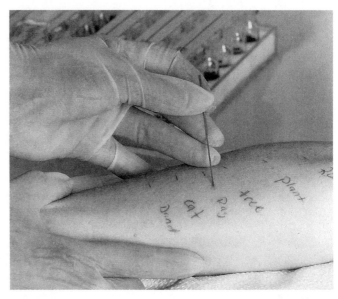

FIGURE 8–5 Each extract is labeled with ink for identification. The medical assistant uses a sterile lancet to scratch the skin, allowing the extract to enter the epidermis.

Generally the diluted solutions used prevent **systemic** reactions. Intradermal test sites are performed at spaced intervals on the forearm, Figure 8–7, or scapular area. In the event of a severe **adverse** reaction, a tourniquet can be applied proximal to the site when the arm is used. The intradermal test can also be referred to as the *subcutaneous test.* Serum or vaccine is sometimes used in intradermal testing. If the initial test is negative, it is often repeated with a stronger solution. Usually the reaction time is 15 to 30 minutes. Adrenaline

P R O C E D U R E

Perform a Scratch Test

PURPOSE: To determine an allergy-causing substance.

EQUIPMENT: Sterile needle(s) or lancet(s), allergen (extract), cotton balls, alcohol, pen, patient's chart, timer or timepiece, control, and disposable latex gloves

TERMINAL PERFORMANCE OBJECTIVE: Provided with all necessary instruments and supplies and a suitable simulated skin surface (such as an orange), demonstrate each of the steps required in the scratch test procedure. Each step will be observed by the instructor.

1. Assemble all needed items on Mayo table near patient, wash hands, and put on gloves. **CAUTION:** Remember, in order to comply with universal precautions guidelines, gloves must be worn if there is any possibility of coming into contact with blood or any body fluids.

2. Explain procedure to identified patient as you prepare test site with alcohol-saturated cotton ball. Sites most commonly used are upper arm and back. Help patient into comfortable position.

3. Apply small drop of extracts onto site and continue until all extracts are applied.

4. Mark site(s) with initial abbreviation or number of extract in pen if more than one test is to be adminis-

tered. Leave about 1½–2 inches between test sites. **RATIONALE: Adequate area for possible reaction must be allowed. Accurate assessment requires measurement of individual reaction areas, which might come together if placed too close.**

5. Remove sterile needle or lancet from package without contaminating it. Make ⅛-inch scratch in surface of skin.

6. Begin timing 20-minute period.

7. Discard disposables and gloves in proper receptacle, return items to proper storage area, and wash hands.

8. As soon as 20-minute time period is up, check each site after cleansing with alcohol-saturated cotton ball. *Note: Be careful not to wipe off the identification of the extract until after interpretation of reaction has been made by tester or physician.*

9. Compare reaction of site with package insert drawings or measure in centimeters. *Note: This step cannot be realistically carried out when a simulated surface is used. However, until the new medical assistant gains experience on the job, the physician will probably make this comparison personally. Cold packs or ice bag may be applied to site to relieve itching.*

10. Record test results on patient's chart and initial.

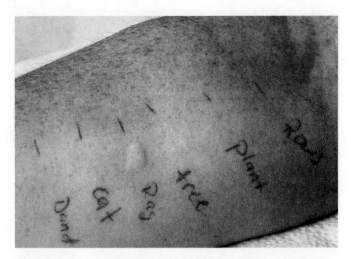

FIGURE 8–6 After timing skin tests for 20 minutes, note the reaction on the patient's chart. Pictured is a +3 wheal reaction to ragweed.

(**Epinephrine**) should be administered about an inch above the site by order of the physician if severe reaction occurs.

In performing an intradermal test, a fine-gauge needle (usually 26 G and ⅜ to ⅝ inch long) is used. The antigen is introduced into the dermal layer of the skin in minute dosages of 0.01 to 0.02 cc by sterile technique. The area will appear as a small blister from the fluid raising the skin. The reaction period is up to 30 minutes, and the interpretation of the results is the same as in the scratch tests. Some antigens, such as fungi and bacteria, produce delayed reactions from 24 to 48 hours after administration.

Intradermal tests are sometimes used by physicians to determine medication sensitivity or immunization needs. Follow the procedure for intradermal injections in Chapter 10.

Patch Test The patch test is done to determine the cause of **contact dermatitis**. A patch consisting of a gauze square saturated with the suspected allergy-causing substance is placed on the surface of the skin and secured with nonallergenic tape, Figure 8–8. The arm is the usual site of choice

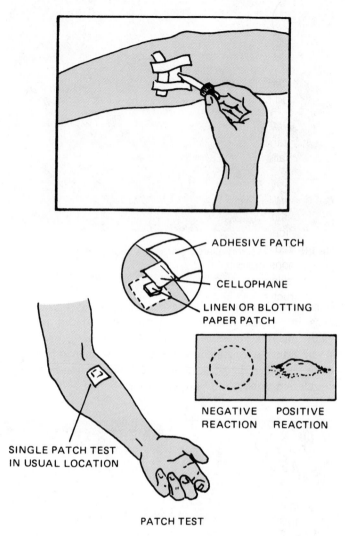

PATCH TEST

FIGURE 8–8 Patch test application. Instruct the patient to keep the patch dry and in place until the results are read by the physician.

Avoid blood vessels.

FIGURE 8–7 The forearm is the most common area for up to 14 sites for intradermal skin tests.

for convenience. The results are read after a 24-hour and then a 48-hour period. A control is thought necessary and should be placed on the arm near the patch if the substance of the patch test is not a known skin irritant. Redness or swelling of the area indicates a reaction, and its interpretation is based on grading similar to that for scratch and intradermal tests.

Nasal Smear A helpful aid for years in the diagnosis of allergies has been a smear done with nasal secretions to observe the **eosinophil** count. If there are many and they are clumped together, there is a strong indication of allergy. This is a simple means of screening for an allergy and is usually the first step in the testing program.

Complete Chapter 8, Unit 1 in the workbook to help you meet the objectives at the beginning of this unit and therefore achieve competency of this subject matter.

Apply a Patch Test

PURPOSE: To determine the causative substance of suspected contact dermatitis.

EQUIPMENT: Commercially prepared paper with suspected substance or gauze saturated with substance, alcohol, cotton balls, gauze squares, nonallergenic tape, pen, patient's chart

TERMINAL PERFORMANCE OBJECTIVE: After practicing with water in lieu of the suspected substance, students will be provided with all necessary supplies, including the suspected substance; using another student as a patient, demonstrate each of the steps required in carrying out the skin patch test, including the 48-hour recheck. The instructor will observe each step.

1. Assemble items on Mayo table next to patient, wash hands, and put on gloves. **CAUTION:** Remember, in order to comply with universal precautions guidelines, gloves must be worn if there is any possibility of coming into contact with blood or any body fluids.

2. Explain procedure while assisting identified patient to comfortable sitting position.

3. Clean test site with alcohol-saturated cotton ball and let air dry.

4. Apply suspected substance to test site and secure with nonallergenic tape. *Note: Usually it is placed near unaffected area in patients with contact dermatitis.* Remove gloves and wash hands.

5. Record date, time, substance, and area tested on patient's chart. Initial.

6. Schedule patient to return in 48 hours.

7. Instruct patient to keep area clean and dry until return appointment.

8. Remove patch; read the results and record. *Note: Discard the patch in biohazardous waste bag.*

PATIENT EDUCATION

During the allergy patient's visit, especially if recently diagnosed as such, giving the patient advice concerning the condition and the prevention of further problems will be well received. The following are a few suggestions for discussion with patients who have allergies.

1. Urge patients to follow the allergy serum desensitizing schedule closely to help build up immunity to the substance to which they are allergic.

2. Advise them to avoid what they are allergic to if at all possible.

3. Instruct patients to read all labels carefully (household products, clothing, consumable products, etc.) to identify possible allergens.

4. Urge them to develop and practice good health habits, such as sensible well-balanced diet, proper rest and exercise.

5. Advise them to take only prescribed medication and to avoid OTC medications unless advised by the physician.

6. If patients have a known severe reaction to a particular substance, remind them to carry their kit with them at all times.

UNIT 2

Cardiology Procedures

OBJECTIVES ....

Upon completion of this unit, you will meet the following terminal performance objectives by verifying knowledge of the facts and principles presented through oral and written communication at a level deemed competent by the instructor or employer and will demonstrate the specific behaviors as identified in the terminal performance objectives of the procedures, observing all aseptic and safety precautions in accordance with health care standards.

1. Explain the reasons for performing an ECG.
2. Describe the electrical conduction system of the heart.
3. Describe the reason for mounting an ECG tracing.
4. Apply limb and chest electrodes properly.
5. Perform a routine 12-lead ECG.
6. Define *artifacts* and list their causes on an ECG.
7. State the purpose of a Holter monitor and explain the procedure to a patient.
8. Demonstrate the procedure for proper hookup of a Holter monitor.
9. State the purpose of defibrillation.

10. Describe cardiac stress testing and discuss the proper placement of the electrodes.
11. State the purpose of cardiac stress testing.
12. Discuss patient education regarding the heart.
13. Spell and define, using the glossary at the back of the text, all the words to know in this unit.

WORDS TO KNOW ....

amplifier	interpretive
arrhythmia	interval
artifacts	limbs
atrial depolarization	mechanical
augmented	multichannel
cardiology	precordial
computerized	Purkinje
countershock	reliable
current	repolarization
defibrillator	sedentary
electrocardiogram	segment
electrocardiograph	simultaneous
electrode	somatic
electrolyte	standardization
galvanometer	stylus
Holter monitor	trace
impulse	treadmill
interference	voltage
intermittent	

FIGURE 8–10   The portable single-channel Burdick Elite II (Courtesy of Siemens Burdick, Inc.)

In family and general practice, internal medicine, and **cardiology**, a procedure frequently used in the diagnosis of heart disease and dysfunction is the **electrocardiogram**. This procedure is painless and safe, and patients should be told so to eliminate apprehension.

You will obtain the electrocardiogram (recording) (EKG/-ECG) by operating the **electrocardiograph** (machine). Figures 8–9 through 8–11 show three widely used models of ECGs.

Through a process of electrical transmission, this machine **traces impulses** of the heart on paper to create a permanent record of its activity.

All muscle movement produces electrical impulses. The ECG is a recording of the electrical impulses of the heart muscle. To accomplish this, **electrodes**, some of which are shown in Figure 8–12 (a, b, and c), and in Figure 8–13, the various

FIGURE 8–9   The portable E200 electrocardiograph (Courtesy of Siemens Burdick, Inc.)

FIGURE 8–11   The multichannel Burdick E350 (Courtesy of Siemens Burdick, Inc.)

FIGURE 8–12 (a) Limb electrode and strap (Courtesy of Siemens Burdick, Inc.)

FIGURE 8–13 (a) Presaturated electrolyte pads (Courtesy of Siemens Burdick, Inc.)

FIGURE 8–12 (b) Blue Max electrodes (Courtesy of Siemens Burdick, Inc.)

FIGURE 8–13 (b) Electrolyte lotion (Courtesy of Siemens Burdick, Inc.)

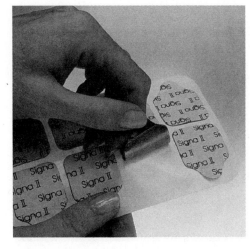

FIGURE 8–12 (c) Signa II disposable sensors (Courtesy of Siemens Burdick, Inc.)

FIGURE 8–13 (c) Electrolyte used with defibrillator. (Courtesy of Siemens Burdick, Inc.)

types of **electrolyte** are pictured for use with metal electrodes, are placed on the patient's **limbs** and chest, which pick up the electrical **current** produced by the contractions of the heart. These minute impulses are transmitted to the electrocardiograph by metal tips (or clips) of the patient cable (wires) attached to the electrodes. Figure 8–14 displays Astro-Clips sometimes referred to as the "universal clip" because they can be used with most types of electrodes. The current enters the electrocardiograph through the wires to reach the **amplifier**, which enlarges the impulses. They are transformed into **mechanical** motion by the **galvanometer**. The **stylus** produces a printed representation on ECG paper. ECG paper is made for the different types of machines, standard, single, and **multichannel**, Figure 8–15. As the heated stylus moves against the tracing paper, the impulses given off by the heart are recorded. The tracing paper should be handled carefully to protect it from being accidentally marked. Dot matrix paper makes tracings easy to read and copy because they are clear and legible.

Some ECGs are mounted onto permanent folders for filing, Figure 8–16. The ECG trimmer is a handy tool for cutting the ECG tracings in preparation for mounting, Figure 8–17.

The ECG is interpreted by the physician, usually the one who ordered the procedure. Some physicians prefer to have a cardiologist interpret the ECG and send the results in the form of a written report with a copy of the tracing. The physician will read the ECG and compare the measurement, rate, rhythm, duration of the electrical waves, **intervals**, and **segments** with known normal ECG readings.

Path of Electrical Impulses ....

The heart is a four-chambered pump that produces minute electrical current by muscular contraction, Figure 8–18. An electrical impulse originates in the modified myocardial tissue of the sinoatrial (SA) node, causing the atria to contract, Figure 8–19. This contraction is the beginning of **atrial depolarization,** which is the first part of the cardiac cycle. The first

impulse as recorded on the graph paper is termed the P wave. The impulse continues through the heart tissue to the atrioventricular (AV) node, to the bundle of His, and spreads to the **Purkinje** fibers. These fibers cause the muscles of the ventricles to contract and produce the QRS complex of waves on the ECG paper. The T wave on the graph paper follows, representing the **repolarization** of the ventricles, or the time of recovery before another contraction.

FIGURE 8–15 (a)   ECG blush-coat paper (Courtesy of Siemens Burdick, Inc.)

FIGURE 8–15 (b)   Single-channel paper (Courtesy of Siemens Burdick, Inc.)

FIGURE 8–15 (c)   Multichannel paper (Courtesy of Siemens Burdick, Inc.)

FIGURE 8–14   Astro clips (Courtesy of Siemens Burdick, Inc.)

FIGURE 8–16 Various types of mounts for ECG tracing paper for patient's permanent record (Courtesy of Siemens Burdick, Inc.)

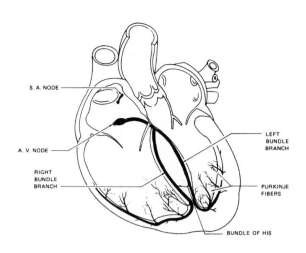

FIGURE 8–18 Anatomy of the heart

FIGURE 8–17 ECG trimmers used to process tracings for mounting (Courtesy of Siemens Burdick, Inc.)

Routine Electrocardiograph Leads ....

The routine ECG consists of 12 leads, or recordings of the electrical activity of the heart from different angles. The first three leads are called standard, or bipolar, leads and are labeled with Roman numerals I, II, and III. These leads are obtained by placing limb electrodes on the fleshy part of the upper outer arms and the inner lower calves, Figure 8–20. Lead I records the electrical voltage difference between the right arm and left arm. Lead II records the difference between the right arm and left leg. Lead III records the voltage difference between the left arm and left leg, Figure 8–21.

The augmented leads are the next three in the standard 12-lead ECG. They are aV_R, aV_L, and aV_F. Augmented voltage right arm (aV_R) is the recording of the heart's voltage difference between the right arm electrode and a central point between the left arm and the left leg. Augmented voltage left

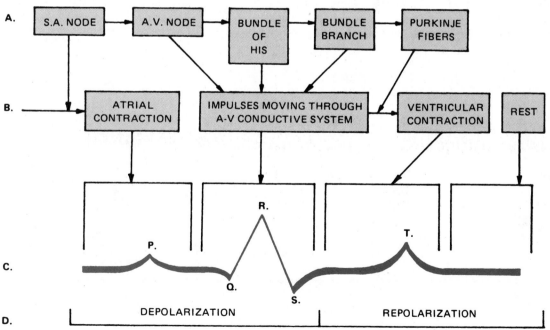

FIGURE 8–19
Diagrammatic representation of cardiac impulses on ECG tracing: (a) Course of electrical impulses. (b) Cardiac muscle reaction to impulses. (c) ECG tracing of impulse waves. (d) Phases of cardiac cycle (Courtesy of Siemens Burdick, Inc.)

arm (aV$_L$) is the recording of the heart's voltage difference between the left arm electrode and a central point between the right arm and the left leg. Augmented voltage left leg or foot (aV$_F$) is the recording of the heart's voltage difference between the left leg electrode and a central point between the right arm and left arm. The term *augmented* means to become larger. Since these three leads are produced by such small impulses, the amplifier of the ECG machine augments their size sufficiently so they can be recorded on the graph paper.

The six standard chest, or **precordial**, leads are obtained by moving the electrode to the anatomical positions shown in Figure 8–22.

The lead selector switch must be set for each different chest lead to obtain the correct code. Some electrocardiographs have an automatic lead marker to identify each of the 12 standard leads as the selector switch is turned. Others require the operator to mark each lead of the ECG. A standard marking code is recommended for use either with the manual or automatic method. Some physicians prefer other codes. It is best to follow the policy where you are employed.

Interference

As with any procedure, a full explanation must be given to the patient to gain cooperation. Providing privacy and adequate draping of the patient during the procedure will ease patient apprehension and avoid chills. The patient must be relaxed for a good tracing to be obtained, as any movement of the patient may cause **interference** on the tracing. Shivering from nervousness or cold can produce muscle voltage artifacts for example. This additional activity is called **somatic** tremor. Arm electrodes should be placed close to the shoulders of the upper outer arms to decrease the possibility of muscle voltage **artifacts**, Figure 8–23, page 441.

LEAD ARRANGEMENT AND CODING

STANDARD LIMB LEADS

LEAD MARKING CODE	LEAD	ELECTRODES CONNECTED	COLOR CODE		
				BODY	INSERT
•	LEAD 1	LA and RA	RL	GREEN	LT. GREEN
	LEAD 2	LL and RA	LL	RED	LT. RED
			RA	WHITE	LT. GRAY
	LEAD 3	LL and LA	LA	BLACK	LT. GRAY

AUGMENTED LIMB LEADS

LEAD MARKING CODE	LEAD	ELECTRODES CONNECTED	COLOR CODE		
				BODY	INSERT
••	aVR	RA and (LA-LL)	RL	GREEN	LT. GREEN
	aVL	LA and (RA-LL)	LL	RED	LT. RED
			RA	WHITE	LT. GRAY
	aVF	LL and (RA-LA)	LA	BLACK	LT. GRAY

CHEST LEADS

LEAD MARKING CODE	LEAD	ELECTRODES CONNECTED	COLOR CODE		
				BODY	INSERT
•••	V$_1$	V$_1$ and (LA-RA-LL)	V$_1$	BROWN	RED
	V$_2$	V$_2$ and (LA-RA-LL)	V$_2$	BROWN	YELLOW
	V$_3$	V$_3$ and (LA-RA-LL)	V$_3$	BROWN	LT. GREEN
••••	V$_4$	V$_4$ and (LA-RA-LL)	V$_4$	BROWN	LT. BLUE
	V$_5$	V$_5$ and (LA-RA-LL)	V$_5$	BROWN	ORANGE
	V$_6$	V$_6$ and (LA-RA-LL)	V$_6$	BROWN	VIOLET

V$_1$ Fourth intercostal space at right margin of sternum
V$_2$ Fourth intercostal space at left margin of sternum
V$_3$ Midway between position 2 and position 4
V$_4$ Fifth intercostal space at junction of left midclavicular line
V$_5$ At horizontal level of position 4 at left anterior axillary line
V$_6$ At horizontal level of position 4 at left midaxillary line

FIGURE 8–20 Proper placement of electrodes for the standard routing 12-lead ECG and lead marking codes (Courtesy of Siemens Burdick, Inc.)

Limb leads

Lead I
Lead II
Lead III
Precordial leads

Augmented limb leads

Lead aV$_R$
Lead aV$_L$
Lead aV$_F$

V$_6$
V$_5$
V$_1$ V$_2$ V$_3$ V$_4$

FIGURE 8–21 Voltage difference between leads (Courtesy of Siemens Burdick, Inc.)

V$_1$	Fourth intercostal space at right margin of sternum.
V$_2$	Fourth intercostal space at left margin of sternum.
V$_4$	Fifth intercostal space at junction of left midclavicular line.
V$_3$	Midway between position V$_2$ and position V$_4$.
V$_5$	At horizontal level of position V$_4$ at left anterior axillary line.
V$_6$	At horizontal level of position V$_4$ at left midaxillary line.

FIGURE 8–22 Recommended positions for precordial ECG leads (Courtesy of Siemens Burdick, Inc.)

Other artifacts which may appear on the ECG, called *AC interference,* are caused by electrical activity. The latest models of electrocardiographs have sensitive filtering devices that eliminate most of the interference, but it is still recommended that a room with a minimum of electrical wiring be used for the ECG procedure. All power cords should be kept away from the patient, and the patient table should be away from the wall to eliminate the possibility of electrical interference from the wall. The patient must be properly connected with the electrodes and properly grounded. Using good technique will also reduce AC interference. The sources of artifacts from different leads is shown in Figure 8–24.

A wandering baseline can be caused by corroded or improperly applied electrodes or by an unequal amount of electrolyte on the electrodes. Another cause is improperly cleaned skin. Oils, creams, and lotions should be removed from the patient's skin with alcohol or the conduction of electrical impulses will be impaired. An interrupted baseline is caused by an electrode becoming separated from the wire or by a broken lead wire. Follow the manufacturer's instructions for repairing the electrocardiograph.

To ensure a good ECG further the operator must use clean electrodes. Metal electrodes should be cleaned with a mild detergent solution after each use and with scouring powder and a cloth as needed. The rubber straps should also be washed with a mild detergent solution after each use. A proper

P R O C E D U R E

Obtain a Standard 12-Lead-Electrocardiogram

PURPOSE: To obtain a graphic representation of the electrical activity of the patient's heart

EQUIPMENT: Electrocardiograph, ECG paper, four metal limb electrodes and straps, [or disposable pregelled adhesive electrodes as appropriate for use with patient cable of ECG machine — lead wires with snaps, clips, or tips (use chest strap if necessary) to attach to electrodes], patient cable, electrolyte (pads, cream, or gel), chest strap, treatment table, pillow, drape sheet, tissues, paper towels, ECG mount, footstool, tongue depressor, patient's chart, pen, disposable razor

TERMINAL PERFORMANCE OBJECTIVE: Provided with an electrocardiograph and all essential equipment and supplies and using other students as patients, demonstrate each of the steps required in obtaining a standard 12-lead ECG reading. The instructor will observe each step. *Note: The specified disrobing may be simulated.*

1. Plug in ECG machine to outlet away from known electrical interference. Plug in patient cable wire to machine. Assemble electrodes and attach to straps. Apply electrolyte pads and set aside. Turn machine on. Wash hands.
2. Ask identified patient to disrobe from waist up and remove clothing from lower legs. Provide privacy and show patient where to put belongings. Explain procedure.
3. Assist patient onto treatment table and cover with drape sheet. Ask patient to lie down. Pull out leg rest. Adjust pillow under patient's head for comfort.

4. Apply chest strap by placing hard plastic end under patient's left side and weighted end against right side of patient's chest. Recover chest with drape sheet.
5. Place arm electrodes (with electrolyte) on fleshy outer area of upper arm with connectors pointing toward shoulders. Straps should be moved one space tighter than relaxed. Leg electrodes (applied with electrolyte) should be placed on fleshy inner area of lower leg near calf, connectors pointing toward upper body. **RATIONALE: Placement of electrodes eliminates friction from examining table and body movement.** If gel or cream is used, use a small amount, the size of a dime, and spread with tongue depressor. *Note: Especially when disposable electrodes are used, it is very important to use a tongue depressor or gauze square to rub sites vigorously to increase circulation and promote better contact of the electrodes.*
6. Connect lead wire tips to appropriate electrodes by screwing tightly into place with all pointing down, or by snapping or clipping electrodes securely in place. *Note: Power cord and patient cable must not be allowed to touch.*
7. Place chest electrode (electrolyte side up) under chest strap and secure until needed, or attach all 6 pregelled disposable adhesive chest electrodes V1 through V6 (shaving dense chest hair as necessary for placement of electrodes), Figure 8–27.
8. Turn lead selector switch to STD and adjust stylus to center of graph paper.

FIGURE 8–27 (a) Chest lead electrode held in place with a chest strap (Courtesy of Siemens Burdick, Inc.)

FIGURE 8–27 (b) Adhesive pregelled disposable electrodes (Courtesy of Siemens Burdick, Inc.)

9. Move record switch to 25-mm/second position and run for a few seconds to adjust centering of stylus. Make standardization mark 2 mm wide and 10 mm high. Then turn machine off, or with computerized electrocardiograph (single and multichannel), press "auto" and run the 12-lead ECG; and proceed to appropriate instructions for steps 13 though 17.

10. Turn lead selector switch to lead I and run 8 to 12 inches of tracing. Proceed in same manner for leads II and III. Run 4 to 6 inches each of leads aVR, aVL, and aVF. *Note: Lead selector switch should be allowed a second or two to pause between leads to allow for adjustment.* **RATIONALE: This permits steadier centering of tracing.** Standardization should appear at beginning of each lead if requested by physician; otherwise at beginning of tracing and whenever sensitivity switch is changed to either reduce or enlarge size of cardiac cycles. *Note: Each lead should be marked accordingly, either manually or automatically by the machine.*

11. Turn lead selector switch either to V of V1 depending on machine you are using. Place chest electrode in proper position and standardize. Run 4 to 6 inches of recording. Turn switch to AMP OFF when changing electrode positions. **RATIONALE: This allows stylus to remain steady.** Move chest electrode to V2 for second chest lead and run 4 to 6 inches of recording, then to V3, and so on. *Note: Turn the run switch to AMP off after each of the chest or precordial leads.*

RATIONALE: Allows the stylus to adjust to next lead by pausing a few seconds so that centering is certain and standardized as instructed. *Note: Mark each lead.*

12. Turn lead selector switch back to STD slowly, one lead at a time, to avoid stripping of dial gears. Run recording out until baseline only appears and turn machine off.

13. Tear off tracing from machine. *Note: Immediately mark it with patient's name, age, day's date, and your initials.* Roll or loosely overlap tracing back and forth, carefully secure with paper clip, and set aside. *Note: This is not required with computerized ECG Figure 8-27 (c).*

14. Remove tips of lead wires from limb electrodes by unscrewing ends. Remove chest electrode and strap and limb straps and electrodes from patient. Clean sites with a warm wet paper towel and dry. Discard used towels in proper receptacle.

15. Assist patient to sitting position and then down from table when ready. Assist patient in dressing if necessary.

16. Change table paper and pillow cover and discard used disposables. Wash hands.

17. Placing tracing in patient's chart, initial ECG order and place in appropriate area for physician to read, or mount tracing on desired form and place in patient's chart for physician to review. *Note: Record any unusual findings or observations on patient's chart.*

A

B

FIGURE 8–23 ECG interference: (a) Somatic tremor, or involuntary muscle movement. (b) AC (alternating current) (Courtesy of Siemens Burdick, Inc.)

amount of electrolyte must be used with each electrode to provide maximum electrical conduction. Individual packets of pretreated disposable pads are available for convenience.

Many offices and clinics still use a standard electrocardiograph with the metal electrodes and limb straps. All of the **computerized**-channel ECG machines require the disposable electrodes and electrolyte pads. These are widely used because of their convenience. Because they are obviously more expensive, you should use them wisely and avoid unnecessary waste.

Standardization ....

The **standardization** of the ECG is necessary to enable a physician to judge deviations from the standard. The usual standardization mark is 2 mm wide and 10 mm high. This

LOCATION OF SOURCE OF ARTIFACTS

Leads 1, 2, and 3 can be helpful in locating the source of interference. Refer to the triangle. Notice that each limb electrode is involved in recording two of the three leads. This means that if an artifact is observed in two leads but not in the third, the artifact is probably caused by a condition at or near the electrode that is common to the two leads. Examples: tremor on leads 1 and 3 and not on lead 2 indicates that the left arm is the probable source since it is common to leads 1 and 3. Similarly, a large amount of AC interference appearing in leads 1 and 2 and a smaller amount in lead 3, would most likely indicate that the AC source is near the right arm. If interference problems cannot be readily solved, contact your Burdick dealer or The Burdick Corporation for the name of your nearest Burdick field representative. They have equipment to help you find the interference source and can offer suggestions to eliminate or reduce the problem.

FIGURE 8–24   Sources of artifacts from leads (Courtesy of Siemens Burdick, Inc.)

mark should begin each lead to provide a **reliable** reading. If the tracing is too large, the sensitivity button should be turned down to ½ to produce a standardization mark 5 mm high and 2 mm wide. If the tracing is too small, the sensitivity button can be turned up to 2, making the impulse 20 mm high and 2 mm wide. You must pay close attention to the tracing as it is being run to make adjustments as needed. Figure 8–25, shows the standardization marking from and electrocardiograph with the sensitivity dial set at ½, 1, and 2 as well as damping of stylus.

The stylus should be centered on the paper. The baseline will allow you to observe the centering and make adjustments as necessary. The temperature of the stylus can be adjusted to control the thickness of the line.

The tracing paper is normally run at a speed of 25 mm/second. If the ECG cycles are too close together, the speed can be changed to 50 mm/second, Figure 8–26. This adjustment should be noted in pen on the tracing.

The physician may order a standard 12-lead ECG with a rhythm strip. This simply means that you should record a long strip, usually 12 inches, or for a period of seconds (generally 30, or however long the physician orders for the rhythm strip) of lead II in addition to the standard tracing. This gives the physician a better look at the rhythm of the heartbeat and how often an irregularity occurs.

Any obvious abnormality should be brought to the physician's attention immediately if the patient is experiencing pain or discomfort at the time it is observed.

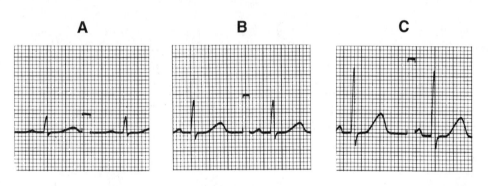

A   **B**   **C**

FIGURE 8–25 (a) Standardization markings with the sensitivity dial set at (A) ½ (to reduce) (B) 1 (normal) (C) 2 (to enlarge) (Courtesy of Siemens Burdick, Inc.)

A   **B**   **C**

CORRECT   OVER-DAMPED   UNDER-DAMPED
Too much stylus pressure   Too little stylus pressure
and/or   and/or
too little stylus heat   Too much stylus heat.

FIGURE 8–25 (b)   (A–C) Damping of the stylus is affected by stylus pressure and temperature. Follow the instructions in the operations manual to adjust the amplitude of the pulse to 10 mm so that the standardization mark looks like the one in Figure 8–25 (a) correct. (Courtesy of Siemens Burdick, Inc.)

FIGURE 8-26 ECG paper: Lead II run at 25 mm/sec (a) and lead II run at 50 mm/sec (b) Lead II is also known as a rhythm strip.

The ECG is an extremely important procedure. Every detail must be performed accurately.

It is extremely important that the patient be relaxed and comfortable during the ECG procedure. Reassure the patient by answering any questions. Explain that the machine does not "put electricity" into the body. Your calm, efficient manner will help the patient relax.

The computerized electrocardiographs have many time-saving features. They have **simultaneous** 12-lead **interpretive** analysis. Dates are not only printed out, but also stored in its memory. The entire ECG tracing is generated in about 1 minute. There is no time involved in mounting. A manual mode provides additional leads, such as the rhythm strip of lead II which may be run from 10 seconds to however long the physician requests. These machines are relatively lightweight and can be easily moved if necessary.

The ECG can detect damage from previous heart attacks, enlargement of the heart muscle, disturbances in the rhythm, and other abnormal conditions. It is usually recommended for patients between the ages of 35 and 40 to establish a base reading. Physicians may then refer to this ECG in the event of later problems. Most often an ECG is performed along with the routine annual physical examination every 5 to 10 years after a baseline normal reading has been establish-

FIGURE 8-27 (c) A representation of an EKG tracing. The newer computerized machine format prints all twelve leads simultaneously. Note: the machine will also diagnose the EKG by means of an on-board computer. (From Lindsey & Rayborn, *The Professional Medical Assistant: Clinical Practice,* Copyright 1993, Delmar Publishers Inc.)

ed. Some physicians prefer to have a tracing more often, even annually, for patients who have a history of hypertension, who are smokers, who are obese, or who have a high serum-cholesterol level. Another factor in heart problems is a **sedentary** life-style, which is usually accompanied by obesity.

tant monitors the patient's blood pressure while he exercises on the treadmill. The purpose of this test is to detect the unknown cause of the patient's heart trouble. Even with ECGs and other diagnostic tests the physician cannot predict future heart attacks.

Stress Tests ....

ECG stress tests are done by some physicians on a routine basis for patients with a high risk of developing heart disease. They are more often done in a limited manner for patients interested in starting a strenuous exercise program or those who continue to have heart pain even after a routine ECG has been read as normal. Figure 8–28, illustrates the BaseLine prep kit and instructions for cardiac stress testing. The stress test ECG is done while a patient is exercising either on a bicycle or **treadmill** under careful supervision. Figure 8–29, page 446 shows a physician reading the computerized printout of a stress test in progress. The medical assis-

Holter Monitoring ....

Patients who have normal routine ECGs but still have **intermittent**, or irregular, chest pain or discomfort are often tested over a period of 24 hours or more with a device known as a **Holter monitor**. This method of recording the electrical activities of a patient's heart for a period of time is also referred to as an ambulatory (walking) or "24-hour ECG." The ECG electrodes are attached to the patient's chest wall. A portable cassette recorder (monitor) is attached to a belt worn around the patient's waist. Figure 8–30, page 446, shows the anatomical placement of electrodes. During the prescribed period, usually 24 hours, the patient's heart action is recorded. The patient is asked to keep a diary of all activities

P R O C E D U R E

Holter Monitoring

PURPOSE: To detect chest pain and cardiac arrhythmias; to evaluate chest pain and cardiac status following pacemaker implantation or after an acute myocardial infarction; and to determine correlation of symptoms and activity.

EQUIPMENT: Disposable razor and shaving cream, alcohol and swabs, pregelled adhesive electrodes, lead wires, appropriate batteries and tape recorder, standard ECG, diary for patient, belt for recorder, nonallergenic adhesive tape to secure electrodes PRN, drape sheet, patient's chart, pen

TERMINAL PERFORMANCE OBJECTIVE: With all equipment and supplies provided, demonstrate the steps of the procedure for hooking up a patient for the Holter monitor. The instructor will observe each step.

1. Explain procedure to identified patient. Ask patient to remove clothing from the waist up (provide a drape sheet). Assist patient to sit at the end of the examination table.
2. Wash hands and assemble equipment and supplies on Mayo table near patient.
3. Test Holter monitor for proper working order and replace with new batteries if indicated. **RATIONALE: Batteries must function for entire test period.**
4. Use shaving cream and razor to remove chest hair if necessary. **RATIONALE: Smooth area provides optimal skin contact.** Rinse and dry electrode sites and clean with alcohol swabs.

5. Rub each site vigorously with gauze square or skin rasp and apply electrodes and lead wires carefully, making sure there is good skin contact. Use extra tape to secure electrodes and wires. Refer to Figures 8–30 and 8–31, page 446.
6. Place the belt around the patient's waist and advise patient in care of recorder and about precautions (refer to text). Assist patient in dressing to help avoid disturbing wires and electrodes. Remind patient not to take a tub bath or shower during 24-hour period.
7. Instruct patient to go about routine daily activities but to be sure to note in diary any symptoms or problems experienced, (time it occurred and how long it lasted). **RATIONALE: Accurate reporting and recording is essential to correct interpretation of ECG findings when compared with activity taking place when symptoms occurred.**
8. Record date and time that monitor began on patient's chart and in the patient's diary, and initial.
9. Give patient diary to take with him or her and arrange a return appointment time.
10. When patient comes in for appointment the next day, assist in disrobing; remove electrodes and wires, clean electrode sites, and place cassette from recorder in computerized ECG for printout of tracing. Place diary and recording of ECG in patient's chart for evaluation by physician and initial.

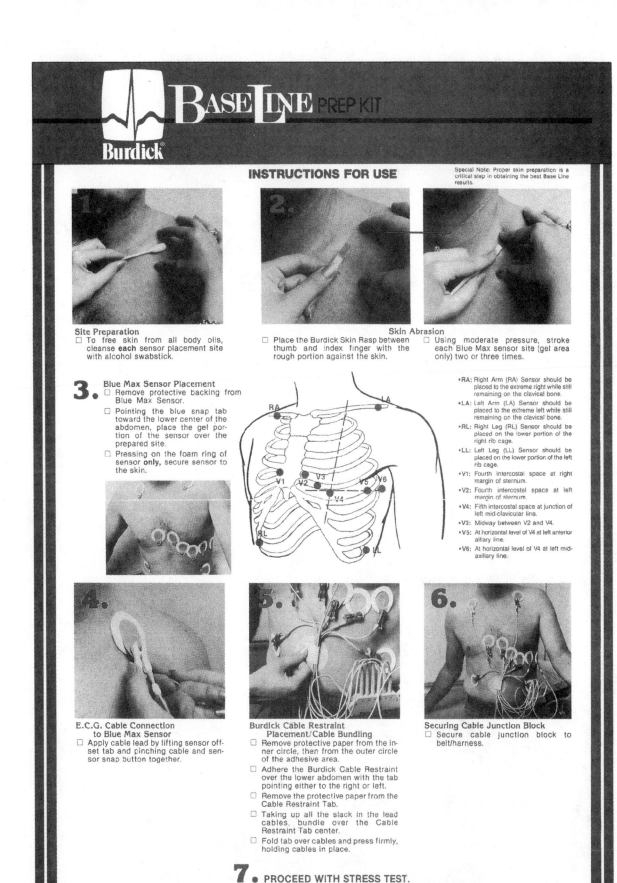

BASE LINE PREP KIT
Burdick®

INSTRUCTIONS FOR USE

Special Note: Proper skin preparation is a critical step in obtaining the best Base Line results.

1. Site Preparation
☐ To free skin from all body oils, cleanse **each** sensor placement site with alcohol swabstick.

2. Skin Abrasion
☐ Place the Burdick Skin Rasp between thumb and index finger with the rough portion against the skin.
☐ Using moderate pressure, stroke each Blue Max sensor site (gel area only) two or three times.

3. Blue Max Sensor Placement
☐ Remove protective backing from Blue Max Sensor.
☐ Pointing the blue snap tab toward the lower center of the abdomen, place the gel portion of the sensor over the prepared site.
☐ Pressing on the foam ring of sensor **only,** secure sensor to the skin.

- RA: Right Arm (RA) Sensor should be placed to the extreme right while still remaining on the clavical bone.
- LA: Left Arm (LA) Sensor should be placed to the extreme left while still remaining on the clavical bone.
- RL: Right Leg (RL) Sensor should be placed on the lower portion of the right rib cage.
- LL: Left Leg (LL) Sensor should be placed on the lower portion of the left rib cage.
- V1: Fourth intercostal space at right margin of sternum.
- V2: Fourth intercostal space at left margin of sternum.
- V4: Fifth intercostal space at junction of left mid-clavicular line.
- V3: Midway between V2 and V4.
- V5: At horizontal level of V4 at left anterior axillary line.
- V6: At horizontal level of V4 at left mid-axillary line.

4. E.C.G. Cable Connection to Blue Max Sensor
☐ Apply cable lead by lifting sensor off-set tab and pinching cable and sensor snap button together.

5. Burdick Cable Restraint Placement/Cable Bundling
☐ Remove protective paper from the inner circle, then from the outer circle of the adhesive area.
☐ Adhere the Burdick Cable Restraint over the lower abdomen with the tab pointing either to the right or left.
☐ Remove the protective paper from the Cable Restraint Tab.
☐ Taking up all the slack in the lead cables, bundle over the Cable Restraint Tab center.
☐ Fold tab over cables and press firmly, holding cables in place.

6. Securing Cable Junction Block
☐ Secure cable junction block to belt/harness.

7. PROCEED WITH STRESS TEST.

FIGURE 8–28 BaseLine prep kit instructions for stress testing (Courtesy of Siemens Burdick, Inc.)

and note any pain or discomfort experienced during this monitoring. Figure 8–31, shows the medical assistant giving instructions to the patient about recording any problems. The patient is instructed to press the "event button" when any cardiac symptoms are experienced. At the end of the test period, the patient returns to have the electrodes and monitor removed. The cassette is then placed in a computerized analyzer for a permanent printout of the results (or sent to a laboratory for interpretation). Evaluation of the 24-hour tracing reveals any cardiac **arrhythmias**, chest pain, and the effectiveness of cardiac medications, and correlates any symptoms with the patient's activity at the time they occurred. You should instruct patients to carry on with all routine daily activities during this test. Advise patients to take a "sponge bath" and not to get into a tub or shower while conducting this monitoring heart test. Ask patients to avoid using electric blankets or being around metal detectors, magnets, and high-voltage areas because these might interfere with the recording. This method of monitoring is also used in evaluating the status of recovering cardiac patients. Another version of this test permits the patient to activate the recording device only when experiencing symptoms. This patient-activated monitor can be worn for several days.

Many medical offices, clinics, and emergency centers are equipped with a **defibrillator**, Figure 8–32. These units are designed to provide **countershock** by a trained individual to convert cardiac arrhythmias into regular sinus rhythm. Part of your routine duties may be to check this, and other equipment and supplies, to ensure that they are in proper working order

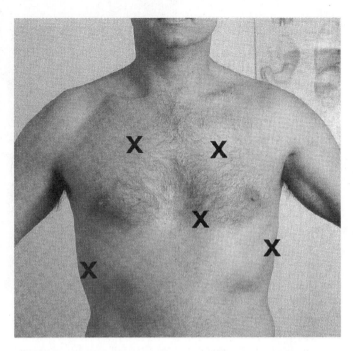

FIGURE 8–30 Anatomical placement of chest electrodes for Holter monitoring

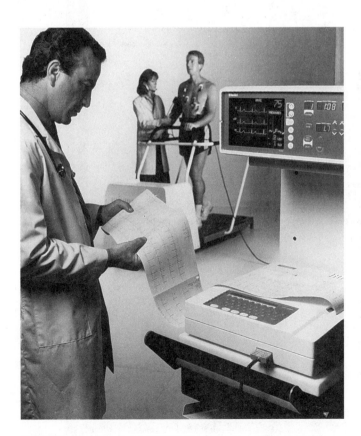

FIGURE 8–29 The Extol 350 ST Stress system (Courtesy of Siemens Burdick, Inc.)

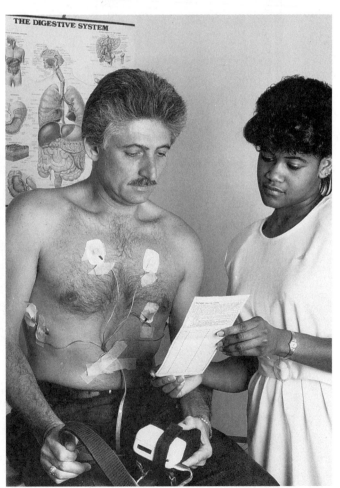

FIGURE 8–31 The medical assistant shows the patient the diary and gives instructions regarding the Holter monitor before securing it around his waist.

FIGURE 8–32 The Medic IV defibrillator and Cor-gel (electrolyte gel) (Courtesy of Siemens Burdick, Inc.)

and that everything is ready in case of a cardiac emergency. Employers offer in-service training periodically to all employees in assisting with emergency procedures. All employees should have current cardiopulmonary resuscitation (CPR) certification.

Complete Chapter 8, Unit 2 in the workbook to help you meet the objectives at the beginning of this unit and therefore achieve competency of this subject matter.

UNIT 3

Diagnostic Procedures

PATIENT EDUCATION

During the time you spend with patients in performing electrocardiographic testing and its instruction, you will have ample opportunity to give patients some of the following suggestions.

1. Remind them to eat a low-fat, low-cholesterol diet, and keep their salt intake at a minimum.
2. Advise them to get proper rest and exercise and keep their weight at an acceptable level.
3. Instruct cardiac patients to take their prescribed medication regularly and to report any problems they may experience to the physician immediately.
4. Remind them to keep their scheduled appointments and make a list of questions for the doctor to review with them at that time.
5. Advise them not to take OTC medications.
6. Urge them not to use tobacco and to avoid alcoholic beverages.

OBJECTIVES

Upon completion of this unit, you will meet the following terminal performance objectives by verifying knowledge of the facts and principles presented through oral and written communication at a level deemed competent by the instructor or employer and will demonstrate the specific behaviors as identified in the terminal performance objectives of the procedures, observing all aseptic and safety precautions in accordance with health care standards.

1. Describe a spirometry test and state the purpose of it.
2. Instruct a patient about the spirometer and demonstrate how to use it.
3. Explain what magnetic resonance imaging (MRI) is.
4. List reasons for contraindication of the MRI.
5. Describe ultrasound and state the purpose of it.
6. Explain the patient preparation for ultrasound procedures.
7. Explain the reason for a Hemoccult sensa test and the procedure to be followed.
8. Perform and interpret a Hemoccult sensa slide test.
9. Discuss patient education concerning the procedures in this unit.
10. Spell and define, using the glossary at the back of this text, all the words to know in this unit.

WORDS TO KNOW

claustrophobia	noninvasive
diaphanography	oscilloscope
echocardiography	sonogram
echoes	sophisticated
electromagnetic	spirometer
implants	thermography
magnetic resonance imaging (MRI)	transducer
	transillumination
maturity	ultrasonic scanning

Vital Capacity Tests

Vital capacity is defined as the greatest volume of air that can be expelled during a complete, slow, unforced expiration following a maximum inspiration. Vital capacity should equal inspiratory capacity plus expiratory reserve. Vital capacity is usually reported in both absolute values and statistically derived values based on the age, sex, and height of the patient. The statistical value is reported as a percentage.

Several devices are used to measure the capacity of the lungs. Many physicians prefer to use the hand-held **spirometer**, which comes with vital capacity charts.

Vital capacity testing is performed to evaluate patients who are suspected to have pulmonary insufficiency. The spirometer is an instrument used to test the capacity of the lungs. Vital capacity testing aids in the diagnosis of and degree of functional or obstructive abnormalities. It also helps the physician find the cause of dyspnea and evaluate the effectiveness of medication and therapy.

When scheduling patients for these tests of vital capacity, it is important to advise them to eat lightly and not to smoke for at least 6 hours before the appointment. Patients should refrain from routine breathing treatment, and medication should not be taken until after the test is completed.

In preparing to perform this diagnostic procedure, instruct the patient regarding the necessary steps and demonstrate the use of the spirometer. Routine measurements, such as, height, weight, and vital signs should be taken and recorded on the patient's chart. Showing the patient how to hold the instrument and what is expected will yield a more accurate test result. Disposable mouthpieces are used to prevent disease transmission. Most spirometers are computerized and have a printout of the results within minutes of administering the test. You should type in the patient's name, age, height, race, sex, account number, and any other information if applicable, before you start the test.

Figure 8–33 pictures the medical assistant coaching a patient through the procedure. A clip is placed on the patient's nose to force the expired air out of the lungs directly into the mouthpiece (make sure patient's mouth is sealed around the mouthpiece) and into the spirometer. Instruct the patient to stand up straight and to take in a slow deep breath. Coach the patient to expel all the air from the lungs quickly until she or he cannot exhale any more, within approximately 15 seconds. Give the patient a couple of practice runs before beginning the official test because it is an awkward procedure for most people. Follow each of the expirations with a few seconds of resting for the patient. Watch for signs of stress, dizziness, coughing, or other problems the patient may have during the test. Generally three to five expirations are tested. The results are analyzed by the computerized instrument, and the diagnostic data are printed for evaluation by the physician. Test results below 80% are usually considered abnormal. This spirometry reading is placed in the patient's chart, along with a notation of any symptoms or problems the patient may have had during

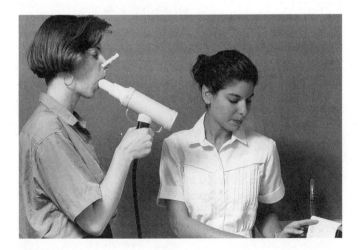

FIGURE 8–33 The medical assistant operates the computerized spirometer while the patient blows exhaled air from the lungs into the disposable mouthpiece.

the test, and your initials. Spirometry tests should not be performed when the patient has been diagnosed with angina, acute coronary insufficiency, or recent myocardial infarction. Allow the patient to sit and relax to wait for consultation with physician. Instruct the patient to resume medication and therapy routine as directed by the physician.

You may be instructed to schedule patients for further pulmonary function studies to be performed by a pulmonary and thoracic specialist. More **sophisticated** equipment may be necessary to evaluate a patient's condition.

Sonographic Studies

Sonograms are records obtained by **ultrasonic scanning**. Ultrasonography is a technique in which internal structures are made visible by recording the reflections, or **echoes**, of ultrasonic sound waves directed into the tissues. These high-frequency sound waves are conducted through the use of a **transducer** (a hand-held instrument resembling a microphone). While the transducer is held against the body area to be tested, it sends sound waves through the skin to various organs. As the echoes are sent back, the transducer picks them up and changes them into electrical energy. This energy is transmitted into an image on a monitor, or printed out on paper in wavy lines. The picture formed on the screen represents a cross section of the organ. Photos of these images are taken for permanent records. The physician interprets these images to aid in the diagnosis and treatment of the patient. **Echocardiography** is a technique used to examine the heart: **echoes** are converted into electrical impulses, which create a picture of the tissues being examined on an **oscilloscope**.

Ultrasonography is useful in examination of the abdominopelvic cavity to locate aneurysms of the aorta and other blood vessel abnormalities. The size and shape of internal organs can also be determined with ultrasound. It can be of value in the identification of cysts and tumors of the eye and in the detection of pelvic masses and obstructions of the urinary tract. In obstetrics and gynecology, where the radiation of X-ray examinations is avoided, ultrasound is useful in the diagnosis of multiple pregnancies and in determining the size, **maturity**, and position of the fetus. Patient preparation may vary but usually the patient is instructed to drink a large amount of water, up to a quart. This will distend the bladder and help to push the uterus into place as well as increase the conduction of the sound waves. Sonograms are not useful in viewing the lungs, for echoes are not created by structures containing air.

When scheduling patients for this type of study, you should give them a few important instructions. They should avoid eating foods that produce gas and drink plenty of fluids (specific amounts are required for certain tests) as mentioned earlier, for example, in determining the size of the fetus, Figure 8–34. Explain to the patient that he or she will be asked to lie down on an examination table and that the procedure lasts approximately 45 minutes to an hour. It is an accurate and painless diagnostic tool. A gel or lotion is used to produce better sound

(1) ABDOMINAL ULTRASOUND: Take nothing by mouth after midnight. No breakfast on the morning of the examination.

(2) PELVIC ULTRASOUND: Drink 24–30 ounces of fluid 1 hour before the examination. Do not urinate after drinking the fluid.

(3) FETAL ULTRASOUND: Drink 24–30 ounces of fluid 1 hour before the examination. Do not urinate after drinking the fluid.

FIGURE 8–34 Preparation for ultrasound

wave conduction and to allow the transducer to glide more easily across the skin.

Besides being a diagnostic procedure, ultrasound is used in the treatment of diseased or injured muscle tissue. Sound waves vibrate into the tissues producing heat, which helps to relieve inflammation and pain. It also increases circulation, which speeds up healing of injured muscle tissues. Another common use of ultrasound is in dentistry. Sound vibrations make it possible for tartar to be painlessly removed from the teeth.

Specific in-service training is necessary before using this instrument because the patient can be burned if precautions are not followed precisely.

Other uses are being discovered as research continues in this field. Other methods besides ultrasound and X rays are used to detect masses and cysts in the body. One such method is called **thermography**. As the name implies, thermography is a measurement of the "heat" patterns given off by the skin. This method is sometimes used to detect masses and cysts in breast tissue. Changes in the images produced are usually suggestive of a problem with breast tissue. A "hot spot" pattern may detect a breast mass. When this is the case, mammography is the next step in determining the diagnosis.

Another method to detect breast tissue masses and cysts is **diaphanography**. A bright light, or **transillumination**, is shown through the breast tissue. This means of examination can show a difference between a solid tumor and a cyst in breast tissue. However, very small cancers are not detected by this method, and again, mammography is the next diagnostic test to determine the patient's condition.

MRI—Magnetic Resonance Imaging ....

A technique to view the structures inside the human body is called **magnetic resonance imaging** (MRI). This method allows physicians to examine a particular area of the body without exposing the patient to X rays or surgery. This **noninvasive** procedure, which may take from 30 to 60 minutes, requires that the patient lie on a padded table that is moved into a tunnel-like structure, Figure 8–35.

There is no advance patient preparation required for this examination. The MRI procedure becomes an *invasive* procedure only when an intravenous contrast medium is adminis-

FIGURE 8–35 Magnetic resonance imaging (MRI system) (Courtesy of GE Medical Systems.)

tered to the patient under certain conditions. This *contrast-enhanced* technique is done during the last series of images of the examination to detect certain pathologies. The patient may resume normal activity following the procedure. There are no known harmful effects to the patient from this imaging technique.

The MRI scans all planes of a body structure, without moving the patient, to produce an image processed by a computer, Figure 8–36. Radio signals are sent from the scanner that are influenced by strong magnetic fields to which the body responds. Figure 8–37 shows an image of the lumbar spine in the sagittal plane. Note the herniated disc and the clarity of the image. The MRI has reduced a great number of diagnostic exploratory surgeries. It is most useful in helping to diagnose brain and nervous system disorders, cardiovascular disease, cancer, and diseases of the visceral organs. MRI is also used to help monitor the effectiveness of treatment. Since the MRI uses a strong **electromagnetic** field, it is extremely important that any metal objects be removed before the procedure is performed. The technician will request that the patient remove all metallic objects including jewelry, hairpins, and nonpermanent dentures before being placed in the tunnel for the MRI. Patients should be inter-

FIGURE 8–36 Magnetic resonance imaging system. The scan is shown on the computer screen on the console in the foreground (Courtesy of GE Medical Systems.)

FIGURE 8–37 MRI scan showing a herniated disc in the lumbar spine (Courtesy of GE Medical Systems.)

viewed thoroughly regarding their health history. Inform the patient that at the facility where the MRI will be performed, they will generally be asked to sign a consent form prior to the procedure. Female patients should refrain from even wearing mascara since tiny metallic flakes may be present in it. During the procedure, these minute pieces of metal may become hot and burn the patient.

During the process the many repetitive noises sound like clanging and banging, humming, and whirring. This is just the sound of the electromagnetic field. There are no sensations of pain and no known side effects. The patient must be still and relax for the test to be properly completed. The technician observes the patient during the entire time. Patients may speak to the technician by the use of a microphone inside the tunnel.

The MRI procedure is contraindicated in patients who have pacemakers, metallic **implants**, are in the first trimester of pregnancy, are severely claustrophobic, or obese. The **claustrophobia** can be handled by counseling or the use of a sedative administered by a physician before the procedure is begun.

 P R O C E D U R E

Perform a Hemoccult Sensa Test

PROCEDURE: To determine the presence of occult blood in the stool.

EQUIPMENT: Hemoccult Sensa slide(s) prepared by patient, developer, timer or timepiece, patient's chart, pen

TERMINAL PERFORMANCE OBJECTIVE: Provided with all necessary equipment and supplies and using samples obtained from own stool, demonstrate each step in the Hemoccult sensa testing procedure.

1. Wash hands and assemble items needed for testing on counter.
2. Open test side of Hemoccult Sensa paper slide.
3. Remove cap from bottle of developer.
4. Place two drops of developer on each of the sections of reagent paper slide: A, B.

5. Immediately begin timing for one minute. At 30 seconds watch closely for any change of color which may be developing. Read at 60 seconds.
6. Compare test with control color and read results.
7. Place one drop of developer between positive and negative control. Read within 10 seconds.
8. Record test results on patient's chart as either positive or negative. *Note: Positive reading means that there is occult blood in the stool. Negative means that no occult blood is present. If first slide is negative and second and third are positive, record as:*

    Hemoccult Sensa slides: 1. neg
                                   2. pos
                                   3. pos

and initial.
9. Discard test in biohazardous bag.

Hemoccult® Sensa® Tests ....

Hemoccult sensa is the trademark for a **guaiac reagent** strip test used to detect the presence of **occult** blood, Figure 8–38. The test may detect bleeding in the digestive tract that is otherwise not detectable. It is a diagnostic aid in the detection of cancer of the colon. Hemoccult sensa tests are usually given routinely to patients aged 40 and over following a complete physical exam or if the patient's symptoms indicate their use. Hemoccult sensa slides are recommended for both men and women who have a personal or family history of colorectal cancer, polyps, or ulcerative colitis. It is also advised as a

PROCEDURE
HEMOCCULT® SLIDES

Identification
Write, or have patient write his name, age, address, phone number, and date specimen was collected in space provided on front of each slide.

Preparation

1. Collect small stool sample on one end of applicator.
2. Apply thin smear inside box A.
3. Reuse applicator to obtain second sample from different part of stool. Apply thin smear inside box B.
4. Close cover. Return slide to physician.
CAUTION: Protect from heat.

Development of Test

1. Open flap in back of slide and apply two drops of Hemoccult® Developer to guaiac paper directly over each smear.
2. Read results within 60 seconds.
ANY TRACE OF BLUE ON OR AT THE EDGE OF THE SMEAR IS POSITIVE FOR OCCULT BLOOD.

Development of Performance Monitors®

1. Apply ONE DROP ONLY of Hemoccult® Developer between the positive and negative Performance Monitors®.
2. Read results within 30 seconds.
A BLUE COLOR WILL APPEAR IN THE POSITIVE PERFORMANCE MONITOR®, AND NO BLUE WILL APPEAR IN THE NEGATIVE PERFORMANCE MONITOR®, IF THE SLIDES AND DEVELOPER ARE FUNCTIONAL.

IMPORTANT NOTE: Follow the procedure exactly as outlined above and on the preceding page. Always develop the test, read the results, interpret them and make a decision as to whether the fecal specimen is positive or negative for occult blood BEFORE you develop the Performance Monitors®. Do not apply Developer to Performance Monitors® before interpreting test results. Any blue originating from the Performance Monitors® should be ignored in the reading of the specimen test results.

READING AND INTERPRETATION OF THE HEMOCCULT® TEST
the world's leading test for fecal occult blood

Negative Smears*

Sample report: negative
No detectable blue on or at the edge of the smears indicates the test is negative for occult blood.
(See **LIMITATIONS OF PROCEDURE**.)

Negative and Positive Smears*

Positive Smears*

Sample report: positive
Any trace of blue on or at the edge of one or more of the smears indicates the test is positive for occult blood.

FIGURE 8–38 Hemoccult® Sensa® test (Courtesy of SmithKline Diagnostics, Inc.)

screening for people who have a personal history of inflammatory bowel disease. Bleeding may be caused by peptic ulcers, hemorrhoids, polyps, and other conditions of the bowel tract. It can also be an early symptom of cancer of the colon. This test was designed to help detect hidden blood in the stool early enough for corrective measures to be taken. Since cancer of the colon is one of the leading cancer killers in the United States, it makes sense to follow the simple, easy-to-use screening test that could help save one's life. Instruct patients how to collect specimens at home and to return them in the double-layered, leak-proof mailing enve-

PATIENT EDUCATION

The patient is advised to avoid eating red meat and foods known to cause digestive tract distress for 48 hours prior to the test and until the specimens are collected. Patients should also avoid processed meats and liver and all raw fruits and vegetables. Instruct patients not to take iron supplements, or vitamin C (in excess of 250 mg a day), aspirin, or other nonsteroidal antiinflammatory medications for a week before and during collection of specimens. Advise patients to eat well-cooked pork, fish, and poultry; cooked fruits and vegetables; and high-fiber foods, such as breads and cereals. Smears of three consecutive bowel movements are requested for testing. The patient should complete the information label on each of the paper Hemoccult sensa slides, filling in the time and date that the samples were obtained. The test kit contains a flushable paper sheet to cover the water in the toilet. (Advise the patient to flush the toilet prior to placing this tissue on top of the water.) This will allow the stool to fall onto the tissue making it easier to obtain the specimens. Remind the patient that the stool samples should be taken from two separate sections with the wooden stick. The sticks should be disposed of in a plastic bag in a waste receptacle, not in the toilet.

lope as soon as possible; otherwise people have a tendency to forget.

The Hemoccult sensa test is easy to complete. It requires proper lighting to compare the color change of the reagent paper to the control. Two drops of developer are applied to each stool smear, A and B, and one drop to the control area. If the test area turns blue compared with the positive control, then the Hemoccult sensa is reported as positive. Further studies will then be ordered by the physician to determine where in the colon the bleeding is occurring.

Intestinal bleeding may be intermittent (not all the time). Giving the patient three slides with smears of two sections of stool for each increases the detection of the presence of blood

in the bowel tract. Ask patients to follow the instructions printed on the envelope carefully.

Complete Chapter 8, Unit 3 in the workbook to help you meet the objectives at the beginning of this unit and therefore achieve competency of this subject matter.

UNIT 4
Diagnostic X-ray Examinations

OBJECTIVES

Upon completion of this unit, you will meet the following terminal performance objectives by verifying knowledge of the facts and principles presented through oral and written communication at a level deemed competent by the instructor or employer and will demonstrate the specific behaviors as identified in the terminal performance objectives of the procedures, observing all aseptic and safety precautions in accordance with health care standards.

1. Instruct patients in the preparation for radiological studies.
2. Discuss the importance of diet in preparation of X rays.
3. Explain why pregnant women should not have X rays.
4. Discuss X rays that require no preparation.
5. Discuss the importance of patient education in scheduling a mammography.
6. Spell and define, using the glossary at the back of the text, all the words to know in this unit.

WORDS TO KNOW

absorb	fluoroscope
artifact	iodine
compression	intravenous pyelogram (IVP)
computerized transaxial tomography (CTAT)	kidneys, ureters, bladder (KUB)
conjunction	lesion
contract	mammography
contrast	planes
cystoscope	radiation
diagnostic	radioactive
distends	radiograph
electromagnetic radiation	radiologist
electron	radiopaque
enema	residual barium
evacuants	retrograde
evacuate	roentgen
flatus	therapeutic
flexible	

FIGURE 8–39 Chest X ray. AP view of the chest.

Radiological Studies ....

Radiological studies are made by the use of X rays (**roentgen rays**), which are high-energy **electromagnetic radiation** produced by the collision of a beam of **electrons** with a metal target in an X-ray tube. An X-ray photograph is taken of the requested part of the patient's body, and a permanent film picture is made. Patients must follow preparation instructions for certain radiological studies. Bone studies do not require preparation and are performed to aid in the diagnosis of tumors, fractures, and other disorders and diseases. Chest X rays do not normally need advanced preparation, Figure 8–39. **Therapeutic** X rays are used in the treatment of cancer. Following are the most commonly ordered radiological studies for which you may be responsible in scheduling and preparing patients.

Gallbladder—Cholecystogram

The gallbladder stores bile that is produced in the liver to break down fat in the digestive process. When the gallbladder malfunctions, the patient experiences abdominal discomfort (nausea) and pain. The cholecystogram enables the physician to diagnose the cause of the patient's distress.

In preparation for this study of the gallbladder, the patient must follow a prescribed diet and take prescribed medication (a **contrast** medium) to make the gallbladder visible on the X-ray film, Figure 8–40. Generally the day before the exam, the patient is advised to avoid drinking alcoholic and carbonated beverages because these drinks may produce **flatus** (gas). Unless otherwise specified by the physician, you should remind patients to take their regularly prescribed medication(s).

Upper GI Series—Barium Swallow

For this study the patient must drink the chalky-tasting contrast medium, barium, during the examination while the **radiologist** observes the flow of the substance directly by means of a **fluoroscope**. The contrast medium is a mixture of barium and water, usually flavored to increase palatability. Radiologic films are taken for a permanent record of the upper digestive tract. During the study the patient is positioned so that different angles of the digestive organs can be seen.

The physician observes the functioning of the esophagus, stomach, duodenum, and small intestine as the barium passes. Such disorders or diseases as hiatal hernias, peptic or duodenal ulcers, and tumors may be diagnosed as a result of the upper GI series.

Lower GI Series—Barium Enema

In this examination, barium sulfate is the contrast medium. It is introduced into the colon by an enema tube, and the radiologist observes the flow into the lower bowel. Many physicians order a barium enema with air-contrast. This procedure **distends** the barium-filled colon with air to make the structures more visible by fluoroscopy. Permanent radiographs are taken periodically during the procedure. This study is helpful in diagnosing diseases of the colon, tumors, and **lesions**.

The barium enema procedure generally takes several minutes and produces discomfort and some pain. Patients should be told to breathe through the mouth slowly and deeply to help relax the abdominal muscles. A strong urge to defecate is normal, and patients often cannot resist the urge. After several films have been taken the patient generally is allowed to use the toilet. Then the study of the lower bowel is completed.

Patients should be encouraged to drink plenty of liquids for

---

1. Two days prior to exam, starting at 6 P.M. take 1 tablet of Oragrafin every 5 minutes until 6 tablets have been taken.
2. On day prior to exam, repeat step 1.
3. Day prior to exam, take 4 oz of Neoloid or 3 Dulcolax 5 mg tablets from 2–4 P.M.
4. Evening before exam, eat a fatfree meal—dry toast, tea, fruit, jello.
5. Nothing by mouth after midnight.
6. No breakfast.

FIGURE 8–40   Preparation for gallbladder series

PATIENT EDUCATION

Undergoing radiological studies can be frightening to some patients. Assure the patient that the studies are done in a controlled environment. Always provide clear and concise oral *and* written instructions for examinations that require advance preparation. Be sure that the patient understands the necessary preparations. Answer all questions. Emphasize the importance of being on time for the radiological appointment to avoid unnecessary delays, since some examinations are very long.

If the patient is not familiar with the facility where the X-ray studies are scheduled, give specific instructions (and a map) of how to get there and where to park. Patients appreciate this courtesy. Often, this information is printed on the appointment or information sheet the facility provides to medical offices and clinics for referral appointments.

It is of vital importance that you advise all female patients who are of childbearing age to inform you if they are pregnant, or could possibly be, if X rays are considered as a part of the assessment of their condition. X rays are contraindicated in pregnant females, especially in the first trimester because radiation is damaging to the fetus. During triage you should always ask females for the date of the last menstrual period (LMP) for documentation in their chart. This will help in preventing any misunderstanding concerning a possible pregnancy. Other **diagnostic** exams can be performed that are safe for the fetus during this time as necessary.

ESOGAGUS, UPPER GI SERIES

1. Nothing by mouth after midnight.
2. No breakfast.

IF SMALL BOWEL

1. Day prior to exam—Take 4 oz. of Neoloid or 3 Dulcolax 5 mg tablets from 2–4 P.M.
2. Nothing by mouth after midnight.
3. No breakfast.

FIGURE 8–41 Preparation for upper GI series

the next few days to help evacuate the **residual barium** sulfate in the lower colon.

Intravenous Pyelogram In studies of the genitourinary system, the **intravenous pyelogram (IVP)** requires that the patient prepare with laxatives, enemas, and fasting, Figure 8–43. The IVP consists of an intravenous injection of **iodine**, the contrast medium, to define the structures of the urinary system. A **retrograde** pyelogram is a study of the urinary tract

PATIENT EDUCATION

Most patients with gallbladder trouble already know they should avoid fatty foods. The usual preparation for a cholecystogram is a nonfatty evening meal the night before the scheduled appointment. Foods which are permitted are fresh fruits and vegetables, lean meat (broiled), toast, bread, jelly, and coffee or tea. Fatty foods will cause the gallbladder to contract and empty the contrast medium, which the patient usually takes following the evening meal.

The medication is usually in pill form, with directions to swallow 1 tablet every 5 minutes with a minimum amount of water until all are consumed. Repeating this a second night is necessary to define the gallbladder sufficiently. This takes approximately half an hour. Spreading the consumption of the contrast medium out over this period of time allows the gallbladder to **absorb** the substance. The patient is instructed to eat or drink nothing after midnight the night before the cholecystogram is performed. In addition to these preparations, many physicians request an **enema** or laxative or both to help remove fecal material and gas which could cause shadows, blockages, or other **artifacts**.

Often when the series of **radiographs** is completed, patients are told to return after a meal containing fats to observe radiographs that show how the gallbladder functions during digestion of fats.

PATIENT EDUCATION

Preparation requires that the patient eat a light evening meal and then only clear liquids, Figure 8–41. The patient should have nothing to eat or drink from midnight until after the X ray series the next day. Prescribed medications are allowed, taken with water. Dairy products, carbonated beverages, and alcohol are not permitted. The digestive tract should be clear of all foods to avoid blockage of or shadows on the anatomical structures to be observed.

Constipation may result from the barium and patients should be advised to drink plenty of clear liquids to help relieve it. You should also mention that their stool may appear lighter than usual from the white barium and that this should not be a cause for concern. Laxatives are ordered only by the physician. Patients should phone the medical office if any problem arises.

done by inserting a sterile catheter into the urinary meatus, through the bladder, and up into the ureters. The **radiopaque** contrast medium then flows upward into the kidneys. This diagnostic test is usually done in **conjunction** with **cystoscopy**. Patients should be tested prior to the examination to determine the possibility of an allergic reaction to the iodine medium. A voiding cystogram may be ordered in conjunction with an IVP. In this case the contrast medium is injected into the bladder by catheter, and no special patient preparation is needed.

KUB The **kidneys, ureters, bladder (KUB)** test is an X ray of the patient's abdomen, sometimes termed "flat plate of abdomen," Figure 8–44. This requires no patient preparation and is used in the diagnosis of urinary system diseases and disorders. It may also be useful in determining the position of

PATIENT EDUCATION

Patients must prepare for this study by precisely following instructions, usually beginning the day before the appointment. The instructions generally include laxatives and enemas to clear the bowel of fecal matter and gas. The patient should eat lightly, avoid dairy products, and drink plenty of clear liquids to encourage more comfortable **evacuation**. Patients should have nothing to eat or drink past midnight the night before the X ray, Figure 8–42. On the day of the appointment, the patient should have an enema 2 hours before the scheduled appointment.

BARIUM ENEMA OR COLON EXAMINATION.

a. Beginning the morning of the day before the examination, change to an all liquid diet*, as outlined below. Do not take any more solid food until after the examinations.

b. At 12:30 PM., or 1/2 hour after lunch on the day before the examination, drink entire contents of a bottle of Citrate of Magnesia (10 oz.).

c. At 1:00 PM., drink one glass of fluid.

d. At 3:00 PM., take 2 Dulcolax tablets with a large glass of water.

e. At 4:00 PM., drink one large glass of fluid.

f. At 5:00 PM., or as close as possible, liquid dinner.

g. At 6:00 PM., drink one large glass of fluid.

h. Bedtime—drink one large glass of fluid.

i. You may have one cup of coffee, tea, or water on the morning of the examination.

*ALL LIQUID DIET
You may have any of the following: Coffee, tea, carbonated beverages, clear gelatin desserts, strained fruit juice, bouillon, clear broths, tomato juice. Do not drink milk of any kind.

Please call office if you have any questions regarding above instructions.

FIGURE 8–42 Preparation for barium enema

FIGURE 8–44 Radiological X ray of kidneys, ureters, and bladder (KUB); no patient preparation is necessary.

an intrauterine device (IUD) or in locating foreign bodies in the digestive tract. In some cases surgery is indicated to remove an object which may block the normal digestive flow, but many small objects are easily passed with solid foods, especially in young children, whose internal structures are more **flexible**. The physician ultimately makes this decision in patient care.

Mammography Mammography aids in the diagnosis of breast masses, some of which may be as small as 1 cm in size or less. Women who practice self-examinations regularly each

month and find lumps in breast tissue early have a much better cure rate if a malignancy is found. Breast self-examination (see Chapter 6, Unit 1) and regular examinations by the physician should be strongly reinforced to female patients in addition to their scheduled mammography. The American Cancer Society recommends a baseline mammography between the ages of 35 to 39 for all women; between ages 40 and 49 every 1 to 2 years; and, over age 50 every year. At any time a lump is found, patients should be advised to see the physician at once for examination. This procedure requires the patient to move into various positions so that different angles

---

ALL LIQUID DIET

You may have any of the following: coffee, tea, carbonated beverages, sherbet, clear gelatin desserts, strained fruit juice, bouillon, clear broths, tomato juice. Do not drink milk of any kind.

1. Day prior to exam—4 oz. of Neoloid or 3 Dulcolax 5 mg tablets from 2–4 P.M.

2. Liquids only after midnight.

FIGURE 8–43 Preparation for intravenous pyelogram (IVP)

To ensure the best results for your mammogram, please follow these procedures prior to your appointment:

a. BE SURE TO NOTIFY OUR PERSONNEL IF YOU ARE PREGNANT.

b. Please shower or bathe as close to your appointment time as possible.

c. Do not use deodorants, powders, perfumes, and etc. on the breast or underarm areas.

d. You will only have to undress to the waist, so wear an easily removable top such as a blouse.

FIGURE 8–45 Instructions for mammography

The medical assistant should schedule the mammography during the first week following the patient's menstrual cycle, since the breasts must be compressed firmly during the procedure to obtain a satisfactory image for diagnostic purposes, Figure 8–46. During this time the patient would experience less discomfort. Since this procedure is often very uncomfortable and even sometimes painful, there are other suggestions that may be helpful in reducing the discomfort. For instance, it is advisable to tell patients to omit caffeine from their diets for 7 to 10 days prior to this examination to reduce the possible effects of swelling and soreness that caffeine often produces. **Compression** of the breasts during this procedure allows less radiation to be used. It also produces a much clearer picture of the breast tissue. Following this exam, some areas of the breast(s) may sometimes become temporarily discolored. However, it does not damage the breast tissue and should not be alarming. At the advice of the physician, a mild analgesic may be taken to relieve any discomfort or aching that may be experienced by the patient.

Explaining these details to the patient and requesting her cooperation with the radiology technician during this procedure will be most helpful in obtaining a quality mammogram for diagnostic study by the physician. It is also important to let the patient know when the results will be available so she will not have to endure unnecessary worry. Remind patients again of the importance of breast self-examinations on a continuing basis. Mammography is not a substitute for this important means of detection.

FIGURE 8–46 Breasts are compressed by the plates during mammography.

of the breast tissue may be X rayed. The X-ray pictures are called mammograms. Patients are usually advised to wear slacks or a skirt for ease in preparation for the procedure, Figure 8–45, since it is necessary to undress from the waist up for the examination. The only preparation required is that the patient wash the chest and underarms and rinse and dry thoroughly. No deodorants or powders are to be used the day of the mammography because the film on the skin from these substances could interfere with the radiograph. As a courtesy to patients, you should remind them to take soap, deodorant, and a fresh blouse with them.

Body Scans Rapid scanning of single-tissue **planes** is performed by a process that generates images of the tissue in "slices" about 1 cm thick. This method of radiology is called the CAT (computerized axial tomography) scan, or **computerized transaxial tomography (CTAT)**. These procedures can be performed in seconds and aid in the diagnosis of diseases and disorders of the breast or other internal organs.

The branch of medicine that uses radionuclides in the diagnosis and treatment of disease is nuclear medicine. Almost any organ of the body may be viewed and recorded by having the patient ingest, or be injected with, radioactive material.

Uptake studies refer to procedures in which patients ingest a **radioactive** substance under careful supervision and return within 24 hours to have the amount of radioactive substance in a particular organ measured. The radioactive thyroid uptake determines the function of the thyroid gland, for example. Tumors of the thyroid may also be determined by this method. In female patients pregnancy should be determined prior to the radioactive thyroid uptake, for it is seriously damaging to the fetus, especially within the first trimester of pregnancy.

Complete Chapter 8, Unit 4 in the workbook to help you meet the objectives at the beginning of this unit and therefore achieve competency of this subject matter.

Mr. Right . . .

documents procedures and their results following their completion and initials. He completes follow-up reports of results in an efficient manner and shows respect for the confidentiality of patient information. He always remembers to advise patients of risks or precautions concerning procedures including X ray precautions regarding pregnancy.

Employment advancement: Excellent

Ms. Wrong . . .

documents procedures and results when she remembers to do it, just as she often forgets to send out follow-up reports. She is careless about leaving patient records out for anyone to see, which violates patients' confidentiality and privacy. She occasionally remembers to advise patients about risks and precautions concerning procedures before they are performed. She usually remembers to tell pregnant women about the dangers of X rays to the fetus.

Employment outlook: Poor

REFERENCES

Diagnostic Tests, Nurse's Ready Reference, Springhouse PA: Springhouse Corporation, 1990.

Mosby's Medical, Nursing, and Allied Health Dictionary, 3d ed. St. Louis: C.V. Mosby, 1990.

C H A P T E R   9
Surgical Procedures

As a clinical medical assistant, you may assist with a variety of sterile procedures. Maintaining medical asepsis is vital to preventing the transmission of diseases *before, during,* and *following* any of the invasive surgical procedures performed in the medical office or clinic. In compliance with universal precautions, proper barriers, such as latex gloves, gown, face mask, and shield, must be worn to protect the health care staff from possible contamination while performing these procedures. All disposable waste must be placed in a plastic biohazardous bag or sharps container and discarded properly to prevent disease transmission.

Setup for various procedures may vary slightly according to the physician's preference. However, sterile technique will always remain the same for any invasive procedure. The basic information for assisting both the physician and patient is covered in this chapter.

OBJECTIVES ....

Upon completion of this chapter, you will meet the following terminal performance objectives by verifying knowledge of the facts and principles presented through oral and written communication at a level deemed competent by the instructor or employer and will demonstrate the specific behaviors as identified in the terminal performance objectives of the procedures, observing all aseptic and safety precautions in accordance with health care standards.

1. Explain scheduling, preop and postop instructions of patients for minor office surgery.
2. Discuss the importance of obtaining the consent form for the surgical procedure.

3. Demonstrate the skin preparation procedure for the surgical site.
4. Prepare the treatment room and minor surgical tray setup.
5. Discuss various procedures that require sterile technique.
6. Demonstrate the procedure for assisting with minor surgery.
7. Demonstrate how to put on and remove sterile gloves properly.
8. Discuss proper care of surgical instruments.
9. Demonstrate the proper way to remove sutures.
10. Discuss important information that should be recorded on the patient's chart.
11. Spell and define, using the glossary at the back of the text, all the words to know in this chapter.

WORDS TO KNOW ....

anesthesia

anesthesiologist

anesthetic

biopsy

coagulation

contaminate

cryosurgery

electrocautery

electrocoagulation

fenestrated

hemophilia

histology

hypoallergenic

incision and drainage
   (I & D)

polyp

postoperative (postop)

preoperative (preop)

suture

taut

wart

The medical assistant is usually responsible for **scheduling** minor office surgery. Surgery may include removal of a sebaceous cyst, **wart,** or foreign object; circumcision; vasectomy; skin biopsy; **incision and drainage (I & D);** out-patient dilation and curretage; (D & C) or insertion of an IUD.

You must be mindful of the amount of time required for each type of surgical procedure you schedule. Advise patients as you make their appointments how long they should plan to be at the doctor's office on the day of their minor surgery. Depending on the type of procedure being performed, patients may need to make arrangements for someone to bring them for the appointment and take them home. Occasionally patients do not feel well enough following a surgical procedure to drive or travel alone and should have some assistance for at least a few hours. Because it is unpredictable how an individual patient may react to even a minor surgical procedure, it is best to advise *all* patients to arrange for assistance to ensure their safety and well-being. Ask patients about any allergies or other former reactions. You should also advise them about possibly taking appropriate time off from work or arranging for home care, depending on the procedure scheduled.

You must first be sure that the patient understands the procedure and the instructions regarding **preoperative (preop)** and **postoperative (postop)** care. Most medical facilities have printed instructions for patients. This eliminates any misunderstandings, and patients feel more at ease knowing they can refer to it. Patients should be advised of the **appropriate** clothing to be worn on the day of the surgery. Loose-fitting clothing, or clothing easy to put on and take off, and not their "Sunday best" should be suggested as appropriate for the anatomical area of surgery. It is a good practice to phone the patient the day prior to the appointment, not only to reassure the patient and answer any questions but to confirm the physician's schedule.

The day before the scheduled surgery, you should get all the necessary surgical instruments and supplies ready.

All surgical instruments must be properly labeled and autoclaved. Most of the instruments will already have been sterilized, as is usual after each use. The basic setup for most minor

surgical procedures includes the following sterile items: scalpel handle and blades, hemostats (straight or curved), needles holder, needles and **suture** material (catgut synthetic or silk), suture scissors, thumb forceps, probe, gauze squares, sponges, vial of anesthetic medication, syringes, needles, towels, and bandages. Some of these supplies may be wrapped and sterilized together. Items that need to be added are dropped onto the sterile field after the wrap has been carefully unfolded on the Mayo table by sterile technique. Autoclaved items remain sterile if they have been properly processed and have been protected from moisture for 30 days. To ensure sterility, packages should be checked before use for any tears or other signs of tampering.

Most items used today are disposable and come already sterile in the manufacturer's packaging. To ensure sterility, you must make sure that the package has not been torn or punctured. The sterilization of the product is guaranteed only to a certain date marked on the package, and this date must be checked.

A variety of minor **invasive** surgical procedures are performed in the medical office, and each requires several instruments. Figure 9–1 shows an example of a surgical instrument tray setup and supplies commonly used in minor office procedures. You must become familiar with the physician's preference for particular items and the way they are to be arranged for use. Until you are certain about the details of a particular procedure, you may want to keep a notebook handy for reference.

When the patient arrives for the surgery the consent form, an example of which is shown in Figure 9–2, must first be explained to the patient and completed. You should allow the

PATIENT EDUCATION

Preop

In scheduling, advise the patient of:
1. Approximate length of time for the procedure
2. Appropriate clothing to wear at the appointment
3. Amount of time to fast as instructed by the physician
4. Arranging for someone to accompany him or her
5. Anticipated time to take off work or arranging for home care.

When patient arrives for the appointment
1. Provide written instructions regarding the surgical procedure and follow-up care
2. Explain the surgical consent form and obtain the patient's signature
3. Answer any questions concerning the procedure
4. Ascertain if the patient has any allergies to any medications, including topical preparations, and adhesive tapes.

FIGURE 9–1 An example of a surgical setup tray

FIGURE 9–3 Hyfrecator electrocautery unit (Courtesy of Birtcher, Los Angeles CA)

patient time to ask any questions about the procedure and answer them adequately. The patient's signature must be on the consent form and filed in the chart. If the patient is a minor, or incompetent, the person **authorized** to give consent must sign for the patient following an explanation of the procedure and answering any questions. The patient's vital signs should be taken, and any complaints or problems should be recorded on the patient's chart. The patient should then empty the bladder before being positioned and draped for the procedure.

Most procedures are performed under local **anesthesia.** A physician always administers the **anesthetic.** Large group practices may have a qualified **anesthesiologist** on staff or a nurse-anesthetist. A careful medical history must be taken from the patient to determine possible allergic reactions. This helps avoid complications during and after the procedure.

If the patient discloses a family history of **hemophilia,** a serious blood-clotting disease, or is himself a hemophiliac you should bring it to the physician's attention immediately. This information should be marked in red ink on the patient's chart. Hemophilia is a sex-linked hereditary trait that occurs mostly in males. Patients who have this diagnosis must have surgery of any type *only* at a completely equipped, well-staffed medical–surgical hospital for their safety and well-being.

In procedures requiring that a **biopsy** be taken for analysis, careful labeling and handling of the specimen is vital. The laboratory provides a formalin solution container for preservation of the tissue specimen. This container is sterile, and the specimen must be placed directly in the solution with sterile transfer forceps. A completed lab request form must accompany the specimen for analysis.

In certain surgical procedures, such as in removing warts or **polyps,** an **electrocautery** device may be used. Often this is used to control bleeding of the surgical site by **electrocoagulation.** Controlled high-frequency current is applied by the physician to the surgical area to **coagulate** the blood to close the incision. If the reusable tips are preferred by the physician for surgical procedures, they must be autoclaved to prevent possible cross-contamination. Disposable tips are available. Figure 9–3 illustrates a Hyfrecator.

Another method used in removing skin tags, warts, and other skin disorders and growths, is by **cryosurgery.** Often certain gynecological treatments and surgical procedures are performed with this instrument. This process uses subfreezing temperature to destroy or remove tissue. Generally the substances used are solid carbon dioxide or liquid nitrogen. It is sometimes referred to as cold cautery.

CONSENT TO OPERATE

Date _____ Time _____ A.M. P.M.

1. I authorize the performance upon _____
   of the following operation _____
   to be performed under the direction of Dr. _____
2. The following have been explained to me by Dr. _____
   A. The nature of the operation _____

   B. The purpose of the operation _____

   C. The possible alternative methods of treatment _____

   D. The possible consequences of the operation _____

   E. The risks involved _____

   F. The possibility of complications _____

3. I have been advised of the serious nature of the operation and have been advised that if I desire a further and more detailed explanation of any of the foregoing or further information about the possible risks or complications of the above listed operation it will be given to me.
4. I do not request a further and more detailed listing and explanation of any of the items listed in paragraph 2.

   Signed _____
   (Patient or person authorized
   to consent for patient)

Witness _____

FIGURE 9–2 Surgery consent form

PROCEDURE

Prepare Skin for Minor Surgery

PURPOSE: To remove hair from surgery site to prevent infection and to clean the skin and apply antiseptic solution to reduce microbial growth.

EQUIPMENT: Small basin for soap solution, 4 x 4 inch gauze squares (sponges), safety razor and blades, scissors, antiseptic soap solution, emesis basin for disposables, gooseneck lamp, sterile drape sheet or towels (or **fenestrated** drape sheet), sterile latex gloves, Mayo table, sterile forceps and container, sterile water for irrigation, Figure 9–4.

FIGURE 9–4 Example of skin prep tray

TERMINAL PERFORMANCE OBJECTIVE: Provided with all necessary equipment and supplies and other students to act as patients, demonstrate each of the steps required in the skin prep procedure. *Note: In the instructional setting, preparing the forearm may be sufficient; moreover, the shaving process may be demonstrated by using a razor with no blade.*

1. Wash and glove hands, and assemble all needed items. **CAUTION:** Remember, in order to comply with universal precautions guidelines, gloves and other protective barriers must be worn if there is any possibility of coming into contact with blood, or any body fluids.

2. Identify patient. **RATIONALE: Speaking to the patient by name and checking chart ensures that you are performing the procedure on the correct patient.**

3. Explain procedure to patient. Ask patient to remove necessary clothing. Explain where patient should put belongings. Assist patient if necessary.

4. Assist patient into proper position on treatment table and drape with sheet or light bath blanket as directed by physician.

5. Position Mayo table over patient near surgical site. Adjust gooseneck lamp to light area to be shaved.

6. Place gauze squares in soapy solution and use one at a time to soap area to be shaved. After use discard each into emesis basin, Figure 9–5 (a, b).

7. When skin prep site is covered by scalp hair, beard, or pubic hair, use scissors to clip hair in preparation for shaving. *Note: Use caution when clipping hair with scissors and in shaving with razor to avoid both self-injury and harm to the patient.* If reusable razor is used, very carefully place new razor blade in razor to prevent self-injury. Shave hair by placing razor against skin at about a 30-degree angle, Figure 9–6. Hold skin **taut** for easier shaving. Shave in direction hair grows. Wipe soap and hair from razor with tissue. Swish razor through soapy water, shake excess water from it, and shave next area.

8. Remove all soap and hair from area by wetting sterile gauze square with sterile water. Dry area with sterile gauze squares.

FIGURE 9–5(a) Remove the transfer forceps from the container without touching the sides.

9. Apply antiseptic solution to surgery site with gauze square held by transfer forceps. *Note: Begin application in center of site and move outward in a circular motion,* see Figure 9–5 (b). **RATIONALE: This pattern of continuous movement ensures total coverage without contamination from untreated areas.**

10. Cover the prepared area with sterile drape sheet or towel until physician is ready to begin. *Note: Instruct patient not to touch sterile field (either the sterile field of surgical site or instrument tray setup).*

11. Discard disposable items and return other items to proper storage area. Remove gloves and wash hands.

12. Attend to patient's comfort. Patients are usually apprehensive about even most minor surgical procedures. Reassurance at this time is most important.

FIGURE 9–5(b) Apply all solutions in this pattern to the skin. Prepping the skin with antiseptic solution should begin at the center of the incision site and proceed outward in one continuous circular motion as shown.

FIGURE 9–6 Angle for shaving a surgery site

Skin Preparation

Preparation of the area of skin that will be affected by the surgical procedure is called skin prep. Because body hair encourages **microbial** accumulation, it is usually shaved. The skin cannot be completely sterilized or the cells would be destroyed, but an **antiseptic** is used to reduce microbial growth.

Many physicians still prefer the use of a stainless steel razor with disposable blades, but there are also disposable skin-prep kits that contain all the necessary items for this procedure. If a reusable razor is preferred for hair removal in preparation for the surgery site, it must be autoclaved to prevent possible disease transmission. A new blade must be used for each patient. To protect yourself and the patient from possible disease transmission, you should wear latex gloves during the skin prep procedure. Practice in the procedure for this skill is necessary to become proficient.

You must be extremely careful to avoid nicking the patient's skin. Microorganisms can enter the body through a break in the skin, and an infection could develop from carelessness. If this should happen, the physician must be notified immediately.

When assisting with accupuncture procedures, preparation of the skin is simply to use an antiseptic, such as alcohol (if the skin is obviously dirty, you should wash the area with soap and water and dry before proceeding). Acupuncture is used for treating a variety of conditions. The most common use is pain control.

Sterile Gloves

If the physician wishes you to assist directly with the surgical procedure, sterile gloves must be worn. Dressing changes should also be performed wearing sterile gloves to protect both yourself and the patient. In addition, you may assist with the repair of lacerations resulting from injury, needle biopsies, and the insertion of IUDs. All of these procedures require sterile technique.

A thorough surgical scrub should be performed for 6 minutes. If it has been within 48 hours since the last surgical scrub was performed, 3 minutes is sufficient.

Assisting with Procedures

Assisting with surgical procedures requires basic knowledge in several areas. The medical assistant should learn anatomy and physiology, medical terminology, and the names and uses of the instruments used in minor office procedures. You should also develop skills in human relations. With experience, you will become more sensitive and aware of the patient's needs. The more knowledge you acquire about procedures and the items necessary to perform them, the more perceptive you will be in assisting the physician.

The following procedures in assisting with minor surgery and suture and skin staple removals are valuable skills that require self-discipline and personal integrity. Keeping a sterile field is of monumental importance for the well-being of the patient. It is also of utmost importance for medical–legal reasons. If sterile technique is not practiced, and infection can result. Patients are very much aware of their rights. You must respect the medical profession and the patient in practicing these skills to the very best of your ability.

Assisting with surgical procedures requires you to be efficient in completing many details. Of primary concern is patient education in both preoperative and postoperative care.

Put on Sterile Gloves

PURPOSE: To protect both patient and medical assistant from contamination.

EQUIPMENT: Package of sterile latex gloves of proper size

TERMINAL PERFORMANCE OBJECTIVE: After practicing with clean gloves, each student will be provided with a package of sterile latex gloves; standing in front of a clean, clear counter surface, demonstrate the correct method of putting on sterile gloves. **CAUTION:** Remember, in order to comply with universal precautions guidelines, gloves and other protective barriers must be worn if there is any possibility of coming into contact with blood, or any body fluids. The instructor will observe each step.

1. Remove wristwatch, rings, and other jewelry from hands and wrists and perform surgical scrub using nail brush. Thoroughly dry hands with sterile towels. *Note: Hands are now clean but unsterile.*

2. Tear seal and open package of sterile gloves as you would open a book, Figure 9–7(a). Place on clean counter surface with cuff end toward your body. *Note: Do not touch inside of package.* **RATIONALE: Hands would contaminate inside of sterile package.**

3. Grasp glove for your **dominant** hand by fold of cuff with finger and thumb of your nondominant hand, Figure 9–7(b). Insert dominant hand, carefully pulling glove on

with other hand, keeping cuff turned back. *Note: Dominant hand is now gloved and sterile, Figure 9–7(c).*

4. Place gloved fingers under cuff of other glove and insert nondominant hand, Figure 9–7(d). Put glove on by pulling on inside fold of cuff, Figure 9–7(e). Avoid touching thumb of dominant hand to outside cuff of other glove where it has been contaminated.

5. Now both hands are gloved and sterile. Place fingers under cuffs to smooth gloves over wrists, Figure 9–7(f) and smooth out fingers for better fit. *Note: Check for tears and holes,* Figures 9–7(g(1) & (2)). **RATIONALE: Any break in the integrity of the glove would not maintain sterility.**

6. Keep hands above waist level. Do not touch anything other than items in sterile field. *Note: Contact with any nonsterile object or surface will contaminate gloved hand(s) requiring removal and regloving.*

7. Remove gloves by pulling glove off dominant hand with thumb and fingers, Figure 9–7(h). Hold outside cuff and pull glove off inside-out. Slip ungloved hand into palm of gloved hand and slip glove off inside-out, Figure 9–7(i). *Note: Be careful not to touch contaminated side of gloves when removing.*

8. Deposit gloves in biohazardous waste bag.

9. Wash hands.

FIGURE 9–7(a) Open the package out by pulling on the center paper folds.

FIGURE 9–7(b) Grasp the fold of the inside cuff of the glove with the thumb and fingers of your dominant hand.

FIGURE 9–7(c) Insert your nondominant hand into the glove and pull the glove on with your dominant hand by the turned-down cuff.

FIGURE 9–7(d) Insert the fingers of your gloved nondominant hand under the folded-down cuff of the glove and insert your dominant hand.

FIGURE 9–7(e) Place the gloved fingers of your nondominant hand under the folded-down cuff of the glove to pull the glove of your dominant hand up over the cuff of the gown.

FIGURE 9–7(f) Place the gloved fingers of your dominant hand (palm down) under the cuff of your gloved nondominant hand to push over the cuff of the gown.

FIGURE 9–7(g) (1) Check the gloves for tears, holes, and imperfections.

FIGURE 9–7(g) (2) Inspect both palm-sides-up and down for proper fit.

FIGURE 9–7(h) Pull the glove from your nondominant hand by grasping the outside of the glove and hold with your gloved dominant hand.

FIGURE 9–7(i) Slip your ungloved hand under your gloved hand (at the base of the palm) and fold over the glove held in your hand and slip off of the hands into the biohazard bag.

P R O C E D U R E

Assist with Minor Surgery

PURPOSE: To assist physician in the performance of a surgical procedure and to provide support for the patient.

EQUIPMENT: Basic sterile setup: needle and syringe, needle holder, appropriate suture, scalpel handle and blade, thumb forceps, surgical scissors, hemostats, retractor, 2 or 3 pairs of latex gloves, gauze squares, cotton-tipped applicators, alcohol pad, fenestrated sheet or towels, towel clamps, bandages; bandage scissors, tape, ordered anesthetic, antiseptic (small glass container for antiseptic solution), plastic biohazardous waste bag (and waste receptacle), patient's chart, pen, **histology** request form for laboratory analysis if a biopsy is indicated, Mayo tray table

TERMINAL PERFORMANCE OBJECTIVE: Provided with all necessary equipment and supplies, with the instructor role-playing as physician and the students role-playing as patients, demonstrate (insofar as possible) each of the steps required in assisting with minor surgery. The instructor will observe each step. *Note: Some steps will need to be simulated in the instructional setting.*

1. Wash hands.
2. Assemble appropriate equipment and supplies on counter or table near Mayo tray. Position the Mayo tray table next to treatment table and check condition and expiration dates of sterile items. **RATIONALE: If an item is expired or package shows signs of improper condition, items may no longer be sterile.**
3. Bring scheduled patient into treatment room. Advise patient to empty bladder. **RATIONALE: This ensures patient's comfort during procedure. Anxiety often results in the urge to void.** When patient returns, take vital signs and record. **RATIONALE: Vital signs must be within acceptable limits to proceed with procedure.** Explain procedure to patient and obtain signature on consent form. **RATIONALE: A signature on consent form is absolutely essential before any invasive procedure is performed.** If biopsy is to be taken, complete lab request form for histology analysis.
4. Instruct patient to disrobe as necessary for procedure and advise where to place belongings. Assist patient if needed. Allow privacy and ask patient to let you know when ready for positioning.
5. Assist patient to treatment table and into desired position for surgery. Perform skin prep procedure. Give

patient support and understanding and answer any questions at this time. Drape patient appropriately.

6. Place sterile towel on Mayo tray by holding the underneath sides of it (the top side must be untouched). Open all sterile items (as ordered by physician for scheduled surgery) carefully by holding them at the tabs; drop them onto the sterile field without touching them.

7. Put on sterile latex gloves. **CAUTION:** Remember, in order to comply with universal precautions guidelines, gloves and other protective barriers must be worn if there is any possibility of coming into contact with blood, or any body fluids. Arrange instruments and other sterile items in the order that they will be used in the procedure. *Note: Do not reach, cough, sneeze, wave, talk, or cross over the sterile field or it will become contaminated. Carefully cover field with a sterile towel until physician is ready to begin.* Remove gloves and wash hands.

8. When physician is ready to begin the surgical procedure, remove the sterile towel from the prepared sterile setup. Assist physician by handing sterile gloves, use alcohol prep to wipe the top of the anesthetic vial, and hold it for physician to draw out the amount needed, Figure 9–8.

9. If you are to assist with surgical procedure, wash hands and put on sterile latex gloves. Hand instruments and other sterile items to physician as needed, mop excessive blood with gauze sponges PRN. *Note: If a biopsy is to be performed, special care must be taken to preserve the specimen. According to physi-cian's preference, the tissue may be placed on a gauze square to be handled later or deposited directly into an open specimen container. Label and attach completed laboratory requisition when procedure is completed.* You may assist the physician in suturing the incision by clipping each individual suture after the knot is tied by the physician, Figure 9–9. You should perform any other assistance as directed by physician during the procedure PRN. If additional sterile items are needed during the procedure, open the package and hand to physician for removal, or drop onto the center of the sterile field. Table 9–1 describes various surgical instruments used in minor office procedures.

10. When surgery is completed, assist in (or perform) cleaning and bandaging the surgery site, remove gloves, and wash hands. Tend to the patient by helping into sitting position to regain balance, and when stable, from the table. Assist in dressing if necessary.

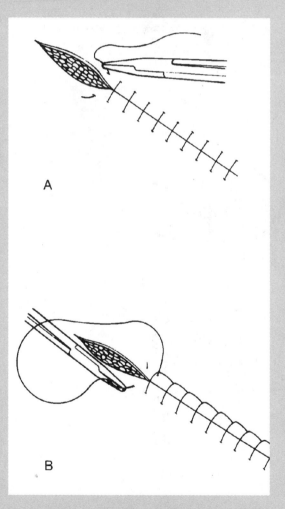

FIGURE 9–9 Two examples of suturing techniques: (a) interrupted (individual) sutures and (b) continuous sutures.

FIGURE 9–8 Hold the anesthetic solution in a convenient position so the physician can fill the syringe without contamination. (From Simmers, *Diversified Health Occupations*, 3rd ed. Copyright 1993, Delmar Publishers Inc.)

Give patient education regarding any return visit, care of surgery site, and any other orders from physician. Ask patient if allergic to adhesive, if so use **hypoallergenic** tape to secure bandage.

11. Put on gloves to clean up treatment table, discard disposable items in biohazardous bag, place instruments in detergent solution to soak after rinsing with cold water, remove gloves and wash hands, restock room.

TABLE 9–1
Instruments Used in Minor Office Surgical Procedures

Figure* Number	Category: Description	Use
	Operating Scissors:	
A	*Deaver* 5½ inches (14 cm) straight, sharp-sharp	Cut tissue and suture
B	*Sistrunk* 5½ inches (14 cm) slightly curved	Same
C	*Deaver* 5½ inches (14 cm) straight, sharp-blunt and curved, sharp-blunt	Same
	Bandage Scissors:	
D	*Lester* 5½ inches (14 cm) sidecurved	Cut dressings, tape
E	*Knowles finger* 5½ inches (14 cm)	Same
F	*Spencer suture* 3½ inches (8.75 cm)	Cut suture
G	*Littauer stitch* 5½ inches (14 cm)	Same
	Petit-Point Hemostats:	
H	*Mosquito* 4¾ inches straight-curved	Grasp tissue to hold, clamp, or pull out of the way
I	*Mosquito* 3½ inches straight-curved	Same
	Towel Forceps:	
J	*Backhaus* (clip) 3½ inches (8.75 cm)	Grasp towels, dressing; hold drape towels in place (use caution—will puncture skin)
K	*Jones* (clip) 3 inches	Same
L	*Knife Handle* #3 5 inches (12.5 cm) holds blades 10, 12, 15	Accept blades
M	*Blades*	Cut tissue
	Sponge-Holding Forceps:	
N	*Foersfer* 7 inches (18 cm) straight-smooth jaws or serrated	Pick up and hold dressings
	Needle Holders:	
O	*Brown* 5¼ inches (13.5 cm)	Grasp suture needle
P	*Collier* 5 inches (13 cm)	Same
	Dressing and Tissue Forceps:	
Q	*Thumb* 4 inches (10 cm) serrated	Pick up dressings, delicate tissue
R	*Tissue* 4½ inches (11 cm) 1 x 2 teeth	Grasp tissue securely for control during dissection or suturing
S	*Adson serrated*, extra delicate, 0.8 mm-wide tip	Pick up delicate tissue
T	*Semken dressing* 4¾ inches (12 cm) serrated	Pick up dressings
U	*Cushing* 7¼ inches (18.5 cm) serrated handle, scraper end, bayonet, 1 x 2 teeth	Close skin
V	*Plain splinter* 3½ inches (8.75 cm)	Remove splinters
W	*Judd-Allis tissue* 6 inches (15 cm)	Grasp tissue

*See pages 566-567 in the Appendix for these illustrations.

P R O C E D U R E

Remove Sutures

PURPOSE: To remove suture(s) from healing laceration or incision.

EQUIPMENT: Sterile: thumb forceps, suture-removal scissors (or staple extractor), gauze squares, latex gloves, cotton-tipped applicators, butterfly or steristrip closures; antiseptic solution, hydrogen peroxide, basin with warm soapy water, bandages, tape, towels, biohazardous waste bag, bandage scissors, patient's chart, pen

TERMINAL PERFORMANCE OBJECTIVE: Provided with all necessary equipment and supplies, and using a mannequin or model as the patient, demonstrate the steps required to remove sutures. The instructor will observe each step. Simulation should be made by the instructor.

1. Wash hands and move Mayo table next to treatment table, or to where patient will be during the procedure.
2. Assemble all necessary items on Mayo table tray, Figure 9–10. Ask if patient is allergic to adhesive, if so use hypoallergenic tape to secure bandage, (ask also about allergies to topical preparations, such as povidone-iodine mixture, or any medications).
3. Bring scheduled patient to treatment room. Ask patient about healing condition of incision or laceration, take vital signs, and record on patient's chart. (If sutures resulted from a laceration injury, ask appropriate questions regarding where and when injury occurred and when a tetanus booster was administered (file ER report in chart). Record.
4. Ask patient to remove appropriate clothing for inspection of healing incision (offer to help PRN).

FIGURE 9–10 Example of a suture-removal tray setup

5. Assist patient to treatment table and into required position and drape appropriately. Explain procedure and answer any questions.
6. Put on gloves and remove bandage. **CAUTION:** Remember, in order to comply with universal precautions guidelines, gloves and other protective barriers must be worn if there is any possibility of coming into contact with blood, or any body fluids. Clean incision with antiseptic solution using cotton-tipped applicators. *Note: If bandage has stuck to the incision (record condition of site on chart: excessive blood, or drainage), apply gauze squares that have been soaked with the soapy warm water solution, or hydrogen peroxide, to the area for a few minutes to loosen the bandage from the sutures and scab.* This will make removal of the bandage easier. (Pulling off a stuck bandage may reopen the wound, or pull out sutures). Either result would be very painful. Advise physician that the incision site is ready to be checked.
7. After physician orders suture removal, open sterile package containing the necessary instruments on the Mayo tray and proceed. Grasp the knot of the suture-material with thumb forceps and gently, but firmly, pull up making just enough space to place the suture removal scissors to clip the suture as close to the skin as possible, Figure 9–11, page 470. Pull the suture with the forceps (back) toward the healing incision so that no **stress** is put on it. **RATIONALE: Pulling the suture away from the site could possibly pull the incision open. CAUTION:** Do not pull a suture that has been on the surface of the skin (exposed to the outside) through the path of the suture being removed, or infection may develop. Continue in this manner until all sutures are removed.
8. Apply antiseptic solution to site and allow to air dry. Apply steristips or butterfly closure if necessary for support during healing process, and bandage.
9. Remove gloves and wash hands.
10. Instruct patient to keep the bandage clean and dry for 24 to 48 hours, or as directed by physician. **RATIONALE: A dirty or wet dressing allows microorganisms to enter the tiny openings where sutures were removed until they are healed.** Advise patient to avoid undue stress for appropriate amount of time for the anatomical area. Give patient education regarding home care and follow-up appointment if ordered by physician.

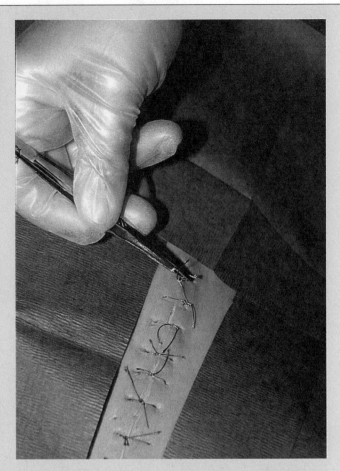

FIGURE 9–11 Suture removal. (a) Grasp the suture knot with thumb forceps, and place the curved tip of the suture-removal scissors just next to the skin under the suture and clip. (b) Gently pull the suture knot up and toward the incision with the thumb forceps to remove (pulling the suture away from the incision may reopen it).

11. Record on progress notes in patient's chart: (1) anatomical area of incision or laceration; (2) condition of site; (3) number of sutures removed; (4) type of antiseptic applied; (5) support closures applied; (6) type of bandage applied, and your initials. Be sure to include the ER report if sent from facility where injury was treated, and record date of tetanus booster if applicable.

Note: If skin staples (or clips) are to be removed, the physician will usually perform the procedure. However, you may be instructed to do so. Basically, skin staples are removed in the following manner: Follow Steps 1 though 6 above and proceed to

Place the sterile staple extractor under staple (one at a time) and squeeze handles of extractor completely closed, Figure 9–12. (Explain to patient that a tugging sensation may be felt.) Lift staple away from skin and place in biohazardous waste container. Continue process until all are removed. Resume procedure above with Step 8.

FIGURE 9–12 Removal of a staple. Staple extractor reforms the staple (clip). Then the staple is lifted from the incision.

Many physicians prefer to perform minor surgical procedures first on the day's schedule. The doctor may require that patients fast for a certain period before the procedure. Fasting lessens the possibility of nausea and vomiting, which some patients may experience during and following any type of surgery. It is best to check with the doctor regarding preference in preop instructions.

Often patients are apprehensive about even the most minor surgical procedure. You must display confidence, concern, and understanding to each individual about the particular procedure. Allow enough time following the explanation of the procedure for the person to think about what was said. Offer to answer patients' questions even if they do not ask.

Make sure that return appointment visits are confirmed and reminder cards are given to patients before they leave the office. Phoning patients the next day is an excellent way to follow-up and reassures them that you and the physician are genuinely concerned about their progress. It will also bring to the physician's attention any problems that could be eliminated early. If patients do have complaints, it is best to have the physician check the problem as soon as possible.

Advise patients about symptoms that may occur following the surgery and to report them immediately to the physician.

Follow-up visits are essential so that assessment of progress can be made by the physician and for the removal of sutures. In general, you should advise all patients who have had any

minor surgical procedure to limit their activity for at least a couple of weeks, or however long the physician has ordered according to the procedure performed.

Specific instructions, such as soaking or applying topical medications, will be given by the physician for certain individual cases. Physicians generally instruct patients (or teach you how to instruct patients) about packing or special bandaging procedures, such as with ingrown toenail removals. Physicians may prescribe an analgesic for any minor pain and discomfort the patient may experience following the procedure.

Patients usually see the family or general practitioner for suture removal following laceration repair from an injury or from a diagnostic procedure, such as heart catheterization. You may have this duty to perform. It is vital that you check the emergency room report regarding the number of sutures put in, so you can be sure to remove all of them. Check the report also for a tetanus booster and record on the patient's chart to bring the immunization record up to date. Before you remove the sutures, check the number of days that the physician who put them in recommended, and ask your physician-employer to inspect the healing wound. Physicians generally order additional closure materials to cover healing incisions or lacerations following suture removal, Figure 9–13. This procedure gives support to the wound and offers the patient more flexibility. Additionally, physicians advise using an elastic bandage to offer more protection and support of surgical areas of the extremities, especially for pediatric and physically active patients. Application of an elastic wrap increases circulation of the area, which hastens the healing process.

Until you are confident in assisting with various office surgeries, it is suggested that you keep a notebook or file cards to help you learn the instruments and steps required for each procedure.

Complete Chapter 9 in the workbook to help you meet the objectives at the beginning of this chapter and therefore achieve competency of this subject matter.

PATIENT EDUCATION

Usual care of the patient:
1. Keep the site clean and dry
2. Place no stress on the area
3. Drink plenty of fluids
4. Get proper rest
5. Eat a sensible well-balanced diet
6. Return for the follow-up appointment

Patients should report to the physician any of the following:
1. Unusual pain, burning, or other uncomfortable sensation
2. Swelling, redness, or other discoloration
3. Bleeding or other discharge
4. Fever above 100°F (37.7°C)
5. Nausea and vomiting
6. Any other problem or symptom

Following suture removal, patients should be advised to
1. Keep the site dry for at least 24 hours
2. Cover the area to keep it clean
3. Apply supportive bandaging PRN
4. Report any sign of infection immediately to the physician

FIGURE 9–13 (a) Use the transfer forceps with sterile gauze to apply antiseptic. (b) Apply a steristrip closure to the center of the incision. (c) Apply closures to each side for evenness. (d) Apply closures parallel to the incision for support.

MEDICAL-LEGAL
ETHICAL HIGHLIGHTS

Ms. Right . . .

explains the procedure to the patient prior to obtaining written consent from the patient for any procedures that involve risk. She provides printed information about the procedure for the patient to take home. If a third party is responsible for payment, she obtains a written contract.

  Employment advancement: Excellent

Miss Wrong . . .

often forgets to obtain a written consent form and third party contract for procedures involving risk. She tells the patient about the procedure and says not to worry about anything, that everything will be all right. She never gives out printed information because she can never remember where she put it.

  Employment advancement: Poor

REFERENCES

J. Jamner Surgical Instruments, Inc., 1991, 9 Skyline Drive, Hawthorne, New York 10532.

Mosby's Dictionary of Medical, Nursing and Allied Health, 3d ed. St. Louis: C. V. Mosby, 1990.

Procedures, The Nurse's Reference Library, Nursing 83 Books, Springhouse, PA: Intermed Communications, 1983.

Taber, Clarence W. *Taber's Cyclopedic Medical Dictionary,* 14th ed. Philadelphia: F. A. Davis, 1983.

CHAPTER 10

Medications

UNIT 1
Prescription and Nonprescription
Medications

UNIT 2
Methods of Administering
Medications

UNIT 3
Injections and Immunizations

Administering medications is one of the most sensitive and important duties that the medical assistant will perform.

You must first become familiar with the medications which are most frequently given to patients. Knowing the properties of the medications will help in answering patients' questions and recognizing common side effects that patients may exhibit. The *Physicians' Desk Reference*, or PDR, and the *Physicians' Desk Reference for Nonprescription Drugs* will become valuable resources. Because these resources are frequently referred to, they should be kept in a central accessible place for use by all members of the health care team. You should also become familiar with the many terms and abbreviations used in administering medications. Some of the most common ones are included in this chapter and in the Appendix.

The laws may vary from state to state in regard to your administering medications. You should check with your employer about this matter. Some physicians prefer always to administer medications to patients themselves, thereby lessening this possible medical–legal concern.

A review of basic math skills will be helpful in preparing medications. The areas in which to practice are addition, subtraction, multiplication, division, fractions, decimals, percentages, and ratio–proportion. Refer to Table 10–5, page 482, for examples of these math problems. Accuracy and care must always be taken in assisting with and administering medications to patients.

UNIT 1

Prescription and Nonprescription Medications

OBJECTIVES

Upon completion of this unit, you will meet the following terminal performance objectives by verifying knowledge of the facts and principles presented through oral and written communication at a level deemed competent by the instructor or employer and will demonstrate the specific behaviors as identified in the terminal performance objectives of the procedures,

Throughout this chapter you should be mindful of all medical–legal and ethical implications. Listed below are a few important reminders.

1. Secure medications or prescription pads in locked storage.
2. Report theft of medications or prescription pads to the authorities.
3. Dispose of expired medications properly.
4. Obtain and file written consent from patients for experimental drugs.
5. Give printed information about and obtain written consent for immunizations.
6. Record medication refills on patient's chart.
7. Keep narcotics records accurate and up to date.
8. Keep physician's narcotics registration current and on file.

observing all aseptic and safety precautions in accordance with health care standards.

1. Demonstrate how to use PDRs for both prescription and nonprescription medications.
2. Explain how to properly phone in prescriptions to a pharmacist.
3. Demonstrate how to write a prescription as ordered by the physician.
4. Discuss the drugs that are under federal regulation according to category, or Schedules I through V.
5. Define abbreviations commonly used in regard to medications.
6. Demonstrate how to record medications properly on the patient's chart.
7. Explain how to categorize medications used in the medical office.
8. Discuss medical, legal, and ethical concerns regarding medications.
9. Spell and define, using the glossary at the back of the text, all the words to know in this unit.

WORDS TO KNOW

accuracy
administer
Drug Enforcement
    Administration (DEA)
dispense
expertise
facility
license
narcotic
over the counter (OTC)

Physician's Desk Reference
    (PDR)
pharmaceutical
pharmacology
prescribe
prescription
reference
resource
vial

Commonly Prescribed Medications

Because of the nature of each type of medical practice, certain medications will be more commonly prescribed than others. It is a good idea to keep a list of these medications handy with the most often questioned information. This list should include the usual dosage and possible side effects. The entire staff should become knowledgeable about these medications.

The list in Table 10–1 is meant as an introduction. The common names of some of the drugs are listed. Consulting a **PDR** or other resource for complete information is suggested.

**P A T I E N T
E D U C A T I O N**

Many patients are very anxious about receiving medication, whether by mouth or by injection. Careful and complete explanation of the procedure and the need for medications is essential in calming the patient. The patient must understand when and how to take prescribed medications to receive the full benefits of these medications. Some medications are to be taken before meals or after meals, with certain fluids or excluding certain fluids, and in the presence or absence of certain foods or other medications. Carefully explained verbal and written instructions are essential for the patient's compliance. The patient must understand that the medication dosage cannot be changed without first consulting the physician.

TABLE 10–1
Selected Drug Classifications

Classification	Action	Examples
Analgesic	An agent that relieves pain without causing loss of consciousness	acetaminophen (Tylenol) aspirin ibuprofen (Advil, Motrin)
Anesthetic	An agent that produces a lack of feeling. May be local or general depending on the type and how administered.	morphine, lidocaine HCl (Xylocaine) procaine HCl (Novocain)
Antacid	An agent that neutralizes acid	Amphojel, Gelusil, Mylanta, Aludrox
Antianxiety	An agent that relieves anxiety and muscle tension	benzodiazepines: diazepam (Valium) and chlordiazepoxide HCl (Librium)
Antiarrhythmic	An agent that controls cardiac arrhythmias	lidocaine HCl (Xylocaine) propranolol HCl (Inderal)
Antibiotic	An agent that is destructive to or inhibits growth of microorganisms	penicillins (Pentids, Duracillin, Polycillin, Pipracil, Augmentin) cephalosporins (Reflin, Mandol, Rocephin)
Anticholinergic	An agent that blocks parasympathetic nerve impulses	atropine, scopolamine, trihexyphenidyl HCl (Artane)
Anticoagulant	An agent that prevents or delays blood clotting	heparin sodium, dicumarol, warfarin sodium (Coumadin)
Anticonvulsant	An agent that prevents or relieves convulsions	carbamazepine (Tegretol) phenytoin (Dilantin) ethosuximide (Zarotin)
Antidepressant	An agent that prevents or relieves the symptoms of depression	ethosuximide (Zarotin), monoamine oxidase (MAO) inhibitors: isocarboxazid (Marplan), phenelzine sulfate (Nardil), amitriptyline HCl (Elavil), imipramine HCl (Tofranil)
Antidiarrheal	An agent that prevents or relieves diarrhea	diphenoxylate HCl (Lomotil), Pepto-Bismol, Kaopectate
Antidote	An agent that counteracts poisons and their effect	naloxone (Narcan)
Antiemetic	An agent that prevents or relieves nausea and vomiting	trimethobenzamide HCl (Tigan), Dramamine, Phenergan, Reglan, Marinol
Antihistamine	An agent that acts to counteract histamine	diphenhydramine HCl (Benadryl), Dimetane, Seldane
Antihypertensive	An agent that prevents or controls high blood pressure	methyldopa (Aldomet) clonidine HCl (Catapres) metoprolol tartrate (Lopressor)
Antiinflammatory	An agent that counteracts inflammation	naproxen (Naprosyn), aspirin, ibuprofen (Advil, Motrin)
Antimanic	An agent used for the treatment of the manic episode of manic–depressive disorder	lithium
Antineoplastic	An agent that kills or destroys malignant cells	busulfan (Myleran) cyclophosphamide (Cytoxan)
Antipyretic	An agent that reduces fever	aspirin, acetaminophen (Tylenol)
Antitussive	An agent that prevents or relieves cough	codeine, dextromethorphan
Bronchodilator	An agent that dilates the bronchi	isoproterenol HCl (Isuprel) albuterol (Proventil)
Contraceptive	Any device, method, or agent that prevents conception	norethynodrel, mestranol (Enovid-E 21), Ortho-Novum 10/11-21; 10/11-28 Triphasil-21

TABLE 10–1
Selected Drug Classifications (continued)

Classification	Action	Examples
Decongestant	An agent that reduces nasal congestion and/or swelling	oxymetazoline (Afrin) epinephrine HCl (Adrenalin) phenylephrine HCl (Neo-Synephrine) pseudoephedrine HCl (Sudafed)
Diuretic	An agent that increases the excretion of urine	chlorothiazide (Diuril) furosemide (Lasix) mannitol (Osmitrol)
Expectorant	An agent that facilitates removal of secretion from bronchopulmonary mucous membrane	guaifenesin (Robitussin)
Hemostatic	An agent that controls or stops bleeding	aminocaproic acid (Amicar), Humafac, vitamin K
Hypnotic	An agent that produces sleep or hypnosis	secobarbital (Seconal); chloral hydrate ethchlorvynol (Placidyl)
Hypoglycemic	An agent that lowers blood glucose level	insulin; chlorpropamide (Diabinese)
Laxative	An agent that loosens and promotes normal bowel eliminations	bisacodyl (Dulcolax), Metamucil powder
Muscle relaxant	An agent that produces relaxation of skeletal muscle	methocarbanol (Robaxin), Norflex, Paraflex, Skelaxin, Valium
Sedative	An agent that produces a calming effect without causing sleep	amobarbital (Amytal) butabarbital sodium (Buticaps) phenobarbital
Tranquilizer	An agent that reduces mental tension and anxiety	chlorpromazine HCl (Thorazine), Mellaril, Haldol
Vasodilator	An agent that produces relaxation of blood vessels; lowers blood pressure	isorbide dinitrate (Isordil) nitroglycerine
Vasopressor	An agent that produces contraction of muscles of capillaries and arteries; elevates blood pressure	metaraminol (Aramine) norepinephrine (Levophed)

(From Rice, *Principles of Pharmacology for Medical Associates,* Copyright 1989, Albany, NY; Delmar Publishers. Used with permission)

Pharmaceutical References ....

The PDR is a valuable **resource** that the medical assistant should keep handy in the medical office. The purpose of the PDR is to provide accurate, reliable, and current information about all prescribed medications and related products. You may need to consult the PDR for the proper spelling, strength, or other information concerning medications, which are not given frequently, to assist the physician in accurately prescribing medications.

One of your responsibilities may be to order the current edition of the PDR so that the practice may keep abreast of the newest **pharmaceuticals** approved by the Food and Drug Administration (FDA). This reference book is published annually. A supplement with the latest information is sent to subscribers quarterly. There are nine sections:

1. Manufacturers' index (white)
2. Product name index (pink)
3. Product classification index (blue)
4. Generic and chemical name index (yellow)
5. Medications in color and actual size for identification assistance
6. Product information section (white, alphabetically)
7. Diagnostic product information (green)
8. Listings of poison control centers
9. Guide to management of drug overdose

Guidelines for using the PDR

1. The pink section alphabetically lists the brand of (if described) generic names of medicines and products. The manufacturer of the product appears next with either one or two page numbers. The first page number refers you to the picture section for identification of the product and the next page number is for the information about the product in the white section.
2. The yellow section alphabetically lists the generic or chemical names of the products with the manufacturer listed beside it and the pages on which information may be obtained.

3. The blue section contains products in alphabetical order according to their classification.

4. The green section contains current information about diagnostic products also listed in alphabetical order.

Note: The medical assistant should become familiar with the PDR's contents page with each new edition to become proficient in assisting the physician with needed information. The *Physicians' Desk Reference for Nonprescription Drugs* is also another valuable resource that can be of great assistance in identifying **over-the-counter (OTC)** medicines that patients use for self-medication. The format of this reference book is almost identical to the PDR for prescription products. A section on patient education material and support groups is also included, besides diagnostic home use products.

Getting familiar with the arrangement of both PDRs will prove its worth very quickly when a difficult situation is encountered in the medical practice.

Many other sources of information about **pharmacology** are used by physicians. Most offices have more than one **reference** for this purpose. The *National Formulary,* the *Pharmacopoeia of the United States of America* (USP), and the *Pharmacopoeia Internationalis* are three.

Writing Prescriptions ....

A **prescription** is a written order for a particular medication or treatment for a particular patient by a **licensed** physician. It is a legal document. Most prescriptions are hand-written by the physician, especially those for **narcotics.** However, some physicians delegate the task of writing the information on the prescription blank to the medical assistant. The physician will then check the prescription and sign it. Any medication that is **prescribed** must be recorded on the patient's chart. Figure 10–1 shows examples of prescription blanks. When the physician prescribes only one medication for a patient, the single medication prescription pad is used. Physicians use the multiple medication prescription pads for those patients whose condition requires several medications to be prescribed at a time. This eliminates having to write in the patient's name, date, and so forth on each single prescription order. It also saves the doctor from having to sign each individual sheet.

The prescription should contain the

■ Date
■ Patient's full legal name and complete address
■ Rx symbol (means recipe, or "take thou")
■ Name of drug and amount
■ Pharmacist's instructions
■ Patient's instructions
■ Signature of physician
■ Physician's full name, address, and phone number
■ Physician's DEA number

This standard information helps the pharmacist fill the prescription. It is much easier for pharmacists today to fill prescriptions because of prepared and prepackaged medications.

Although it is rare, however, some medications must still be prepared by the licensed pharmacist from the directions on the prescription. When phoning in prescriptions, you must give the pharmacist all the information that the prescription contains. To ensure

FIGURE 10–1 Sample prescription blanks for single medication (a) and multiple medications (b)

FIGURE 10–2 Examples of instructions and warning labels for prescription medications.

Form DEA – 224
(Jun 1990)

OMB No. 1117-0014

APPLICATION FOR REGISTRATION
UNDER
CONTROLLED SUBSTANCES ACT OF 1970

Please PRINT or TYPE all entries.

No registration may be issued unless a completed application form has been received (21 CFR 1301.21).

RETAIN Copy 3. Mail Orig. and 1 copy with FEE to:

UNITED STATES DEPARTMENT OF JUSTICE
DRUG ENFORCEMENT ADMINISTRATION
CENTRAL STATION
P. O. Box 28083
WASHINGTON, D.C. 20038 - 8083
For INFORMATION, Call: (202) 307 7255

See "Privacy Act" Information on reverse

NAME		
PROPOSED BUSINESS ADDRESS		
CITY	STATE	ZIP CODE

THIS BLOCK FOR DEA USE ONLY

● FEE MUST ACCOMPANY APPLICATION

REGISTRATION CLASSIFICATION: Submit Check or Money Order Payable to the **DRUG ENFORCEMENT ADMINISTRATION** in the Amount of $ 60.00 (3 year registration period)

1. BUSINESS ACTIVITY: *(Check ONE only)*

A ☐ RETAIL PHARMACY   B ☐ HOSPITAL/CLINIC   C ☐ PRACTITIONER *(Specify Medical Degree, e.g., DDS, DO, DVM, MD, etc.)*   D ☐ TEACHING INSTITUTION *(Instructional purposes only)*

2. SCHEDULES: *(Check ☑ all applicable schedules in which you intend to handle controlled substances. See Schedules on Reverse of Instruction Sheet.)*

SCHEDULE II ☐ NARCOTIC
SCHEDULE II ☐ NONNARCOTIC
SCHEDULE III ☐ NARCOTIC
SCHEDULE III ☐ NONNARCOTIC
SCHEDULE IV ☐
SCHEDULE V ☐

3. ☐ CHECK HERE IF YOU REQUIRE ORDER FORMS.

4. **ALL APPLICANTS MUST ANSWER THE FOLLOWING:**

(a) Are you currently authorized to prescribe, distribute, dispense, conduct research, or otherwise handle the controlled substances in the schedules for which you are applying, under the laws of the **State** or jurisdiction in which you are operating or propose to operate ?

☐ YES - **State** License No. _____
☐ Not Applicable   ☐ Pending

☐ YES - **State** Controlled Substance No. _____
☐ Not Applicable   ☐ Pending

(b) Has the applicant ever been convicted of a crime in connection with controlled substances under State or Federal law, or ever surrendered or had a Federal controlled substance registration revoked, suspended, restricted or denied, or ever had a State professional license or controlled substance registration revoked, suspended, denied, restricted or placed on probation ?   ☐ YES   ☐ NO

(c) If the applicant is a corporation (other than a corporation whose stock is owned and traded by the public), association, partnership, or pharmacy, has any officer, partner, stockholder or proprietor been convicted of a crime in connection with controlled substances under State or Federal law, or ever surrendered or had a Federal controlled substance registration revoked, suspended, restricted or denied, or ever had a State professional license or controlled substance registration revoked, suspended, denied, restricted or placed on probation ?   ☐ YES   ☐ NO   ☐ NOT APPLICABLE

IF THE ANSWER TO QUESTIONS 4(b) or (c) is YES, include a statement using the space provided on the REVERSE of this part.

● ATTACH CHECK HERE ●

5. CERTIFICATION FOR FEE EXEMPTION
☐ CHECK THIS BLOCK IF INDIVIDUAL NAMED HEREON IS A FEDERAL, STATE, OR LOCAL OFFICIAL.

The Undersigned hereby certifies that the applicant herein is an officer or employee of a Federal, State or local agency who, in the course of such employment, is authorized to obtain, dispense, or prescribe controlled substances or is authorized to conduct research, instructional activity or chemical analysis with controlled substances, and is exempt from the payment of this application fee.

_____   _____
Signature of Certifying Official   Date

_____
Print or Type Name

_____
Print or Type Title

_____
Name of Institution or Agency

WARNING: SECTION 843(a)(4) OF TITLE 21, UNITED STATES CODE, STATES THAT ANY PERSON WHO KNOWINGLY OR INTENTIONALLY FURNISHES FALSE OR FRAUDULENT INFORMATION IN THIS APPLICATION IS SUBJECT TO IMPRISONMENT FOR NOT MORE THAN FOUR YEARS, A FINE OF NOT MORE THAN $30,000.00 OR BOTH.

Mail the Original and 1 copy with FEE to the above address. Retain 3rd copy for your records.

SIGN HERE ▶

_____
Print or Type Name Here - Sign Below

_____
Applicant's Business Phone No.

_____   _____
Signature of applicant or authorized individual   Date

Title (If the applicant is a corporation, institution, or other entity, enter the TITLE of the person signing on behalf of the applicant (e.g., President, Dean, Procurement Officer, etc...))

FIGURE 10–3   Example of a DEA physician registration form

TABLE 10–2
Schedules of Controlled Substances

Drug Category	Potential for Abuse (Addiction)	Medical Use	Potential for Dependence	Example
Schedule I	High	—Unaccepted —Limited to research	High	Heroin, LSD, marijuana, peyote
Schedule II	High	—Accepted —Tightly restricted	Severe psychic or physical	Amphetamines, morphine
Schedule III	Less than I or II Low to moderate	Current	High psychological	Certain opioids, barbiturates and some depressants
Schedule IV	Low	Acceptable	Limited physical and psychological	Phenobarbital propoxyphene
Schedule V	Low	Acceptable	Limited physical and psychological	Small amounts of codeine in cough preparations and analgesics

TABLE 10–3
Abbreviations and Symbols Commonly Used in Administering Medications

Abbreviation	Meaning	Abbreviation	Meaning
@	at	CAP(S)	capsule(s)
aa	of each	cc	cubic centimeter
ac	before meals	comp	compound
ad	up to	contra	against
AD	right ear	coq	boil
adde	add, let it be added	DC, Disc	discontinue
ad lib	as much as needed, as desired	dil	dilute
agit	shake, stir	div	to be divided
agNo₂	silver nitrate	dos	doses
alt dieb	alternate days	dr, 3	dram
alt hor	alternate hour	EENT	eye, ear, nose and throat
alt noc	alternate nights	elix	elixir
am	morning	emul	emulsion
ante	before	et	and
aq	water	ext	extract
aq bull	boiling water	f, ft	make, let there be made
aq com	tap water, common water	Fe	iron
aq dist	distilled water	fl	fluid
aq ferv	hot water	G	gauge
aq frig	cold water	garg	gargle
aq susp	water suspension	GI	gastrointestinal
AS	left ear	g, G	gram
AU	in each ear, both ears	GR	grain
Ba	barium	gt	drop
bid, BID	twice a day	gtt	drops
BSA	body surface area	GU	genitourinary
/c, c	with	guttat	drop by drop

Abbreviation	Meaning	Abbreviation	Meaning
h	hour	prn, PRN	as necessary, whenever necessary
H_2O_2	hydrogen peroxide	pt	patient
hs	bedtime, hour of sleep	pulv	powder
IM	intramuscular	qd	every day
inj	injection	qh	every hour
IV	intravenous	q (2,3,4) h	every (2,3,4) hours
k	potassium	qid, QID	four times a day
kg	kilogram	qns	quantity not sufficient
L	liter, left	qod, QOD	every other day
lb, LB(S)	pound(s)	qs	quantity sufficient
•	minim	rep	let it be repeated
M	mix	R	right
μg, MCG	microgram	Rx, ℞	take, recipe
M et f pil	mix and make into pill	/s, s̄	one-half
M et f pulv	mix and make into powder	sat	saturated
M et sig	mix and label	sc, sub cu, SC, Subc	subcutaneous (under the skin)
mg, MG	milligram	Sig, Sig, S	write on label, give directions
mL, ML	milliliter	sol	solution
noct	night	ss, s̄s̄	one-half
non rep	do not repeat	stat, STAT	immediately
NPO	nothing by mouth	suppos	suppository
o h	every hour	syr	syrup
o m	every morning	T, tbsp	tablespoon
OS	left eye	TAB	tablet
OD	right eye	tid, TID	three times a day
OU	in each eye, both eyes	tr, tinct	tincture
oz, ℥	ounce	tsp	teaspoon
pc	after meals	u	unit
pil	pill	ung	ointment
po	by mouth		

accuracy, you should ask the pharmacist to repeat the information. This practice will help avoid dangerous misunderstandings.

When patients have their prescriptions filled by a pharmacist, the container often has an instruction label on it. Pharmacists frequently use one or more of these labels to alert the patient of special instructions or warnings regarding a particular medication ordered by the doctor. Warning labels are made in a variety of bright colors to attract attention to their messages, Figure 10–2.

All physicians who prescribe, **dispense,** or **administer** medications in the United States must register with the U.S. Department of Justice, **Drug Enforcement Administration (DEA),** under the Controlled Substances Act of 1970. A form must be filled out, with the physician's state license number and signature, and accompanied by a standard fee, Figure 10–3. If the physician moves the medical practice, this change of address must be reported in writing to the nearest DEA field office. Registration must be renewed every 3 years. The certificate must be filed at the registered location and be available for inspection by officials on request. If the physician practices medicine in one or more locations, as long as it is within the same state, individual registration must be filed for each address only if controlled substances are administered or dispensed at each place. If prescriptions only are written at other locations, registration needs to be filed with the DEA just for the primary location. Physicians must be in compliance with these requirements of the 1984 Diversion Control Amendments to administer, dispense, or prescribe any controlled substance. A current printed schedule of controlled substances is enclosed with the application and this

TABLE 10–4
Commonly Used Weights and Measures

Units of Volume				Units of Weight			
1	liter	= 1000	milliliter	1	gram	= 1000	milligrams
0.001	liter	= 1	milliliter	0.001	gram	= 1	milligram
	or			1	kilogram	= 1000	grams
	1		cubic centimeter	0.001	kilogram	= 1	gram

Commonly used metric measurements

Volume		Weight	
0.1	liter = 1 deciliter	0.1	gram = 1 decigram
0.01	liter = 1 centimeter	0.01	gram = 1 centigram
0.001	liter = 1 milliliter	0.001	gram = 1 milligram
10.0	liter = dekaliter	10.0	grams = 1 dekagram
100.0	liters = 1 hectoliter	100.0	grams = 1 hectogram
1000.0	liters = 1 kiloliter	1000.0	grams = 1 kilogram

Metric units, divisions, and multiples

Volume Equivalents		Weight Equivalents	
Metric	Apothecaries'	Metric	Apothecaries'
1 milliliter =	15 or 16 minims	0.06 gram or 60 milligrams =	1 grain
4 milliliters =	1 dram	1 gram or 1000 milligrams =	15 grains
30 milliliters =	1 ounce	500 milligrams =	7½ grains
500 milliliters =	1 pint	4 grams =	1 dram
1000 milliliters =	1 quart	30 grams =	1 ounce

Equivalency chart for volumes and weights

Volume	Weight
60 minims = 1 (fluids) dram	60 grains = 1 dram
8 drams = 1 (fluids) ounce	8 drams = 1 ounce
16 drams = 1 pint	12 ounces = 1 pound
2 pints = 1 quart	

Apothecary measurements

should also be kept on file. Table 10–2 lists the drugs that are under federal control according to their actual or potential level for abuse or addiction in five categories or schedules.

Since there is no medical use for any of the drugs in Schedule I, prescriptions are prohibited. Drugs in Schedule II must have a written or typed prescription order with the physician's personal signature and DEA registry number. These medications may not be refilled. If a genuine emergency situation arises, the doctor may phone in a limited amount of medication to the pharmacist for the patient. To comply with DEA regulations a written, signed prescription order must be presented to the pharmacist within 72 hours for the controlled substance. In Schedule III of controlled substances, medications may be ordered by phone or written prescription presented to the pharmacist. Five refills may

TABLE 10–5
Review Examples of Math Problems

Addition

```
   876
   493
 + 521
  1890
```

Subtraction

```
  691        581
 - 98       - 98
  593        483
```

Fractions   numerator / denominator

Addition   ⅖ + ⅘ = ⁶⁄₅ = 1⅕

⅕ = ³⁄₁₅	1⅞ = 1³⁵⁄₄₀
+ ⅓ = ⁵⁄₁₅	+ 7⁷⁄₁₀ = 9²⁸⁄₄₀
⁸⁄₁₅	10⁶³⁄₄₀ = 11²³⁄₄₀

Multiplication

```
    437
  x  25
   2185
   874
 102,925
```

To Prove
Divide your answer by 437

```
          25
 437)10,925
      874
     2185
     2185
```

Division

```
        56.80
 70)3976.00
    350
     476
     420
     560
     560
```

To Prove
Multiply your answer by 70

```
   56.80
 x    70
 3976.00
```

Subtraction   ⅗ – ⅓ = ⁹⁄₁₅ – ⁵⁄₁₅ = ⁴⁄₁₅
3⁷⁄₁₆ – 2⅛ = 3¹⁴⁄₃₂ – 2⁴⁄₃₂ = 1¹⁰⁄₃₂ = 1⁵⁄₁₆

Multiplication   ⅖ x ⁷⁄₁₆ = ⅕ x ⅞ = ⁷⁄₄₀
⅕ x ⁷⁄₁₀ = ⅕ x ⁷⁄₁₀ = ⁷⁄₅₀

Division   ¹⁄₁₂ ÷ ⅔ ÷ = ¹⁄₁₂ x ³⁄₂ = ⅛
1¼ ÷ 3 = ⁵⁄₄ x ⅓ = ⁵⁄₁₂

Decimals

Addition	Subtraction	Multiplication	Division
87.43	796.37	394.75	272.52 ⅕
+ 39.57	– 55.62	x 68.29	35)9538.27
127.00	740.75	3552.75	70
		7895	2538.27
		315800	2450.00
		236850	088.27
		26,957.4775	70
			18.27
			17.5
			0.77
			7

Percentages   To find out what percent (%) one number is to another, use the number following the word "of" as a denominator and make a fraction. Divide the numerator by the denominator, for example:

25 is what percent of 35?

²⁵⁄₃₅ = ⁵⁄₇ = 0.70 = 70%

```
 7)5.00
   4 9
     10
```

Ratio   Ratios show how one quantity relates to another and are separated by a colon (:), for example:

20 : 100 = ²⁰⁄₁₀₀ = 0.20 parts or 20%

Proportion   A set of two equal ratios is a proportion. In the equation a double colon (::) separates each of the equal ratios, for example:

To mix a cleaning solution knowing the correct portions for a small amount you can find out how much baking soda to use to make a larger amount, using x for the unknown amount.

½ cup baking soda : 16 oz water :: x amount of baking soda : 32 oz water

$$½ : 16 :: x : 32$$
$$0.5 : 16 :: x : 32$$
$$16x = 32 \times 0.5$$
$$16x = 16$$
$$x = 1 \text{ cup baking soda}$$

be ordered within a 6-month period. Schedule V medications are subject to state and local regulations. A written prescription for these medicines is not necessarily required.

Recording Medications

You will be expected to read and record many types of medications. Memorizing the commonly used abbreviations and symbols given in Table 10–3, page 479, will prepare you to carry out this responsibility. Another useful reference is the list of equivalent weights and measures given in Table 10–4, page 481. These will be needed in ordering medications. An extended list of these is given in the Appendix.

Basic math skills should be among your many areas of **expertise.** These skills may mean monetary savings to your employer, because there are competitive prices for everything, including medical supplies and medications. When ordering injectables, for instance, you may find that a multiple-dose **vial** is more economical for the needs of the practice than a single-dose vial. Determining what is cost-effective for the practice and shopping for the best values will make you an asset to the practice. Table 10–5 provides examples of the common math problems you may encounter in determining costs, dosages, and other mathematical calculations in the medical setting.

Pharmaceutical representatives will undoubtedly visit the medical **facility** from time to time, bringing detailed information concerning prices and the newest products. These representatives are always willing to answer questions. Many of these companies offer support in the area of education for members of the American Association of Medical Assistants.

Storing Medications

In storing medication, "a place for everything and everything in its place" is the rule. Many necessary forms, prescription blanks, and records must be kept. Commonly used medications must be rotated according to their expiration dates. The most practical way to store medications is to categorize them by their classification as in Table 10–1, page 475. Medications may also be stored alphabetically. Labeling shelves increases efficiency, as do pull-out shelves.

Complete Chapter 10, Unit 1 in the workbook to help you meet the objectives at the beginning of this unit and therefore achieve competency of this subject matter.

U N I T   2
Methods for Administering Medications

OBJECTIVES

Upon completion of this unit, you will meet the following terminal performance objectives by verifying knowledge of the facts and principles presented through oral and written communication at a level deemed competent by the instructor or employer and will demonstrate the specific behaviors as identified in the terminal performance objectives of the procedures, observing all aseptic and safety precautions in accordance with health care standards.

1. List and describe the various methods of medications.
2. Demonstrate how to instruct patients in the method of medication ordered by the physician.
3. Explain how to apply a transdermal patch medication properly.
4. Discuss precautions in applying a transdermal patch medication.
5. Identify each time and explain the importance of checking medications prior to administration.
6. Discuss patient education to females regarding vaginal medications.
7. List considerations regarding drug action in the body.
8. Spell out and define, using the glossary at the back of the text, all the words to know in this unit.

WORDS TO KNOW

BSA (body surface area)	ointment
buccal	parenteral
douche	salve
infusion	sublingual
interaction	suppository
nomogram	tolerance

Administering Medication

There are many methods of medicating patients, and even though you may not administer every type, you should know something about each one. You will also assist in the preparation of different types of medications for patients and in the instruction of patients in specific directions for taking medications. The methods of administering medications are oral, including **sublingual** and **buccal;** by inhalation; **topical,** including **transdermal;** vaginal; rectal and urethral; and by injection.

When administering any medication to a patient you should follow a standard format checklist to make certain that you are accurate and efficient. Develop the habit of using the checklist that follows to help you to achieve this standard of quality patient care. Before you administer the medication always be sure that you have the correct

1. Patient
2. Medication
3. Dose or amount
4. Route and method

It is common practice, and sound advice, when giving any medications to follow these precautions:

- Compare the medication order to the container when taking the container from storage.
- Compare the medication order to the container when preparing the medication.
- Compare the medication order to the container before administering the medication.
- Compare the medication order to the container when returning the container to storage.

This practice ensures accuracy in giving any medication.

If there is ever a chance that a medication was given in error, the necessary action must be taken immediately. Admitting such a mistake is not a pleasant experience, but it is necessary for the well-being of the patient. Reporting the error to the physician at once is essential.

Properly instructing the patient about how a medication should be taken is extremely important. If the patient does not understand the directions or the need for carrying out the physician's orders, then the medication will be virtually useless and may be dangerous because the patient may not take it or may take it incorrectly. Patients who are given medication that may induce drowsiness should be made aware of the dangers of driving or operating machinery while taking the medication. Even though the physician may give these instructions to patients, you should make sure the information is clearly understood before the patient leaves the office. You should be mindful of recording all medications given to patients, including sample packages. On the patient's chart, record the name of the medication, the strength, directions for use, and how many dispensed. Writing the directions for use for the patient will eliminate possible confusion for the patient. Package inserts enclosed with all medication contain the necessary information. This same information is found in the PDR. If there is any further question, the PDR should be consulted.

5. Technique
6. Time and schedule

It may seem unlikely that one would make a mistake and administer a medication to a patient in error. However, care must be taken in identifying the patient for whom the medication is intended before it is administered or such a mistake is possible. Many offices and clinics care for so many patients in the course of the daily schedule, with multiple family members being seen in the same treatment room for example, that if particular attention is not paid, an error could result.

Reading the label of the ordered medication and the amount or dose when you obtain it from storage, as you prepare it, just before you administer it, and finally again, after you have administered it, will safeguard you from committing an error. If an error is made, necessary steps must be taken immediately in reporting it to the doctor for emergency care to be given if necessary.

The route or method of administering medication is equally important. Carefully reading the order provides instruction in how the physician wants the medication to be administered, that is, topical—applying a cream or other preparation to the skin; by injection—intramuscular, subcutaneous, intradermal; transdermal—skin patch; or orally—buccal or sublingual. All of these are certainly very different.

Technique refers to how the method is administered, that is, the skill in giving the different types of injections; the manner in which you apply a topical preparation; or the way in which you administer an inhalation treatment to a patient.

Attention must be given to time and schedule in administering medicines. For example, immunizations must be given within a certain time frame for maximum effectiveness in the immunity process of the patient. What time a medication is administered is also important to the well-being of the patient. For instance, some medicines should not be taken when the stomach is full, and some should not be taken when the stomach is empty. Checking the time the patient has eaten last is important. Also check the expiration date of the medication to be sure of its quality strength.

FIGURE 10–4 Means of administering oral medication: (a) medicine cups. (b) capsules, tablets (unscored and scored), and pills

PROCEDURE

Obtain and Administer Oral Medication

PURPOSE: To obtain the ordered oral medication and administer it to the patient.

EQUIPMENT: Ordered oral medication (for practice, any tiny candies), medicine cup (disposable), disposable paper cup filled with water, medicine tray

TERMINAL PERFORMANCE OBJECTIVE: Provided with all necessary equipment and supplies, and using other students as patients, demonstrate the steps required to obtain the ordered oral medication and administer it to the patient. The instructor will observe each step.

1. Obtain medication from storage area and read label carefully, comparing it with order. *Note: Work in a well-lighted area and avoid distractions.*
2. Calculate dosage if necessary and wash hands.
3. Take bottle cap off and place inside up on counter. **RATIONALE: The counter top is considered contaminated and must not come into contact with inside of cap. Likewise, touching inside of bottle or cap will result in contamination.** Read label of medication container.
4. If in pill or capsule form, pour desired amount into cap. Then pour medication into medicine cup. If liquid medicine, pour directly into measuring device to calibrated line of ordered amount. *Note: Hold measuring device at eye level with thumbnail placed at desired amount, Figure 10–5.* Syrup or liquid medications may also be given in disposable plastic measuring spoons. Liquids should be poured from the opposite side of the bottle's label to prevent the contents from dripping and discoloring the label.
5. Place medication container on tray and ordered dose in medicine cup. Place cup of water on tray for patient to take with medicine. Read label of container again.
6. Take medication tray to patient and confirm patient's identification. Explain procedure.
7. Give patient medication and offer cup of water. Observe patient taking medicine and report any reaction or problem to physician.
8. Discard any disposables and return medication container and tray to proper storage area. *Note: Read label of medication container again.*
9. Record information on patient's chart and initial.

FIGURE 10–5 Pour liquids at eye level with your thumbnail held at the point of the amount needed.

Most oral medications are intended for absorption in the small intestine. The remaining methods are **parenteral,** or intended for absorption outside the digestive system.

Oral Administration One of the most common methods of administering medications is the oral method. These medicines are in the form of pills, tablets, capsules, lozenges, syrups, sprays, and other liquids, which are swallowed, Figure 10–4. These medications are usually given to patients as prescriptions, although they may be administered in the office. For example, an analgesic may be given to a patient while in the office for relief of pain. Sabin (immunization against polio) is given orally to infants and children in the medical office by the physicians or the medical assistant. Medicine which is given or sold to patients to be taken home is said to be dispensed.

Oral medications have many advantages. An obvious one is their convenience. If a patient exhibits an intolerance or an adverse reaction to an oral medication, the remedy may be to just discontinue the medicine. The reaction to a single oral dose would certainly be much less dangerous than if the medication were given by injection. They are also easily stored and are economical for the medical practice and the patient.

Sublingual and Buccal. The sublingual method of administering medication involves placing the medication, usually tiny tablets, under the tongue. This introduces the medication immediately into the bloodstream. An example is nitroglycerine, which is usually prescribed for patients who suffer from angina. Tiny tablets are also administered by the buccal method, that is placed in the mouth between the gum and the cheek. The medication is then absorbed through the mucous membranes. Patients should avoid eating, drinking, or chewing while the medication is in place. Instruct patients how to use these medications properly because sublingual and buccal medications should not be swallowed whole or their intended action would be delayed and ineffective.

Inhalation Administration Medications given to patients by the inhalation method are in the form of gases, sprays, fluids, or powders to be mixed with liquid and used with equipment that will produce a mist or vapor. These are breathed into the respiratory tract. The patient usually self-administers the medication at home. After being instructed properly, the patient should feel comfortable in doing so. Manufacturers prepare instruction material on the proper use and care of their equipment. You should keep a file of these for the most commonly prescribed medications.

A form of inhalation medication that should be kept in every medical practice is oxygen. Although it isn't given often in most practices, it should be available for emergency use. Many companies offer instruction in the use and care of such equipment. They also offer various home oxygen treatment programs for patients who need this treatment daily. Setting aside a time when instruction in this service could benefit the entire medical staff would be advantageous.

Topical Administration Topical medications are used in treating diseases or disorders of the skin by application to the skin in some form. They come in sprays, lotions, creams, **ointments,** paints, **salves,** wet dressings, and adhesive patches.

Topical medications must be applied as instructed for maximum effect. For example a patient should apply a medication to reduce itching with gentle single strokes. If the medication is rubbed into the skin vigorously, the itching will increase from the heat produced from the friction, which increases the circulation.

The patch type of medication, commonly called a *transdermal patch,* is a convenient method of choice for medicating patients for many medical conditions. It is painless, and ensures patient compliance. The patch is placed on the skin according to the directions of the pharmaceutical company. It then releases minute dosages of the desired medicine into the patient's tissues, which carry it into the circulatory system. The patient receives timed-release treatment without worrying about when to take the medication. Patients return as scheduled or as indicated to have the patch changed or removed. The effectiveness of the medication is then evaluated. Patients are also instructed to apply the transdermal patch themselves. When applying the transdermal patch, one must be extremely careful when handling it to avoid getting the medication on the fingers. A priming dose of medication is in the adhesive edge of the patch. The medication intended for the patient can also be absorbed by the person who applies it. If one is not careful to wash the hands with soap and water immediately after application of the transdermal medicating patch, the effects could be undesirable or even dangerous to the one who applied it. Traces could also be transferred to any person you may touch, which could also present problems. Wearing disposable gloves when applying transdermal patches is a suggested practice, especially when

FIGURE 10–6 (A) The Transderm-Nitro skin patch is applied once a day. It helps prevent the pain of angina by delivering a steady level of nitroglycerin to the body. The patch provides medication without interfering in a patient's daily activities. (Courtesy of Ciba-Geigy.)

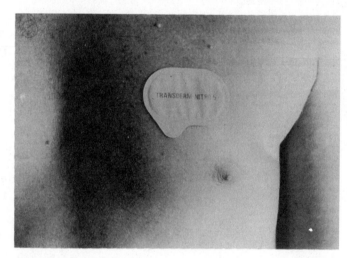

FIGURE 10–6 (B) When applied to the skin, Transderm-Nitro delivers nitroglycerin at a constant and predetermined rate through the skin directly into the bloodstream. One patch gives 24-hour protection against the pain of angina pectoris due to coronary artery disease. (Courtesy of Ciba-Geigy.)

FIGURE 10–6 (C) The Transderm-Nitro is a multilayer unit. It consists of a backing layer, a reservoir of nitroglycerin, a rate-controlling membrane, and an adhesive layer which has a priming dose of nitroglycerin. (Courtesy of Ciba-Geigy.)

CAUTIONS

If your physician has prescribed "under-the-tongue" nitroglycerin tablets in addition to Nitro-Dur II, you should sit down before taking the "under-the-tongue" tablet. If dizziness should occur, notify your physician. This may be an indication that the "under-the-tongue" tablet dosage needs to be reduced.

POSSIBLE SIDE EFFECTS

The most common side effect experienced by people taking nitroglycerin is headache. Your physician may tell you to take a mild analgesic to relieve the headache.

Some people may experience dizziness. This is due to a slight decrease in blood pressure, which is usually experienced when a person changes position, from lying flat to sitting upright or from sitting to standing. If this occurs, sit down until the dizziness stops, then notify your physician. He may wish to reduce your Nitro-Dur II dosage.

In some people, nitroglycerin preparations may cause the skin to feel flushed or the heart to beat faster. If this should occur, notify your physician; again, he may wish to change your Nitro-Dur II dosage.

Nitro-Dur II is a unique drug that depends on direct contact with the skin to work. For this reason, the skin should be reasonably hair-free, clean and dry.

INSTRUCTIONS FOR USE
PLACEMENT AREA

☐ Select a reasonably hair-free application site. **Avoid** extremities below the knee or elbow, skin folds, scar tissue, burned or irritated areas.

APPLICATION

☐ Wash hands before applying.

☐ Hold the unit with brown lines facing you, in an up and down position.

☐ Bend the sides of unit away from you.

☐ Then bend the sides toward you, until the clear plastic backing "snaps" down the middle.

☐ Peel off both halves of the clear plastic.

☐ Apply the sticky side of the unit to the selected body site.

☐ Wash hands to remove any drug.

☐ It is important to use a different application site every day.

REMOVAL

☐ Gently lift unit and slowly peel away from skin.

☐ Wash skin area with soap and water. Towel dry. Wash hands.

SKIN CARE

1. After you remove Nitro-Dur II, your skin may feel warm and appear red. This is normal. The redness will disappear in a short time. If the area feels dry, you may apply a soothing lotion.

2. Any redness or rash that does not disappear should be called to your physician's attention.

OTHER INFORMATION

1. Allow Nitro-Dur II to stay in place for 24 hours unless otherwise instructed by your physician.

2. Showering is permitted with Nitro-Dur II in place.

3. Apply your Nitro-Dur II the same time every day, preferably before going to bed. This allows it to adhere firmly to your skin while you are sleeping, when body movement is minimal.

4. Nitro-Dur II should be kept out of reach of children and pets.

5. Store at controlled room temperature—15-30° C (59-86° F). Do not refrigerate.

6. Nitro-Dur II is boxed so that you have a 30-day supply. Be sure to check your supply periodically. Before it runs low, you should visit your pharmacist for a refill or ask your physician to renew your Nitro-Dur II prescription.

7. It is important that you do not miss a day of your Nitro-Dur II therapy. If your schedule needs to be changed, your physician will give you specific instructions.

8. Nitro-Dur II has been prescribed for you. Do not give your medication to anyone else.

9. Nitro-Dur II is for prevention of angina; not for treatment of an acute anginal attack.

10. Notify physician if angina attacks change for the worse.

If you have any questions about Nitro-Dur II, ask your physician or pharmacist.

FIGURE 10–7 Transdermal infusion system for the administration of nitroglycerin (Courtesy of Key Pharmaceuticals.)

FIGURE 10–8 (A) Estraderm, a low-dose estrogen skin patch. Less than 2 inches in diameter, the wafer-thin patch contains 17-β estradiol, which is identical to the estrogen produced naturally before menopause. The patch releases small amounts of medication at a relatively constant and controlled rate through the skin directly into the bloodstream. It relieves such menopausal symptoms as hot flashes, night sweats, and vaginal dryness. The patch is worn on a dry, non-oily part of the trunk of the body. (Courtesy of Ciba-Geigy.)

1. A SEALED BACKING THAT HOLDS THE DRUG IN THE SYSTEM.
2. A RESERVOIR CONTAINING ESTRADIOL.
3. A MEMBRANE THAT CONTROLS THE RELEASE OF ESTRADIOL.
4. A NON-ALLERGENIC ADHESIVE THAT KEEPS THE PATCH ON THE SKIN.
5. A PROTECTIVE PEEL STRIP.

FIGURE 10–8 (B) The Estraderm skin patch is a multilayered unit. (Courtesy of Ciba-Geigy.)

a potential adverse reaction is possible for the person who applies the patch.

Several commonly prescribed medications are available as transdermal patches. Figure 10–6, page 486, shows the once-a-day Transderm-Nitro patch to help control the pain of angina. The instructions for use of another transdermal nitroglycerin infusing system are shown in Figure 10–7, page 487. Figure 10–8 shows a skin patch containing a low dosage of estradiol, a form of the hormone estrogen. The medication is used to relieve menopausal symptoms, such as hot flashes, night sweats, and vaginal dryness. Figure 10–9 shows the instructions for the use of a transdermal system of administering scopolamine for the prevention of nausea and vomiting due to motion sickness. You should remind patients that medications to prevent motion sickness should be taken or applied 4 hours before travel for effectiveness.

Transdermal patches containing timed-release amounts of nicotine have become popular as a means of quitting the cigarette habit. These are intended to curb the craving for smoking. Patients may obtain a prescription for the patches, which supply decreasing doses of nicotine over a 3-month period. The patch is changed every 24 hours. They are relatively

expensive, but the initial expense is a sound investment in the long run for good health. It is extremely important to determine the amount of nicotine the patient consumes daily before the patient begins this program. Patients who have been trying to quit the habit may already have reduced their nicotine intake. The daily dose of nicotine for the first month of transdermal patches must be carefully prescribed so the patient will not get too much nicotine. Excessive amounts of nicotine can produce unpleasant side effects including insomnia, heart palpitations, and tachycardia. Patients should also be warned against smoking while wearing the patches or these same side effects can occur with the risk of a heart attack. Consultation with each patient is necessary to establish individual needs.

How to Use Transderm Scōp

Transderm Scōp may be kept at room temperature until you are ready to use it.

1. Plan to apply one Transderm Scōp disc at least 4 hours before you need it. **Wear only one disc at any time.**
2. Select a hairless area of skin behind one ear, taking care to avoid any cuts or irritations. Wipe the area with a clean, dry tissue.
3. Peel the package open and remove the disc (Figure 1).
4. Remove the clear plastic six-sided backing from the round system. Try not to touch the adhesive surface on the disc with your hands (Figure 2).
5. Firmly apply the adhesive surface (metallic side) to the dry area of skin behind the ear so that the tan-colored side is showing (Figure 3). Make good contact, especially around the edge. Once you have placed the disc behind your ear, do not move it for as long as you want to use it (up to 3 days).
6. *Important:* **After the disc is in place, be sure to wash your hands thoroughly with soap and water to remove any scopolamine. If this drug were to contact your eyes, it could cause temporary blurring of vision and dilation (widening) of the pupils**

(the dark circles in the center of your eyes). This is not serious, and your pupils should return to normal.
7. Remove the disc after 3 days and throw it away. (You may remove it sooner if you are no longer concerned about motion sickness.) After removing the disc, be sure to wash your hands and the area behind your ear thoroughly with soap and water.
8. If you wish to control nausea for longer than 3 days, *remove* the first disc after 3 days and place a new one *behind the other ear,* repeating instructions 2 to 7.
9. Keep the disc dry, if possible, to prevent it from falling off. Limited contact with water, however, as in bathing or swimming, will not affect the system. In the unlikely event that the disc falls off, throw it away and put a new one behind the other ear.

This leaflet presents a summary of information about Transderm Scōp. If you would like more information or if you have any questions, ask your doctor or pharmacist. A more technical leaflet is available, written for your doctor. If you would like to read the leaflet, ask your pharmacist to show you a copy. You may need the help of your doctor or pharmacist to understand some of the information.

(Figure 1)

system
disposable backing

(Figure 2)

tan-colored system

(Figure 3)

FIGURE 10–9 Transderm Scop is a prescription transdermal system that administers scopolamine for the prevention of nausea and vomiting associated with motion sickness. The disc is placed behind the ear several hours before traveling and prevents symptoms for up to 3 days. (Courtesy of Ciba-Geigy.)

Vaginal Administration Vaginal medications are applied as creams, **suppositories,** tablets, **douches,** foams, ointments, tampons, sprays, and salves, Figure 10–10.

Considerations of Drug Action ....

Several considerations may affect how the body responds to a drug. These are age, weight, and **body surface area (BSA),** method of administration, **tolerance,** allergies, time, and **interaction.** Pediatric and geriatric patients, and some individuals, usually require a smaller dose than an average adult. To achieve a specific blood level of a medication, the dosage must be calculated according to the patient's weight. Special medications, such as chemotherapy drugs, are determined by the BSA, which is derived by plotting the patient's height and weight on a **nomogram.** The different methods of administering medications and the rate at which the body uses them varies. Medications given by injection are circulated in the bloodstream rapidly; transdermal patch **infusion** systems deliver small amounts of medication in a sustained timed-release manner; oral medicines take considerable time before they are absorbed by the small intestines, and so on for each of the methods. If a patient has to take a particular medication for a long period, a tolerance may develop. An increase in the amount or a change in medicine may be necessary for the desired effect to take place. An allergy to a medication may occur at any time in an individual. Careful attention must be given to the medical history and to the patient's responses during the interview. Further, the medical assistant must be alert to notice any notations in red ink signifying allergies. Many patients take several medications daily. Helping the patient determine what to take medicine with and when to take it will encourage the desired result.

Complete Chapter 10, Unit 2 in the workbook to help you meet the objectives at the beginning of this unit and therefore achieve competency of this subject matter.

FIGURE 10–10 Suppositories: vaginal and rectal

U N I T   3

Injections and Immunizations

OBJECTIVES ....

Upon completion of this unit you will meet the following terminal performance objectives by verifying knowledge of the facts and principles presented through oral and written communication at a level deemed competent by the instructor or employer, and will demonstrate the specific behaviors as identified in the terminal performance objectives of the procedures, observing all aseptic and safety precautions in accordance with health care standards.

1. Correctly identify the parts of a syringe and needle.
2. Name the tissue layers and sites of injection for intradermal, intramuscular, and subcutaneous injections.
3. Demonstrate how to administer intradermal, intramuscular, and subcutaneous injections properly.
4. Demonstrate how to reassure an apprehensive patient in preparation for an injection.
5. Demonstrate how to recap a needle properly after filling a syringe from a vial or an ampule.
6. Demonstrate the proper way to discard a used needle and syringe.
7. List and explain the immunization schedule for normal infants and children and adults.
8. Explain the importance of informing patients, or the responsible party for a minor, verbally and in writing, of both the benefits and the risks of immunizations before they are administered.
9. Discuss the importance of patient education regarding medications.
10. Demonstrate how to instruct patients in self-administration of insulin injections.
11. Identify the various sites for administering insulin injections.
12. Spell and define, using the glossary at the back of the text, all the words to know in this unit.

WORDS TO KNOW ....

ampule	epiglottis	intradermal
anaphylactic	flu	intramuscular
antitoxin	haemophilus	intravenous
attenuated	hepatitis B	lethal
booster	HIB/Hib	measles
catarrhal stage	immunization	meningitis
cholera	immunoglobulin	mumps
debridement	incubation	paroxysmal stage
decline stage	influenza	pertussis
diphtheria	inoculate	photophobia
disciplinary	insulin	polio

retardation	series	trimester
risk	subcutaneous	typhoid
rubella	tetanus	vaccine
rubeola	toxin	vial
sensitivity	toxoid	Z-tract

Injections ....

You will be helping to prepare and possibly to administer medications in the form of injections. Since this method of medication introduces the substance directly into the tissues, where it quickly enters the patient's bloodstream, extreme caution must be practiced. The proper technique must be learned under supervision. Latex gloves should be worn to administer an injection. Medication should only be given to patients when a physician is available nearby should the patient exhibit any adverse reaction. There is always a possibility of **anaphylactic** shock. Refer to Chapter 8, Unit 1 for symptoms of anaphylactic shock. In the event that this situation occurs, the physician should be notified to administer the immediate treatment of injecting epinephrine just above the initial injection site. Following the injection into the muscle or subcutaneous tissue, the area should be massaged. This is to aid in speeding the distribution of the epinephrine into the circulatory system as fast as possible. You should keep taking the patient's vital signs until the patient is stable. Provisions should always be made for emergency situations. Even though the patient's past history reveals no **sensitivity** to a particular drug, there is no guarantee of what the next dose may do.

The term *hypodermic* simply means under the skin. You must become familiar with the parts of the syringe and needle as well as proficient in handling them. Figure 10–11 pictures a needle and syringe with labeled parts. Practice with different types of syringes and needles; filling the syringe with varying amounts of sterile water from a **vial** and **ampule** will

FIGURE 10–11 A hypodermic needle and 3-cc syringe

General Guidelines for Teaching Patients about Medications

The following are general considerations patients need to know about taking prescribed medication:

1. Take only the medicine that has been prescribed by the physician for you.
2. Never share your medicine with anyone else, not even family members.
3. Take your prescribed medication when and only as directed, not more or less, to maintain proper blood level for its desired effect in your treatment.
4. Keep *all* medicines (or any chemicals) out of the reach of children.
5. Phone the physician's office immediately if you experience any reaction (regardless of how minor) to any medication or immunization.
6. Report any OTC or home remedy medication that you are taking to the physician.
7. Eat a well-balanced diet and include plenty of fluids while taking your medication. (Avoid foods or beverages that you have been instructed to stay away from because they may interfere with the action of the medicine).
8. Refrain from alcoholic beverages or any other drugs (both OTC and home-remedy type) that are not prescribed by the physician while you are taking prescribed medication to avoid dangerous side effects.
9. Women should report to the physician if they are pregnant, plan to become pregnant, or are nursing mothers before taking any medication.
10. Never save some of your prescription for a later date (i.e., antibiotics, take only as directed).
11. Throw old medicines away—flush down the toilet—after they are 6 months old.
12. Direct questions that patients have regarding diet, activity, dosage, or any concern about their medications to the physician's attention immediately.
13. To avoid confusion and gain compliance, explain to patients that generic products and brand name products are the same.
14. Caution patients about taking medications that could cause them to become sleepy, interfere with their concentration, or affect their ability to operate machinery or drive.

give you confidence. Use an orange to practice inserting different needle lengths at different angles of injection, Figure 10–12. This should be done under supervision for instruction, practice, evaluation, and correction in developing proper technique. While becoming proficient in handling the syringe and needle confidently, and thereafter, one must use caution to avoid dangerous needle sticks. It is recommended that to prevent injuries needles *never* be recapped. Used needles and syringes should be discarded intact in the biohazardous sharps waste container. Even though you are strongly urged to never recap needles, in reality it may be necessary in certain circumstances to do so. For your safety you should recap a needle by placing your nondominant hand behind your back, and holding the syringe and needle intact "scoop" the cap onto the needle, Figure 10–13. Secure the cap onto the hub of the syringe by pressing the tip against a hard surface. Keeping your other hand behind you will lessen the chance of being tempted to use it to recap the needle, the point at which most needle sticks occur. Some needle and syringe units have a shield that locks into place over the used needle to prevent injury to the user.

Injectible medications also come in single-dose, prefilled, disposable sterile syringes and cartridges. This method guarantees an accurate dosage and is also convenient and time-saving. The single-dose units are assembled by inserting the cartridge into a reusable injector as illustrated in Figure 10–14.

In injecting medications, technique is extremely important.

If injections are given carelessly, injury to the nerves, blood vessels, and tissues can occur, as can infection. These can lead to legal action. When proper technique is used, however, giving medications by injection can be a minimally painful experience for the patient.

You can help relieve the patient's anxiety by explaining the procedure. Being honest with patients is most important. In the case of children's immunizations, for example, it is far better to explain that the injection will hurt for a minute, than to say

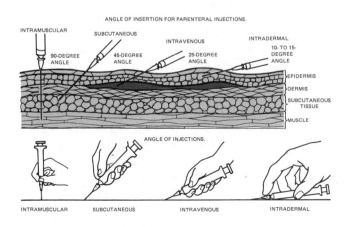

FIGURE 10–12 Angle of injections

FIGURE 10–13 (a) Keeping one hand behind your back, "scoop" the cap onto the needle carefully so it does not become contaminated. (b) Secure the cap onto the hub of the syringe by pressing the tip against a hard surface.

it won't hurt at all. You may give the child a simplified explanation of the disease for which the immunization is meant. This may help the child understand how it is really better in the long run to hurt for a minute rather than to suffer the dreaded disease. If the child shows extreme apprehension, it is advisable to have assistance in restraining the child before proceeding with the injection. Instructing parents in how they can explain injections to their children can be helpful. Unfortunately, many parents use injections as disciplinary threats. This is not an acceptable practice. It not only creates anxiety for the child but makes the work of the health care team more difficult. Some pharmaceutical companies provide badges of courage or other awards to pediatric patients who display bravery in receiving their immunization injections. This gives the child a sense of pride in good behavior and makes future visits much easier for all concerned.

Authorization forms should be in order before immunizations are administered to minors. You should allow sufficient time for parents (or those responsible for the child) to read the information regarding the vaccine and have all questions answered before obtaining the authorization signature. This form must be filed in the patient's chart.

The site to be injected should be free from restricting clothing. Patients should be asked to remove these items of clothing while the medication is being prepared.

Follow correct gloving procedure before you begin to administer the injection. Proper preparation of the skin at the site of injection is necessary before and after injecting the medication, since microorganisms can enter the body through a break in the skin. Alcohol is the antiseptic usually used, because it is least irritating to the skin and is economical.

Proper disposal of used needles and syringes is also of vital importance in preventing possible accidents to the medical and custodial staff of the facility and avoiding transmission of dis-

ease. Nondisposable needles and syringes must be properly sanitized and autoclaved before using again. Disposable syringes and needles should be used only once and discarded properly. Keep the needle guard on the needle until just before you are ready to administer the injection (again, this is a situation where recapping a needle may be necessary. Remember to scoop the cap onto the needle; do not use your other hand or you risk a needle stick, besides risking contamination of the needle before it is to be used for injecting the patient.) Afterward dispose of the entire syringe and needle intact in the biohazardous sharps container according to universal precautions recommendations. *Do not recap.* Remove latex gloves before washing your hands.

Before you can become proficient in injecting medications, you must first learn to withdraw medications into the syringe accurately. Medications for injection are available in single-dose and multiple-dose ampules or vials.

Intradermal Injections Intradermal injections are used in allergy and tuberculin testing. The intradermal injection is administered just under the surface of the skin with a fine-gauge needle, 26G or 27G. The needle is generally ⅜ to ⅝ inch in length, and the angle of the insertion into the skin 10 to 15 degrees, Figure 10–18. The sites for this type of injection are usually the anterior forearm and the mid back area. Proper positioning of patients is vital for the accuracy of results as well as for the patient's comfort. Intradermal injections themselves go very quickly, but the patient must be observed for 20 minutes or more after the administration. Make sure the patient's forearm is supported on the treatment table while sitting comfortably, or have the patient lie on the treatment table.

A small wheal should develop at the site of the injection to give evidence that the medication is in the dermal layer of the skin. Very small amounts of medication, from 0.01 to 0.05 cc,

TUBEX® Injector

NOTE: The TUBEX® Injector is reusable: do not discard.

DIRECTIONS FOR USE:

Ribbed Collar
Plunger
Plunger Rod
TUBEX® Sterile Cartridge-Needle Unit

To load a TUBEX® Sterile Cartridge-Needle Unit into the TUBEX® Injector

CLOSE   OPEN

1. Turn the ribbed collar to the "OPEN" position until it stops.

2. Hold the Injector with the open end up and fully insert the TUBEX® Sterile Cartridge-Needle Unit.

Firmly tighten the ribbed collar in the direction of the "CLOSE" arrow.

CLOSE

3. Thread the plunger rod into the plunger of the TUBEX® Sterile Cartridge-Needle Unit until slight resistance is felt.

The Injector is now ready for use in the usual manner.

Ribbed Collar
Plunger Rod
Plunger
E.S.I. DOSETTE® Sterile Cartridge-Needle Unit

To load an E.S.I. DOSETTE® Sterile Cartridge-Needle Unit into the TUBEX® Injector

CLOSE   OPEN

1. Turn the ribbed collar to the "OPEN" position until it stops.

2. Hold the Injector with the open end up and fully insert the E.S.I. DOSETTE® Sterile Cartridge-Needle Unit.

Firmly tighten the ribbed collar in the direction of the "CLOSE" arrow.

CLOSE

3. Thread the plunger rod into the plunger of the E.S.I. DOSETTE® Sterile Cartridge-Needle Unit until slight resistance is felt.

---

4. Engage the needle-cap assembly by pulling the cap down over the silver cartridge hub. The needle is fully engaged when the silver hub is completely covered.

The Injector is now ready for use in the usual manner.

To administer

Method of administration is the same as with conventional syringe. Remove needle cover by grasping it securely; twist and pull. Introduce needle into patient, aspirate by pulling back slightly on the plunger, and inject.

To remove the empty TUBEX® or DOSETTE® Cartridge-Needle Unit and dispose into a vertical needle disposal container

1. Do not recap the needle. Disengage the plunger rod.

2. Hold the Injector, needle down, over a vertical needle disposal container and loosen the ribbed collar. TUBEX® or DOSETTE® Cartridge-Needle Unit will drop into the container.

OPEN

3. Discard the needle cover.

To remove the empty TUBEX® or DOSETTE® Cartridge-Needle Unit and dispose into a horizontal (mailbox) needle disposal container

1. Do not recap the needle. Disengage the plunger rod.

2. Open the horizontal (mailbox) needle disposal container. Insert TUBEX® or DOSETTE® Cartridge-Needle Unit, needle pointing down, halfway into container. Close the container lid on cartridge. Loosen ribbed collar; TUBEX® or DOSETTE® Cartridge-Needle Unit will drop into the container.

3. Discard the needle cover.

The TUBEX® Injector is reusable and should not be discarded.

Used TUBEX® or DOSETTE® Cartridge-Needle Units should not be employed for successive injections or as multiple-dose containers. They are intended to be used only once and discarded.

NOTE: Any graduated markings on TUBEX® or DOSETTE® Sterile Cartridge-Needle Units are to be used only as a guide in mixing, withdrawing, or administering measured doses.

Wyeth-Ayerst does not recommend and will not accept responsibility for the use of any cartridge-needle units other than TUBEX® or E.S.I. DOSETTE® Cartridge-Needle Units in the TUBEX® Injector.

FIGURE 10–14   Directions for using the TUBEX "Hands-Off" injector. Note that latex gloves should be worn when administering any injection. (Courtesy of Wyeth-Ayerst Laboratories.)

P R O C E D U R E

Withdraw Medication from Ampule

PURPOSE: To withdraw an ordered amount of medication into a syringe from an ampule.

EQUIPMENT: Ampule of medication (sterile water for injection), medication tray, sterile gauze square, sterile needle and syringe

TERMINAL PERFORMANCE OBJECTIVE: Provided with all necessary equipment and supplies, demonstrate each of the steps required to withdraw medication (sterile water for instructional purposes) from an ampule; the procedure will be repeated three times, each time withdrawing a specific quantity of fluid as predetermined by the instructor.

1. Place sterile gauze square over middle of ampule and hold ampule between thumb and index finger of one hand, Figure 10–15. **RATIONALE: Sterile gauze will keep any fragments of glass from flying.**

2. Flick pointed end of ampule with index finger to release medication into bottom of ampule before opening.

3. Grasp tip of ampule and snap it off. Discard tip.

4. Make sure that syringe and needle are secured by turning barrel to right while holding needle guard. Remove guard.

5. Expel air from syringe by pushing down on plunger. Insert tip of needle into solution while holding ampule in upright position. *Note: Do not touch the rim of ampule to maintain sterile technique.*

6. Draw back plunger quickly and steadily to fill syringe with medication, Figure 10–16. Keep needle point below meniscus level of liquid to avoid air bubbles entering syringe. *(Note: If air bubbles do enter, turn syringe pointing up and gently tap the barrel to free the bubbles to the top. Gently push plunger up to release the air bubbles.)*

7. Replace needle guard by gently scooping it onto the needle to maintain sterility and safety. Place filled syringe on medication tray.

8. Discard ampule and gauze in proper receptacle.

FIGURE 10–15 Snap open the ampule using sterile gauze for protection from possible flying glass fragments.

FIGURE 10–16 Keep the needle point below the meniscus of the liquid with the ampule upright.

P R O C E D U R E

Withdraw Medication from Vial

PURPOSE: To withdraw an ordered amount of medication into a syringe from a vial.

EQUIPMENT: Multiple- and single-dose vials (sterile water for injection), alcohol-saturated cotton balls, sterile needle and syringe, medication tray

TERMINAL PERFORMANCE OBJECTIVE: Provided with all necessary equipment and supplies, demonstrate each of the steps required in withdrawing medication (sterile water for instructional purposes) from multiple- and single-dose vials; the procedure will be repeated three times, each time withdrawing a specific quantity of fluid as predetermined by the instructor.

1. Calculate dosage if required and wash hands.
2. Use alcohol-saturated cotton ball to clean rubber-topped vial.
3. Secure needle onto syringe by holding needle guard and turning barrel of syringe to right.
4. Remove needle guard and pull back on plunger to fill syringe with same amount of air as medication that has been ordered. **RATIONALE: This prevents vacuum from forming in vial and thus makes it easier to withdraw solution.**
5. Hold syringe by barrel between thumb and fingers and with other hand hold vial upside-down, Figure 10–17. Insert needle into rubber top and push plunger in, expelling air into vial.
6. Pull back on plunger so desired amount of medication will flow into syringe, keeping needle below level of solution to avoid air bubbles. *Note: Air takes up space where medication should be, and the dosage would not be correct if air remained.* To release air bubbles if they appear, flick barrel of syringe with finger in quick, hard motion. They will be released into hub of syringe. Push plunger carefully to make sure they are out of needle. Withdraw needle from vial.

FIGURE 10–17 Hold the vial upside-down at eye level and insert the needle into the rubber-topped vial.

7. Let go of plunger. Hold barrel of syringe and pull needle out of vial, keeping syringe in vertical position. Check for air bubbles. Replace needle guard by carefully scooping it onto the needle to keep needle sterile and for safety.
8. Keep medication with loaded syringe on medication tray to ensure proper identification. Place alcohol-saturated cotton ball with syringe to administer medication.

are administered by this method. The patient should be watched carefully and any reaction reported to the physician at once. The speed of the reaction and the size of the wheal should be recorded. Most allergy testing is done under the direct supervision of the physician. In the event of a hypersensitive reaction, a preparation of epinephrine may be injected by order of the physician.

Subcutaneous Injections Subcutaneous injections are used to administer small doses of medication, usually not more than 2.0 cc. The injection is most often given in the upper outer part of the arm (deltoid area), abdominal area, or upper thigh

(midvastus lateralis area), Figure 10–20, page 498. The length of the needle ranges from ½ to ⅝ inch and the gauge from 25G to 27G. Subcutaneous injections are administered at a 45-degree angle of insertion. Many medications, including allergy injections, insulin, and immunizations are administered by the subcutaneous method. Refer to Chapter 8, Unit 1 for specific details in giving allergy injections. The patient should be asked to sit or lie on the treatment table for safety.

Intramuscular Injections As the name suggests, **intramuscular** (IM) injections are made into muscle tissue. The most common sites for this method of injection are the deltoid (upper outer arm), gluteus medius (upper outer portion of the hip), ventrogluteal (lateral outside portion of the hip), and vastus lateralis (midportion of the thigh), Figures 10–21 and 10–22, page 499. Proper positioning of patients is important. For injections in the deltoid area, the patient should be sitting. If the site is the gluteus muscle, ask the patient to lie in the prone position on the treatment table with the toes pointed inward, or to lean over the treatment table and stand on the noninjection-site leg. This will allow the muscle to relax and make the procedure much easier. For injection of the vastus lateralis site, the patient may be sitting or lying in the horizontal recumbent position.

The site of injection must be recorded so that injection sites can be rotated. This practice is necessary when patients receive injections routinely, so the possibility of muscle tissue damage is reduced.

In the administration of IM injections, the needle is from 1 to 3 inches in length or longer, for it must penetrate many layers of tissue. The angle of injection is 90 degrees. IM injections are indicated when large doses of medication or irritating substances must be given. Dosage may vary from 0.5 to 3.0 mL. Medications given by IM method are absorbed quickly by the rich blood supply of the muscle tissue.

The gauge of the needle ranges between 18G and 23G to accommodate the density of the substance. In giving injections intramuscularly to pediatric patients, the gauge and length of the needle may be smaller.

10°

FIGURE 10–18 Intradermal injection

For injecting substances that may be irritating or cause discoloration of the subcutaneous tissues, the **Z-tract** IM method is used. Tissue is displaced by holding it to the side of the injection site. Following injection of the medication, the tissue is moved back over the site blocking any residual substance. Using this technique prevents the irritating medication from following the path of the needle and leaking out into the tissues. After Z-tract IM administration, the injection site should not be massaged because this action would encourage the irritating substance to circulate into the subcutaneous tissues.

Intravenous Injections The **intravenous,** or IV, method of injection is used by the physician usually in an emergency situation. You are not qualified to administer medications by this method but may prepare medications to be given intravenously. IV medications have an immediate effect on the patient for they are introduced directly into the bloodstream. Needles are 1 to 1½ inches in length and are usually 20G to 21G. Intravenous preparations vary in amount from a few milliliters to much larger doses, which are given by IV drip. The items needed are needle and syringe, medication, tourniquet, alcohol-saturated cotton balls, adhesive bandage, and IV stand if necessary.

Usually you will draw up medication into the syringe for an intravenous injection. After filling the syringe, be sure to recap the needle carefully by the scoop method to avoid contaminating the needle. You then place the vial or ampule on the medication tray so that the physician can check to be certain it is correct. You may be asked to stay with the patient while waiting for the emergency squad or ambulance to transport the patient to the hospital. Observing the patient for signs of distress and reactions to the administered medication is an important responsibility. The physician must be notified immediately of any complications. All information should be recorded on the patient's chart.

The medical assistant is often the one who will give instruction to the diabetic patient in the technique of self-administration of daily **insulin** injections. You may be of great help in demonstrating the proper method of filling a syringe, preparing the injection site, and acquiring skill in injecting the insulin. Figure 10–23, pages 500–501, shows a step-by-step self-injection outline for the patient who needs daily insulin injection. Generally, the physician teaches the patient initially about diet, dosage, and the different types of insulin. You may be delegated to do follow-up patient education in this area. Since the insulin-dependent diabetic patient must self-administer this injection at home at least once each day, you should instruct the patient to follow a pattern of rotation of injection sites, an example of which is shown in Figure 10–24, page 503. Explain to the patient to number each area of the body that is injected each time in the boxes in an alternating rotation pattern. This method offers the patient the means to develop his or her own personal schedule. Printed patient education material for patients is available from most pharmaceutical companies to help patients gain an understanding of their diabetes. You may also want to refer patients

P R O C E D U R E

Administer Intradermal Injection

PURPOSE: To inject liquid solutions of 0.01 cc and 0.05 cc into the dermal layer of tissue for allergy and immunity testing of patients.

EQUIPMENT: Medication (sterile water for injection in vial/ampule), cotton balls, adhesive bandage (or hypoallergenic tape), sterile needle and syringe (needle is usually ⅜ to ⅝ inch length and 25G to 27G), medication tray, alcohol, patient's chart, pen, latex gloves

TERMINAL PERFORMANCE OBJECTIVE: Provided with all necessary equipment and supplies, demonstrate each of the steps required in administering an intradermal injection; three injections will be administered to a latex training arm with the instructor observing each step. The dosage amount will be determined by the instructor each time.

1. Wash and glove hands. **CAUTION:** Be extremely careful when using the "scoop" method for recapping the needle by always placing the hand you are not using behind your back so you will not be tempted to help with the procedure. Prepare syringe with ordered amount of medication. Replace needle guard by carefully scooping it onto the needle. *Note: Read label of medication and compare with order.*

2. Place medication tray near patient. Compare medication order with patient's chart, identify patient, and explain procedure.

3. Use alcohol-saturated cotton ball to clean injection site. Allow alcohol to air dry. Do not blow on the area to dry. **RATIONALE: The area may be contaminated by microorganisms in the exhaled air.**

4. Remove needle guard. Hold patient's skin taut between thumb and fingers to steady area to be injected. With other hand insert needle at a 10- to 15-degree angle of insertion and slowly expel medication from syringe by depressing plunger. *Note: Bevel of needle should be up; this allows the material to produce a wheal by infiltrating the dermal layer of the skin.*

5. Remove needle quickly by the same angle of insertion and wipe site with alcohol-saturated cotton ball. *Note:*

Do not massage injection site. **RATIONALE: Massaging distributes the material throughout the tissues.**

6. Observe patient and time reaction. Give patient instructions as ordered and answer any questions. Determine if patient is allergic to adhesive before applying a bandage. Hypoallergenic tape is recommended.

FIGURE 10–19 Discard the entire used syringe and needle intact into a sharps biohazardous container to prevent dangerous needle sticks.

7. Wash and prepare any reusable items for sterilization. Discard any disposable items and gloves into biohazardous waste bag. (Place entire syringe and needle intact into the biohazardous sharps container according to universal precautions recommendations, Figure 10–19.) Wash hands. Return medication and tray to proper storage area.

8. Record information and initial.

---

to educational programs held at local hospitals or through the American Diabetes Association.

Immunizations ....

Our immune system acts immediately in response to invasion of disease-causing microorganisms. If the exposure to the disease is slight and our susceptibility is low, our immune response may defend us from coming down with the disease itself. However, if we are susceptible to the disease, meaning our resistance is low, we come down with the disease, experience the symptoms, and are sick. Antibodies are produced to protect us, making us resistant to further attacks of the specific pathogen that has made us sick. For instance, if one gets mumps, the body produces antibodies to destroy the mumps-causing organisms. After recovery

FIGURE 10–20 Subcutaneous injection

from this illness, antibodies against mumps will protect one from coming down with mumps again. This is a process which is called *natural immunity*.

Artificial immunity is produced by administering **immunizations** or **vaccines** made from the dead or harmless infectious agents that trigger the immune response in the body to manufacture antibodies against the particular disease-causing agent. Occasionally, one has a slight reaction during this process by experiencing mild symptoms of the disease or having a slight fever. In this process one becomes immune (resistant) to the disease. The immunization schedule, Table 10–6, page 502, is the recommendation of public health officials in the United States against the usual childhood diseases (UCHD) and suggested vaccines for adults (especially high-**risk** patients). Immunization schedules may vary in other countries for infants, children, and adults. You should make sure that the patient does not have an active illness or fever before administering any immunization. If the patient is ill, the vaccine should be rescheduled when the patient is well. Also check the patient's health and medical history to be sure the patient has no past history of convulsions or allergies of any kind. If an allergy is known, bring it to the attention of the physician *before* the vaccine is administered. You may want to look the immunization up in a medications reference book for con-

FIGURE 10–22 IM sites: ventrogluteal and vastus lateralis

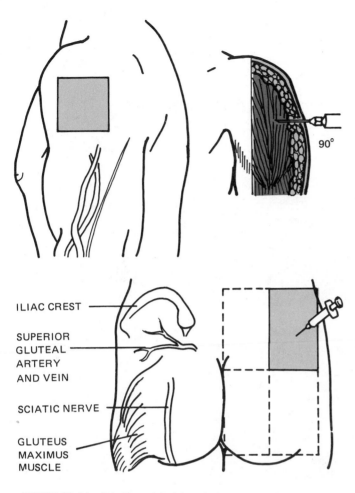

FIGURE 10–21 IM sites: deltoid and gluteus medius

traindications, precautions, and warnings. It is strongly advised that the parent of patient be made aware of the benefits and risks of all vaccines. Sufficient time should be given to the responsible person to read printed material after a verbal explanation is given regarding the vaccine(s). An opportunity must be provided for any questions of the parent or patient to be answered by the doctor before administration of immunization(s). When more than one dose of a vaccine is necessary to reach adequate immunization against a particular disease, such as the DPT injections, it is referred to as a primary **"series."** Each of these should be given with at least 6 to 8 weeks between each dose within a reasonable period of time. The primary series requires a **booster** for the immunization to be most effective and complete. In years past, these diseases were dreadful illnesses, which often caused death and affected children and adults. In the following text is a brief description of each of the diseases, the symptoms, the method of transmission, **incubation** period, and its treatment. This is to help you in answering questions about the diseases in the immunization schedule when patients ask "why" they need to have the vaccine. Childhood illnesses, which can be largely prevented with immunizations, are increasing in great numbers. Over half the young population in the nation is unprotected from these preventable diseases. It is strongly urged that

you provide patient education in this extremely important matter. Encourage the adult caregivers to immunize their young loved ones against these potentially fatal childhood diseases. Be ready to answer their questions concerning the risks versus the protection that is provided with vaccines. Certainly a short period of discomfort is well worth the minor suffering to gain protection from a potentially fatal disease.

The anatomy and physiology section of this text (Chapter 4) provides information regarding pneumonia and influenza, which are diseases affecting the respiratory system. A brief description follows.

Influenza. Commonly referred to as "the **flu**," **influenza** is a disease caused by a myxovirus that affects the respiratory tract. It is spread by direct contact, by droplet infection from the vapor of coughing and sneezing from an infected person, and by indirect contact from handling soiled items (such as used tissues) of the patient. The incubation period is between 1 and 4 days. Symptoms include sudden onset of fever, chills, sore throat, cough, muscle aches and pains, general malaise, and weakness. Treatment for the flu consists of bed rest, increased intake of fluids, antipyretics, and mild analgesics. Immunization against some strains of influenza is recommended for high-risk patients, such as the elderly, those with chronic illness, respiratory distress, or other conditions that warrant protection from infectious disease.

Pneumonia. This is an acute inflammation of the lungs. Eighty-five percent of pneumonia cases are caused by the

Preparing and Injecting the Dose of Insulin

Preparing the Dose of Insulin

1 Wash your hands.

2 Gently roll the insulin bottle several times to mix the insulin. Be sure it is completely mixed. Do not shake bottle. Flip off the colored protective cap on the bottle, but **do not** remove the rubber stopper.

3 Wipe top of bottle with alcohol swab.

4 Remove the needle cover. Draw air into the syringe by pulling back on the plunger. The amount of air should be equal to your insulin dose.

5 Put the needle through rubber top of insulin bottle. Push plunger in. The air injected into the bottle will allow insulin to be easily withdrawn into syringe.

6 Turn bottle and syringe upside down in one hand. Be sure tip of needle is in insulin. Your other hand will be free to move the plunger. Draw back on plunger slowly to draw the correct dose of insulin into syringe.

7 Check for air bubbles. The air is harmless, but too large an air bubble will reduce the insulin dose. To remove air bubbles, push insulin back into the bottle and measure your correct dose of insulin.

8 Double-check your dose. Remove needle from bottle. Cover needle with guard or lay syringe down so that needle does not touch anything.

FIGURE 10–23 Instructions for self-administration of insulin (Courtesy of Eli Lilly and Company.)

Injecting the Dose of Insulin

1 Cleanse the skin where the injection is to be made.

2 With one hand, stabilize the skin by spreading it or pinching up a large area of skin. Pick up syringe with other hand and hold it as you would a pencil. Insert needle straight into the skin (90° angle). Be sure to insert needle all the way.

3 Push the plunger all the way down, using less than five seconds to inject the dose.

4 Hold alcohol swab near the needle and pull needle straight out of skin. Press alcohol swab over injection site for several seconds.

5 Use disposable syringe only once to ensure sterility of syringe and needle and accuracy of dose. Destroy syringes as directed.

6 If you are taking more than one injection a day, use a new syringe every time, unless recommended otherwise by your physician, nurse-educator, or pharmacist, and follow the same steps.

Any change of insulin should be made cautiously and only under medical supervision.

Humulin®
human insulin
(recombinant DNA origin)

ILETIN® **I**
beef-pork insulin

ILETIN® **II**
purified pork insulin
purified beef insulin

FIGURE 10–23
(Continued)

pneumococcus bacterium, *Streptococcus pneumoniae*. Pneumonia may also be caused by other bacteria, as well as by a virus, rickettsia, and fungi. The pneumococcus bacterium disease (pneumonitis) is spread by droplet infection and direct contact with an infected person. The incubation period is only a few hours after exposure to the bacterium. The symptoms are abrupt in onset and include severe chills, high fever, headache, chest pain, dyspnea, rapid pulse, cyanosis, and cough with blood-stained sputum. Bed rest, increased fluid intake, analgesics, antipyretics, and in many cases oxygen, are necessary for successful treatment of the patient. Pneumovax

is a vaccine to protect high-risk patients from contracting the disease.

Haemophilus influenza Type B. Hemophilus, or **haemophilus,** also known as **Hib** and **HIB,** is a disease caused by the small gram-negative, nonmotile parasitic bacterium, *Haemophilus influenzae,* that leads to severe destructive inflammation of the larynx, trachea, and bronchi. The disease is transmitted by droplet airborne infection. Incubation is from 1 to 3 days. The symptoms are sudden onset of fever, sore throat, cough, muscle aches, weakness, and general malaise. General care is bed rest, increased fluid intake, antipyretics, antibiotics, and analgesics as necessary. Because this particular disease affects infants and small children, immunization is recommended to this population. Each year this illness attacks 1 in every 200 infants in the United States; the most at-risk group is between the ages of 6 months and 5 years. With the rise in popularity of day care centers, immunization against the Hib bacterium is a most sensible way to prevent this often resistant-to-antibiotic disease from spreading through the very young population in the United States. Complications of this childhood disease include **meningitis,** which could result in damage to the nervous system, or in mental **retardation; epiglottitis,** could cause a child to choke to death if immediate treatment is not given; and joint infections, and forms of crippling arthritis. The Hib vaccine is administered in a series of three subcutaneous or intramuscular injections at ages 2, 4, and 6 months, see Table 10–6. A booster is given at age 15 months.

Measles, Mumps, and Rubella (MMR). The MMR vaccine protects children from three childhood diseases. **Measles** is medically termed **rubeola.** It is also referred to as "old-fashioned," and 10-day, measles. It is spread by direct contact, droplet infection, and by indirect contact from infected items of a patient. It has a 10- to 21-day incubation period. In the prodromal stage (earliest) the patient exhibits fever, malaise, runny nose, cough, sometimes conjunctivitis, and progresses with loss of appetite, **photophobia,** sore throat, and eventually Koplik's spots (the red skin rash). The cause is the rubeola virus, which is an acute and highly contagious viral disease involving the respiratory tract. Complications of measles can result in deafness, brain damage, and pneumonia. Treatment for measles is bed rest, increased fluid intake, antipyretics, antibiotics, cough medicine, and calamine lotion. The patient should be kept in isolation to prevent transmission to others. Quiet activity is suggested for the patient during recovery time, usually a few days.

Mumps is an acute contagious febrile disease that causes inflammation of the parotid and salivary glands. Parotitis is transmitted by droplet infection or direct contact with an infected person. The usual incubation period is from 14 to 28 days. Symptoms include chills and fever, headache, and pain below and in front of the ear(s) for 5 to 7 days' duration. Another symptom is pain between the ear and the angle of the jaw with drinking or eating acidic substances. Bed rest and a soft diet, including increased fluid intake, is recommended. Application of cold packs to control swelling of the glands of the neck, and in males, of the testicles in orchitis, is advised.

Rubella, also called German measles or 3-day measles, is an acute contagious viral disease characterized by an upper respiratory infection. If a female acquires rubella during the

TABLE 10–6
Immunization Schedule of Normal Infants and Children

Age	Vaccine(s)
Birth to 2 months	Hepatitis B
2 months	DTP-1, (diphtheria, tetanus **toxoid,** and pertussis vaccines) Hib *Haemophilus influenzae* - type B OPV-1 (oral, attenuated poliovirus vaccine)
Between 2 and 4 months	Hepatitis B
4 months	DTP-2, Hib OPV-2
6 months	DTP-3, Hib
12 to 15 months	Hepatitis B
15 months	MMR 1 (measles, mumps, rubella), Hib
18 months	DTP-4 OPV-3 (completes primary series)
4–6 years	DTP-5, MMR 2 OPV-4
14–16 years	Td (adult tetanus and diphtheria toxoid) (should be repeated every 10 years)

Adult Immunizations	
Td	every 10 years (more often if severe or dirty injury or laceration)
Pneumovax	Once administered at age 60–65
Influenza A and B	Annually, age 65 and older
Hepatitis B	One series of three injections

P R O C E D U R E

Administer Subcutaneous Injection

PURPOSE: To inject aqueous solutions of 0.5 to 2.0 cc into the subcutaneous tissue.

EQUIPMENT: Medication (sterile water for injection in vial or ampule), alcohol, cotton balls, adhesive bandage (hypoallergenic tape), sterile needle and syringe (needle is usually ½ to ⅝ inch, 25G), latex gloves

TERMINAL PERFORMANCE OBJECTIVE: Provided with all necessary equipment and supplies, demonstrate each of the steps required in administering a subcutaneous injection; three injections will be administered to a latex training arm with the instructor observing each step. The dosage amount will be determined by the instructor each time.

1. Compare orders with medication and wash and glove hands. **CAUTION**: Prepare syringe and place it on medication tray.
2. Compare medication order with patient's chart, identify patient, explain procedure, and ask patient to remove clothing if necessary.
3. Use alcohol-saturated cotton ball to clean injection site. Remove needle guard.
4. Hold patient's skin taut between thumb and fingers of one hand and with other hand hold syringe securely.
5. Insert needle (bevel down) at a 45-degree angle with a steady penetration. Let go of patient's skin.
6. With one hand hold barrel of syringe while pulling back on plunger slightly with other hand to make sure a blood vessel has not been penetrated. If no blood appears in syringe, proceed by slowly pushing down on plunger to expel medication into tissues. *Note: If blood appears in syringe, pull needle out carefully at angle of entry. Discard medication, syringe, and needle. Replace with new syringe and medication.* **RATIONALE: Blood in the needle indicates the possibility of the needle placement being within a blood vessel. Medication injected directly into the bloodstream causes rapid absorption and may cause undesirable as well as dangerous results.**

7. Pull needle out at angle of insertion and wipe injection site with alcohol-saturated cotton ball. Replace with dry one and gently massage area. **RATIONALE: Massaging the site helps distribute medication throughout the tissue.**

8. Observe patient for possible reaction and report to physician if a reaction occurs. Extra caution must be taken when giving desensitizing allergy injections. Reactions may take 15 to 20 minutes to develop. Instruct patient to wait for a full 20 minutes in case of a possible reaction. Answer any questions. Determine if patient is allergic to adhesive before applying a bandage. Hypoallergenic tape is recommended.

9. Discard all used disposable items. (Place entire syringe and needle in sharps container.) Wash and sterilize all reusable items, remove gloves, and wash hands. Return medication and tray to proper storage area.

10. Record information and initial.

---

first **trimester** of pregnancy, fetal abnormalities may result. You should remind female patients in childbearing years of this concern and encourage them to be tested for a rubella antibody titer, or to be vaccinated before becoming pregnant. *Females should not be vaccinated during pregnancy.* Be sure to determine whether a patient is pregnant before administering the vaccine. Rubella is transmitted by droplet infection and by direct contact. The incubation period is from 12 to 23 days. Symptoms include slight fever, sore throat, drowsiness and malaise, swollen glands and lymph nodes, arthralgia, and a diffuse fine red rash, Figure 10–26. Treatment is bed rest, liquids, antipyretics, and sponge baths. Complications of rubella can result in blindness, deafness, brain damage, heart defects, enlarged liver, and bone malformation.

Diphtheria. This acute infectious disease is caused by *Corynebacterium diphtheriae,* a gram-positive, nonmotile, nonspore-forming, club-shaped bacillus. **Diphtheria** diagnosis is confirmed by throat culture. Transmission is by direct and indirect contact. The incubation period is between 2 and 5

FIGURE 10–24 Selection and rotation of insulin injection sites

P R O C E D U R E

Administer Intramuscular Injection

PURPOSE: To inject large amounts of medication, 0.5 cc to 3.0 cc, and oil-based substances or irritating solutions which are more easily tolerated in the muscle tissue.

EQUIPMENT: Medication (sterile water for injection in vial or ampule), cotton balls, alcohol, adhesive bandage (or hypoallergenic tape), sterile needle and syringe (needle usually is 1 to 3 inches length, 18G to 23G), medication tray, patient's chart, pen, latex gloves

TERMINAL PERFORMANCE OBJECTIVE: Provided with all necessary equipment and supplies, demonstrate each of the steps required in administering an intramuscular injection; three injections will be administered to a latex training arm with the instructor observing each step. The dosage amount will be determined by the instructor each time.

1. Wash and glove hands. **CAUTION:** Prepare syringe with ordered amount of medication. Replace needle guard. Place medication on tray. *Note: Read label of medication and compare with order.*

2. Compare medication order with patient's chart. Identify patient and explain procedure. Ask patient to remove any clothing if necessary.

3. Use alcohol-saturated cotton ball to clean injection site. *Note: Allow alcohol to dry. Remove needle guard.*

4. Secure a large area of skin (to accommodate large amount of medication) between thumb and fingers of one hand. With other hand, grasp syringe midway as you would a dart and hold over site at 90-degree angle. Insert needle quickly with firm and steady action. *Note: Avoid force when injecting to keep bruising to a minimum.* Pull back plunger to make sure a blood vessel has not been penetrated. If no blood is seen in barrel of syringe, proceed by pushing down on plunger and expelling medication into muscle. *Note: If blood appears in syringe barrel, pull out needle at angle of insertion. Discard syringe, needle, and medication and begin again with new syringe and medication.* **RATIONALE: Blood in the needle indicates the possibility of the needle placement being within a blood vessel. Medication injected directly into the bloodstream causes rapid absorption and may cause undesirable as well as dangerous results.**

5. Pull needle out at angle of insertion carefully and quickly. Wipe injection site with alcohol-saturated cotton ball and gently massage area. **RATIONALE: Massaging the site helps distribute medication throughout the tissue.**

6. Observe patient for any reaction and report to physician if needed. Determine if patient is allergic to adhesive before applying a bandage. Hypoallergenic tape is recommended.

7. Discard disposable items. (Place entire syringe and needle in sharps container.) Wash and sterilize reusable items, remove gloves, and wash hands. Return medication and tray to proper storage area.

8. Record information and initial.

---

days. Symptoms include headache, malaise, fever, and sore throat with a yellowish white or gray membrane. Treatment consists of adequate liquids and a soft diet, antibiotics, bed rest, and in some cases a tracheostomy. The Schick test is an interdermal injection of a minute amount of the diphtheria toxin used to determine the degree of immunity to the disease. Little or no reaction indicates immunity (the presence of antibodies).

Pertussis. Whooping cough, or **pertussis,** is an acute infectious disease characterized by respiratory drainage, then a peculiar paroxysmal cough, which ends in a whooping inspiration (sounds like a shrill trumpeting cry; the name comes from the whooping crane that makes this sound). This disease is most common in children under 4 years of age, although it can affect children of all ages if they have not been immunized against it. Pertussis is caused by the small, nonmotile, gram-negative bacillus, *Bordetella pertussis.* It is transmitted by direct and indirect contact. The incubation period is from 7 to 14 days. Symptoms of whooping cough include: in the **catarrhal stage**—an increase in leukocyte count marked by lymphocytosis, respiratory drainage, sneezing, slight fever, dry cough, irritability, loss of appetite; in the **paroxysmal stage**—violent cough with whooping inspiration sounds, forceful vomiting that can evoke hemorrhaging from various portions of the body from the straining; and in the **decline stage**—decline in coughing and return of appetite. A trace cough may last for several months to 2 years.

Because some infants have notable reactions to the pertussis vaccine, including nonstop crying for hours, some physicians withdraw this immunization from the child's schedule after the child experiences an unpleasant reaction the first time. Other physicians prefer to give the vaccine in minute doses of 0.1 cc a week for 5 weeks. The vaccine is of course a part of the DPT (diphtheria, pertussis, and tetanus). This gives the child a much smaller dose to tolerate and offers more protection from the disease than not having any

P R O C E D U R E

Administer Intramuscular Injection by Z-Tract Method

PURPOSE: To inject irritating substances deep into the muscle layer of tissue. These irritating substances would cause tissue discoloration and irritation if given in the subcutaneous tissues from leakage in following the path of the needle when administered. The site of injection is in the gluteal muscle of the buttocks (upper outer quadrant; for some medications the deltoid muscle may be used). Dose is from 0.5 cc to 3.0 cc.

EQUIPMENT: Medication (sterile water for injection in vial/ampule), cotton balls, alcohol, adhesive bandage (or hypoallergenic tape), sterile needle and syringe (needle usually is 2 to 3 inches, 19G to 21 G), sterile gauze square, medication tray, patient's chart, pen, latex gloves

TERMINAL PERFORMANCE OBJECTIVE: Provided with all necessary equipment and supplies, demonstrate each of the steps required in administering a Z-tract intramuscular injection using a clinical mannequin; three injections will be administered with the instructor observing each step. The dosage will be determined by the instructor.

1–3. Same as for intramuscular injection. See Figure 10–25.
4. Use gauze square to securely hold patient's skin at injection site to one side to displace skin and tissues until injection is completed. Insert needle into gluteal muscle of buttocks or deltoid at a 90-degree angle, holding syringe as you would a dart. First and second fingers may be used to aspirate while thumb and ring finger hold syringe near needle end. If no blood is seen in barrel of syringe, proceed by expelling medication into muscle. Wait a few seconds before removing needle. *Note: If blood is seen in barrel of syringe, pull needle out quickly at angle of insertion.* Discard syringe, needle, and medication and begin again with new syringe and medication. **RATIONALE: Blood in the needle indicates the possibility of the needle placement being within a blood vessel. Medication injected directly into the bloodstream causes rapid absorption and may cause undesirable as well as dangerous results.** *Note: Read package insert of medication carefully. There may be additional instructions for certain medications.* Some Z-tract injection instructions suggest that 0.5 cc of air be in syringe to follow medication to prevent leakage from needle track.

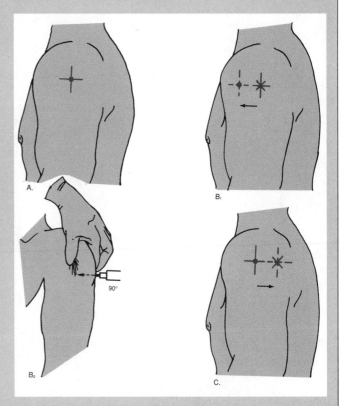

FIGURE 10–25 (a) The upper outer arm (deltoid muscle) shows the site for the Z-tract injection at the +. (b) (1) Skin (tissue) is moved over to the left and *held*. (2) During administration of a 90-degree IM injection into the muscle. (c) A few seconds after the injection is given the skin is released to cover the path of the needle preventing leakage of medication into the subcutaneous tissues. The X shows where the actual puncture site occurred; beneath the + is actually where the medication is in the muscle.

5. Pull needle out at angle of insertion and let go of skin quickly so that displaced tissue will cover needle track and prevent it from leaking into surrounding subcutaneous tissues. Cover injection site with alcohol-saturated cotton ball and hold it in place for a few seconds. *Note: Do not massage area.* **RATIONALE: Massage causes distribution of the medication, which is undesirable with Z-tract injections due to the tissue irritating properties of the medication.**
6–8. Same as for intramuscular injection.

FIGURE 10–26 Eleven-month-old infant with rubella (postnatal). This infant has a typical discrete macupapular erythematous rash indistinguishable from that seen in other viral illnesses.

immunity toward pertussis at all. DT (diphtheria and tetanus) is given to those who cannot tolerate the pertussis vaccine.

Tetanus. This acute, potentially fatal, infectious disease affects the central nervous system. **Tetanus** was commonly referred to as "lockjaw." Motor nerves transmit impulses from the infected central nervous system to muscles. The infection is caused by the bacillus, *Clostridum tetani,* the **toxin** of which is one of the most **lethal** poisons known. The bacillus is found in superficial layers of the soil. It is a normal inhabitant of the intestinal tracts of horses and cows. Tetanus affects only wounds that contain dead tissue, transmitted commonly in puncture wounds, abrasions, lacerations, and burns. There is a short incubation period of 3 to 21 days, and a longer one of 4 to 5 weeks. The symptoms of tetanus are stiffness of the jaw, esophageal, and sometimes the neck muscles. Progressing rigidity follows soon with fixed jaw (thus lockjaw), altered voice, fever, painful spasms of all body muscles, irritability, and headache. Immediate cleaning

of the wound and **debridement** are necessary initially in treatment. Maintaining an airway is vital as well as administering **antitoxin.** Additionally, treatment consists of sedation, controlling muscle spasms, maintaining fluid balance, administering penicillin G, and performing tracheostomy and providing oxygen as necessary. The patient must be in a quiet room to prevent the triggering of muscle spasms.

Hepatitis B. This is a highly contagious, potentially fatal, form of viral hepatitis. It is caused by the **hepatitis B** virus (HBV). It has been known as "serum hepatitis." Hepatitis B is transmitted by contaminated serum in blood transfusions or by using contaminated needles or instruments. It has an incubation period of 14 to 50 days. The symptoms are slow at onset with fever, malaise, loss of appetite, nausea, and vomiting, progressing to include jaundice, weakness, dark urine, and whitish stool. Bed rest and a forced-fluid diet are recommended. Alcohol and fats should be eliminated from the patient's diet. The hepatitis B vaccine is urged for all who may be at risk, especially *all health care workers.* OSHA standards indicate that employees who may be exposed to bloodborne pathogens must be offered the three-series HBV within 10 working days of employment. Those who refuse to be vaccinated must sign a declination form. Follow-up evaluation must be conducted in confidence by an accredited laboratory for the employee and at no cost to the individual. Hepatitis B is thought to be widespread everywhere, and immunization is strongly urged to protect the country's population and to prevent a massive epidemic.

Mothers who have the disease are advised to have their newborns **inoculated** within the first 12 hours after birth along with an additional injection of hepatitis B **immunoglobulin.** Screening of all pregnant women is also advised. Patients who have experienced anaphylactic reaction to yeast or the hepatitis B injections should alert their physician before being immunized against the disease.

The American Academy of Pediatrics recommends that newborn infants receive the series of three hepatitis B immunizations. The first dose is recommended to be given to neonates anywhere from birth to a month old. Many hospital neonatal nurseries provide the first dose which is given before the infant leaves the hospital. The second dose of the hepatitis B vaccine is advised to be scheduled between the ages of 2 and 4 months; the third, between the ages of 12 and 15 months. The usual recommended time between the doses of the hepatitis B immunization series is 1 month between the first and second injection, and 5 months between the second and third injection.

Other vaccines. All of the immunizations mentioned thus far are vaccines administered by injection. As with any parenteral administration of medications, it is important to instruct the patient to relax as much as possible during the procedure. Tense or tight muscles around the site of injection

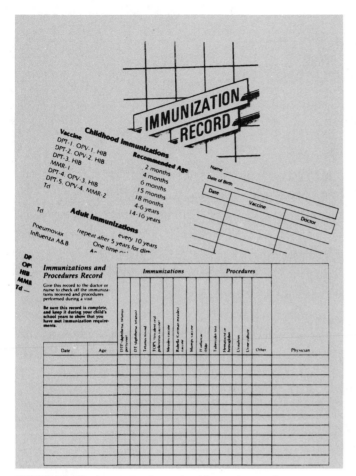

FIGURE 10–27 Immunization schedule and records

will not only make the procedure itself an unpleasant experience, but will have the aftereffect of creating unnecessary soreness in the area. Becoming proficient in technique, besides developing a good rapport and educating the patients you serve, is fundamental.

A vaccine administered orally is the **polio** immunization. It is kept frozen until just before it is to be administered. It should never be refrozen. As you can see in the immunization schedule, this vaccine is administered to infants and young children. It is made from the pathogenic microorganisms and is **attenuated,** which makes it less virulent. The disease it protects against is known as infantile paralysis, or poliomyelitis, which is the acute infection and inflammation of the gray matter of the spinal cord caused by the poliovirus. As the name suggest, children are more susceptible than adults. It is transmitted by the oral–fecal route. Incubation is usually from 7 to 12 days (and can be from 5 to 35). The symptoms begin with fever, malaise, headache, nausea and vomiting, slight abdominal discomfort, and gen-

eral paralysis (if respiratory muscles are involved it is likely to be fatal). Treatment consists of relieving symptoms, bed rest, mild analgesics, sedatives as necessary, fluid and salt balance, laxatives or enemas as necessary to relieve constipation, oxygen, respirator, and tracheostomy if necessary. Physical and occupational therapy are needed as the patient recovers.

Remind patients to protect themselves and their families against all of these diseases to prevent the return of epidemics. There are other diseases, such as **cholera** and **typhoid,** for which there are vaccines to prevent dangerous epidemics that have the potential to wipe out entire populations. Many underdeveloped countries have such situations even today. Immunizations other than what appears in the schedule in Table 10–6 are not recommended on a routine basis in most Western countries. Health officials advise immunizations as determined necessary. Travel to some countries requires immunizations against particular diseases before entry is permitted. To provide up-to-date immunization information by country, computer databases have been established. One such program containing health information for travelers on over 200 countries is available from Immunization Alert, in Storrs, Connecticut. Current information may also be obtained at local and state health departments. You should provide the patient with a card or booklet to record accurately each immunization, including the month, day and year for each, Figure 10–27, as well as recording each vaccine on the patient's chart. Any reaction, no matter how slight, must also be recorded on the patient's chart. Remind patients to make appointments and carry the immunization record (or a copy) with them at all times.

There is continuing research and development of vaccinations against many infectious diseases. With the available vaccines one might think that these illnesses would be rarely experienced in developed countries and be a problem only in severely poverty-stricken areas. Unfortunately, children in general (in developed countries and in third-world nations) are not being vaccinated adequately because of inadequate education, poor living conditions, and lack of funding for vaccines. There are many places in the world where people in these third world nations are still constantly fighting a losing battle against communicable diseases. Deaths from them are staggering in number. Many parents think that these diseases are no longer a risk and therefore don't immunize their children or themselves. Patient education and community involvement is the key to eliminate this ongoing problem.

Complete Chapter 10, Unit 3 in the workbook to help you meet the objectives at the beginning of this unit and therefore to achieve competency of this subject matter.

MEDICAL-LEGAL ETHICAL HIGHLIGHTS

Mrs. Right . . .
makes sure that all prescription pads are secured at all times to prevent theft. She keeps accurate records of narcotics and reminds the physician about keeping the narcotics registration current. In the event of theft of any medication or prescription pad, she reports it immediately to the proper authorities. When patients agree to take experimental drugs, she obtains written consent. She disposes of all expired medicines properly. She explains about immunizations to patients and obtains written consent from them. She remembers to record medication refills on the patients' records.

Promotion outlook: Excellent

Ms. Wrong . . .
never concerns herself about securing prescription pads, and therefore, wouldn't even know if one were missing. She pays no attention to recording refills of prescriptions on the patient records, saying that the patient should tell the doctor that they got more medicine when they come in for the next appointment. Her haphazard narcotics records and the physician's narcotics registration forms are always misplaced so she doesn't know if they are accurate or current. She rarely obtains a written consent form from patients for experimental drugs or for immunizations. She pays no attention to expiration dates on medicines she prepares or puts away.

Promotion outlook: None

REFERENCES

American Medical Association Family Medical Guide, rev. ed. New York: Random House, 1987.

Code of Federal Regulations and Drugs 21, 1990.

Erickson, Belle. *Nurse's Clinical Guide Dosage Calculations.* Springhouse, PA: Springhouse Corporation, 1991.

Flodin, Kim C. *Immunizations Update, Child (*November 1992).

Miller, Benjamin F., and Keane, Claire Brackman. *Encyclopedia and Dictionary of Medicine, Nursing and Allied Health,* 3d ed. Philadelphia: W. B. Saunders, Co., 1983.

Morbidity and Mortality Weekly Report (MMWR), 32, no. 1 (January 14, 1983).

Mosby's Medical, Nursing, & Allied Health Dictionary, 3d ed. St. Louis: C. V. Mosby Co., 1990.

Physician's Desk Reference. Oradell, NJ: Medical Economics, updated annually.

Physician's Desk Reference for Nonprescription Drugs. Oradell, NJ: Medical Economics, updated annually.

Physician's Manual. U. S. Department of Justice, DEA, Government Printing Office, Washington, DC, revised 1990.

Taber, Clarence W. *Taber's Cyclopedia Medical Dictionary*, 14th ed. Philadelphia: F.A. Davis, 1983.

OSHA Bloodborne Pathogens Final Standard: Summary of Key Provisions. Occupational Safety and Health Administration, U. S. Department of Health and Human Services, Government Printing Office, Washington, DC, 1993.

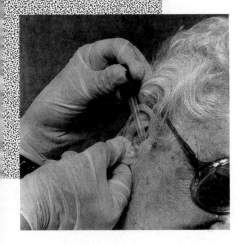

C H A P T E R   1 1

Medical Emergencies

UNIT 1
Safety in the Medical Office

UNIT 2
Medical Office Emergency Procedures

UNIT 3
First Aid Care of Accidents and Injuries

The emergency situations a medical assistant is most likely to encounter will depend on the employer's practice. However, if an accident occurs near a physician's office the victim may appear in your waiting room with an injury which does not fall within your practice area. You must know how to evaluate the situation and respond in the manner expected from a member of a health care team. This chapter will present guidelines for preventing accidents and describe emergency procedures and first aid care of accident victims.

U N I T   1

Safety in the Medical Office

OBJECTIVES ....

Upon completion of this unit, you will meet the following terminal performance objectives by verifying knowledge of the facts and principles presented through oral and written communication at a level deemed competent by the instructor or employer.

1. Identify potential office hazards.
2. List steps to take in accident-proofing an office.
3. Describe methods of fire prevention in the office.
4. Explain why fire, earthquake, and severe weather drills are needed.
5. Discuss steps of an evacuation procedure and include the manner in which it should be carried out.
6. Explain where a fire extinguisher should be affixed and why.
7. Spell and define, using the glossary at the back of the text, all the words to know in this unit.

WORDS TO KNOW ....

accessible	drill
ambulate	extinguisher
conceal	evacuation
concise	procurement
crisis	volatile
disaster	

Reports of injuries reveal that a large percentage occur in the home. A medical office may also present dangers for employees and patients. As described in Chapter 3, you should do a daily check of the waiting room to be sure all electrical wires, furniture, and carpet are in good repair. No throw rugs should be on the floor.

All medications should be in a locked cupboard or in drawers not easily **accessible** to patients. Spills of any kind should be cleaned up immediately. Any medications dropped must be located and destroyed. File drawers and cupboard doors should be closed when not in use to avoid both head injuries and falls from tripping over them. All equipment cords should be **concealed** where people will be moving about. No prescription blanks should be left where they could be forged and used illegally for drug **procurement**

A very young child should never be left unattended. Patients who are ill are sometimes unsteady when they attempt to **ambulate**; always assist these patients as needed. Never leave ill or elderly patients unattended on an examination table.

Learn to give clear, **concise** instructions to patients. When you position the patient for examinations your instructions are important in obtaining the desired results and in maintaining the safety of the patient moving about on the table.

Be sure office staff knows when the autoclave is in operation so that burns will not result from touching the machine.

Computers need to be situated so that glare is not present on the screen. Employees using computers or word processors should rest their eyes by looking away from the screen at regular intervals.

If chemicals are kept in the office for laboratory work, care must be taken to store them properly. Some chemicals become **volatile** when kept beyond the expiration date, so these dates need to be carefully monitored.

Fire prevention is of utmost importance for the safety of everyone. There are rare exceptions to the "no smoking" regulations in medical and public facilities. Even though this is true, there is still a possibility of the danger of a match, lighter, or cigarette dropped into furniture, a planter, or trash container by someone looking for an ashtray. Some facilities provide ashtrays just outside the entrance for this very reason. However, you should keep an eye on it for people tend to use this ashtray as a trash disposal as well. This can become a prime setting for a fire to start. Ashtrays should be emptied often and the contents (possibly smoldering smoking materials) flushed down the toilet.

Fire **extinguishers** should be affixed on a wall closest to the lab or kitchen area where the potential for a fire is the greatest. It should be checked periodically by the fire department for effectiveness. Each employee should be instructed in the proper use of it in case of fire.

Electrical outlets which do not work should be checked by an electrician, as a defective outlet may cause a fire. Frayed wires of any electrical appliance or office equipment must not be used until repaired. Do not attempt to tape or fix a frayed wire for the danger of fire or shock to you and others is too great. Coffee pots boil dry and can burn, as can boiling water sterilizers. Some office procedure manuals require that all electrical appliances be unplugged each night.

The office should have an established policy so that all employees know what to do in the event of a fire or severe weather warning, such as a tornado alert. Natural **disasters** are certainly unpredictable and can claim many lives if necessary steps are not taken immediately. **Evacuation** from a building of all persons is necessary in cases of fire, possible explosions, or other similar dangers. Exit signs should be clearly posted. All stairways and hallways should be free from clutter to allow safe passage. In an earthquake (and in a tornado), however, it is advisable for persons to take shelter in a door frame or under a sturdy structure and *not* go outside. For example, in areas of the country where earthquakes are known to occur, children in school settings are taught to immediately get under their desks for shelter from falling objects. Going outside may result in being struck by objects, electrical power lines, and falling trees and buildings. Electrical power is usually disrupted during such a situation or severe storm. Never use an elevator in any threatening situation because the power could be cut off at any time and those in the elevator could be trapped or killed. Some medical facilities, such as hospitals, clinics, and group practices, have emergency generators. A generator is a machine that changes mechanical energy into electrical power. They are used for emergency situations on a temporary basis.

Routine **drills** psychologically prepare you for sensible and safe actions should an emergency situation occur. A practical time to review drill procedures is at staff meetings or during orientation of a new employee. Studies have shown that those who are prepared have a greater chance of surviving a **crisis** than those who did not know what to do or how to act. Keeping a calm and commanding attitude and acting in an efficient manner helps to reduce panic in a stressful situation. This will allow others to follow your example in leading them to safety. It is not practical to decide at the time of such an emergency what to instruct your patients and the employees to do. Each member of the health care team should have specific tasks to accomplish in such emergencies. Complete Chapter 11, Unit 1 in the workbook to help you meet the objectives at the beginning of this unit and therefore achieve competency of this subject matter.

UNIT 2
Medical Office Emergency Procedures

OBJECTIVES ....

Upon completion of this unit, you will meet the following terminal performance objectives by verifying knowledge of the facts and principles presented through oral and written communication at a level deemed competent by the instructor or employer, and will demonstrate the specific behaviors as identified in the terminal performance objectives of the procedures, observing all aseptic and safety precautions in accordance with health care standards.

1. Describe the universal emergency medical identification system.
2. Assemble and maintain an emergency tray of appropriate drugs and equipment.
3. Describe the symptoms and first aid for

- bee, wasp, and hornet stings
- bites, animal and human
- burns
- convulsions
- diabetic coma and insulin shock
- dislocations
- fainting
- foreign bodies
- fractures
- heart attack
- heat and cold exposure
- hemorrhage
- poisoning
- respiratory emergencies
- shock
- sprains and strains
- stroke
- wounds

4. List the symptoms of substance abuse (drugs and alcohol).
5. List methods of obtaining local emergency services.
6. Discuss the purpose of applying heat and cold packs.
7. Discuss the importance of following universal precautions in caring for injuries.
8. Spell and define, using the glossary at the back of the text, all the words to know in this unit.

WORDS TO KNOW ·······································

activate	forge
antihistamine	incision
aspiration	ingest
cessation	molten
complicated	perfusion
confront	prophylactic
convulsion	psychopathic
delirium tremens	rotate
diaphoresis	shock
emetic	superficial
exogenous	syncope
flushed	universal

A medical emergency is any situation in which an individual suddenly becomes ill or has an injury in circumstances calling for swift and decided action. You should first identify the person if at all possible and determine who to contact as next of kin. If the patient is conscious you should try to obtain

FIGURE 11–1 Universal emergency medical identification symbol

information regarding the illness or injury. If the patient is unconscious you should check for a **universal** emergency medical identification symbol, Figure 11–1. This symbol, designed by the American Medical Association, is worn like a dog tag around the neck, wrist, or ankle. If you find this symbol, you should check for an identification card, which will tell you the health problem the patient has, Figure 11–2. You should encourage patients who have serious heart conditions, diabetes, allergies, or a laryngectomy to wear such a symbol.

As part of your preparation for an emergency, you and your employer should list the supplies and equipment that would be necessary to handle an emergency that could come under your care. Then set aside a place in the office where these items will always be ready for use. All employees in the office should know where the items are and how they are to be used. You should have a supply of sterile dressings, bandage material, and adhesive tape; easily **activated** hot and cold packs; disposable syringe and needle units with adrenaline, narcotics, and **antihistamines**. Adrenaline (epinephrine) is available in cartridge units ready for use. Other supplies include: ipecac, an effective **emetic**; tubes of glucose for use in diabetic patients suffering from a severe hypoglycemic reaction; and an oxygen tank with a mask. Oxygen tanks should be routinely checked monthly to determine how much oxygen is still available. If the amount is insufficient during an emergency, an unfortunate situation could result. Only disposable face masks and tubing

EMERGENCY
I am a laryngectomee (no vocal cords).
I breathe through an opening in the neck, not through the nose or mouth.
If artificial respiration is necessary:
1. Keep neck opening clear of all matter.
2. Don't twist head sidewise.
3. Apply oxygen only to neck opening.
4. Don't throw water on head.
5. Mouth-to-opening breathing is effective.

FIGURE 11–2 Emergency medical identification card

should be used for each patient. They should be used only once and discarded in the proper receptacle. Any supplies used should be replaced immediately. A backup supply must be available at all times. **Rotate** the supplies so that you use older supplies first, and be careful to check dates on medications to be sure they have not expired.

First Aid for Sudden Illness and Injuries ....

Bee, Wasp, and Hornet Stings Bees, wasps, and hornets cause deaths every year. If the victim of a sting is not sensitive to the sting, the result may only be a painful swelling with redness and itching. When several stings are received at one time, the victim may become quite ill. The patient may develop severe hives or edema of all tissues.

When a patient is severely allergic to stings, they can cause acute illness with shortness of breath. The patient may become restless, complain of headache, or have mottled blueness of the skin. In the cases where shortness of breath is not apparent, the victim may appear to be in shock and have severe nausea, vomiting, and blood may be evident in diarrhea. The severely allergic patient should always have a special emergency kit close at hand when there is any possibility of a sting. Refer to Chapter 8 for discussion about anaphylactic shock and stings. If there is evidence of anaphylactic shock, epinephrine should be given as a life-saving measure.

A honeybee leaves the stinger in the skin, and it should be immediately removed by scraping it out carefully with a sharp object. Never grasp the stinger with your fingers or a tweezers, as that would inject more of the venom. Apply commercial meat tenderizer to site. Wasps, hornets, and yellow jackets retain their stingers and can sting repeatedly.

Bites An animal bite may tear skin and cause a bruise. The bite is dangerous because of the possibility of infection and rabies. The animal should be held for observation for at least 15 days to see if it is rabid. The bite must be reported to the police or local health authorities, who will examine the animal for rabies. The wound should be thoroughly cleansed with an antiseptic soap and rinsed well. The area should be bandaged and immobilized, and the victim should be examined by a physician as soon as possible. The decision must be made regarding the use of antirabies serum. If the skin is broken and the animal cannot be tested, antirabies serum should be used. When the animal can be observed for 15 days and is found to be free of rabies, no serum is necessary.

There is also concern regarding human bites because of AIDS, hepatitis B, staph or other infections. The only way AIDS could be transmitted in this manner is if the bite breaks the skin and the person doing the biting has bleeding gums. It is still necessary to cleanse the wound thoroughly, cover with a sterile bandage, and have a physician examine the patient. Patients who have sustained such a bite from another person should be advised to have a series of three injections to be immunized against hepatitis B.

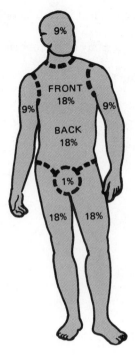

FIGURE 11–3 (A) Diagram for use in calculating the extent of burns or other injuries for an adult

Burns The severity of a burn is determined by the amount of skin surface and the layer of skin involved, Figures 11–3(a) and (b) and 11–4. Any amount involving 15% of the total body surface (TBS) is considered a serious or critical burn. Burns occur as a result of radiation from the sun or a heat lamp, or contact with electricity, chemicals, or heat. A first-degree burn is a **superficial** injury resulting in reddening of the skin and severe pain. A sunburn or contact with boiling water or steam may cause this type of burn. It will heal without special treatment.

Treating the area with cold water or ice packs should stop the pain and may even keep the burn from progressing into deeper tissue layers. The application of butter or ointments will hold the burn in and cause more pain as well as being a problem to remove. In treatment of burns a physician may use an antiseptic ointment, which can easily be washed off.

A second-degree burn, which affects 30% of the TBS of an adult (20% of TBS of a child), involves both reddening and blistering because the burn extends into deeper layers of skin. The leakage of plasma and electrolytes from the capillaries damaged by the burn into the surrounding tissues raises up the epidermis to form blisters. Patients should be cautioned to refrain from breaking blisters as this opens up the area to infection. Blisters will heal more quickly if they are opened by a physician, who would first paint the area with an antiseptic and then open them with a sterilized needle. The area should then be covered with a sterile gauze pad bandaged in place. First aid for a second-degree burn would involve treatment for **shock,** removal of any jewelry as edema may be severe, as much fluid as the patient can take, and covering the burn area with a sterile dressing. A victim of severe sunburn would be encouraged to soak in a tub of cold water and take large amounts of fluid. Pain medication as advised by the physician, may be taken to ease

Relative percentages of areas affected by growth

	At birth	1 yr	5 yr	10 yr	15 yr	Adult
A: Half of head	9½%	8½%	6½%	5½%	4½%	3½%
B: Half of thigh	2¾%	3¼%	4%	4¼%	4½%	4¾%
C: Half of leg	2½%	2½%	2¾%	3%	3¼%	3½%

FIGURE 11–3 (B) Lund and Browder chart for estimating the extent of burns. Because this chart takes proportional age–size differences into account, it can be used for infants and children, as well as for adults. (Adapted with permission from *Surgery, Gynecology, & Obstetrics* 79:352, 1944.)

FIGURE 11–4 Layers of skin in relation to degree of burn

painful burns. Some medications increase the danger of exposure to the sun. It is important to warn patients of this potential problem. Pharmacists generally place a warning label on the patient's prescription bottle.

Third-degree burns involve the epidermis, dermis, and subcutaneous tissues and require surgical care. They affect 10% to 15% of the TBS. The patient should receive immediate treatment for shock. No first aid can be given to the burn area except for clothing burned to the tissue should be removed only under sterile conditions in surgery by the physician. Cover the area with a sterile dressing.

Some physicians use the term fourth-degree burn for burns involving all the layers of skin, muscle, and even bone. This can result from an industrial injury, such as contact with **molten** metal. The intense heat of a burning building or a chemical fire could cause this type of burn.

An electrical burn may result from contact with electrical power lines or lightning. The circuit breaker should be cut off and the electric power company should be called immediately. In the case of an electrical burn, the primary aid is to remove the victim from the contact with the power source. This can best be done by the use of a wooden stick or cloth or special heavy gloves used to pull the victim away from the electrical power source. The rescuer could also be injured if contact is made with the electrical source. Depending on the total voltage that the victim has come in contact with, the articles used to free the victim can still conduct electricity. There should be immediate care for shock and cardiopulmonary resuscitation (CPR) if breathing or pulse is absent.

Chemical burns are treated by removing any clothing from the area and then flooding the area with water for at least 15 minutes. The one exception to the rule of immediate flooding with water is a carbolic acid burn, which should be flooded first with alcohol and then with water. A dry chemical should be brushed off carefully before flushing the patient's skin because some chemicals, such as lime, are activated by water. These burns should all be covered with a sterile dressing after thorough washing with water. A chemical burn of the eye should be flooded with water continuously for at least 20 minutes. A physician should always examine and treat eye burns immediately. Any other acid burn to the skin should be flushed with water for at least 5 minutes.

Convulsions **Convulsions** may occur when the patient has high body temperature, head injuries, brain disease, or brain disorders, such as epilepsy. A convulsion is a severe involuntary contraction of muscles that causes the patient first to become rigid and then to have uncontrollable movements. The patient becomes unconscious and may be injured during the seizure. The face and lips may become cyanotic, and the patient may stop breathing. The patient may also lose bladder and bowel control and bite the tongue. When the convulsion has stopped, the patient may be confused and complain of headache.

During the convulsion do not restrain movement. You should move objects that might cause injury. If possible, put a padded tongue depressor or soft object between the teeth to prevent biting the tongue. However, do not force any object between the patient's teeth or it could cause vomiting, **aspiration,** or spasm of the larynx. Keep the head turned to the side to prevent choking from profuse salivation. Never attempt to force the mouth open or pour water over the face. Allow the patient to rest or sleep after the seizure is over. Artificial respiration should be given if necessary. Emotional support should be given as the patient regains composure because this situation can cause the person to feel awkward.

Diabetic Coma and Insulin Shock   Diabetic patients may present emergency situations by going into diabetic coma or insulin shock, Table 11–1. A diabetic coma is caused by an increased amount of sugar in the blood. This may be caused by eating sweets or failing to take insulin. The patient may complain of confusion, dizziness, weakness, or nausea. Vomiting may occur. Respiration may be rapid and deep. The skin may be dry and **flushed.** The patient's breath has a sweet or fruity odor, which may be evident some distance away. The patient can lapse into unconsciousness and die from this condition if not treated immediately. The patient should be transported by ambulance to the nearest hospital for immediate care.

Insulin shock may occur from an excess amount of insulin in the body. This can happen if food is not eaten regularly in measured amounts, if the patient vomits after taking insulin, or if too much insulin is taken. The patient may have muscle weakness, anxiety, mental confusion, and a rapid and irregular heartbeat. The patient may be hungry and have **diaphoresis.**

The skin will be cold, pale, and moist. The patient may lapse into a coma and may develop convulsions. The patient should be given some form of sugar. Sweetened orange juice or tubes of glucose are often used. The sugar should control the shock but if it does not the patient must be transported at once to a hospital.

You must be alert to the possibility of diabetic coma or shock in a known diabetic patient with the above symptoms. If the patient can talk, ask if insulin or food has been taken. This will give you a better idea of the need for treatment of coma or shock. If you do not know the diagnosis, it is safer to give a spoon of sugar, because insulin shock can cause brain damage, which is not reversible. Recent studies indicate that by placing a very small amount of sugar under the tongue of an unconscious person it may be absorbed rapidly in the blood stream.

Dislocations   At least half of all dislocations involve the shoulder, but dislocations are possible of any freely moving joint. When a bone end slips out of the socket or when the capsule surrounding a joint is stretched or torn, a dislocation is likely to occur. There is usually severe pain and obvious deformity of the joint area. There may be loss of function of the affected limb. There is also noticeable swelling. Dislocations are best treated by a physician. The only first aid measure is to immobilize the dislocation during the trip to the medical office or hospital. Treat all sprains, strains, and dislocations as if they were fractures. Splint the injured limb in the position in which you find it to avoid additional injury to the accident victim.

TABLE 11–1
Causes and Symptoms of Diabetic Coma and Insulin Shock

Diabetic Coma or Acidosis	Insulin Shock or Reaction
Causes	
Too little insulin	Too much insulin or oral hypoglycemic drug
Too much to eat	Too little to eat
Infections, fever	An unusual amount of exercise
Emotional stress	
Symptoms	
Skin: Dry and flushed	Moist and pale
Behavior: Drowsy	Often excited
Mouth: Dry	Drooling
Thirst: Intense	Absent
Hunger: Absent	Present
Vomiting: Common	Usually absent
Respiration: Exaggerated, air hungry	Normal or shallow
Breath: Fruity odor of acetone	Usually normal
Pulse: Weak and rapid	Full and bounding (gives patient feeling of heart pounding)
Vision: Dim	Diplopia (double)
First aid: Keep patient warm	If conscious, give patient sugar or any food containing sugar (fruit juice, candy, crackers, etc.)
Obtain medical help immediately.	Obtain medical help immediately.

Fainting A temporarily diminished supply of blood to the brain may cause fainting. The medical term for fainting is **syncope.** A patient who feels faint should lower the head between the legs or lie down with feet elevated to improve the blood circulation to the head. The patient who is about to faint may be pale, perspiring, have cold clammy skin, and complain of dizziness or nausea. Another term or slang phrase you may hear to describe the strange color which some patients turn before they get sick and vomit or pass out is "turning green." An emesis basin should be handy in case the patient vomits. Each examination room should be supplied with capsules of aromatic spirits of ammonia, which can easily be broken and used to arouse the patient. These should not be held directly under the nose but passed back and forth about 6 inches under the nose. The patient should be kept in a reclining position until fully recovered and then may be given sips of water. The patient should regain consciousness within 5 minutes from a simple fainting episode. If not, the physician should check the patient. You should keep checking the patient's vital signs to determine that the patient is stabilized before allowing the patient to leave. Realize that in this situation, too, the patient needs emotional support.

Foreign Bodies Foreign bodies are substances or objects which become lodged in any part of the human body where they do not belong. It is fairly common for a speck of dirt, soot from a fire, or an eyelash to lodge in the eye, for example. Always wash your hands before touching the eyes. A foreign body under the lower lid can usually be seen easily and can be removed with a bit of cotton or a fold of tissue moistened with sterile water. If a foreign body is under the upper lid, it may be

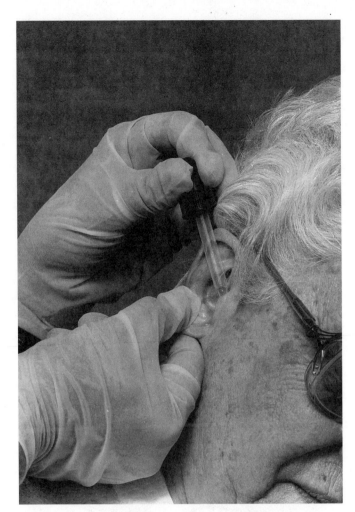

FIGURE 11–6 After the patient's head is tipped to the side, insert eardrops by pulling back on the earlobe to straighten the external canal.

FIGURE 11–5 Remove a foreign object from the upper eyelid by turning the eyelid back over a cotton-tipped swab or the stem of a wooden kitchen match.

possible to remove it by pulling the upper lid over the lower lid. If this procedure is not successful it may be necessary to grasp the eyelashes and carefully turn back the upper lid over a cotton swab, Figure 11–5. When the object is located it may be removed with a folded piece of sterile gauze moistened with sterile water. Any object lodged on the cornea should be removed by a physician. A sterile compress should be placed over both eyes to keep the eye from moving until a physician can examine it. A sterile eye irrigation solution should be kept on hand for just this type of emergency. Use it to continuously flush the affected eye for 20 minutes to prevent further tissue damage, or to remove a foreign substance (such as dust). Refer to Chapter 6 for the procedure regarding eye irrigation.

First aid for an object lodged in the ear consists of placing several drops of warm olive oil, mineral oil, or baby oil into the ear, pulling back on the earlobe to straighten the external canal, while the head is leaning toward the uninjured side, Figure 11–6. Then let the oil run out and see if the object will come out with it. Never try to dig an object out of the ear; damage can be done to the eardrum. If first aid measures are not successful, a physician should examine the patient.

You may get a call from a parent who is frightened because a child has swallowed a small object. It is best for the physician to perform a fluoroscopic examination to see if the object is in the stomach. If the object is not sharp it will probably pass on through the intestinal tract and be eliminated in normal fashion.

Splinters can generally be removed with a needle if at home or with a splinter thumb forceps in the office, Figure 11–7. The skin should be washed with soap and water. The needle should be held over a flame until it is thoroughly heated and then cooled before making a slit over the splinter. The splinter forceps should be wrapped and sterilized in the autoclave. Lift the end of the exposed splinter with the needle and remove by grasping with a pair of tweezers. If a splinter or thorn is under a fingernail it is best to have a physician remove it. After the

FIGURE 11–8 Remove a fish hook by cutting the barb (a) and cutting the shank (b)

FIGURE 11–7 To remove a splinter: (a). Clean area around splinter, (b). Heat needle in flame and let cool, (c). Cut the skin over the splinter, (d). Lift the splinter partially out, (e). Remove the splinter with tweezers.

splinter or thorn is removed the area should again be washed with soap and water and covered with an adhesive bandage.

One of the hazards of fishing or of being around individuals who are casting for fish is that hooks can become embedded in fingers, backs, scalps, or any part of the anatomy that is exposed. It is best for a physician to use a local anesthetic for such removal. If you do not have a physician near at hand, you should push the barb through the flesh and then cut it off with a pair of nipper pliers, Figure 11–8. After this is done you can back out the remainder of the hook. The other possibility is to cut off the shank of the hook and pull out the barbed end. After the hook is removed, the area should be carefully cleaned and a dry dressing applied. If the removal is done away from the office, the patient should be seen by a physician for a tetanus toxoid booster or tetanus antiserum as needed. The physician may also prescribe an antibiotic.

Fractures Fractures are breaks in bone caused by trauma or bone disease. In a *closed*, or *simple, fracture* there is no open wound. In an *open*, or *compound, fracture* there is an open wound. First aid for an open fracture is to control bleeding and to splint without moving the bone ends. The patient may also need to be treated for shock. You should check the PMS (pulse, and motor and sensory reflexes). Capillary refill of the distal area to all fracture sites on an injured limb will be impaired. To ensure good **perfusion** and nonimpaired neurologic function, treatment must be administered as soon as possible. A fracture can be diagnosed only by an X ray unless bone ends can be seen in an open wound or severe deformity is present. A physician is the only person who should attempt to straighten, or reduce, a fracture.

In addition to the fractures described in Chapter 4, Unit 5, you may have patients with extracapsular fractures, where the bone is broken just outside the joint; intracapsular fractures, where the bone is broken inside the joint; fracture dislocations, where the break is **complicated** by the end of the bone being out of the joint; pathologic fractures, or breaks at the site of a bone tumor or bone disease; longitudinal fractures, where the break is parallel with the bone; transverse fractures, where the break runs across the bone; and oblique fractures, where the break slants across the bone.

Heart Attack

Heart Attack When you are **confronted** with a patient who is complaining of severe chest pain, it is extremely important for the physician to diagnose whether the patient is suffering from a heart attack or indigestion. Other terms for a heart attack are coronary thrombosis, coronary occlusion, and myocardial infarction. The cause is usually a blockage of one or more of the coronary arteries. The patient may also complain of pain radiating down one or both arms and a tightness of the chest or pain radiating into the left shoulder and jaw (mandible). The pulse is usually rapid and weak. The patient may be perspiring profusely, have cyanotic lips and fingernails, and may be anxious and agitated.

Never allow such a patient to walk or carry objects, such as a heavy purse or coat. If you have a wheelchair, help the patient into the chair. In the absence of a wheelchair, use any chair with rollers to move the patient to an examination room. Most cardiac patients prefer to have the head elevated.

The physician may want you to administer oxygen or prepare an injection for the patient. If the patient is using a medication, such as nitroglycerine, it should be given immediately. The patient should be quickly but calmly transported to a hospital if the physician is not in the office. If the physician is in, he or she will want an electrocardiogram done immediately, so you should loosen clothing and connect the ECG at once. Treat for shock by maintaining body heat. If the patient should stop breathing, start artificial respiration, and if there is no pulse, start CPR. These procedures will be discussed under respiratory emergencies. Always have the emergency tray with IV equipment ready for the physician.

Heat and Cold Exposure

Heat and Cold Exposure Elderly patients are especially vulnerable to excessive exposure to heat, and you should recognize the differences between heatstroke and heat exhaustion. The patient suffering from heatstroke will have a red, dry face. The skin will be hot and dry, and the temperature may be very high. The pulse will be strong, and respirations may be loud and difficult. The pupils of the eyes will be dilated but equal. The patient may have muscle tenseness or even convulsions. Treatment is bed rest with head elevated and the use of cold packs. The patient may be given normal saline infusion to force fluids.

In heat exhaustion the face is pale, cool, and moist. The skin is cool and clammy with profuse perspiration. There may be slight temperature elevation. The pulse is weak and rapid, and the respirations are quiet and shallow. The muscles may be tense. The pupils of the eyes are normal. The patient should be put in recumbent position with head lowered and warmth maintained for treatment of shock. If the patient is conscious, salt tablets may be given along with fruit juices in large amounts. If the patient is unconscious, an IV isotonic saline solution may be required.

The patient who is exposed to high temperatures for a long period in industry or at home may suffer from heat cramps. These patients may have diaphoresis and should drink large amounts of water. The problem is that they lose a large amount of body salt. The patient will complain of severe muscle cramps of the abdomen and legs and may also complain of faintness, dizziness, and exhaustion. First aid is designed to replace salt by taking salt tablets or drinking a solution of one teaspoon of table salt in a quart of water. If there is a problem with nausea when the patient uses salt tablets or table salt, a coated salt tablet may be given, or the patient may be encouraged to drink cool water with the salt tablets. Ice water should not be taken.

Exposure to freezing temperatures will often result in frostbite. The body parts most often damaged by cold are the hands, feet, ears, and nose. Symptoms that might indicate damaged tissue are a tingling sensation with numbness followed by pain and redness of the skin. If exposure is continued, the patient may complain of burning and itching. Sensation may be completely lost. The first aid required is to warm the part as quickly as possible by placing it in water with a temperature of 103° to 107° (39° to 41°C). This will help to reduce tissue damage. Never rub frostbite because this will cause tissue damage. Hot tea or coffee will help because they are both cardiac stimulants and vasodilators, ie. (they dilate blood vessels, thereby increasing circulation). The patient should not be allowed to smoke because smoking constricts blood vessels and decreases circulation.

Hemorrhage

Hemorrhage It is important to understand what the different sources of bleeding are to determine the seriousness of hemorrhage. Arterial bleeding will produce bright red blood in spurts. If the ruptured artery is a large branch, death can occur in 3 minutes or less. Bleeding from a vein will produce a steady flow of dark red blood. It is important to control this bleeding quickly because of the danger of an air bubble getting into the bloodstream and causing a blockage in the heart. Any bleeding from capillary damage will produce a steady ooze from the wound area. This type of bleeding will often clot without first aid measures being taken.

Internal bleeding causes symptoms you should be able to recognize. They are similar to those of shock. The patient may have a rapid weak pulse, shallow breathing, cold clammy skin, dilated pupils, dizziness, faintness, thirst, restlessness, and a feeling of anxiety. Internal hemorrhage might need to be controlled by surgery. The patient must be kept in a recumbent position with strictly limited movement until the physician takes over care.

Internal bleeding may be difficult to detect unless it leads to external signs. The patient who coughs up bright red blood may have a lung hemorrhage. Vomiting bright red blood could mean the patient has an ulcer that has started bleeding. If the patient is coughing up what looks like coffee grounds it could indicate chronic slow bleeding into the stomach. If the patient notices coal-black stools there is probably a loss of blood in the intestines. If the patient has a rectal hemorrhage it is likely to be from a lesion in the lower colon. A patient with severe abdominal pain from trauma may have a ruptured internal organ, such as a kidney, liver, or spleen.

Epistaxis (nosebleed) may be the result of excessively dry air over a prolonged period, hypertension, injury, or simply blowing the nose too hard. First aid for epistaxis is to elevate the head and pinch the nostrils closed for at least 6 minutes. Keep the patient in a sitting position with the head tilted forward so that the blood trickling down the throat will not be aspirated. The use of a cold compress over the nasal area or on the back of the neck may be helpful. A piece of gauze may be placed between the lips and gums with pressure against this area for several minutes. Specially treated gauze is best to use for nasal packing because cotton is difficult to remove. A physician should be consulted if bleeding is not easily controlled. Sometimes the addition of humidity to the air will relieve the patient who has recurrent epistaxis.

If a pregnant patient experiences vaginal bleeding, you need to determine the kind of flow. If there is gushing blood, the patient should lie down immediately with feet elevated, and an emergency squad should be called. If there has been discharge of clots or tissue substance, this should be taken to the hospital for analysis. Your employer will let you know how these emergencies should be handled.

Poisoning
Poison is not only **ingested**, it is absorbed, inhaled, injected, and produced by bites and stings.

If you get a call regarding a possible ingestion of poison, you should always ask what was taken, how much was taken, and the time it was taken. You should know the location and the telephone number of the local Poison Control Center so that you can direct callers to the best source of help. If an antidote is on the label of the poison, the patient should be given the antidote only after approval or order of the Poison Control Center or the physician. It is usually safe to dilute the poison with water or milk. If the substance is one which should be removed after diluting you may use ipecac or large amounts of warm water or activated charcoal to induce vomiting. The area at the back of the tongue known as the gag reflex may be touched to cause vomiting also. If table salt is available you may add a small amount to warm water to induce vomiting. The patient should *not* be encouraged to vomit if a strong alkali, acid, or petroleum product has been ingested.

For poisoning from plants, such as mushrooms or from bacteria-contaminated shellfish, the emergency treatment is to keep the patient as quiet as possible and induce vomiting.

Poisoning by inhalation may be caused by the use of cleaning fluids and sprays in a poorly ventilated area. Carbon monoxide poisoning may be caused by a faulty exhaust system in an automobile. First aid for inhalation poisoning is pulmonary resuscitation and immediate care in a hospital.

Poisoning by injection is usually the result of drug abuse. The patient may exhibit symptoms from confusion to excitement to hallucinations to convulsions. These patients need hospitalization for proper treatment.

Patients who are sensitive to insect stings may suffer anaphylactic shock and die if proper measures are not taken. They may show a decrease in blood pressure and difficulty breathing (dyspnea). They should be kept quiet and medical help obtained at once. The stinger should be brushed off. Any attempt to squeeze the stinger will inject more poison into the skin.

Many patients suffer from contact with poison ivy, poison sumac, and poison oak. A person who is sensitive to these poisons may not need to touch the plant but merely to pet a dog or cat which has come in contact with it. The patient will complain of reddening of the skin and blister formation that itches and is easily spread to other portions of the body. The physician may need to prescribe antihistamines (for relief of severe itching) and ointments (effective in clearing up the inflammation).

Respiratory Emergencies
One of the most common medical emergencies is an obstructed airway. The obstruction must be cleared away immediately as brain damage may result in 4 minutes from lack of oxygen. A person who is choking signals by placing the hand at the throat, Figure 11–9. Such an individual may make no sound but simply fall from the chair if nothing is done.

The method used to relieve an obstructed airway is a manual thrust, or subdiaphragmatic abdominal thrust, also known as the Heimlich maneuver. You should stand behind the victim and reach around the waist. Clench one hand to make a fist and grasp your fist with your other hand. Place the thumb side of the fist against the midline of the victim's abdomen between the waist and the rib cage, Figure 11–10. Thrust fist inward and upward six to ten times in a quick, firm movement to move air out of the lungs and with enough force to dislodge the obstruction. A chest thrust may be used if the victim is pregnant or has a problem with **exogenous** obesity. Chest thrusts are exerted downward. The abdominal thrust may be performed on an unconscious victim by sitting astride the victim's thighs. The

FIGURE 11–9 Universal distress signal for choking (From Hegner & Caldwell, *Nursing Assistant*, 6th ed. Copyright 1992, Delmar Publishers Inc.)

FIGURE 11–10 Hand placement for abdominal thrust (From Hegner & Caldwell, *Nursing Assistant*, 6th ed. Copyright 1992, Delmar Publishers Inc.)

heel of one hand is placed on the midline of the breastbone (sternum). The second hand is placed on top of the first, and the thrust is inward and upward. A choking victim who is alone may use the abdominal thrust with the fist or may thrust against a chair back or any hard object of adequate height.

If the thrusts have dislodged the obstruction but not expelled it from the victim's mouth, then the finger sweep is performed. Open the victim's mouth by tilting the head back (do not use the former head tilt; use the modified jaw thrust) with one hand and moving the jaw forward to lift the tongue away from the back of the throat. Insert the index finger of the first hand along the side of the cheek and sweep deeply into the mouth in a hooking action. Be careful not to push an obstruction deeper into the throat. If it is possible to dislodge an obstruction, be sure to remove it from the mouth. If dentures are worn it is helpful to remove them. If the patient has vomited it is extremely important to turn the patient on the side and jut the jaw to keep an open airway and prevent inspiration of vomited material into the lungs.

A patient suffering from severe edema of the vocal cords as a result of an allergic reaction to food or stings of bees or wasps must be hospitalized as quickly as possible.

The victim of a drowning must receive artificial respiration immediately. This can be given before the patient is taken from the water if there is help to support the patient while mouth-to-mouth resuscitation is given. Any surviving drowning victim needs to be hospitalized for followup of delayed reactions which are apt to occur. Poisoning by toxic gases, such as carbon monoxide, or suffocation may also require immediate artificial respiration.

The patient suffering from an asthma attack might have severe difficulty breathing. The physician must determine the treatment needed but you can be helpful in attempting to calm the patient. Remove the patient to a clean air environment. Emotional upset may start a severe asthmatic attack.

Some medications will cause a slowing or **cessation** of breathing. Electric shock may cause respiratory paralysis. The victim must be moved away from the source of the electricity

and then be given artificial respiration and CPR if necessary.

All medical assistants should take a standard first aid course and a course in CPR. The following procedures are for review purposes only and should not be used as the primary means of learning these skills.

CPR must be learned by taking a course from a certified instructor. Procedures are constantly being refined, and the procedure you learn should be the one you practice. There is currently a recommendation that a one-way valve facepiece be used in a health care environment as a guard against HIV transmission. If that is not possible, the mouth-to-nose method is recommended. According to the American Heart Association, two-person CPR is no longer used or taught to basic emergency care providers. The exception to the teaching or the practice of two-person CPR is to persons in an advanced training program.

The CPR procedure has some variations when used for a child or infant. Infants are generally considered to be under 1 year of age and children ages 1 to 8. Adult procedure would be used for anyone over 8.

Shock Shock may be associated with many different kinds of injuries and is a serious depressor of vital body functions. Symptoms include a rapid, thready, weak pulse; shallow, rapid respirations; dilated pupils; ashen color; and cool clammy skin. All of these result from decreased blood volume, due to diminished cardiac output and the blood pressure drops. It is possible for shock to cause death even when the injury causing the shock is not life-threatening. First aid measures include placing the patient in a recumbent position with feet elevated unless there is a head injury, in which case the patient is kept flat. If the patient has difficulty breathing or has a chest injury, the head and shoulders should be elevated. It is best to place a blanket under and over the patient to maintain body warmth but not to overheat.

Anaphylactic shock is an acute allergic reaction to a foreign substance, which may include certain foods, bee stings, or injections of therapeutic or **prophylactic** substances. The

Give Mouth-to-Mouth Resuscitation

TERMINAL PERFORMANCE OBJECTIVE: In a simulated situation, using a training manikin, demonstrate the procedure in the course taught by a certified instructor by explaining each step as it is being demonstrated with 100% accuracy. Remember that you must follow universal precautions even in emergency situations when you may come into contact with blood or body fluids.

1. Position victim on back and use finger sweep of mouth to remove any foreign material.
   Note: This may be accomplished with your finger alone or with a gauze sponge if these are available.
   RATIONALE: This procedure is necessary to clear mouth area for mouth-to-mouth contact.
2. Use modified jaw thrust, thereby moving tongue from back of throat. **RATIONALE: This opens victim's airway and determines whether victim is breathing independently.** Continue with procedure if there are no breath sounds.
3. Pinch victim's nostrils together with fingers of one hand while leaving other hand on forehead to keep the head tilted. **RATIONALE: This prevents escape of air through nose.**
4. Take a deep breath and then seal your mouth over victim's and breathe two times into the victim's mouth. Refill your lungs after each breath. *Note: This forces air into lungs for oxygen and carbon dioxide exchange. Breathe at a rate of 1 to 1½ seconds for each breath. Note:*
   a. *If mouth is injured, hold it shut and blow into nose.*
   b. *With small child, place your mouth over mouth and nose and blow into both, adjusting the force of your breaths for the size of the child.*
5. Turn your head to one side and listen for return of air. Watch chest for movement.
6. Repeat this cycle of blowing and listening with approximately 12 breaths per minute for adults and 20 for children until breathing is fully restored or another medical helper takes over or physician is in charge. *Note: Number of breaths corresponds to average number of breaths per minute for adults and children.*

---

patient will have severe difficulty breathing, blueness of the skin, and may have convulsions. The emergency supplies of epinephrine and oxygen should be immediately available for use by the physician or by the medical assistant under the direction of the physician. No patient should be given an allergy injection and then be allowed to leave the office immediately as anaphylactic shock may result from these injections. Patients may also have severe reactions to penicillin and other medications.

Sprains and Strains
Strains are the result of overuse of a muscle or group of muscles. They may be caused by improper lifting or by slipping while moving a heavy object. First aid is to rest the injured muscles in a comfortable position. Application of ice and then heat will help to relieve muscle strain. The physician may prescribe an analgesic or muscle relaxant.

Sprains are injuries to ligaments surrounding a joint. They are usually the result of twisting the joint and are sometimes so severe that a fracture may also occur. The injured extremity should be immobilized as soon as possible with a splinting device to avoid further injury to the person. Figure 11–14 shows an example of a preformed splint to immobilize a knee. Treatment is to elevate the sprained area and apply ice for the first 24 hours. The ice should be applied as soon as possible after the injury takes place. An elastic bandage is helpful but should not be put on too tightly. Temporary support may be given to an ankle by use of a cravat bandage, which may be applied over the shoe. (Note: A cravat is a folded, triangular bandage.)

Applying Heat and Cold Treatments. In the treatment of injuries physicians often order the application of a heat or cold pack, Figure 11–15. The physician will give specific instructions concerning the length of time it should be applied and where to apply the treatment.

Many offices and clinics today use disposable hot and cold packs because of their convenience. These plastic packs contain chemicals that are activated by either squeezing the bag and mixing the contents to produce cold, or by bending a metal disc to initiate heat. Many of these disposable packs are reusable by boiling or freezing them, which is of further convenience to the patient. With either of these packs it is recommended that the pack be placed in a cloth covering or a cloth or disposable towel be placed next to the area to protect the skin. If the physician requests moist heat or cold treatment, you should use a clean moist cloth towel between the plastic pack and the skin. Moisture better facilitates conduction of cold to tissues. Moist heat is less likely to cause burns of the skin or to dry it. It also provides deeper penetration to tissues. Unless otherwise ordered by the physician, the pack should be left in place for 20 minutes at a time. The maximum is 30 minutes. Generally

Give Cardiopulmonary Resuscitation

TERMINAL PERFORMANCE OBJECTIVE: In a simulated situation, using a training manikin (Figure 11–11), demonstrate the procedure in the course taught by a certified instructor by explaining each step as it is being demonstrated with 100% accuracy. Remember even in emergency situations you must follow universal precautions when you may come into contact with blood or body fluids.

1. Position manikin on its back on blanket on floor.
   Note:
   a. *Victim must always be in recumbent position on firm surface (floor or ground).*
   b. *Never practice this procedure on a person.*
2. Gently shake victim and ask "Are you OK?" Call for help. **RATIONALE: Call to another person, phone 911 or local emergency service before beginning resuscitation, or ask someone else to summon assistance while you are attempting to revive the victim. This should always be done so that you will not forget with a real patient.**
3. Place one hand on forehead to tilt head back and use your other hand to lift chin, Figure 11–12. **RATIONALE: This opens airway.**
4. Check for breathing by putting your ear close to victim's nose and mouth and watch chest for rise and fall. Check for 3 to 5 seconds.
5. If victim is not breathing, keep airway open, pinch nose, seal your mouth over victim's, and breathe twice into victim's mouth. Refill your lungs after each breath.
   Note:
   a. *Watch chest for evidence that air is entering lungs.*
   b. *Request that someone get help if victim is not breathing.*
6. Check for carotid pulse by placing your index and middle fingers into natural groove at side of neck. Take at least 5 to 10 seconds to locate pulse. Check carefully as pulse will probably be weak.
7. If victim has a pulse, continue mouth-to-mouth respirations at rate of one breath every 5 seconds (12 times per minute). *Note: Correct timing can be obtained by counting one, one thousand; two, one thousand; three,*

FIGURE 11–11 Chris Clean CPR training manikins with disposable parts

FIGURE 11–12 Basic CPR for adults: (a). After opening the airway, look, listen, and feel for breathing; if the victim is not breathing, give two slow, full breaths. (b). Palpate the carotid pulse for at least five seconds to determine whether or not the heart is beating. (c). Use smooth, even motions to compress the chest straight down, about 1 to 2 inches in an adult. (From Hegner & Caldwell, *Nursing Assistant,* 6th ed. Copyright 1992, Delmar Publishers Inc.)

one thousand; four, one thousand; and breathe. Go to Step 16.

8. If victim does not have a pulse, chest compression must be started. Locate lower margin of victim's rib cage and follow it to notch where ribs meet sternum in center of chest.
9. Place index finger on lower end of sternum.
10. Heel of hand closest to head is then placed on lower sternum next to index finger of first hand.
11. Place heel of hand which located notch over hand on sternum and lock fingers. Hold fingers high, away from body.

12. Rise on your knees so your shoulders are directly over hands on victim's sternum. Lock your elbows and keep arms straight.
13. Use a smooth, even motion to push straight down on chest and compress about 1 to 2 inches for a count of 15 compressions. A count of one and, two and, three and, etc. will help you obtain correct rate. (The rate of compressions is 80 to 100 times per minute.)
14. After administering 15 compressions, give victim two mouth-to-mouth respirations or ventilations *Note: Do this without moving from your position beside body.*
15. Repeat four cycles of compressions and respirations before pausing to check for breathing and presence of carotid pulse.
    a. If no pulse is felt, resume compressions and respirations.
    b. Check every few minutes or when second rescuer arrives.
16. You must not discontinue CPR unless victim recovers, someone takes over for you, a physician pronounces victim dead, or you become so exhausted that you cannot continue.
17. Use alcohol or benzalkonium chloride (Zephiran) to clean manikin. To sanitize the manikins used in training for CPR, you should use a solution of 1/4 cup bleach to a gallon of water. It is recommended that manikins with disposable mouthpieces and air bags be used in training for CPR, as shown in Figure 11–11, page 521, to prevent disease transmission. Manikins that have no disposable parts must be carefully and faithfully cleaned after each use with a clean gauze pad soaked in a liquid chlorine bleach and water solution, or with rubbing alcohol. The soaked gauze pad should remain on the area for at least 30 seconds and then wiped clean. It should be dried with a clean gauze pad.

the standard instruction is 20 minutes on and 10 minutes off. This may be repeated to increase circulation, but constant hot or cold is never advised.

Application of cold decreases local circulation temporarily, bacterial growth, and body temperature. It also is a temporary anesthetic, relieves inflammation, helps control bleeding, and reduces swelling. The average temperature produced by a cold pack is between 50° and 80°F (10°–26.7°C). Cold applications are used in burns, sprains, strains, and bruises and in the initial treatment of injuries to the eye.

Heat applications are used to increase tissue temperature, circulation, and the rate of healing. When heat is applied to an injured area, pain decreases. The average temperature produced by a hot pack is between 105° and 120°F (40.6°– 49°C). Heat treatments are used to relieve congestion in deep muscle layers and visceral organs and muscle spasms.

Stroke   For a patient who has suffered a cerebrovascular accident (CVA), loosen the clothing and be sure the patient is positioned so as not to choke on excess saliva. The common terms for a CVA are stroke, apoplexy, or cerebral thrombosis. A CVA is the result of a ruptured blood vessel in the brain. A CVA can also be caused by an occlusion of a blood vessel. The patient may have a light stroke with very little damage or an immediate paralysis in the form of sagging muscles on one side of the face or inability to use an arm or leg. One entire side of the body may be paralyzed. The patient may complain of numbness. The pupils of the eyes may be unequal in size. There may be mental confusion, slurred speech, nausea, vomiting, or difficulty in breathing and swallowing. Avoid any unnecessary movement of the patient. Keep in mind that the patient who appears to be unconscious or unable to speak may be able to hear what is being said.

Give Cardiopulmonary Resuscitation to Infants and Children

TERMINAL PERFORMANCE OBJECTIVE: In a simulated situation, using a training manikin, demonstrate the procedure as taught by a certified instructor by explaining each step as it is being demonstrated with 100% accuracy. Remember even in emergency situations you must follow universal precautions when you may come into contact with blood or body fluids.

1. Gently shake infant or child or tap bottom of foot to check for consciousness. Place infant or child on back on firm surface. **RATIONALE: Calling to another person, phoning 911 or local emergency service before beginning resuscitation summons assistance while you are attempting to revive the victim.** Send someone for help if the child does not respond.

2. Tip victim's head back and lift chin to open airway, Figure 11–13. *Note: Be careful not to tip head too far back as this can cause obstruction of airway in infant.*

3. Listen and watch for breathing. Place ear by mouth to listen. Also feel for breath on cheek and watch chest for breathing.

4. If no breathing is observed, give two slow breaths, 1 to 2 seconds each.
   a. For infants, cover nose and mouth with your mouth and breathe gently.
   b. For a child, cover mouth and pinch nostrils and carefully give two slow breaths.

5. For a child, check carotid pulse as for an adult. For an infant, check pulse over brachial artery by putting your middle fingertips on inside of upper arm halfway between elbow and shoulder. At the same time, keep airway open. *Note: Child's pulse should be checked at brachial artery for no longer than 10 seconds.*

6. If pulse is present, continue giving an infant one breath every 3 seconds and a child one ventilation every 4 seconds. Go to Step 8.

7. If no pulse is present, start cardiac compression. For an infant, use two fingers to compress middle of sternum to 1 inch at rate of 100 per minute. For a child use adult hand position, but use only the heel of one hand. Compress 1 to 1½ inches at rate of 80 to 100 times per min-ute. Give one breath for every five compressions.
   a. Be sure infant or child is on a firm surface or is being supported in back while administering compressions.
   b. Correct rate for infants could be counted as one, two, three, four, five, breathe.
   c. Correct rate for child would be one and two and three and four and five and breathe.

8. Do 10 cycles of compression and breath, and then check for breathing and pulse. *Note: Do not take more than five seconds for this check.*

9. If there is no pulse, give one breath and continue cycle until help arrives.

10. To sanitize the manikins used in training for CPR, use a solution of ¼ cup bleach to a gallon of water, or according to manufacturer's instructions.

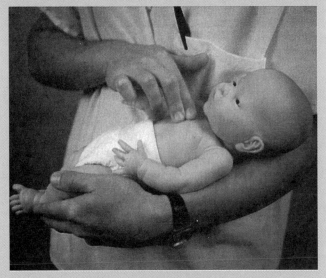

FIGURE 11–13 Basic CPR for infants (From Hegner & Caldwell, *Nursing Assistant,* 6th ed. Copyright 1992, Delmar Publishers Inc.)

FIGURE 11-14 Preformed splint; knee immobilizer. (From Lindsay, *The Professional Medical Assistant Clinical Practice*, Copyright 1993, Delmar Publishers Inc.)

FIGURE 11-15 Examples of disposable heat and cold packs before the chemicals are activated.

Wounds

You should be able to recognize and treat many types of wounds. Abrasions involve a scrape of the epidermis with dots of blood and possibly the presence of foreign material, such as dirt or gravel. First aid is to carefully clean the area with soap and water, apply an antiseptic solution or ointment, and cover with a dressing. If the abrasion resulted from contact with rusty metal or an unusually dirty object, a tetanus toxoid or antitoxin may be required.

A wound caused by a sharp object that leaves a clean cut is called an **incision** and may need sutures to close. Some people prefer to use tape for closure rather than sutures. The area must be carefully cleaned with soap and water, and an antiseptic may be applied before covering with a sterile dressing. A laceration is a tearing of body tissue and is more difficult to clean and suture properly. Special care must be taken to avoid infection. In the first aid care of an incision or laceration, the

first concern must be to control bleeding. This is accomplished with direct pressure to and elevation of, Figure 11–16. If direct pressure is not effective, indirect pressure on the appropriate pressure point should be used, Figure 11–17. The injured extremity should be immobilized as soon as possible with a splinting device to avoid further injury to the person. Figure 11–14 shows an example of a preformed splint to immobilize a knee. A puncture wound is one made with a pointed object, such as an icepick, knife, or nail. First aid is to clean the wound area and if necessary enlarge the hole with a probe to allow for irrigation with antiseptic solutions. A puncture wound may also be the result of an animal bite or human bite. It is usually possible to identify the type of bite by looking at the shape of the wound. For example, a snake bite would show a two-fang wound; it generally would be treated with a tourniquet tight enough to prevent venous return. Ice packs might also be used to prevent absorption of venom. Treatment must be given at once. A human bite is identified by the shape of the denture and needs to be carefully cleaned. An animal bite may result in a laceration. Any bite, human or animal, that breaks the skin should be seen by a physician. It is also important to report animal bites to the health department authorities so that the animal can be confined and checked for rabies. The bite should be cleaned thoroughly by washing with soap and water and dressed and the person should be treated for shock. If the animal shows evidence of rabies, a full 14 days of vaccine injections is necessary to protect the patient. A gunshot wound entrance will be a small deep puncture site with evidence in some cases of powder burns. This type of wound needs to be treated by a physician. First aid would be to keep the patient in shock position and carefully monitor vital signs while taking measures to control hemorrhage. Gunshot or stab wounds must be reported to the police. The location of either of these wounds would dictate the first aid measures to be taken. If a lung puncture is suspected, do not remove the object; send the patient immediately to an emergency facility.

Substance Abuse

Drug dependency is an increasing problem that can often create emergency situations. You need to know the symptoms associated with the various substances abused so that appropri-

FIGURE 11–16 Direct pressure

ate questions may be asked in taking a history from family members, see Table 2–4 in the Substance Abuse unit of Chapter 2, pages 41–43.

The authorities are greatly concerned about marijuana use because marijuana is often contaminated by addition of other substances. It may also be a stepping stone to more serious substance abuse. The effects of marijuana are swings from an unreasonable feeling of well-being, to disorientation in time, confusion, and irritability. The individual may lose the ability to accomplish anything requiring effort or concentration. Chronic asthma and bronchitis may also result.

The LSD user is described as experiencing sudden changes in the physical sense, and more acute sensory impressions. These individuals sometimes seem to be happy and sad at the same time. The effects are not always the same, and users describe "good trips" and "bad trips." These individuals may lose all sense of proportion and judgment and fancy themselves as having unusual powers. The user of LSD may develop strong **psychopathic** tendencies.

The chronic cocaine abuser may have elevated blood pressure, rapid pulse, dilated pupils, and may be nervous and apprehensive.

Amphetamines are powerful central nervous system stimulants and require a prescription for purchase, but there is considerable black market production of lookalikes. The illegal user of this type of drug develops a dependency and requires larger and larger amounts to obtain the desired "high." Abuse of this drug may cause hallucinations severe enough to require hospitalization. Large doses make patients irritable and may create difficulty in speaking clearly. Amphetamines also affect blood pressure and respirations, and cause arrhythmia of the heart. The pupils may be dilated, and excess sweating, headache, and diarrhea may be experienced.

Barbiturates are also addictive. They lower blood pressure and respiratory rate and the patient may suffer from mental disorientation, slurred speech, and staggering gait. An overdose of a barbiturate may cause death. The sudden withdrawal of barbiturates may cause nausea, delirium, convulsions, and death.

Alcohol dependence may result in emergency situations because of accidents in which alcoholics are involved. Alcohol acts as a depressant on the central nervous system and becomes addictive. The patient may develop grand mal epilepsy or **delirium tremens** when alcohol is withdrawn.

You must be aware of the problems of narcotic addiction. It is important to keep any narcotic supply in the office locked in a cabinet at all times. Physicians are careful to regulate the narcotics prescribed for a patient, but patients may see more than one physician for the purpose of obtaining narcotic prescriptions. You should be certain prescription pads are not left where they can be stolen and the name of the physician **forged**. It is also important to keep syringes and needles where patients cannot easily obtain them. You should be able to recognize chronic narcotic abusers. Some might have scars over the veins used for injecting substances, such as heroin or crack cocaine. The addict may attempt to cover up pin-point pupils

FIGURE 11–17 Pressure points: (A), temporal artery (B), carotid artery (C), subclavian artery (D), facial artery (E), brachial artery (F), radial artery (G), femoral artery (H), dorsalis pedis

by wearing dark glasses. These individuals may have ulcerated areas at the injection sites and also frequently suffer from hepatitis from using dirty needles. To prevent being infected with HIV, hepatitis B, or other bloodborn diseases, you should always remember to use universal precautions when caring for all patients.

Emergency Services ....

You should be able to contact the service that will be able to give the most help in an emergency. Contact the fire and police departments before you need them to find out what help is available and the quickest way to obtain that help. Find out what information must be reported in an emergency. The list of emergency numbers should be posted by every phone in the office and on a card on the emergency supply tray. All office staff should be aware of this information. The card kept on the tray can be handed to a family member to call for help while you administer first aid to the patient or assist the physician in this care.

If all emergency care fails and the patient should die in the office and the physician is not there at the time, the medics may be called to pronounce the patient dead. Arrange, if possible, for the body to be removed from the office through a back door and not the waiting room. The police must be notified, and usually they notify the coroner who will pick up the body for postmortem examination. A copy of the death certificate should be filed in the deceased patient's chart. It is important to find out what the procedure is in the area where you are working. The local statutes dictate the procedure to be followed.

Complete Chapter 11, Unit 2 in the workbook to help you meet the objectives at the beginning of this unit and therefore achieve competency of this subject matter.

U N I T 3
First Aid Care of Accidents and Injuries

OBJECTIVES ································

Upon completion of this unit, you will meet the following terminal performance objectives by verifying knowledge of the facts and principles presented through oral and written communication at a level deemed competent by the instructor or employer, and will demonstrate the specific behaviors as identified in the terminal performance objectives of the procedures, observing all aseptic and safety precautions in accordance with health care standards.

1. Demonstrate the proper method of cleaning a wound.
2. Demonstrate the application of a dressing and recurrent-turn bandages.

P R O C E D U R E

Prepare Basic Suture Setup

TERMINAL PERFORMANCE OBJECTIVE: Provided with all necessary equipment and supplies, demonstrate all steps required in the basic suture setup procedure. The instructor will observe each step. Remember even in emergency situations you must follow universal precautions when you may come into contact with blood or body fluids.

1. Wash your hands. **CAUTION:** Remember, in order to comply with universal precautions guidelines, gloves must be worn if there is any possibility of coming into contact with blood or any body fluids.
2. Assemble local anesthetic as directed by physician, sterile dressings and bandages, tape, and appropriate drape.
3. On a sterile towel, assemble sterile gloves, syringe and needle, hemostats, scissors, sponges, suture and needle holder, and forceps.
   Note:
   a. Your office procedure manual should list necessary items.
   b. As you gain experience, you should also have your own reference cards to help you remember various procedures.
4. You may be instructed to bandage area when suturing is completed. **CAUTION:** Remember, in order to com-

ply with universal precautions guidlines, gloves must be worn if there is any possibility of coming into contact with blood or any body fluids.
   Note:
   a. Always hold dressing material by edges which will not touch wound.
   b. In bandaging, be careful to make bandage snug enough to hold dressing in place but not so tight that circulation is impaired or patient is uncomfortable.
5. You are usually expected to give patient instructions for follow-up care. Have follow-up instructions in printed form. **RATIONALE: Patient's are often nervous and upset following trauma and may not understand or remember the instructions.**
6. Make an appointment for suture removal.
7. Note: If gloves were worn they may have been removed following step #4 if it was necessary for you to schedule the appointment. Be certain to reglove to clean up examining room.
8. Discard contaminated materials and gloves in biohazardous waste bag.
9. Wash hands.
10. Record and initial prodedure on patient's chart.

Clean Wound Areas

TERMINAL PERFORMANCE OBJECTIVE: Provided with all necessary equipment and supplies, and using other students as patients, demonstrate the steps in this procedure for cleansing wounds. The instructor will observe each step. Remember even in emergency situations you must follow universal precautions when you may come into contact with blood or body fluids.

1. Assemble basin, mild detergent with warm water, sterile gauze sponges, sterilized sponge forceps,. and latex gloves, and sterile water for irrigation.
2. Wash your hands thoroughly with soap and water. Put on latex gloves. **CAUTION:** Remember, in order to comply with universal precautions guidelines, gloves must be worn if there is any possibility of coming into contact with blood or any body fluids.
3. Grasp several gauze sponges with sponge forceps.
4. Dip into warm detergent water. *Note: Make certain water is at a comfortable temperature.*
5. Wash wound and wound area to remove microorganisms and any foreign matter.
Note: Be careful not to injure patient further with instrument. Wash wound area with sponges only. Work from inner to outer area 2 to 3 inches around wound as you would for surgical prep. **RATIONALE: This will prevent bringing microorganisms from surrounding skin into open wound.**
6. Irrigate wound thoroughly with sterile water.
7. Blot wound dry with sterile gauze.
8. Cover with dry sterile dressing and bandage in place.
9. Advise patient to call physician immediately if evidence of infection should develop. *Note: Patient should be told to watch for redness, swelling, and sensation of pain or fever. Typed instructions should be given to patient for follow-up care.*
10. Clean up work area. Place all blood-stained materials and gloves in the biohazardous waste bag and into proper receptacle for safe disposal.
11. Wash hands.

Apply Bandage in Recurrent Turn to Finger

TERMINAL PERFORMANCE OBJECTIVE: Provided with all necessary equipment and supplies and using other students as patients, demonstrate the steps in the procedure for recurrent turn. The instructor will observe each step. Remember even in emergency situations you must follow universal precautions when you may come into contact with blood or body fluids.

This procedure will show you how to bandage after the wound area has been covered with a dressing.

1. Wash hands. **CAUTION:** Remember, in order to comply with universal precautions guidlines, gloves must be worn if there is any possibility of coming into contact with blood or any body fluids.
2. Assemble supplies: dressing, scissors, bandage, antiseptic or medication as ordered.
3. Carefully open dressing without contaminating and place over injury area.
4. Secure dressing with bandage of gauze, which is started at the proximal end of the finger on the palm side and then directly over the finger to the proximal end on the back of the hand and repeated several times.
5. Hold recurrent turns in place with spiral turns.
6. Secure by tying off at gauze proximal end of finger. The tying off may be accomplished by using a figure-eight turn.
   a. From the finger take the end of the bandage diagonally across the back of the hand to the wrist.
   b. Circle the wrist once or twice.
   c. From the opposite side of the wrist, continue back to finger and loop.
   d. Repeat the figure eight several times and tie off at wrist, or tape in place. *Note: It is difficult to tear and handle tape while wearing gloves.*
7. Discard contaminated materials and gloves in biohazardous waste bag.
8. Wash hands.
9. Record and initial procedure on patient's chart.

3. Demonstrate the application of a dressing and open-spiral bandage.
4. Demonstrate the application of a dressing and closed-spiral bandage.
5. Demonstrate the application of a dressing and figure-eight bandage to the hand.
6. Demonstrate the application of a cravat bandage to the head.
7. Demonstrate the application of a triangular bandage to the head.
8. Demonstrate the application of a sling.
9. Demonstrate the application of tube gauze.
10. Demonstrate fitting and instruction in the use of crutches.
11. Demonstrate fitting and instruction in the use of a cane.
12. Demonstrate instruction in the use of a walker.
13. Demonstrate movement of a patient from a wheelchair to and from an examination table.
14. Spell and define, using the glossary at the back of the text, all the words to know in this unit.

WORDS TO KNOW ....

axilla   friction   recurrent

Human skin cannot be sterilized, but the microorganisms that may be harmful can be washed off with soap and water using **friction** at the skin surface. The procedure of cleaning a wound is usually the responsibility of the medical assistant. If bleeding has been severe, no attempt should be made to clean the area because the patient will need medical care. A pressure bandage should be applied securely and the patient taken for emergency medical care immediately. If the office or clinic policy is to treat such emergencies, you should notify the appropriate staff and follow the procedure quickly to prepare for treatment of the patient. When the wound does not bleed excessively and does not involve tissues below the skin, the area should be thoroughly cleaned.

If a wound is superficial and will heal well with simple cleaning and protection from contamination, there is no need for sutures. Some clean cuts may be closed with adhesive steristrips or butterfly closures. You will be responsible for having suture setup packets sterilized and ready for use when the physician needs them. The emergency patient who needs suturing may come to the office with a pressure dressing in place to control hemorrhage. You should wait for instructions from the physician before removing a pressure dressing. You may question the patient or a relative to find out what caused the wound and how large and deep it is. You should also inquire about the most recent tetanus immunization booster and record the information on the patient's chart. The physician will write the orders for the necessary immunization(s) the patient may need. You should not proceed with any medication or injection until the order has been written by the physician.

An injury to fingers or toes or an amputation can be effectively bandaged with the use of a nonstick dressing over the wound area which is held in place with **recurrent** turns, Figure 11–18.

FIGURE 11–18   Recurrent turn on a finger (From Simmers, *Diversified Health Occupations*, 3rd ed. Copyright 1993, Delmar Publishers Inc.)

FIGURE 11–19 Application of a bandage in an open spiral

Apply Bandage in Open or closed Spiral

TERMINAL PERFORMANCE OBJECTIVE: Provided with all necessary equipment and supplies and using other students as patients, demonstrate the steps in the procedure for application of open- and closed-spiral bandage. The instructor will observe each step. Remember even in emergency situations you must follow universal precautions when you may come into contact with blood or body fluids.

This procedure will show you how to bandage after the wound area has been covered with a dressing.

1. Wash hands. **CAUTION:** Remember, in order to comply with universal precautions guidelines, gloves must be worn if there is any possibility of coming into contact with blood or any body fluids.
2. Assemble needed supplies.
3. Carefully open dressing, without contaminating, and place over wound area.
4. Anchor bandage by placing end of bandage on bias at starting point.
5. Encircle part, allowing corner of bandage end to protrude.
6. Turn down protruding tip of bandage.
7. Encircle part again.
8. Continue to encircle area to be covered with spiral turns spaced so that they do not overlap. *OR* Form closed spiral by continuing to encircle with overlapping spiral turns until all open spaces are covered.
9. Complete bandage by tying off or taping in place.
    Note:
    a. *Tape should be long enough to hold bandage snugly in place.*
    b. *Tape should be applied to run in opposite direction from body movement.*

   c. *Tearing adhesive tape is difficult while wearing gloves. You may find it necessary to remove gloves and discard them into proper container.* (See Figure 11-20.)
10. If gloves were removed, reglove to clean up area.
11. Discard contaminated materials and gloves in biohazardous waste bag.
12. Wash hands.
13. Record and initial procedure on patient's chart.

FIGURE 11-20 Tearing adhesive tape is much simpler when holding the edge of the strip between the thumbnails and forefingers and using a quick rotary motion of the hands in opposite directions.

P R O C E D U R E

Apply Figure-Eight Bandage to Hand and Wrist

TERMINAL PERFORMANCE OBJECTIVE: Provided with all necessary equipment and supplies and using other students as patients, demonstrate the steps in the procedure for applying a figure-eight bandage to hand and wrist. The instructor will observe each step. Remember even in emergency situations you must follow universal precautions when you may come into contact with blood or body fluids.

This procedure will show you how to bandage after the wound area has been covered with a dressing.

1. Wash hands. **CAUTION:** Remember, in order to comply with universal precautions guidlines, gloves must be worn if there is any possibility of coming into contact with blood or any body fluids.
2. Assemble needed supplies.
3. Apply dressing. Do not contaminate any part will touch wound area.
4. Anchor bandage with one or two turns around palm of hand.
5. Roll gauze diagonally across front of wrist and in figure-eight pattern around the hand as many times as necessary, Figure 11–21.
6. Tie off the at wrist. **CAUTION:** Do not impair circulation.

FIGURE 11–21 Figure-eight bandage

7. Discard contaminated materials and gloves in biohazardous waste bag.
8. Wash hands.
9. Record and initial procedure on patient's chart.

FIGURE 11–22 Folding a triangular bandage to make a cravat bandage (Adopted from Simmers, *Diversified Health Occupations*, Copyright 1993, Delmar Publishers Inc.)

An injury on the arms or legs will require a dressing to be held in place with an open or closed spiral bandage, Figure 11–19.

A wound on the palm or back of the hand may be protected with a dressing and a figure-eight bandage to hold the dressing in place.

When a dressing is needed for the forehead, ears, or eyes, a cravat may be used to hold the dressing in place. A cravat can be made from a triangular bandage, Figure 11–22.

A bandage that is particularly useful in keeping a dressing in place over a large head wound or a burn is the triangular bandage.

A sling is often used to support an arm after a fracture or injury to the shoulder or arm. It is important to learn the correct way to put a sling on a patient and to practice with the patient standing, sitting, and lying down. Care must be taken to elevate the hand properly. You must also be sure that the sling is tied to one side and never over the spine where a knot is extremely uncomfortable.

Triangular bandages may be made from muslin or purchased in individual packages. Some physicians like to use a print material for children. The standard adult sling is about 55 inches across the base and 36 to 40 inches along the sides.

The easiest and probably the quickest way to bandage arms, legs, fingers, and toes is with a tubular gauze bandage,

Apply Cravat Bandage to Forehead, Ear, or Eyes

TERMINAL PERFORMANCE OBJECTIVE: Provided with all necessary equipment and supplies and using other students as patients, demonstrate the steps in the procedure for applying a cravat bandage to the head. The instructor will observe each step. Remember even in emergency situations you must follow universal precautions when you may come into contact with blood or body fluids.

This procedure will show you how to bandage after the wound area has been covered with a dressing.

1. Wash hands. **CAUTION:** Remember, in order to comply with universal precautions guidelines, gloves must be worn if there is any possibility of coming into contact with blood or any body fluids.
2. Assemble needed supplies.
3. Carefully place dressing over wound taking care not to contaminate area which will be over wound.
4. Place center of cravat over dressing, Figure 11–23.
5. Take ends around to opposite side of head and cross

Figure 11–23 Applying a cravat bandage to the head (Adapted from Simmers, *Diversified Occupations,* 3rd ed. Copyright 1993, Delmar Publishers Inc.)

them. Do not tie.
6. Bring ends back to starting point and tie them.
7. Discard contaminated materials and gloves in biohazardous waste bag.
8. Wash hands.
9. Record and initial procedure on patient's chart.

Apply Triangular Bandage to Scalp

TERMINAL PERFORMANCE OBJECTIVE: Provided with all necessary equipment and supplies and using other students as patients demonstrate the steps in the procedure for applying a triangular bandage to the scalp. The instructor will observe each step. Remember even in emergency situations you must follow universal precautions when you may come into contact with blood or body fluids.

This procedure will show you how to bandage after the wound area has been covered with a dressing.

1. Wash hands. **CAUTION:** Remember, in order to comply with universal precautions guidelines, gloves must be worn if there is any possibility of coming into contact with blood or any body fluids.
2. Assemble needed supplies.
3. Carefully place dressing over wound area without contaminating.
4. Fold a hem about two inches wide along base of bandage, Figure 11–24.
5. With hem on outside, place bandage on head so that middle of base is on forehead close to eyebrows and point hangs down back.
6. Bring two ends around head above ears and cross them just below bump at back of head.
7. Draw ends snugly around head and tie them in center of forehead.
8. Steady head with one hand and with other hand draw point down firmly behind to hold compress securely against head. Grasp point and tuck it into area where bandage ends cross.
9. Discard contaminated materials and gloves in biohazardous waste bag.

FIGURE 11–24 Applying a trianguler bandage to the scalp

10. Wash hands.
11. Record and initial procedure on patient's chart.

Apply Arm Sling

TERMINAL PERFORMANCE OBJECTIVE: Provided with all necessary equipment and supplies and using other students as patients, demonstrate the steps in the procedure for applying an arm sling. The instructor will observe each step.

1. Wash hands. **CAUTION:** Remember, in order to comply with universal precautions guidelines, gloves must be worn if there is any possibility of coming into contact with blood or any body fluids.
2. Place one end of bandage over shoulder on uninjured side and let other end hang down over chest, Figure 11-25.
3. Pull point behind elbow of injured arm.
4. Pull end of bandage which is hanging down up around injured arm and over shoulder. Elevate hand 4 to 5 inches above elbow. **RATIONALE: Elevation aids in return circulation, which reduces swelling and dis-**comfort. Tie ends together at side of neck (never over spine).
5. Bring point of bandage at elbow over front of sling and pin to sling with safety pin.

Note:

a. *If pin is not available, twist point until it is snug against the elbow and tie a single knot.*
b. *Be sure ends of finger extend slightly beyond edge of sling.* **RATIONALE: It is necessary to be able to observe fingers for signs of impaired circulation, such as swelling or discoloration.**

FIGURE 11–25 (a). Buckle type of arm sling for support (b). Applying an arm sling

Figure 11–26. This is accomplished with the use of a cylindrical cage applicator. The amount of gauze you expect to use is stretched over the applicator and placed over the extremity.

It is often necessary for a patient to walk with crutches to give a foot, ankle, knee, or leg injury an opportunity to heal. It is important for the crutches to be adjusted to the correct height. This is accomplished by holding the crutches up to the side of the patient and adjusting them so that the underarm pad is 2 to 3 inches below the **axilla.** The handhold should be adjusted so that the hands fit comfortably with the arms extended. The axillary pad and handhold should be foam-padded for comfort. The patient should be instructed to stand on the uninjured foot while swinging the injured leg forward as the crutches are moved forward. Refer to Figure 11–27. The weight of the body should be on the hands and never on the axillary area since pressure there can cause nerve damage.

The patient who needs only a cane for support should have one that is the proper length to fit comfortably in the hand with the arm hanging naturally at the side. Many canes are adjustable; if not, they must be fitted to the correct length. Canes come in a variety of materials and types. An elderly patient usually has less trouble with a quad-base cane. The patient should carry the cane on the strong or uninjured side. The cane should swing forward with the uninjured extremity. Part of the weight is carried by the cane being firmly placed on the floor simultaneously with the uninjured extremity.

A walker is useful for patients who because of age or physi-

A

B

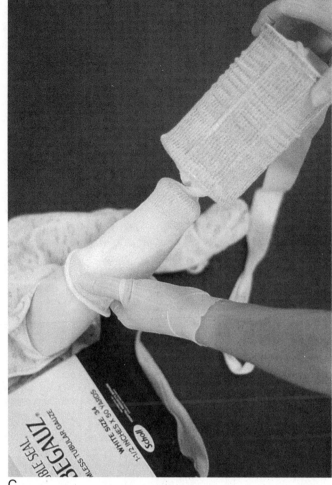

C

FIGURE 11–26 (a) Push the tube-gauze onto the cylinder and allow for an excessive amount. (b) Place the cylinder with tube-gauze over the injured extremity carefully. (c) Hold the end of tube-gauze gently above the injury and pull the cylinder away from the extremity, twisting the gauze. Repeat applications as desired for protection of the wound.

cal condition cannot safely use crutches. The walker may be adjusted to the proper height for the patient. The patient must be cautioned not to step too closely to the walker as it is then difficult to stay balanced. The patient should move the walker forward and then step into the walker while leaning slightly forward on the walker.

When a patient comes to your office in a wheelchair, you need to know how to help that patient from the wheelchair to the examination table and back again.

If you have had to put a patient onto an examination table from a wheelchair, you will need to return that patient to a wheelchair to leave the office.

All of the procedures in this chapter need to be practiced many times so that you feel comfortable and confident when the need arises to use them.

Complete Chapter 11, Unit 3 in the workbook to help you meet the objectives at the beginning of this unit and therefore achieve competency of this subject matter.

Instruct Patient in Use of Crutches

TERMINAL PERFORMANCE OBJECTIVE: Provided with all necessary equipment and supplies, and using other students as patients, demonstrate the steps of this procedure to instruct a patient in using crutches. The instructor will observe each step.

1. Identify patient and confirm physician's orders.
   RATIONALE: Speaking to the patient by name and checking chart ensures that you are performing the procedure on the correct patient.
2. Assemble equipment. Make sure crutches are intact (hand pads and rubber tips), and stable.
3. Stabilize patient upright near wall or chair for support. *Note: Patient must be wearing nonskid shoes or foot coverings.*
   RATIONALE: This helps prevent slipping or falling.
4. Adjust crutches for patient so that the handles of the crutches are comfortable with a 30-degree angle bend

of the elbows with 2 inches between the area under the arm and the top of the crutches.
Note:
a. *Explain to the patient to support his or her weight at the handle and not under the arm.* **RATIONALE: Pressure in the axilla from upper body weight may damage nerves.**
b. *Tell patient to take small steps slowly to avoid getting off balance and possibly falling.*
c. *Instruct patient to stand on his or her uninjured foot while swinging the injured leg forward with crutches.* Crutches should be placed approximately 4 to 5 inches in front and 4 to 5 inches to the side of the patient's heels. Use Figure 11–27 to show the ordered gait for walking safely with crutches.
5. Record procedure on patient's chart.

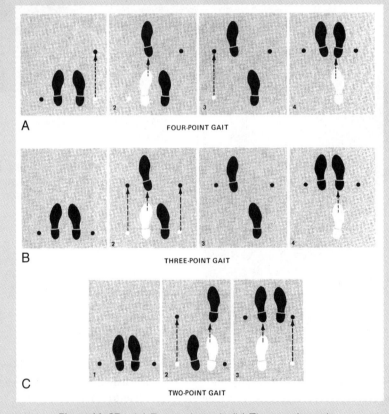

A FOUR-POINT GAIT

B THREE-POINT GAIT

C TWO-POINT GAIT

Figure 11–27 (a) Four-point gait. (b) Three-point gait. (c) Two-point gait. (From Simmers, Diversified *Health Occupations,* 3rd. ed., copyright 1993, Delmar Publishers Inc.)

Instruct Patient in Use of Cane

TERMINAL PERFORMANCE OBJECTIVE: Provided with all the necessary equipment and supplies, and using other students as patients, demonstrate the steps of this procedure for instructing a patient in the use of a cane. The instructor will observe each step.

1. Identify patient and confirm physician's orders. **RATIONALE: Speaking to the patient by name and checking chart ensures that you are performing the procedure on the correct patient.**
2. Assemble equipment. Check cane for intact rubber tip. *Note: Patient must be wearing nonskid shoes or foot coverings.* **RATIONALE: This helps prevent slipping or falling.**
3. Adjust height of cane so that patient's elbow is flexed comfortably at approximately a 25- to 30-degree angle, and that the handle of the cane is positioned just below hip level of the uninjured or strong side.
4. Demonstrate to the patient the gait ordered to safely ambulate by.
   a. moving the cane and injured extremity forward simultaneously,
   b. then moving the strong or uninjured extremity forward. *Note: Observe patient and be alert to assist patient and rescue in case of fall.*
5. Explain to patient how to go up stairs:
   a. Move the uninjured extremity up first.
   b. Then move injured extremity up. Remind patient to use cane for support.
6. Explain to patient how to go down stairs:
   a. Move uninjured extremity down first.
   b. Then move injured extremity down. Remind patient to use cane for support.
7. Instruct patient to take small, slow steps. **RATIONALE: This aids in maintaining balance.** *Note: Answer questions patient may have and give emotional support.*
8. Record and initial on patient's chart.

Instruct Patient in Use of Walker

TERMINAL PERFORMANCE OBJECTIVE: Provided with all necessary equipment and supplies, and using other students as patients, demonstrate the steps in the procedure to instruct a patient in the use of a walker.

1. Identify patient and confirm physician's orders. **RATIONALE: Speaking to the patient by name and checking chart ensures that you are performing the procedure on the correct patient.**
2. Assemble equipment. Check walker for rubber tips, pads at handles, and stability.
3. Stabilize patient upright near wall or chair for support. *Note: Patient must be wearing nonskid shoes or foot coverings.* **RATIONALE: This helps prevent slipping or falling.**
4. The height of the walker should be adjusted so that the handles are at the patient's hip level, and the bend of the patient's elbows is at a comfortable 25 to 30 degree angle.
5. Position the walker with the patient inside it.
6. Instruct patient to pick up the walker and move it slightly forward and walk into it.
   Note:
   a. Instruct patient to keep all four feet of walker on the floor.
   b. Explain to patient not to slide the walker. **RATIONALE: It may slip or catch and cause a fall.**
   c. Instruct patient not to step too close to walker. **RATIONALE: This makes it possible to lose balance.**
   d. Observe patient and be ready to assist in case of possible fall.
7. Record and initial on patient's chart.

Assist Patient from Wheelchair to Examining Table

TERMINAL PERFORMANCE OBJECTIVE: Provided with necessary equipment and using other students as patients, demonstrate the steps in the procedure for assisting patient from wheelchair to examination table. The instructor will observe each step.

1. Unlock wheels of chair and wheel patient to examination room. *Note: Wheelchairs should always be locked in position when sitting still to prevent unexpected movement. This is accomplished by flipping brake on each wheel.*
2. Position chair as near as possible to place you want patient to sit on table.
3. Lower table to chair level. *Note: If this cannot be done, position footstool beside table.* **CAUTION:** If footstool is used, be certain patient steps on squarely to avoid tipping stool.
4. Lock wheels on chair.
5. Fold footrests back. If necessary, assist patient in moving feet.
6. Stand directly in front of patient with feet slightly apart to give a good base.
7. Bend knees and have patient place hands on your shoulders while you place your hands under patient's armpits to assist patient to standing position. Pause in this position for a moment before next step.

8. Maintaining position of hands pivot or side step to position in front of table, Figure 11–28.
9. Place one foot slightly behind you for support and help patient to sitting position on table.
10. If patient still needs support, place one hand around patient's back. Help patient raise legs to table by placing free arm under legs and lifting them as patient turns. *Note: If patient needs to remove clothing get someone to help you. One person balances patient while other removes necessary clothing.*
11. Place pillow under patient's head. Drape patient appropriately. *Note: Never leave a very ill patient alone on a table. There is danger of a fall.*
12. Unlock chair wheels and move chair out of way. *Note: If room is small, it may be necessary to place chair outside examining room.*

FIGURE 11–28
Position of the feet when assisting patient from wheel chair onto examination table

Assist Patient from Examining Table to Wheelchair

TERMINAL PERFORMANCE OBJECTIVE: Provided with necessary equipment and using other students as patients, demonstrate the steps in the procedure of assisting the patient from examination table to wheelchair. The instructor will observe each step.

1. Reposition chair and lock wheels.
2. Assist patient to sitting position on table. Support back if necessary. Lift patient's legs as patient is turned until feet dangle over edge of the table.
3. Ask patient to put hands on your shoulders. Support patient on sides below armpits. Have stepstool in place if table is not lowered to chair height. **CAUTION:** Take

special care to ensure that patient steps squarely on stool when getting down from examining table. Place your feet against legs of footstool, on outside, to maintain its position.
4. Support patient into standing position.
5. Side step or pivot patient to position in front of chair. *Note: Assist patient if necessary in putting on robe or clothing.*
6. Have patient reach back to arms of chair as you help in lowering patient into chair.
7. Adjust footrests.
8. Unlock wheels and return patient to reception room.

Mr. Right . . .

has taken first aid and CPR courses and remains current in certification so he can administer emergency assistance when needed. He keeps the emergency phone numbers updated by each phone in the office. He makes a routine check of the office daily for safety hazards and deals with problems immediately. He makes sure that all exits are free of obstacles and marked clearly. He also makes sure that emergency evacuation routes are visible for the general public.

Promotion outlook: Excellent

Ms. Wrong . . .

doesn't want to renew her certification in CPR or first aid because she doesn't have time. She takes the list of emergency phone numbers with her from phone to phone and frequently misplaces them. Once in a while she looks over the office to see if there are any safety hazards and if the emergency evacuation instructions are still on the wall by the exit, which is blocked with the delivery of supplies from yesterday.

Promotion outlook: Questionable

R E F E R E N C E S

American Red Cross, *Adult CPR,* 1988.
Mosby's Medical, Nursing, and Allied Health Dictionary, 3d ed. St. Louis: C.V. Mosby, 1990.
The Nurse's Reference Library, Procedures, Nursing 83 Books, Springhouse, PA: Intermed Communications, 1983.
Simmers, Louise. *Diversified Health Occupations,* 3rd ed. Albany, NY: Delmar Publishers, 1993.

C H A P T E R 1 2
Employment

UNIT 1
The Job Search

UNIT 2
Getting the Job and Keeping It

A vast array of jobs require either administrative or clinical skills or a combination of both. Physicians in private practice usually have an average of three employees. In group practice, there may be from five to as many as forty or more, depending on the number of physicians and the size of the facility.

In seeking employment, you must be aware of the different opportunities and decide which area of medical assisting you would prefer. Many medical assistants prefer general or family practice because of its variety and challenge; others enjoy the specialty fields with their new developments and rapid change. There are still many health care facilities whose job descriptions specify particular duties, such as medical secretary, office nurse, or receptionist. The generally trained medical assistant should be able to perform the dual role of administrative and clinical assistant and will therefore be a valuable asset to any medical practice.

This chapter will discuss the steps involved in seeking employment in the health care field as well as presenting ideas for being a valuable employee. These job acquisition skills will be useful in other employment fields as well. Showing a genuine interest in others and the desire to work are the first steps in the job search.

U N I T 1

The Job Search

Upon completion of this unit, you will meet the following terminal performance objectives by verifying knowledge of the facts and principles presented through oral and written communication at a level deemed competent by the instructor or employer, and will demonstrate the specific behaviors as identified in the terminal performance objectives of the procedures.

1. Prepare a neat, accurate, and well-organized resumé.
2. Discuss information contained in a resumé and the purpose of each style of resumé.
3. Write a cover letter to accompany a resumé.
4. Reply to a classified ad in the newspaper.
5. Explain employment agency services.
6. List three contacts to assist you in your job search.
7. Define the common abbreviations used in the newspaper "Help Wanted" section.
8. Spell and define, using the glossary at the back of the text, all the words to know in this unit.

aspirations

attribute

chronological

classified

dual

elaborate

fringe

functional

ingenuity

negotiable

resumé

targeted

transcript

The job search begins with the desire to work. A medical assistant with skills in communication and medical office procedures should discover excellent opportunities for employment.

The Resumé..

One of the first steps in presenting yourself for employment is to develop a personal resumé. A **resumé** is an outlined summary of your abilities and experience. It should be complete, accurate, and neatly organized. The resumé will describe to prospective employers your educational background, previous work experience, professional affiliations, community service, personal interests, honors, employment objectives, and whatever else you feel is important for them to know. It need not contain personal information about your marital status, race, religion, age, or any other facts that may be used to discriminate against you illegally. The purpose of the resumé is to inform the prospective employer of how well you measure up to the position for which you are applying.

There are several styles of resumés. You may arrange the information in a variety of ways. Some popular styles include the following: a traditional format in **chronological** order, a listing of your career objective, in a **functional** plan, or in a **targeted** layout. Figure 12–1 (a) through (e) shows an example of each type. Each of these designs is attractive and easy to read. The *traditional (chronological) approach* shows the reader your background information in an organized fashion. It is a good way to highlight your abilities when you are just beginning the job search. The *career objective* style shows your obvious career choice to the reader and is followed by your abilities and qualifications. It is also a frequently chosen style for the novice. A *chronologically arranged* resumé, page 540, shows the prospective employer your employment history in dated order from present (or most recent) back to the beginning of your work experience. You should highlight the responsibilities of each position. Your present job duties

---

P R O C E D U R E

Prepare a Resumé

PURPOSE: To document information concerning education, experience, and abilities for employment consideration.

Items needed: Paper, pen, dictionary, thesaurus, telephone book, typewriter or word processor

1. Write your complete legal name, address, and phone number. This information may be arranged flush left or centered at the top of the page.
   Refer to Figure 12–1 for the particular style of resumé that is appropriate for you and your needs. Use reference materials listed above for accuracy, expression, and correct spelling in composing your resumé.

2. Briefly state your qualifications and abilities, and list the position desired next to the heading of: Job Objective or Job Target.

3. List your educational background, beginning with the most recent or present date. You may note at the bottom of the resumé that you will furnish **transcripts** or certificates on request.

4. List all pertinent employment experience, beginning with the most recent or present date. Include the dates of employment, employer's name, address, and the position you held with a brief description of your responsibilities according to the style of resumé you have selected.

5. List memberships and affiliations in professional organizations. These may be arranged alphabetically or ranked by order of importance.

6. List community service, including volunteer programs and activities as may be appropriate. This is optional.

7. List outside interests briefly as appropriate. This is optional.

8. List references on a separate sheet of paper. State on the bottom of the resumé that references will be furnished on request. You should have at least three references (persons *not* related to you) and no more than five. Permission should be obtained from these persons *before* they are listed.

9. Type the completed resumé on a sheet of bond paper, or use the word processor to enter your information. Underscore (underline) headings for clarity and attractiveness. Check the finished copy for errors (use spellcheck program on your word processor, but don't rely on it exclusively). Ask a reliable person to proofread your resumé. Have a number of copies printed on quality paper for distribution (off-white, beige, or ivory white are preferred colors).

10. Revise and update your resumé to document additional employment experience, educational achievements, certificates, awards, and personal development. Items of lesser importance should be deleted as more important accomplishments are added.

Seth M. Nelson, CMA
4030 Newbank Road
Wheelersburg, Ohio 45794
(614) 555-1212
Qualifications: Certified Medical Assistant
Desired Position: Clinical Medical Assistant
Education:
    1992 to date: Attending evening courses in Nursing, Southern Ohio Technical College, Lucasville, Ohio
                     AAMA National Certification 1990
    1986–87:   Certificate, Ohio Valley Training Academy, Wellston, Ohio. Major: Medical Assisting
    1984:   Diploma, Portsmouth East High School, Portsmouth, Ohio. Major: General Business
EMPLOYMENT EXPERIENCE:
    1990 to date: Administrative Medical Assistant to Wilber Roth, M.D., Rolling Hills, Ohio
    1987–90:   Admissions Clerk, Green Meadows Community Hospital, Green Meadows, Ohio
    1984–87:   Cashier, Garden Inn Restaurant, Hilldale, Ohio
PROFESSIONAL ASSOCIATIONS:
    American Association of Medical Assistants
    Ohio State Society of Medical Assistants
    Scioto County Chapter of Medical Assistants
COMMUNITY SERVICE:
    Red Cross Volunteer
    Big Brothers Association Volunteer
Interests: camping, music, reading, volleyball
References, transcripts and certificates, furnished upon request.

FIGURE 12–1   Sample Resumés   **A.** Traditional (chronological order) format

Jody C. Lawrence
270 Huxley Road
Avondale, Ohio 41234
(614) 555-1212
CAREER OBJECTIVE
    To establish a career as a Medical Assistant in a professional medical practice in both administrative and clinical capacities; To become a Certified Medical Assistant.
EDUCATION
    Independence High School, Major: Business; plan to receive diploma this June
    Southfield Vocational Center, Program Specialty; Medical Assisting; plan to receive vocational certificate this June
EXPERIENCE
    Avondale Civic Center; part-time secretary, 29 East Main Street, Avondale, Ohio 41234
    Southfield Family Practice; externship as Student Medical Assistant, 589 Garfield Avenue, Suite 212, Southfield, Ohio 41239
ACTIVITIES/HONORS
    Cheerleader, all four years, Independence High School
    Class Secretary, Senior year, Independence High School
    Health Fair Committee, Junior and Senior years, Southfield Vocational Center Honor Roll, all four years
    Vocational Industrial Clubs of America, Class Club Treasurer, Senior year, Southfield Vocational Center
SKILLS
    Typing—65 WPM, transcribing, operating: calculator, IBM computer
    Basic clinical laboratory procedures; CPR
INTERESTS
    Cooking, dancing, poetry, softball, swimming

FIGURE 12–1 B.   "Career objective" style

Sharon R. Beach, RMA, CMA
4270 Hilldale Drive
Fernridge, CA 95061
(406) 555-1122

Employment Experience

1989–Present	Fernridge Family Health Center
	Clinical Medical Assistant
	Provide patient education regarding therapeutic diets; assist with minor office surgery; perform ECGs and Holter monitors; phlebotomy and routine diagnostic tests.
1986–1989	Brownsville General Hospital
	Phlebotomist/ECG Technician
1985–1986	Ronald L. Botkin, D.O.—General Practice
	Administrative and Clinical Medical Assistant
	Completed medical insurance claim forms; office correspondence; transcription; basic clinical assisting.

Professional Affiliations/Achievements

1985 to Present	Member American Association of Medical Assistants
1990 to Present	CPR Certification
1990	Certified Medical Assistant Certificate
1992	Registered Medical Assistant Certificate

Education

| 1988 | B.A. Degree; Nutrition, Brownsville University |
| 1985 | Medical Assistant Program Certificate, Baldwin Community College |

FIGURE 12–1 C. Example of chronological resumé

should be emphasized. This will show the employer your strengths. The *functional type resumé* draws attention to the most important areas of your achievements and strengths. You may arrange the information to highlight your abilities but not necessarily in dated order of your employment experience. A *targeted resumé,* page 543, is used for a precise field of employment. It shows the employer your expertise in a particular area. This type of resumé is directed to a specific job title. One that is basic but complete and properly arranged will attract an employer's attention. One that is flashy, too lengthy, or too wordy may well be discarded. A one-page resumé is a preferred length. It should be well-organized and grammatically correct. You should always have someone proofread your resumé because often our own mistakes go unnoticed. Spelling must be correct. There is no need for being **elaborate** in style. A simple typed or printed resumé on quality paper will make the information stand out, which is the sole purpose of it. Describing your objectives clearly will direct the employer's attention to your qualifications for employment. Noting your **aspirations** will give the interviewer some insight as to your long-term goals and your level of ambition. Although the main purpose of the resumé is to communicate your abilities to an employer, it also may spur interest in getting an interview for a specific position. Preparation of a resumé requires you to list experiences systematically that show your valuable **attributes.** Awards and special certificates should be listed along with the reasons for which they were given. These will interest an employer and may be the deciding factor when the final hiring decision is made.

In composing your resumé you should be aware that some items are optional. Realizing that employers are people too will help you decide about including personal information. This section of your resumé can convey your genuine caring for others and good citizenship in your community. Interests and community service are not required, but often communicate a human touch to the reader. Often the employer can relate to the community service organization you have listed (or one similar). It is possible that you may be selected for an interview over others who are just as qualified because you have communicated to the reader that you are a well-rounded person. Employers are often interested in what you do with the other hours of your day besides work. A person who has a balance in life is usually happier, healthier, and more productive and full of life in general.

The Cover Letter

After you have perfected your resumé, you should do the same in composing a cover letter to send with it. It must state *why* you should be hired for the desired position. The cover letter should be addressed to the person who decides who is interviewed and hired. Finding out the name of the office manager or supervisor may be done by making a simple phone call and asking (be sure to get the correct spelling). Personalizing the letter will gain more attention than will the standard form letter. Let the employer know that your skills and qualifications will be an asset. Make the letter simple and direct to convey what makes you special for the job. Be sure to request an inter-

Sharon R. Beach, RMA, CMA
4270 Hilldale Drive
Fernridge, CA 95061
(406) 555-1122

Communication skills:
- Providing patient education regarding therapeutic diets
- Sending referral, follow-up, and other correspondence
- Scheduling appointments

Administrative skills:
- Completing medical insurance claim forms
- Transcribing medical histories and progress notes
- Date entry of patient information

Clinical Skills:
- Phlebotomy and basic diagnostic laboratory tests
- Electrocardiogram and Holter monitor
- CPR and first aid
- Sterile technique and assisting with minor surgery

Employment Experience:

1989–Present	Fernridge Family Health Center
	Clinical Medical Assistant
	Provide patient education regarding therapeutic diets; assist with minor office surgery; perform ECGs and Holter monitors; phlebotomy and routine diagnostic tests
1986–1989	Brownsville General Hospital
	Phlebotomist/ECG technician
1985–1986	Ronald L. Botkin, D.O.—General Practice
	Administrative and Clinical Medical Assistant
	Completed medical insurance claim forms; office correspondence; transcription; basic clinical assisting

Education:

1985	Baldwin Community College
	Medical Assistant Program
1988	Brownsville University
	B.A. Degree; Nutrition

FIGURE 12–1 D. Functional resumé

view and make it clear when and how you can be reached for an appointment to be made. Figure 12–2, page 544, gives sample cover letters.

Both cover letter and resumé must be error-free. Employers eliminate numerous resumés by pitching those with spelling or grammatical errors and tears or smudges, or those that are too wordy or unorganized. Refer to the Appendix in the back of this textbook for spelling reference rules, parts of speech, sentence structure, numbers, and the guide to spacing letters to help you.

Classified Advertisements ....

You may send your resumé to a prospective employer in response to a **classified** ad in the local newspaper. A classified ad is a request for qualified applicants to send information about themselves to a prospective employer. The employer may then request an interview with those who meet the requirements for the position instead of interviewing all per-

sons who may wish to apply. This method of screening saves time for the employer and makes the resumé a most important means of communication. Figure 12–3, page 545, shows abbreviations commonly used in classified advertisements.

In responding to a classified ad, it is customary to write a cover letter to accompany your resumé. This cover letter expresses your desire to be interviewed for the position and describes briefly who you are and what you have to offer.

Public Employment Services ....

All states offer assistance in locating jobs through the state employment service. Local offices of this agency will have job openings on file, including, possibly, the one you are looking for. You simply walk in, fill out the general forms, wait your turn, and then have a conference with an employment counselor. If there are listings which call for your kind of experience and training, you will have immediate leads to begin checking. If no appropriate listings are currently on file, the employment counselor will place your name on file and notify you when listings do materialize. Because this agency is supported by tax dollars, there is no fee for the service.

Private Employment Agencies

Private employment agencies offer similar services. A cover letter and resumé should be sent to the agency explaining your area of expertise and desired employment. Many agencies specialize in the medical field and can give efficient service in locating openings in medical assisting. Many potential jobs are "fee paid," meaning that the employer pays the agency's fee. In general, you should avoid positions which require you to pay the fee. This is too often a means of taking advantage of employees. The decision is obviously yours. You may definitely be interested in a particular position for which you have to pay the fee. Carefully weighing the advantages and disadvantages will help you decide if the cost is worth it to you in the long run. A substantial pay increase is an obvious advantage. If you have been waiting for a certain position to open for a relatively long time, or the position is unique and rarely provides an opening, it may well be a wise choice to secure it by paying a fee. Often arrangements may be made for the fee to be paid in installments. Fees for finding employment positions are generally based on a percentage of the annual wages of an employee.

Other Contacts

A resumé with a cover letter requesting an interview may be sent to many medical offices or health care facilities even if there is no position available. If you ardently wish to be employed in a particular facility, making it known may spark an interest in you as a prospective employee should there be an opening. Introducing yourself through correspondence and specifying your interest in employment should a position become available can be very productive. Employers may keep your letter and resumé on file for as long as a year and respond as the need arises.

Additional information about job opportunities may be obtained at the public library. Many services, periodicals, and books deal with occupational information, and library personnel can be very helpful. Membership in professional associations is quite helpful in the job search, too. Not only may an association's publications include classified ads, but personal contact with other members at meetings may provide invaluable information about job openings. Participation in community service groups can put you in touch with yet another net-

---

Sharon R. Beach, RMA, CMA
4270 Hilldale Drive
Fernridge, CA 95061
(406) 555-1122
Job Target: Clinical Medical Assistant
Abilities:
- Communication skills—patient education
- CPR and first aid
- Phlebotomy
- Basic clinical laboratory skills
- Electrocardiography

Achievements:
- Certified Medical Assistant
- Bachelor's degree in Nutrition
- CPR certification

Employment Experience:

1989–Present	Fernridge Family Health Center
	Clinical Medical Assistant
1986–1989	Brownsville General Hospital
	Phlebotomist/ECG Technician
1985–1986	Ronald L. Botkin, D.O.—General Practice
	Administrative and Clinical Medical Assistant

Professional Affiliations:
- Member—American Association of Medical Assistants

Education:

1985	Baldwin Community College
1988	Brownsville University

FIGURE 12–1 E. Example of targeted resumé

Date

Karla Baker, CMA-A
Office Manager
Hilldale Medical Center
Hilldale, Ohio 45102

Dear Ms. Baker:
My training in medical assisting at Ohio Valley Training Academy has provided me with skills in both administrative and clinical areas. I am very interested in securing a position in your health care facility as a **dual** Medical Assistant. I am nationally certified as my enclosed resumé states.

Please let me know if you wish an appointment for an interview. I can be reached at home on Tuesday and Thursday afternoons and every evening at 555-8131.

Thank you for your consideration.

Sincerely,

Sandy Lynn Beach, CMA

FIGURE 12–2   Sample cover letter for a resumé

4270 Hilldale Drive
Fernridge, CA 95061
(406) 555-1122
March 4, 1992

Ms. Doreen Castle
Office Manager
Hopkin's Medical Clinic
739 Mountainview Way
Great Valley, CA 95068

Dear Ms. Castle:
I read your ad in the local paper about the opening for a full-time clinical medical assistant at Hopkin's Medical Clinic. I feel that my training and experience would make me a worthy candidate for this position. As you will see from my resume, I am a Certified Medical Assistant and have a bachelor's degree in Nutrition.

In addition, my experience in patient education regarding therapeutic diets has helped me to sharpen my communication skills. I also have excellent clinical skills and am current in CPR certification.

I would like to meet with you for an interview at your earliest convenience. Please call me at the number listed above to schedule an appointment. I can be reached at home every evening and on Wednesday afternoons.

Yours truly,

(Miss) Sharon R. Beach, CMA

FIGURE 12–2   Sample cover letter B.

APPT—Appointment	MED—Medical
ASST—Assistant	MGR—Manager
BGN or BEG—Beginning	MOS—Months
COL—College	NEC—Necessary
DEPT—Department	NEG—**Negotiable**
EDUC—Education	OFC—Office
EOE—Equal Opportunity Employer	PD—Paid
	POS—Position(s)
EXP—Experience	PT—Part Time
F—Female	REF—References
FB—**Fringe** Benefits	REQ—Required
FT—Full Time	SAL—Salary
GRAD—Graduate	SEC—Secretary
H—Handicapped	T—Temporary
HS—High School	TRANSP—Transportation
HR—Hour	WPM—Words per minute
HRS—Hours	WK—Week
IMMED—Immediate	WKENDS—Weekends
INT—Interview	W/—With
LIC—License	Yrs—Years
M—Male	

FIGURE 12–3 Abbreviations used in the "Help Wanted" section of the newspaper

work of persons who may have information about job openings. Finally, you should not overlook your friends and acquaintances; the job one of them happens to mention in conversation could turn out to be just the one you have been waiting for. If you have a sincere desire to be employed, a job can be found. However, as most people have realized from time to time, it may take patience, persistence, and **ingenuity** to find it.

Complete Chapter 12, Unit 1 in the workbook to help you meet the objectives at the beginning of this unit and therefore achieve competency of this subject matter.

U N I T   2
Getting the Job and Keeping It

OBJECTIVES

Upon completion of this unit, you will meet the following terminal performance objectives by verifying knowledge of the facts and principles presented through oral and written communication at a level deemed competent by the instructor or employer.

1. Complete a job application form.
2. Discuss the importance of appearance when interviewing or applying for a job.
3. State the purpose of a job interview.
4. Explain the importance of promptness and courtesy in a job interview.
5. Explain the reasons for sending a follow-up letter after an interview.
6. Write a follow-up letter.
7. List the qualities employers regard as most important in employees.
8. Discuss "dos" and "don'ts" in interviewing and applying for a job.
9. List the most important qualities necessary for job advancement.
10. Discuss each of the 15 commonly asked questions on a job interview.
11. Discuss questions that applicants may ask on a job interview.
12. Spell and define, using the glossary at the back of the text, all of the words to know in this unit.

WORDS TO KNOW

apprise	demeanor
arbitrary	negate
competent	reiterate
contemporary	

Application Forms

Filling out an application for employment may be your next step. These forms may range from the simple to the complex. Figure 12–4 shows an example of an application form that asks for a minimal amount of information. Often the information is the same as what is contained on your resume. Remember to take a copy of your resume with you to help you fill out the job application. Some applications are extremely lengthy (several pages). It may be best if this type is taken home to complete as it may take a considerable amount of time. It is not considered proper to ask for a phone directory or any other reference when applying for a job. You are supposed to show that you are prepared. In filling out an application for employment, you must be accurate and honest. Being prepared with dates, names, addresses, phone numbers, and other detailed information will expedite completion of the form. You should also be aware of the impression you may give when you apply for employment. Even if you are merely picking up an application to take home to complete, or returning it after you have completed it, your appearance, including your attitude, will certainly be noticed. You should dress for success any time a prospective employer may see you. Other employees will surely notice you and relay the information to the employer, especially if there is a negative impression given.

Because of the professional setting (medical field) for which you are seeking employment, many employers require that the

EMPLOYMENT APPLICATION FORM

PERSONAL

NAME		DATE_____
(LAST)	(FIRST)	(MI)

ADDRESS—STREET	CITY	STATE	ZIP

PHONE NUMBER	SOCIAL SECURITY NUMBER

POSITION DESIRED:

EXPECTED SALARY OR HOURLY WAGE:

EDUCATION

	NAME OF SCHOOL	ADDRESS	DATE(S)	DEGREE/CERTIFICATE
HIGH SCHOOL				
VOCATIONAL/TECHNICAL				
COLLEGE				
OTHER				

WORK EXPERIENCE—Give present position (or last position held first).

JOB TITLE:	EMPLOYER	ADDRESS	DATES
DUTIES PERFORMED:			
JOB TITLE:	EMPLOYER	ADDRESS	DATES
DUTIES PERFORMED:			

REFERENCES—LIST THREE PERSONS (OTHER THAN RELATIVES) WHO HAVE KNOWN YOU FOR AT LEAST 2 YEARS

NAME/TITLE	ADDRESS	TELEPHONE NUMBER

FIGURE 12–4 Example of an employment application

trust of prospective employees is checked. Among the areas of concern are the person's credit rating, police record, and history of chemical abuse. You may be asked to produce these documents or give authorization for the employer to find out about your personal records before you may be considered for hiring.

Since the job application will probably reach the personnel manager's office before you do, it must speak well for you; it must make a good impression on the person who reads it. Applications must be complete, neat, and legible or they will promptly be discarded. Reading and following the instructions on the form is of utmost importance. Most forms begin with directions to print all information requested. Ignoring basic directions of this nature is not the mark of a good candidate for employment. The application form will provide the employer not only with factual information about you but with many other insights as well.

If you take sufficient time and interest in completing the application you will be more likely to be given a personal interview. Additionally, because of the Immigration Reform Act of 1986, employers are required by federal law to ask you for documents that show both your identity and eligibility to work in the United States. Employers will make copies of your documents and return them to you. Further, the Employment Eligibility Verification Form I-9 must be completed and filed in the employee's record along with other important documents. Employers must verify that you are legally entitled to work in the U.S. All applicants and employers must comply with this law.

The Interview

An interview is a face-to-face meeting between you and your prospective employer. The day of the scheduled interview you should allow sufficient time to get ready. If you chew gum or smoke cigarettes, leave these at home for this trip. Neither has any place in a job interview.

When applying for a job, your appearance is extremely important. Appearance is an outward indication of who you are. Remember what you learned about nonverbal communication. If you are a sincere, **competent,** and dedicated person, then by all means attend to your appearance accordingly. Nonverbal messages, though silent, can speak loudly.

Most employers expect appropriate attire and some require adherence to a very specific policy concerning mode of dress and general appearance.

If you are interviewing for a clinical position, ask beforehand about what type of dress to wear. Your inquiry will most likely be taken as showing genuine interest. Often employers will want to see you dressed in what you perceive as a "uniform" to see how you will look on the job.

Women who prefer to wear business type attire should dress conservatively in a navy, gray, tan, or brown tailored suit. Bright colors, or jewelry, miniskirts, pants, and frilly outfits are not considered professional attire. Men should also follow this advice and dress conservatively, avoiding outrageous ties, jewelry, and fad clothes. Remember that you should make every effort to make a positive impression with the interviewer concerning yourself and your qualifications, not your ability to show off fashions and accessories. It follows that those interested in employment at a facility should conform to the standards set forth. Following fads in fashion is usually not advisable. Trendy looks are for models for the most part. A medical assistant who is more interested in meeting the requirements of the job than in being the center of attention is more appealing to a personnel manager.

The same rules apply to job interviews that have already been mentioned in terms of the job. Since they are important, they will be **reiterated.** All matters concerning personal cleanliness are vital. The following attributes are sure to interfere with or **negate** the possibility of employment: bad breath, dirty or uneven fingernails, dirty or unkempt hair, overpowering aftershave or perfume, unclean teeth, unpleasant or offensive body odor, or untended complexion problems.

The point is this: no matter how well qualified or eager you are, you may not find anyone willing to pay for your services if you fail in certain matters of personal hygiene. Take nothing for granted. Make strict adherence to proper personal grooming a rigid daily rule.

Rushing usually detracts from your appearance and **demeanor.** If the address of the facility is not familiar to you, get directions and plan your time beforehand. (It is a good idea to drive, or have someone take you, a day or two before the scheduled interview to scout out the area to determine the approximate travel time, exact location, parking, bus route, and so forth to avoid getting lost or being delayed because of confusion due to construction or some other problem.) You should arrive about 10 minutes before the appointment. (You may be instructed to arrive up to an hour or more before the interview to complete an application form or to take required preemployment tests.) Arriving too early will make you appear insecure. Being late for almost any reason will make you appear irresponsible and a poor candidate for the position. If you happen to find yourself in this predicament, a telephone call explaining the delay and a sincere apology are in order. Being on time is a sign of reliability, dependability, and conscientiousness.

Introducing yourself with a handshake should initiate a friendly and pleasant conversation. Your manner should tell the interviewer you are happy to be there.

The interview ought to allow sufficient time for each of you to inquire about the other and to discuss the requirements of the position. Often the interviewer will have reviewed your resumé.

You should be prepared to answer questions concerning your career goals and objectives, how you feel about changes, why you decided on this career, your further educational plans, and so on, Figure 12–5. Your answers should be brief, concise, and honest.

In terms of perspective and dimension, the section of the resumé that lists community services is an appealing area to prospective employers. It is an indicator of your concern for others, your involvement, and your enjoyment of working.

Many employers will ask what prompted your interest in a particular service area.

Contemporary federal laws are designed to deal with arbitrary discrimination in hiring practices. Toward this end, you should not be asked questions concerning your age, cultural or ethnic background, marital status, or parenthood. Nevertheless, these issues may come up in the course of your interview. You are not required to provide this information if you choose not to. The purpose of the interview is to ascertain the relevance of your experience and character to the job at hand. Should any of these unrelated issues come up, be careful to analyze the context in which they arose (it could be from something you said). In any case, if you are honestly convinced that you have been denied a job because of **arbitrary** discrimination, be advised that this is illegal, and you have legal recourse.

At some point during the interview, the interviewer may give you a written job description of the position for which you are applying. You will probably be given time to look it over and then asked if you would feel confident about performing the job described. An honest answer is the best. Avoid hedging or bluffing about issues because an experienced interviewer will pick up on your insecurities. Remember that body language tells the rest of the story. If there are one or two duties you have never performed before or one or two pieces of equipment which you know little about, say this but add that you are eager to learn. The employer will appreciate the initiative in your answer. If the job description sounds totally unfamiliar, it is best to say that, too, or if you feel it would be an impossible task. The interviewer will appreciate your openness.

Some positions may have no job description, and the duties involved will be discussed during the interview. Knowing that there are probably as many duties not mentioned as mentioned will give you an idea of the amount of work the job requires.

By the time all of these matters have been dealt with, the interview will be starting to wind down. The interviewer beginning to reach closure will **apprise** you of this by asking you if you have any further questions. If issues of salary, raises, and advancement have not been dealt with previously, this is an appropriate point to mention them. This is also the logical point for you to ask about any other matters you may be uncertain about, Figure 12–6. See Figure 12–7 for the "dos and don'ts" of applying for a job. However, do not drag out this time. Let the interview end smoothly. When it is over, rise and thank the interviewer for his or her time. Firmly shake hands if the interviewer extends a hand, Figure 12–8. Remember to smile and be pleasant and polite as you exit with confidence.

The interviewer may talk to a number of people about a specific job opening in the office. To help the interviewer remember specific facts and traits about each individual, a form such as the one shown in Figure 12–9 may be filled out.

You may be one of many candidates interviewing for a particular job. Therefore, any decision may take some time. Out of courtesy as well as to enhance your image with the interviewer, take the time to compose a follow-up letter shortly

1. What are your qualifications for employment in our facility?
2. Do you have plans for continuing education? If yes, what are your plans?
3. What were your favorite subjects in school and why?
4. Why are you seeking employment with us?
5. What made you decide to enter the medical assisting field?
6. What is your most rewarding experience in life thus far?
7. What are your long-range career goals?
8. What motivates you to do your best?
9. What is the most difficult problem you ever had to deal with? And how did you handle it?
10. What does success mean to you?
11. What relationship should exist between supervisors and those under their supervision?
12. How would you describe yourself?
13. Do you work well under pressure?
14. What are your strengths and weaknesses?
15. What two things are most important to you in a job?

FIGURE 12–5 Fifteen commonly asked questions during interviews

after the interview has taken place. Figure 12–10 offers a sample letter.

What Employers Want Most in Employees

The personal investment that you have made with regard to your education and skills training along with all of the effort you have put forth in producing a resumé and interviewing for employment does not stop with being hired. After securing a position, you must continually endeavor to do your best. An

1. To see a Job Description
2. About Hours—Work Day Schedule
3. Rate of Pay (if not Discussed by the Close of the Interview)
4. Chances for Advancement or Promotion
5. About Continuing Education—In-Service Programs
6. Fringe Benefits:
   a. Health insurance plan
   b. Dental insurance plan
   c. Eye care
   d. Vacation/time off
   e. Membership dues in AAMA
   f. Profit sharing
   g. Retirement plan
   h. Other
7. Evaluations of Job Performance Periodically

FIGURE 12–6 Questions *you,* the applicant may ask during an interview

ARRIVE ON TIME (10–15 minutes early)	BE LATE!
SHOW INTEREST—ENTHUSIASM!	ASK TOO MANY QUESTIONS
	OR
	MAKE EXCUSES
DISPLAY A POSITIVE ATTITUDE	TALK ABOUT PERSONAL PROBLEMS
USE COURTESY	ACT OVER-CONFIDENT
ACT COMPOSED	DRUM FINGERS, SWING LEG, TAP FOOT
DRESS APPROPRIATELY	OVERDRESS
KEEP GOOD POSTURE (SIT STILL AND STRAIGHT)	CHEW GUM/SMOKE

FIGURE 12–7 Reminders in applying for employment

employer will expect you to perform with increasing expertise in your position as you continue to gain experience.

Desirable employee qualities that employers generally rank as most important are listed as follows:

1. Communication skills (oral and written)
2. Cooperation
3. Courteousness
4. Dependability
5. Enthusiasm
6. Initiative
7. Interest
8. Math skills
9. Punctuality
10. Reading skills
11. Reliability
12. Responsibility
13. Time management skills

FIGURE 12–8 A firm handshake at the conclusion of the interview conveys courtesy and mutual respect.

These qualities are fast becoming increasingly more important and are vital in holding a job. Becoming proficient in grammar, including both the written and spoken word, is a must. Speaking in a well-educated manner is necessary for portraying a professional image not only of yourself but also of the facility where you are employed. You become a member of a team of medical personnel who reflect each other to the public you serve. Many evening classes, such as a business English course, offer basic review in grammar. Taking the initiative to improve oneself is admirable. Employers recognize these efforts and for those with ambition, rewards will surely follow.

Attendance is most important as schedules must be constantly changed and reassignments made when an employee is absent, especially when it is unexpected. An absent employee affects everyone as work must be divided among other team members. Scheduling personal appointments should be done on your day off or after working hours. If there is an important engagement for which you need time off from your job, you should ask for a meeting with your supervisor to discuss making arrangements for a day off well in advance of the date. Remember that only when it is *absolutely necessary* should you call in sick. If you are not sure about the office policy regarding this issue, you should ask your employer. Employees have a responsibility to report a personal or serious illness to their supervisor as soon as possible. When an emergency involves an accident or acute medical problem, notification of the circumstance will be received with sympathy and concern. Generally employers are most understanding about illness when the reason is genuine. If child care is a problem, and the reason for absence is due to needing someone to care for children, the supervisor should be made aware of the situation. Often supervisors may be helpful in assisting with information that could be a possible solution to the problem. However, repeated occurrences of calling in "sick" just to take a day off will become annoying and may lead to disciplinary action. Usually offenders are more likely to take off on Mondays and Fridays for long weekends. These are days when schedules are full and all employees are most needed. If one is placed on pro-

INTERVIEW EVALUATION					
Subject	Excellent	Good	Satisfactory	Needs Improvement	Poor
Appearance					
Attitude					
Eye contact					
Self-control					
Voice					
Grammar					
Responses					
Manners					
Resumé					
Comments					
Date					
Employer		Title			
Address		Phone			
Applicant					

FIGURE 12–9 Employers may use a form such as this after an interview to record information about an applicant.

bation and warned about poor attendance practices and the warnings go unheeded, it could ultimately result in the employee's dismissal.

It is equally important to be on time daily. Being prompt is a valuable personal quality appreciated by both employers and patients. Leaving early is not advised unless absolutely necessary and after having obtained the supervisor's permission in advance. When one leaves before the scheduled time it puts an added burden on other team members to finish your job. With each member of the health care team doing what is expected, the work will be shared and the group's efficiency will be noticed by your employer. This makes for a harmonious working relationship among employees. You have studied throughout this text about various patient education materials and guidelines for better health. You must have realized by now that you should be practicing what you are expected to teach patients. This can only help you to feel better about yourself, which will be evident to others with whom you come in contact. In good health you will be more productive, energetic, and display better coping skills. All of the qualities important to employers should also be important to you. The secret to success is simple. Strive toward fulfilling the goals you set and do everything in your power to reach them. Your personal satisfaction is surely one goal that will be realized if you follow this plan.

In addition to these qualities, one in particular that the medical assistant must keep in mind is personal appearance. A medical assistant must continually strive to maintain an impec-

cable appearance; this is essential to ensure job security. Looking your best requires that you compliment your best assets and always keep neat, clean, and attractive to the public eye.

When you obtain employment, you must necessarily dedicate yourself first of all to the task of keeping the job. This is where your work history begins, and it will probably follow you throughout your working life. If the health care field remains your chosen career area and if medical assisting is your point of entry, then you must be determined to become the very best medical assistant you can. Ultimately, your eventual advancement into more responsible medical assisting duties and higher pay will depend largely upon your demonstrated capabilities in performing your administrative and clinical tasks. However, the aforementioned employee qualities will also become significant factors in paving the way for advancement.

Consider this scenario: A physician employs two medical assistants; both are the same age and possess relatively equal administrative and clinical skills. The only differences between the two come down to appearance and attitude. One maintains a considerably nicer appearance than the other, along with a more positive attitude. As the physician's volume of business expands and a promotion and salary increase for one of the positions becomes inevitable, guess which one will likely get the nod from the physician. You do not have to be a genius to figure this one out. In the end, it comes down to common sense. Although clinical competency is crucial to your success as a medical assistant, your personal appearance can contribute to or detract from the overall impression you give to patients, co-workers, and to your employer.

Date

Karla Baker, CMA-A
Office Manager
Hilldale Medical Center
Hilldale, Ohio 45102

Dear Ms. Baker:

Thank you very much for granting me an interview for the Clinical Medical Assistant's position on your staff. The interview was both challenging and stimulating; I found it to be an enjoyable and rewarding experience.

You outlined the duties and responsibilities which come with the position very specifically. This is the type of position for which I have been trained; I feel confident that if I am offered the position, I can handle the responsibilities and become an asset to your staff.

Again, thank you for considering me for this position. I would be most appreciative if you would inform me of your final decision as soon as it is convenient for you.

Sincerely,

Sandy Lynn Beach, CMA

FIGURE 12–10 A follow-up letter

The Employee Evaluation or Review ....

Most employers require that employees have regular, routine, or periodic reviews or evaluations regarding their work performance. The schedule for such reviews may vary from place to place, but usually they are held initially every 3 months for the first year and then every 6 months thereafter. Some physicians or employers prefer to have annual reviews scheduled unless there is a problem or the employee requests it more often. Evaluations should be regarded in a positive light.

These are generally conducted by the supervisor, the office manager of the facility, and sometimes by the physician-employer. Whoever holds this meeting with the employee offers insightful observations about the person. This is done to point out both positive and negative areas of which the employee may or may not be aware. Most facilities hold regular weekly staff meetings where suggestions, problems, and other important information is discussed. It is vital, however, to have private meetings to discuss such personal topics as goals, promotion opportunities, pay increase possibilities and educational pursuits. The review, or evaluation as it is also known, is meant for both employer and employee to provide just such an opportunity. You should use this meeting to your advantage. Let the employer or supervisor know your intentions regarding promotion goals. Ask questions (tactfully) about what has been on your mind (bothering you) regarding policy, dress code, or whatever else you feel is important. You may ask about or schedule your vacation during this meeting. Your supervisor or evaluator may use a form similar to the one shown in Figure 12–11. Usually it will be completed and then offered to you to read. You may be asked to sign it at the bottom indicating that you have read, discussed, and understood the rating on the form. You may request a copy if it is not offered. The original will remain in your employee record and filed with all of the other documents pertaining to your employment. It is a good idea to study the form and heed the rating scale. If you take the review seriously and with an open mind, you will most likely find out some good points and sometimes a couple of not so good things about yourself that you may not have realized before. Try to improve on the not so good things such as poor attendance, poor grammar, or untidy appearance, before the next review. Showing improvement immediately and continuing on with the improvement will only make good points to remark about on the next review. As the old expression says, a word to the wise should be sufficient. If you show a poor attitude, it will only make matters worse. Remember that the supervisor's job responsibilities require that this evaluation be performed. You should not take the suggestions for improvement or reprimands about poor attendance, for instance, as personal insults. Try to remember the old saying "if the shoe fits, wear it," and consider the source of the remark. If you give the remark a chance to sink in and it doesn't, then possibly there is no just cause for it. Try to remain unaccusing and calm and discuss the problem. Chances are it may be a misunderstanding that can easily be

FIGURE 12–11 Example of employee evaluation/review form

talked out in a matter of seconds. Open dialogue and clear communication works wonders and leads to a better working relationship between you and your employer, Figure 12–12. Many positive results are achieved from reviews for both employee and employer.

Time should be allowed during the evaluation (for both employer and employee) to address topics in depth that are difficult to discuss during the work day. Tact and respect should be maintained when bringing up touchy subjects. One in particular is a situation where the employer asks the employee to perform a duty for which there has been no training. Doing a task that you are not trained in or qualified to do is risky for all concerned. Politely explaining to the supervisor (employer) that you do not wish to be difficult but that you do not feel comfortable in performing a procedure for which you are neither trained nor qualified will usually be all that is necessary. The employer should respect your position and either get another who is qualified or perform the task himself or herself. If the situation is not resolved this easily, it may mean that you should seek employment in a facility where you will not have such unreasonable demands made of you.

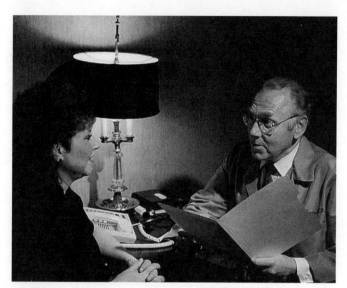

FIGURE 12–12 Employer discussing evaluation review in an open communication

Terminating Employment ....

There are many reasons for terminating employment—relocation, advancement to a more responsible position, a higher paying job, illness, educational pursuits, pregnancy, a change in life-style, among others. There is, however, a major responsibility that an employee has to an employer, that of giving at least a 2-weeks' notice, Figure 12–13. This should be done to give the employer adequate time to fill the position that you will vacate. The notice that you give should be directed to your immediate supervisor, your physician-employer, or other appropriate member of the staff, with carbon copies to whoever else is appropriate at your place of employment. The letter should include the date that will be your last working day. Employers appreciate this considerate gesture, as it allows for a smoother transition of personnel. There is even time for a new person to be hired to work with you so that you may help in the training and explain your job description in more detail.

Employment can also be terminated by the employer. This is an unpleasant experience for both employer and employee. The usual cause for termination initiated by the employer is failure to perform job responsibilities. Deficiencies can include incompetence, being tardy, high absenteeism, failure to get along with coworkers and patients, poor work habits, undependability, dishonesty, poor attitude, and uncooperativeness. On some occasions and in some situations, through employer–employee communication, one may be able to smooth over the conflict and ask if it is possible to change the situation from being fired to accepting a letter of resignation. This is mentioned because misunderstandings *do* happen from time to time. Having a poor work record is something that could follow a person and make it difficult to land another job in the future.

Date

Marlene Blackstone, CMA-A
Office Manager
Sports Medicine Center
7386 Canyon Road
Anywhere, U.S.A. 10000

Dear Ms. Blackstone:

It is with much regret that I submit this letter as my notice of resignation. My employment over the past five years in Sports Medicine has been a most interesting experience for me. I have learned so much in working with such a fine group of professionals. I am grateful for having had this opportunity.

From the date of this letter I am giving my two week notice; my last day will be (insert date).

Since my husband has taken a new position with his company, we are being transferred out of state. I will miss working with everyone at the center.

My thanks to all of you for making my years of employment at the center something that I can look back on with fond memories.

Sincerely,

Patsy J. Keene, CMA

Date

Maxwell S. Mitchell, M.D.
472 Circle Drive
Anywhere, U.S.A. 10000

Dear Dr. Mitchell:

Please accept this as my letter of resignation. During my employment in your practice I have learned a great deal, and I have greatly enjoyed working for you. However, (at this point the writer may choose to add a sentence or two elaborating on the specific reason for leaving).

My X years of employment with you have been a valuable experience for me; thank you for the opportunity to work and learn.

In accordance with your personnel regulations, this letter is also my two week notice; my last day in the office will be (at least two weeks hence).

Sincerely,

Your name and title or position with your signature

FIGURE 12–13 Letters of resignation

Keeping on your toes can prevent this unwanted dilemma from happening. Strive to do whatever is possible to secure a good reference from an employer. You may need it in the future.

Miss Right . . .
does only those procedures which she has been trained to do. She follows the job description for which she was hired and stays within her boundaries. She is an active member of the AAMA and participates in their continuing-education program to stay current in the medical assisting field. She was honest on the employment application form.

Employment advancement: Excellent

Ms. Wrong . . .
does only what she has to do. She stated that she could do many procedures on her employment application form that she really doesn't know anything about. She did it to get this job. She won't take the time to attend any meetings or educational programs because she feels that she knows enough to get by. She ignores her job description and frequently steps out of her boundaries making many other workers upset.

Employment advancement: None

Summary

Requirements for medical assistant's positions will be as varied as the practice of medicine. The medical assistant is the most versatile member of the health care team. Some physicians still hire medically untrained persons as file clerks, secretaries, receptionists, and the like. More physicians recognize the value of employing trained and experienced medical assistants who have a basic background in the administrative and clinical areas of medical office practice. If you have successfully completed a training program, you have established the basis for a rewarding career.

Employers in medical practice have begun to realize the worth of certified medical assistants (CMA). CMAs are usually considered for employment over untrained applicants. Currently, this is more true in some states than others, but certification may well become a nationwide requirement for employment in medical practice as regulations tighten. Keeping yourself up to date by attending continuing-education programs, seminars, meetings, and other informative ways will make you a most valued employee. By opting to become a CMA you will demonstrate that you are knowledgeable in basic entry-level skills. Further, you will demonstrate to a prospective employer that you have pride in the profession as well as in your professional skills.

A Final Note

Throughout this chapter much emphasis has been directed toward securing employment. Although it may seem to you that employers ask the impossible as you review their expectations, you must keep in mind that an employee is paid for work performed. Gainful employment is a mutually agreed to contract which is either written or implied. To assist you in gaining a better understanding of why employers have such expectations, you may find it interesting to know how and where they originated.

The concept of the "work ethic" originated from the sixteenth century's Protestant Ethic. During this time work was considered a sacred task and success in one's work was a sign of divine grace. One was looked down on by society in general if one was thought to have moral flaws, such as being lazy, having no ambition, or other undesirable characteristics. Essentially this ideal has not changed. The work ethics of today are basically the same as the original with some minor changes. The word *responsible* can be substituted for sacred. And being a success in one's work is a sign of *ambition, hard work, and perseverance.* These expectations are fair, realistic, and sensible. It simply means that one should give an honest day's work for an honest day's wages. Taking the responsibility of providing for oneself financially usually makes most people aware of what is necessary to keep a job. Being a part of the health care team means that you have to be a team player!

Our best wishes for a successful and rewarding career in medical assisting!

Complete Chapter 12, Unit 2 in the workbook to help you meet the objectives at the beginning of this unit and therefore achieve competency of this subject matter.

REFERENCES

Burns, William E. "Jobs for the Future." *Industrial Education*, January 1987.

Hess, Beth B. *Sociology*, 3rd ed. New York: Macmillan, 1988.

Jackson, Tom. *The Perfect Resumé for the '90s*, Doubleday, a division of Bantam Doubleday Dell Publishing Group, Inc., 1990.

Shapiro, Robert J. and Maureen Walsh. "The Great Jobs Mismatch." *U.S. News & World Report*, September 7, 1987.

"Why Me? What Every Applicant Needs to Know about the New Immigration Law," *Business & Legal Reports*, booklet, 64 Wall Street, Madison, CT 06443-1513, reorder #54i, 1987.

Appendix

Converting measurements   555
Common household measures and weights   556
Symbols   556
Common medical abbreviations   556
Selected English, Latin, and Greek equivalents   558
Prefixes and suffixes   560
Uniform Care, Stain Removal Chart   562
Grammar and punctuation   563
Instruments used in minor office surgical
  procedures   566
Growth charts   568
Substance analysis request form
  ("Chain of Custody " form)   572

Converting Measurements ....

LENGTH	Centimeters	Inches	Feet
1 centimeter	1.000	0.394	0.0328
1 inch	2.54	1.000	0.0833
1 foot	30.48	12.000	1.000
1 yard	91.4	36.00	3.00
1 meter	100.00	39.40	3.28

VOLUMES	Cubic Centimeters	Fluid Drams	Fluid Ounces	Quarts	Liters
1 cubic centimeter	1.00	0.270	0.033	0.0010	0.0010
1 fluid dram	3.70	1.00	0.125	0.0039	0.0037
1 cubic inch	16.39	4.43	0.554	0.0173	0.0163
1 fluid ounce	29.6	8.00	1.000	0.0312	0.0296
1 quart	946.0	255.0	32.00	1.000	0.946
1 liter	1000.0	270.0	33.80	1.056	1.000

WEIGHTS	Grains	Grams	Apothecary Ounces	Pounds
1 grain	1.000	0.064	0.002	0.0001
1 gram	15.43	1.000	0.032	0.0022
1 apothecary ounce	480.00	31.1	1.000	0.0685
1 pound	7000.00	454.0	14.58	1.000
1 kilogram	15432.0	1000.00	32.15	2.205

Rules for Converting One System to Another ·······························

Volumes
Grains to grams—divide by 15
Drams to cubic centimeters—multiply by 4
Ounces to cubic centimeters—multiply by 30
Minims to cubic millimeters—multiply by 63
Minims to cubic centimeters—multiply by 0.06
Cubic millimeters to minims—divide by 63
Cubic centimeters to minims—multiply by 16
Cubic centimeters to fluid ounces—divide by 30
Liters to pints—divide by 2.1

Weights
Milligrams to grains—multiply by 0.0154
Grams to grains—multiply by 15
Grams to drams—multiply by 0.257
Grams to ounces—multiply by 0.0311

Temperature
Multiply centigrade degrees by $\frac{9}{5}$ and add 32
Subtract 32 from the Fahrenheit degrees and multiply by $\frac{5}{9}$

Household Measures and Weights ···········

1 teaspoon	= $\frac{1}{6}$ fluid ounce or 1 dram
3 teaspoons	= 1 tablespoon
1 dessert spoon	= $\frac{1}{3}$ fluid ounce or 2 drams
1 tablespoon	= $\frac{1}{2}$ fluid ounce or 3 drams
4 tablespoons	= 1 wine glass or $\frac{1}{2}$ gill
16 tablespoons (liq)	= 1 cup
12 tablespoons (dry)	= 1 cup
1 cup	= 8 fluid ounces
1 tumbler or glass	= 8 fluid ounces or $\frac{1}{2}$ pint
1 wine glass	= 2 fluid ounces
16 fluid ounces	= 1 pound
4 gills	= 1 pound
1 pint	= 1 pound

Symbols ·······································

m	minim	s̄	without
ʒ	dram	c̄	with
ʒ	ounce	−	minus, negative, alkaline reaction
O	pint	+	plus, excess, acid reaction, positive
#	pound, number	×	multiply
℞	recipe, prescription	÷	divide
'	foot, minute	=	equals
"	inch, second	>	greater than

°	degree	<	less than
%	percent	∞	infinity
♂	male	↑	increase
♀	female	↓	decrease

Common Medical Abbreviations ···············

a, aa	of each
ac	before meals
ad lib	as desired
A & P	anterior and posterior
aq	aqueous, water
BE, ba.en.	barium enema
BlF	black female
bib	drink
bid BID	twice a day
bm, BM	bowel movement
BlM	black male
BP, B/P	blood pressure
BSA	body surface area
BUN	blood urea nitrogen
c̄	with
C	centigrade
Ca	calcium
CA	carcinoma
CAP(S)	capsule(s)
CBC	complete blood count
cc	cubic centimeter
CCU	coronary care unit
CHF	congestive heart failure
cm³	cubic centimeter
CNS	central nervous system
CO₂	carbon dioxide
comp	compound
COPD	chronic obstructive pulmonary disease
CPR	cardiopulmonary resuscitation
CSF	cerebrospinal fluid
CVA	cerebrovascular accident
cysto	cystoscopy
D & C	dilatation and curettage
Dil, dil	dilute
DOA	dead on arrival
DPT	diphtheria, pertussis, tetanus
dr	dram
dx, Dx	diagnosis
ECG	electrocardiogram
EEG	electroencephalogram
EENT	eye, ear, nose, throat
EKG	electrocardiogram
elix	elixir
ER	emergency room

et	and	NB	newborn
expl lap	exploratory laporatomy	no	number
ext	extract	noxt	at night
		NPO	nothing by mouth
F	fahrenheit	N & V	nausea and vomiting
F	female		
FBS	fasting blood sugar	O	pint
fl	fluid	OB	obstetrics
fl dr	fluid dram	OD	overdose
fl oz	fluid ounce	OD	right eye
Fx	fracture	OP	outpatient
		OR	operating room
GB	gallbladder	os	mouth
GI	gastrointestinal	OS	left eye
g, G	gram	OU	both eyes
GP	general practitioner	oz	ounce
GR	grain		
gtt, Gtt, gtts	drop, drops	Path	pathology
GU	genitourinary	PBI	protein bound iodine
GYN	gynecology	pc	after meals
		Peds	pediatrics
h, hr	hour	per	through, by
HCl	hydrochloric acid	PID	pelvic inflammatory disease
Hgb	hemoglobin	PKU	phenylketonuria
hs	hour of sleep, bedtime	PO, po	by mouth
Hx	history	POL	physician's office laboratory
hypo	hypodermic, under	prn, PRN	as desired, needed
		pro time	prothrombin time
ICU	intensive care unit	Psych	psychiatry
I & D	incision and drainage	pt	patient, pint
IM	intramuscular	pulv	powder
inj	injection	Px, PE	physical examination
I & O	intake and output		
IPPB	intermittent positive pressure breathing	q	every
		qd	every day
IT	inhalation therapy	q 4 h	every 4 hours
IUD	intrauterine device	qh	every hour
IV	intravenous	qid, QID	four times a day
IVP	intravenous pyelogram	qns	quantity not sufficient
		qs	quantity sufficient
K	potassium	qt	quart
KUB	kidney, ureter, and bladder		
		R	right
L	liter, left	Ra	radium
LB(S), lb(s)	pound(s)	RBC	red blood cells
lat	lateral	REM	rapid eye movement
liq	liquid	rep	let it be repeated
LLQ	left lower quadrant	R/O	rule out
LMP	last menstrual period	ROM	range of motion
LUQ	left upper quadrant	ROS	review of systems
		Rx, R$_x$	prescription, take
min	minim		
M	male	s̄	without
μg, MCG	microgram	sig, SIG, S	instructions, directions
mg, MG	milligram	SOB	short of breath
mL, ML	milliliter	sol	solution
mm, MM	millimeter	solv	dissolve
MS	multiple sclerosis		

sos	distress signal
sp gr, SG	specific gravity
ss	half
stat, STAT	immediately
STD(s)	sexually transmitted disease(s)
subq	subcutaneous
syr	syrup
T	temperature
T & A	tonsillectomy and adenoidectomy
TAB	tablet
TIA	transient ischemic attack
tid, TID	three times a day
tinct	tincture
TPR	temperature, pulse, respiration
TUR	transurethral resection
UA	urinalysis
ung	ointment
URI	upper respiratory infection
UTI	urinary tract infection
VD	venereal disease
vin	wine
VS	vital signs
WBC	white blood cells
WF	white female
WM	white male
WNL	within normal limits
wt, Wt	weight

Selected English, Latin, and Greek Equivalents ....

and—et
arm—brachium; brachion (Gr)
artery—arteria
attachment—adhaesio

back—dorsum
backbone—spina
backward—retro
belly—venter
bend—flexus
bile—billis; chole (Gr)
bladder—vesica
blind—obscurus
blister—pustulo
blood—sanguis; haima, aima (Gr)
blood vessel—vena
body—corpus; soma (Gr)
bone—os; osteon (Gr)
bony—osseus
bowels—intestina, viscera

brain—cerebrum
breach—ruptura
breast—mamma; mastos (Gr)
buttock—gloutos (Gr)

cartilage—cartilago; chondros (Gr)
chest—thorax
choke—strangulo
confinement—puerperium
corn—callus, clavus
cornea—cornu; keras (Gr)
cough—tussio
cramp—spasmus

dead—mortuus
deadly—lethalis
dental—dentalis
digestive—pepticus
disease—morbus
dose—potio

ear—auris
egg—ovum
entrails—viscera
erotic—amatorius
exhalation—exhalatio
expell—expello
expire—expiro
external—externus
extract—extractum
eye—oculus; ophthalmos (Gr)
eyeball—pupula
eyelid—palpebra

face—facies
fat—adeps; lipos (Gr)
feel—tactus
fever—febris
finger—digitus
flesh—carnis
foot—pedis; pous (Gr)
forearm—brachium
forehead—frons

gall—bilis
gravel—calculus
gum—gingiva
gut—intestinum

hair—capillus
half—dimidius
hand—manus; cheir (Gr)
harelip—labrum fissum
head—caput; kephale (Gr)
healer—medicus
health—sanitas
hear—audio

heart—cor; kardia (Gr)
heat—calor
heel—calx, talus
hysterics—hysteria

illness—morbus
infant—infas, puerilis
infectious—contagiosus
infirm—debilis
injection—injectio
intellect—intellectus
internal—intestinus
intestine—intestinum; enteron (Gr)
itch—scabies
itching—pruritis

jaw—maxilla
joint—artus; anthron (Gr)

kidney—ren; nephros (Gr)
knee—genu
kneecap—patella

lacerate—lacero
larynx—guttur
lateral—lateralis
leg—tibia
limb—membrum
listen—ausculto
liver—jecur, hepar (Gr)
loin—lapara
looseness—laxitas
lukewarm—tepidus
lung—pulmo, pneumon (Gr)

mad—insanus
male—masculinus
malignant—malignus
maternity—conditio matris
milk—lac
moist—humidus
month—mensis
monthly—menstruus
mouth—os; stoma (Gr)

nail—unguis
navel—umbilicus; omphalos (Gr)
neck—cervis; trachelos (Gr)
nerve—nervus; neuron (Gr)
nipple—papilla
no, none—nullus
nose—nasus; rhis (Gr)
nostril—naris
nourishment—alimentus

ointment—unguentum
orifice—foramen

pain—dolor
patient—patiens
pectoral—pectoralis
pimple—pustula
poison—venenum
powder—pulvis
pregnant—gravida
pubic bone—os pubis
pupil—pupilla

quinsy—angina

rash—exanthema
recover—convalesco
redness—rubor
rib—costa
ringing—tinnitus
rupture—hernia

saliva—sputum
scab—scabies
scalp—pericranium
scaly—squamosus
sciatica—ischias
seed—semen
senile—senilis
sheath—vagina
shin—tibia
short—brevis
shoulder—humerus; omos (Gr)
shoulderblade—scapula
shudder—tremor
side—latus
skin—cutis; derma (Gr)
skull—cranium; kranion (Gr)
sleep—somnus
smell—odoratus
socket—cavum
solution—dilutum
sore—ulcus
spinal—dorsalis, spinalis
spine—spina
spittle—sputum
sprain—luxatio
stomach—stomachus; gaster (Gr)
stone—calculus
sugar—saccharum
swallow—glutio

tail—cauda
taste—gustatus
tear—lacrima
teeth—dentes
testicle—testis; orchis (Gr)
thigh—femur
throat—fauces; pharygx (Gr)
throb—palpito

tongue—lingua; glossa (Gr)
twin—geminus

urine—urina

vagina—vagina; kolpos (Gr)
vein—vena; phleps (Gr)
vertebra—vertevra; spondylos (Gr)
vessel—vas

wash—lavo
water—aqua
wax—cera
weary—lassus
wet—humidus
windpipe—arteria aspera
woman—femina
womb—uterus; hystera (Gr)
worm—vermis
wrist—carpus; karpos (Gr)

yolk—luteum

Prefixes and Suffixes ·····························

a- an-	without, negative
ab- abs-	away from
ad-	toward
adeno-	gland
aero-	air
-aesthesia	sensation
-algia	pain
ambi-	both
angio-	blood vessel
ano-	anus
ante-	before
anti-	against
arterio-	artery
arthro-	joint
auto-	self
bi-	two, twice
brady-	slow
broncho-	bronchial
cardio-	heart
cata-	down
-cele	tumor, cysts
cent-	hundred
-centesis	puncture
cephal-	head
chole-	gall
chromo-	color
-cide	causing death
circum-	around
-cise	cut

co- com- con-	together
colo-	colon
colpo-	vagina
contra-	against
costo-	rib
cranio-	skull
cysto-	bag, bladder
-cyte -cyto	cell
dacry-	tears
de-	from, down
deca-	ten
deci-	tenth
demi-	half
dent-	teeth
derma-	skin
di-	double
dia	through, between
diplo-	double
dis-	negative, apart
dys-	difficult, painful
ecto-	out, on the outside
-ectomy	cutting out
-emesis	vomiting
-emia	blood
en-	in, into
encephalo-	brain
endo-	within
entero-	intestine
epi-	above, over
-esthesia	sensation
ex- exo-	out
extra-	on the outside
fibro-	connective tissue
fore-	before, in front of
-form	form
-fuge	to drive away
galact- galacto-	milk
gastro-	stomach
-gene -genic	origin, formation
glosso-	tongue
gluco- glyco-	sugar, sweet
-gram	a tracing, record
-graph	machine
-graphy	the process
gyne-	woman
hema- hemato- hemo-	blood
hemi-	half
hepa- hepato-	liver
herni-	rupture
histo-	tissue
homo-	same, similar

hydra- hydro-	water	nephr- nephro-	kidney
hyper-	above, increased, over	neu- neuro-	nerve
hypo-	below, under, decreased	niter- nitro-	nitrogen
hyster-	uterus	non- not-	no
		nucleo-	a nucleus
-iasis	condition of		
ictero-	jaundice	o-	ovum, an egg
idio-	peculiar to the individual	ob-	against
ileo-	ileum	oculo-	eye
in-	in, into, not	-ode -oid	form, shape
infra-	beneath	odont-	a tooth
inter-	between	oligo-	few
intra- intro-	within	-ology	study of
-ism	condition, theory	-oma	a tumor
-itis	inflammation of	oophor-	ovary
-ize	to treat by special method	ophthalmo-	eye
		-opia	vision
karyo-	nucleus, nut	orchid-	testicle
kata- kath-	down	-orrhaphy	to repair a defect
kera-	horn, indicates hardness	ortho-	straight
-kinesis	motion	os-	mouth, bone
		-osis	disease, condition of
lact-	milk	oste- osteo-	bone
laparo-	abdomen	-ostomy	to make a mouth, opening
-lepsy	seizure, convulsion	oto-	ear
leuco- leuko-	white	-otomy	incision, surgical cutting
lipo-	fat	oxy-	sharp, acid
lith-	a stone		
-logia -logy	science of, study of	pachy-	thick
-lysis	disintegration	pan-	all, entire
		para-	alongside of
macro-	large, long	path- -pathy	disease, suffering
mal-	bad, poor	ped- (Greek)	child
-mania	insanity	ped- (Latin)	foot
mast-	breast	-penia	too few, lack
med- medi-	middle	per-	through, excessive
mega-	large, great	peri-	around
-megalia -megaly	large, great, extreme	pharyng-	throat
melan-	black	phelebo-	vein
men-	month	-phobia	fear
meso-	middle	-phylaxis	protection
meta-	beyond, over, between, change, transportation	-plasty	operate to revise
		-plegia	a stroke, paralysis
-meter	measure	-pnea	breathing
metro- metra-	uterus	pneumo-	air, lungs
micro-	small	poly-	many, much
mio-	smaller, less	post-	after
mono-	single, one	pre-	before
multi-	many	pro-	before, in behalf of
my- myo-	muscle	procto-	rectum
myel- myelo-	marrow	proto-	first
		pseudo-	false
narco-	sleep	psych-	the mind
naso-	nose	pyelo-	kidney, pelvis
necro-	dead	pyo-	pus
neo-	new	pyro-	heat

re-	back, again	super- supra-	above
reni- reno-	kidney	syn-	with, together
retro-	backward, behind		
-rhage -rhagia	hemorrhage, flow	tele-	distant, far
-rhaphy	a suturing, stitching	tetra-	four
-rhea	flow	-therapy	treatment
rhino-	nose	-thermy	heat
		thio-	sulfur
sacchar-	sugar	thoraco-	chest
sacro-	sacrum	thrombo-	clot
salpingo-	a tube, fallopian tube	thyro-	thyroid gland
		trans-	across
sarco-	flesh	tri-	three
sclero-	hard, sclera		
-sclerosis	dryness, hardness	uni-	one
-scopy	to see	-uria	urine
semi-	half	urino- uro-	urine, urinary organs
septi-	poison, infection		
stomato-	mouth	vaso-	vessel
-stomy	to furnish with a mouth	venter- ventro-	abdomen
sub-	under	xanth-	yellow

Uniform Care—Stain Removal Chart ·······························

Treat stains as quickly as possible.

Check fabric labels for care instructions.

Use an enzyme presoak for protein-based stains, such as blood, milk, fruits, grass (Example: Axion, Biz)

Use prewash spot treatments for greasy stains. (Example: Spray'n Wash, Shout)

Use proper bleach for hard-to-whiten and difficult stains. (Example: Chlorine bleach for whites Clorox.)

Chlorine will fade most colors. Use all-purpose bleach for colored fabrics (Example: Clorox 2.)

Stain	Method for Washable Fabrics
felt-tipped pens	Soak in rubbing alcohol at least 30 minutes, preferably overnight. Wash and add bleach.
blood, milk, egg, chocolate, ice cream	Pretest using an **enzyme presoak**. Use only **cold** water. If the presoak is not enough, work in detergent paste. Wash in warm water. Bleach if needed.
butter, grease, oil, margarine, dressings	Prewash with **prewash spot treatment** or rub a detergent paste into the stain. Launder.
fruits, juices	Use an **enzyme presoak**; bleach if the stain persists or for cherry, peach, pear, plum stains, soak in cool water. For others pour boiling water through the stain. Launder.
chewing gum	Place an ice cube under the gum to harden it. Rub off the excess with a dull knife. If stained, use cleaning fluid.
coffee, tea	Pour boiling water through the stretched fabric. Launder in hot water.
cosmetics	Pretreat with detergent paste. Launder in hot water.
grass	Rub detergent paste into the stain. Launder in hot water. Use appropriate bleach.
ballpoint ink	Rub white petroleum jelly into the stain. Pretest with detergent paste. Launder using bleach if the fabric permits.
mildew	Launder in hot water. Bleach with appropriate bleach.
Scorch, white	Dampen a white cloth with hydrogen peroxide and place on the stain. Place a clean cloth on top. Press.
perspiration	Apply ammonia to wash water for a new stain. Use vinegar on an old stain. Launder.
shoe polish	Pretreat with detergent paste. Launder.

CONSULT YOUR DRY CLEANER FOR ESPECIALLY DIFFICULT STAINS AND CLOTHING LABELED "DRY CLEAN ONLY."

Grammar and Puncuation

Parts of Speech

To proofread for grammar you must remember the eight parts of speech and how they are identified.

1. A **noun** is the name of anything. It may be a person, a place, an object, an occurrence, a quality, a measure, or a state. Examples of words that may be used as nouns are *assistant, laboratory, instruments, office, empathy, manners, kindness,* and *attention.*

   Examples:
   The *assistant* draws *blood* and takes it to the *laboratory.*
   The *assistant* shows *kindness, empathy,* and *attentiveness* to all *patients* in the *office.*

2. A **pronoun** is a word that is used as a noun substitute. The most often used pronouns are *I, me, she, her, you, he, him, who, which, that, one, all, some, everyone, it, their, they, any,* and *nobody.*

3. A **verb** is a word (or word group) that expresses action or state of being. Every sentence must have a verb. Examples of words which may be action verbs are *do, write, speak, hesitate, educate, perform, assist, obtain,* and *attend.* Examples of verbs that may express state of being are *am, are, is, will be, have been, feel, seem,* and *appear.*

4. An **adjective** is a word that describes, limits, or restricts a noun or pronoun.

   Examples:
   The *conscientious* medical assistant reports for work on time.
   She is an *energetic, efficient,* and *dedicated* employee.

5. An **adverb** is a word that **modifies** a verb form, an adjective, or another adverb. The most common ending for adverbs is *ly.* Adverbs should be used to answer questions such as: How? When? Where? How often? To what degree? It is incorrect to say "I did real good on the terminology test." You should say, "I did very well on the terminology test."

   Examples:
   Sometimes the assistant reports *early* at the office and stays *late.*
   Usually when a patient *angrily* confronts an assistant, she should answer *calmly* and *quietly* after the patient has finished talking.

6. A **preposition** shows the relationship of an object to some other word in the sentence. Prepositions *must* have an object. If a pronoun is the object of a preposition, it must be in the objective case.

   Examples:
   Medical supplies arrived *for* the doctor, the nurse and *me.*

   Between you and *me* that physician's handwriting is most difficult to read.
   Some common prepositions include *with, without, for, against, above, below, on, under, through, between, by, during, among, concerning, in, from, to,* and *of.*

7. **Conjunctions** are connectives that join words, phrases, and clauses. Examples are *and, but, or, nor, for, yet, because, if,* and *since.*

8. An **interjection** is a word used to express strong feeling or emotion. Examples are *ouch, hurray, well,* and *oh.* These words are usually followed by an exclamation point or a comma. The following are examples of sentences containing all eight parts of speech:

   Examples:
   Yes! A busy medical practice like theirs always employs efficient and energetic medical assistants.
   Well, a conscientious medical assistant like you will sit confidently for the certification examination and pass it!
   Oh, that emergency patient canceled after he had rested and settled down.

Sentence Structure

When writing letters, write in complete thoughts. A **simple sentence** consists of only one complete thought, that is, one independent clause with a subject and a verb.

Examples:
Physicians examine patients.
Physicians prescribe medication.
The receptionist scheduled appointments.

A **compound sentence** contains two or more independent clauses.

Examples:
The physician dictates letters, and the medical assistant transcribes them.
Administrative medical assistants perform clerical duties, and clinical medical assistants perform nursing skills.
Laboratory technicians analyze specimens, and medical assistants assist with physical examinations.

A **complex sentence** contains one independent clause and one or more dependent clauses. A dependent clause cannot stand alone as a sentence.

Examples:
The doctor, who is off on Thursdays, sees allergy patients in the morning. (an adjective clause)
Patients are sometimes quite apprehensive when they come to the office for diagnostic examination. (an adverb clause)
Physicians require that patients receive proper instructions for diagnostic procedures. (noun clause)

Rule 1. Write *ie* when the sound is *ee*, as in:

achieve   piece
field   shield
grief   yield

EXCEPT after c, as in:

conceive
deceive
perceive
receive

EXCEPTIONS:

leisure
neither
seize
weird

Rule 2. Write *ei* when the sound is not long *e*, especially when the sound is long *a*, as in:

freight   veil
height   vein
sleigh   weigh

EXCEPTIONS:

friend
mischief

Rule 3. The prefixes *mis, il, in, im* and *dis* do not change the spelling of the root word:

mis + spell = misspell
il + legal = illegal
il + literate = illiterate

in + audible = inaudible
im + mature = immature
dis + appear = disappear

Rule 4. Only one word in English ends in *sede*: supersede.
Only three words end in *ceed*: exceed, proceed, and succeed.
All other words of similar sound end in *cede*, as in:

concede
recede
precede

Rule 5. The suffixes *ly* and *ness* do not change the spelling of the root word:

sudden + ness = suddenness
final + ly = finally
truthful + ly = truthfully
lean + ness = leanness

EXCEPTIONS: Words ending in *y* preceded by a consonant change *y* to *i* before any suffix not beginning with *i*:

kindly + ness = kindliness
happy + ly = happily
happy + ness = happiness

Words ending in *y* preceded by a vowel also follow this rule.

FIGURE A Spelling reference rules

A **compound–complex sentence** contains two or more independent clauses plus one or more dependent clauses.

Example:

Medical assistants should seek continuing education because medical technology is constantly changing, and the medical assistant must keep current with new procedures.

Punctuation

A comma or period should appear in front of an ending quotation mark (," ."").

There are four general rules for the use of a **comma**:

1. Use between main clauses connected by *and, but, so, for, or, nor,* and *yet*. If the main clauses are short, no comma is needed.
2. Use following long introductory phrases or clauses that may begin with words such as *after, whenever, if, until, since,* and *once*.
3. Use to separate items in a series.
4. Use to set off nonrestrictive modifiers. A **nonrestrictive phrase** or **clause** is a nonessential phrase or clause. It just adds descriptive or explanatory detail. A **restrictive modifier** restricts or limits the meaning of the noun it modifies.

Example:

The medical assistant, being dedicated to her profession, helps the doctor in countless ways.

The medical assistant, who is a part of the medical team, needs to be especially careful in attending to details.

Apostrophes need your attention. An **apostrophe** is used in **contractions** to signify that one or more letters have been left out. Be sure if you use *it's* that you mean *it is*. *Who's*, meaning *who is*, should not be confused with *whose*, and *there's*, meaning *there is*, is not to be confused with *theirs*.

An apostrophe is also used to signify possession in a noun.

Example:

The medical assistant's pen, pencil, and note pad are always beside the office telephone.

The assistant's stethoscope hangs in the examination room.

Carefully check all **hyphens** at the end of a line to be sure the word is divided correctly. Check your dictionary if you are in doubt.

Two forms of **ellipses** may be used—three and four dots. The three-dot ellipsis is used with spaces on either end, and between the dots, to signify an omission of words.

Example:

"They come in two varieties—the three-dot variety . . . and the four-dot variety."

Rule 6. Drop the *e* from the end of a word before adding the suffixes *al, ed, ing,* and *able*:

    complete—completed—completing
    care—caring
    fine—final
    love—lovable
    observe—observable
    EXCEPTIONS: Words ending in *ce* and *ge* usually keep the silent *e* when the suffix begins with *a* or *o* in order to preserve the soft sound of the final consonant:
    notice + able = noticeable
    change + able = changeable

Rule 7. Keep the final *e* before a suffix beginning with a consonant:

    large + ly = largely
    care + ful = careful
    care + less = careless
    state + ment = statement
    EXCEPTIONS:
    argue + ment = argument
    true + ly = truly

Rule 8. With words of one syllable ending in a single consonant preceded by a single vowel, double the consonant before adding *ing, ed,* or *er*:

    sit + ing = sitting
    hop + ed = hopped
    dip + er = dipper
    run + ing = running
    swim + ing = swimming

Rule 9. If a one-syllable word ends in a single consonant not preceded by a single vowel, do not double the consonant before adding *ing, ed,* or *er*:

    reap + ed = reaped
    heat + ing = heating

Rule 10. To make a word ending in *y* plural, check the letter before the *y*. If it is a vowel, just add *s*:

    birthday—birthdays

    day—days
    ray—rays
    toy—toys
If it is any other letter, change the *y* to *i* and add *es*:
    city—cities   lady—ladies
    study—studies   guppy—guppies
    fly—flies

Rule 11. Most nouns (names of people, places, things, ideas) become plural by adding *s*:

    boy—boys
    dog—dogs
    desk—desks
    window—windows

Rule 12. The plural of nouns ending in *s, x, z, ch,* or *sh* is formed by adding *es*.

    wax—waxes
    dish—dishes
    waltz—waltzes

Rule 13. The plural of most nouns ending in *f* is formed by adding *s*. The plural of some nouns ending in *fo* or *fe* is formed by changing the *f* to *v* and adding *s* or *es*:

    gulf—gulfs
    belief—beliefs
    knife—knives
    life—lives
    half—halves
    loaf—loaves
    thief—thieves
    wolf—wolves

Rule 14. The plural of nouns ending in *o* preceded by a vowel is formed by adding *s*. The plural of nouns ending in *o* preceded by a consonant is formed by adding *es*.

    patio—patios
    ratio—ratios
    tornado— tornadoes
    hero—heroes
    EXCEPTIONS:
    Eskimo—Eskimos
    silo—silos

FIGURE A–1 Spelling reference rules (Continued)

The four-dot ellipsis signifies an omission of words and the end of a sentence with no space between the last letter and the first dot.

Example:
    "The four-dot. . . ."

Capitalization

Capitalize names of persons and places, the first word in a sentence, names of holidays, principal words in titles of major works, and any product or title that might be trademarked. Many medical terms begin with a capital letter because they are names of the physicians who named them. Brand name (proprietary) medications are usually capitalized. Again, use your dictionary when in doubt.

Be especially careful to check every word in a heading or title for correct spelling. Use your medical dictionary or a good general dictionary. Always have these reference books in the office.

Numbers

The use of numbers must be consistent. If you follow a specific reference style book (e.g., *The Chicago Manual of Style*, *CBE Style Manual*, *AMA Manual of Style*), you should follow its instructions for using numerals or spelling out the numbers. Also, follow the rules your employer wishes to be used for your office.

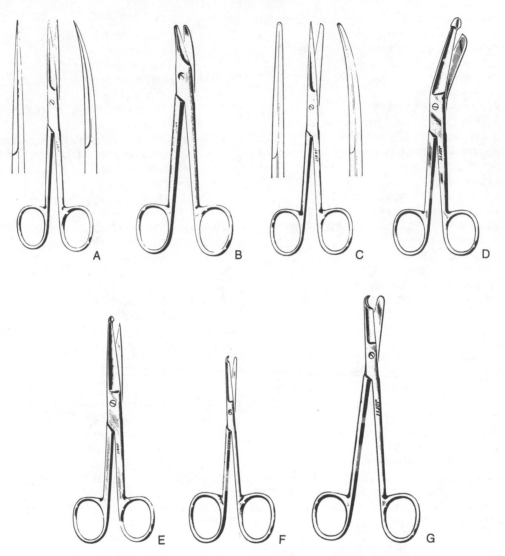

Operating Scissors: (A) Deaver, (B) Sistrunk, (C) Deaver.   Bandage scissors: (D) Lester,
(E) Knowles finger, (F) Spencer suture, (G) Littauer stitch
(Courtesy of J. Jamner Surgical Instruments Inc.)

Petit-point hemostats: (H) and (I) mosquito (Courtesy of J. Jamner
Surgical Instruments Inc.)

Towel forceps: (J) Backhaus, (K) Jones
(Courtesy of J. Jamner Surgical Instruments Inc.)

Needle holders: (O) Brown, (P) Collier
(Courtesy of J. Jamner Surgical Instruments Inc.)

(L) Knife handle, (M) Blades (Courtesy of J. Jamner
Surgical Instruments Inc.)

10 11 12 15 20 21 22 23

Dressing and tissue forceps: (Q) thumb, (R) tissue, (S) Adson,
(T) Semken dressing, (U) Cushing, (V) plain splinter,
(W) Judd-Allis tissue (Courtesy of J. Jamner
Surgical Instruments Inc.)

(N) Foersfer sponge-holding forceps (Courtesy of
J. Jamner Surgical Instruments Inc.)

GIRLS: BIRTH TO 36 MONTHS
PHYSICAL GROWTH
NCHS PERCENTILES*

NAME _____ RECORD # _____

*Adapted from: Hamill PVV, Drizd TA, Johnson CL, Reed RB, Roche AF, Moore WM: Physical growth: National Center for Health Statistics percentiles. AM J CLIN NUTR 32:607-629, 1979. Data from the Fels Research Institute, Wright State University School of Medicine, Yellow Springs, Ohio.

© 1982 ROSS LABORATORIES

DATE	AGE	LENGTH	WEIGHT	HEAD CIRC.	COMMENT

Recommend the formulation you prefer
with the name you trust

SIMILAC®
SIMILAC® WITH IRON
SIMILAC® WITH WHEY
Infant Formulas

The ISOMIL® System of
Soy Protein Formulas

ADVANCE®
Nutritional Beverage

ROSS LABORATORIES
COLUMBUS, OHIO 43216
Division of Abbott Laboratories, USA

G106/JUNE 1983 LITHO IN USA

NAME _____   RECORD # _____

*Adapted from: Hamill PVV, Drizd TA, Johnson CL, Reed RB, Roche AF, Moore WM: Physical growth: National Center for Health Statistics percentiles. AM J CLIN NUTR 32:607-629. 1979. Data from the Fels Research Institute, Wright State University School of Medicine, Yellow Springs, Ohio.
© 1982 ROSS LABORATORIES

DATE	AGE	LENGTH	WEIGHT	HEAD CIRC.	COMMENT

Recommend the formulation you prefer with the name you trust

SIMILAC®
SIMILAC® WITH IRON
SIMILAC® WITH WHEY
Infant Formulas

The **ISOMIL®** System of
Soy Protein Formulas

ADVANCE®
Nutritional Beverage

ROSS LABORATORIES
COLUMBUS, OHIO 43216
Division of Abbott Laboratories, USA

G105/JUNE 1983   LITHO IN USA

Growth chart for boys head circumference, birth to 36 months

GIRLS: 2 TO 18 YEARS
PHYSICAL GROWTH
NCHS PERCENTILES*

NAME _____ RECORD # _____

*Adapted from: Hamill PVV, Drizd TA, Johnson CL, Reed RB, Roche AF, Moore WM: Physical growth: National Center for Health Statistics percentiles. AM J CLIN NUTR 32:607-629, 1979. Data from the National Center for Health Statistics (NCHS) Hyattsville, Maryland.

Ross
Growth &
Development
Program

© 1982 ROSS LABORATORIES

BOYS: 2 TO 18 YEARS
PHYSICAL GROWTH
NCHS PERCENTILES*

NAME _____ RECORD # _____

DATE	AGE	STATURE	WEIGHT	COMMENT

MOTHER'S STATURE _____ FATHER'S STATURE _____

AGE (YEARS)

STATURE

WEIGHT

*Adapted from: Hamill PVV, Drizd TA, Johnson CL, Reed RB, Roche AF, Moore WM: Physical growth: National Center for Health Statistics percentiles. AM J CLIN NUTR 32:607-629, 1979. Data from the National Center for Health Statistics (NCHS) Hyattsville, Maryland.

© 1982 ROSS LABORATORIES

Ross Growth & Development Program

Growth chart for boys height and weight, age 2 to 18 years

USA LABS
ID#

Referred by

Health Care Provider
Address
Phone

**DO NOT WRITE
IN THIS AREA**

C H A I N   O F   C U S T O D Y

STEP 1 — TO BE COMPLETED BY EMPLOYER/COLLECTOR.
DONOR IDENTIFICATION — PLEASE PRINT

LAST NAME

FIRST NAME   M.I.

SOC. SEC. NO. _____ — _____ — _____

EMPLOYEE NO. _____

DONOR I.D. VERIFIED   ☐ PHOTO I.D.

☐ EMPLOYER REPRESENTATIVE

SIGNATURE OF EMPLOYER REP.
REASON FOR TEST (CHECK ONE)
☐ (1) PRE-EMPLOYMENT ☐ (2) POST ACCIDENT ☐ (3) RANDOM

☐ (4) PERIODIC ☐ (5) REASONABLE SUSPICION/CAUSE

☐ (6) RETURN TO DUTY

☐ (99) OTHER (SPECIFY)

TESTS REQUESTED: TOTAL TESTS ORDERED

SPECIMEN   ☐ URINE   ☐ BLOOD   (SUBMIT ONLY ONE SPECIMEN WITH EACH REQUISITION)

STEP 2 — COLLECTOR, FOR URINE SPECIMENS, READ TEMPERATURE WITHIN FOUR MINUTES OF COLLECTION.
CHECK THE BOX IF TEMPERATURE IS WITHIN THE SPECIFIED RANGE ☐ 90°–100°F / 32°–38°C
                                                    OR RECORD ACTUAL TEMPERATURE HERE: _____

STEP 3 — TO BE COMPLETED BY COLLECTOR.   COLLECTION SITE

COLLECTION DATE _____ TIME _____ ☐ AM PM _____
                                                                                    Address

REMARKS _____
                                                                                    City   State   Zip
_____ (_____)
                                                                                    Phone

I certify that the specimen identified on this form is the specimen presented to me by the employee identified in Step 1 above, and was collected, labeled and sealed in the donor's presence.

COLLECTORS NAME PRINT (FIRST, M.I., LAST)   SIGNATURE OF COLLECTOR

STEP 4 — TO BE INITIATED BY THE DONOR AND COMPLETED AS NECESSARY THEREAFTER

PURPOSE OF CHANGE	RELEASED BY SIGNATURE	RECEIVED BY SIGNATURE	DATE
A. PROVIDE SPECIMEN FOR TESTING			
B. SHIPMENT TO LABORATORY			
C.			

COMMENTS:

Self-stick   identification
Labels for sealing specimen:

(123)   (123)   (123)   (123)

SPECIMEN PACKAGE INTEGRITY WAS ☐ ACCEPTABLE ☐ UNACCEPTABLE WHEN RECEIVED IN LAB.

RECEIVER'S INITIALS

FOR OFFICE USE

Glossary

abdomen   the cavity in the body between the diaphragm and the pelvis

abdominal   pertaining to the abdomen

abdominopelvic   pertaining to the anterior body cavity below the diaphragm

abduct   to move away from the midline

ablation   a surgical procedure utilizing a resectoscope inserted into the uterus through the cervix

abnormality   person, thing, or condition that is not normal

abortion   the termination of pregnancy before the stage of viability; spontaneous or induced

absolute   free as to condition, unlimited in power

absorb   to suck or swallow up, to drink in

abstinence   to keep from doing; the act of giving up; to do without

absurd   contrary to sense or reason

accelerator   increasing action or function

accessible   capable of being reached

accommodation   the process of the lens changing shape to permit close vision

accuracy   correctness, exactness

acetylcholine   a hormone released at the parasympathetic and skeletal nerve endings

Achilles tendon   a tendon attaching the gastrocnemius muscle of the leg to the heel

achromatic   colorless, without color

acidosis   a disturbance of the acid-base balance of the body

acquire   to gain by one's own efforts or actions; to get

acromegaly   a chronic condition characterized by enlargement of bones of the extremities and some bones of the head; thickening of facial soft tissues

action potential   the temporary electrical charge within a cell

activate   to make active or more active

acuity   clearness of thought or vision

acute   sharp, severe. Having a rapid onset, severe symptoms and a short course; not chronic

addiction   the state of being governed or controlled by a habit, as with alcohol or drugs

adduct   to draw together toward the midline

adenitis   inflammation of lymph nodes or a gland

adequate   equal to the requirement or occasion, sufficient

adjustments   changes to fit or bring into harmony

administer   to manage; to conduct, as in business

adrenal   pertaining to the adrenal glands, which sit atop each kidney

adrenaline   an internal secretion derived from the adrenal glands; can be commercially prepared from animal glands; acts as a stimulant

adrenocorticotrophic hormone (ACTH)   a hormone secreted by the anterior lobe of the pituitary gland

advantageous   beneficial, profitable

adverse   hostile, opposed, unfavorable; opposite in position or direction

aerobe   a microorganism which can live and grow only in the presence of oxygen

afebrile   without fever

agar   a dried mucilaginous substance, or gelatin, extracted from algae, used as a culture medium

Al-Anon   a support group for family members of alcoholics

Al-Ateen   a support for teenagers with an alcoholic parent

albino   a person who lacks pigment in the skin, hair, and eyes, either partial or total; a person with albinoism

alcoholic   an individual who uses alcohol to excess

Alcoholics Anonymous   an organization formed to assist alcoholics to refrain from the use of alcohol

aldosterone   a mineralocorticoid hormone secreted by the adrenal cortex

alignment   being in proper position

alimentary canal   the intestinal tract, from the esophagus to the rectum, and accessory organs

allege   to state positively but not under oath and without proof; to affirm

allergen   a substance that produces the symptoms of an allergy

allergic rhinitis   inflammation of the nose due to an allergy

allergy   an altered or acquired state of sensitivity; abnormal reaction of the body to substances that are normally harmless to other people

allosteric   a protein found in erythrocytes that transports oxygen in the blood; hemoglobin

alopecia   the loss of hair; baldness

alveoli   microscopic air sacs in the lung

amber   orange-yellow color

amblyopia   lazy eye; a condition characterized by the inward turning of the affected eye

ambulate   to walk, not be confined to bed

amniotic   pertaining to the fluid within the membrane surrounding the fetus

amphetamine   a central nervous system stimulant, often referred to as an "upper"

amplifier   a device on an electrocardiograph which enlarges the EKG impulses

ampule   a small glass container that can be sealed and its contents sterilized

amputate   to cut off, remove a part

anaerobe   a microorganism having the ability to live without oxygen

anal   pertaining to the anus or outer rectal opening

analysis   the examination of anything to determine its makeup; a description of the process or the examination, point by point

analytical   characterized by a method of analysis, a statement of point-by-point examination

anaphalatic shock   reaction from injection of a protein substance to which the patient is sensitized

anaphylaxis   a hypersensitive reaction of the body to a foreign protein or a drug; the term implies symptoms severe enough to produce serious shock, even death

anatomical   pertaining to the anatomy or structure of an organism

anatomy   the study of the physical structure of the body and its organs

anchor   the attachment of a skeletal muscle; the wrapping at the start of a gauze or elastic bandage

anemia   a deficiency of red blood cells, hemoglobin, or both

aneroid   operating without a fluid; when used in reference to a sphygmomanometer, measuring by a dial instead of a mercury column

anesthesia   without sensation, with or without loss of consciousness

anesthesiology   the study of anesthesia

anesthetic   an agent which produces insensibility to pain or touch, either generally or locally

aneurysm   a widening, external dilation due to the pressure of blood on weakened arterial walls

angina   pain and oppression radiating from the heart to the shoulder and left arm; a feeling of suffocation

angiography   a radiological study of an artery using a radiopaque medium

angioplasty   a surgical procedure performed within an artery to enlarge its opening

anorexia   loss of appetite; with anorexia nervosa, loss of appetite for food not explainable by disease, which may be a part of psychosis

antecubital   the inner surface of the arm at the elbow

anterior   before or in front of

antibody   a protein substance carried by cells to counteract the effect of an antigen

antibody-mediated   humoral immunity; when antibodies and complement work together to destroy antigens

anticoagulant   a substance that prohibits the coagulation of blood

antigen   any immunizing agent which, when introduced into the body, may produce antibodies

antihistamine   a class of drugs used to counteract allergic reactions or cold symptoms

antiseptic   an agent which will prevent the growth or arrest the development of microorganisms

antitoxin   a protein that defends the body against toxins

anuria   the absence of urine

anus   the external opening of the anal canal

anxiety   a condition of mental uneasiness arising from fear or apprehension

aorta   the main trunk of the arterial system of the body

apex   the point, tip, or summit of anything; in reference to the heart, the point of maximum impulse of the heart against the chest wall

apical   referring to the apex

apnea   the absence of breathing

aponeurosis   extension of connective tissue beyond a muscle in round or flattened tendons; a means of insertion or origin of a flat muscle

appendectomy   the excision of the appendix

appendicitis   inflammation of the appendix

appendicular   pertaining to the limbs or things that append (attach) to other parts

apprehension   anticipation of something feared, dread; a mental conception

appropriate   correct, suitable

aqueous humor   a watery, transparent liquid which circulates between the anterior and posterior chambers of the eye

arachnoid   a delicate, lacelike membrane covering the central nervous system

ardently   eagerly, passionately, intensely

areola   a ringlike coloration about the nipple of the breast

arrhythmia   without rhythm; irregularity

arteriography   a radiological study of an artery using a radiopaque medium

arterioles   small blood vessels connecting arteries with capillaries

arteriosclerosis   a degeneration and hardening of the walls of arteries

artery   a blood vessel carrying blood away from the heart, usually filled with oxygenated blood

arthritis   inflammation of a joint

articulate   to join together, as in a joint

artifact   something extraneous to what is being looked for, an activity which causes interference on EKGs

ascending   referring to that portion of the colon which ascends from the lower right quadrant to the upper right quadrant of the abdomen

asepsis   a condition free of organisms

aseptic technique   means of performing tasks without contamination by organisms

asphyxiation   suffocation, loss of consciousness as the result of too little oxygen and too much carbon dioxide

aspirate   to remove by suction, to suck into

asthma   an allergic reaction to a substance resulting in wheezing, shortness of breath, and difficulty in breathing

astigmatism   blurring of the vision due to an abnormal curvature of the cornea

asymmetry   lack of same size, shape, and position of parts or organs on opposite sides

atelectasis   lack of air in the lungs due to the collapse of the alveoli of the lungs

atherosclerosis   fatty degeneration of the walls of the arteries

atrial depolarization   the excitement and contraction caused by the SA node at the beginning of the cardiac cycle

atrioventricular   see **A-V node**

atrium   cardiac auricle; the upper chamber of the heart

atrophy   wasting away of a muscle

attenuated   diluted; to reduce virulence of a pathogenic organism

atypical   not characteristic, unusual, abnormal

audible   loud enough to be heard

audiometry   testing of the hearing sense

auditory   pertaining to the sense of hearing; the external canal of the ear

aural   pertaining to the ear; temperature measurement using tympanic infrared scanner

augmented   refers to leads 4, 5, and 6 of the standard 12-lead EKG tracing; these leads are of different voltages

auscultate   to listen for sounds produced by the body

authorization   the giving of authority

autoclave   an apparatus using heat and pressure to sterilize items

autoimmune   a condition wherein the person's antibodies react against their own normal tissues

autologous   given by oneself

automation   behavior in an automatic or mechanical fashion

autonomic   spontaneous; the part of the nervous system concerned with reflex control of bodily functions

autotrophs   microorganisms that feed on inorganic matter

averted   to turn away or aside; to prevent; ward off or avoid

A-V node   atrioventricular node; the beginning of the bundle of His in the right auricle and atrium; nerve fibers responsible for the contraction of the ventricles

axial   pertaining to the spinal column, skull, and rib cage of the skeleton

axilla   the underarm area, armpit

axillary   referring to the underarm area

axon   an extension from a nerve cell

bacteria   unicellular microorganism concerned with the fermentation and putrefaction of matter; disease-causing agent

barbiturate   a sedative or hypnotic drug, also known as a "downer"

Bartholin's glands   two small mucous glands, situated one on each side of the vaginal opening at the base of the labia minora

baseline   the initial information on which additional data is based

basophil   a granulated white blood cell

benign   nonmalignant; not cancerous

benign hypertrophy   nonmalignant enlargement

beriberi   a disease resulting from lack of vitamin B (thiamine)

biceps   the muscle of the upper arm which flexes the forearm

biconvex   the curving out on both sides

bicuspid   heart valve between the left atrium and left ventricle, also known as the mitral valve

bile   a secretion of the liver; a greenish yellow fluid with a bitter taste

bimanual   two-handed; with both hands

binocular   pertaining to the use of both eyes; possessing two eyepieces as with a microscope

biochemistry   the science concerned with the chemistry of plants and animals

biohazardous   any material that has been in contact with body fluid and is potentially capable of transmitting disease

biopsy   excision of a small piece of tissue for microscopic examination

bizarre   odd, unusual, strikingly out of the ordinary

bladder   a membranous sac or receptacle for a secretion; e.g., the gallbladder, urinary bladder

bloodborne   carried by the blood

bloodborne pathogen(s)   disease-causing microorganism(s) present in the blood

blood pressure   the amount of force exerted by the heart on the blood as it pumps the blood through the arteries

body mechanics   the use of appropriate body positioning when moving and lifting objects in order to avoid injury

body surface area (BSA)   the total surface of the human body

bold   prominent, clear; in printing means heavy-faced type

bolus   a mass of masticated food which is ready to be swallowed

booster   a subsequent injection of immunizing substance to increase or renew immunity

Bowman's capsule   part of the renal corpuscle; surrounds the glomerulus of the nephron

brachial   refers to the brachial artery in the arm; the artery used in measuring blood pressure

bradycardia   slow heart rate

brain scan   a diagnostic test using a scanner to measure radioisotopes within the brain

bronchi   the primary divisions of the trachea

bronchiole   small terminal branches of the bronchi which lack cartilage

bronchitis   inflammation of the mucous membranes of the bronchial tree

bruit   an adventitious sound of venous or arterial origin heard on auscultation; usually refers to the sound produced by the mixing of arterial and venous blood at dialysis shunts

BSA   see **body surface area**

buccal   pertaining to the mouth or cheeks; oral cavity

bulbourethral gland   two small glands, one on each side of the prostate gland, terminating in the urethra by way of a duct

bunion   a bursa with a callus formation

bursa   a sac or pouch in connective tissue chiefly around joints

calculate   to compute

calculi   commonly called stones; usually composed of mineral salts

calibrations   a set of graduated markings to indicate values

callus   in fractures, refers to the formation of new osseous material around the fracture site

calorie   a unit for measuring the heat value of food

calyces   plural of calyx

calyx   the cuplike division of the kidney pelvis

cancer   a malignant tumor or growth; specifically the hyperplasia of cells with infiltration and destruction of tissue

cannula a tube or sheath enclosing a trocar (triangular bore needle); after insertion the trocar is removed

capillary a microscopic blood vessel connecting arterioles and venules

carbohydrate an organic combination of carbon, hydrogen, and oxygen as a sugar, a starch, or as cellulose

carbon dioxide a gas found in the air, exhaled by all animals; the chemical formula of which is CO_2

carbon monoxide a colorless, odorless, poisonous gas caused by the incomplete combustion of carbon

carboxyhemoglobin combined carbon monoxide and hemoglobin in red blood cells

carbuncle a staphlococcal infection following furunculosis, characterized by a deep abscess of several follicles with multiple draining points

carcinoembryonic antigen a tumor marker which can be detected in the blood when tested

carcinogenic cancer-causing agents

carcinogenesis the malignant transformation of a cell

carcinoma a malignant tumor from epithelial tissue

cardiac pertaining to the heart

cardiac sphincter the muscle which encircles the esophagus where it enters the stomach

cardinal signs principal signs: temperature, pulse, respiration, and blood pressure

cardiology the study of the heart and its diseases

cardiovascular pertaining to the heart and blood vessels

carotid pertaining to the main artery in the neck

carpal tunnel syndrome the symptoms associated with the entrapment of the median nerve within the carpal bones and the transverse ligament at the wrist

carpals bones of the wrist

cartilage a strong, tough, elastic tissue forming part of the skeletal system; precalcified bone in infants and young children

CAT scan see **computerized axial tomography**

cataract an opacity of the lens of the eye that can result in blindness

catarrhal pertaining to inflammation of mucous membranes; causing severe spells of coughing with little or no expectoration

catheterize to insert a catheter into a cavity (for example, into the urinary bladder to remove urine) to remove a body fluid

caudal pertaining to any taillike structure

caustic capable of burning; an agent that will destroy living tissue

cauterize to burn with an electrical cautery or chemical substance to stop bleeding or excise tissue

cavities a hollow space, such as within the body or organs

cecum the beginning of the ascending portion of the large intestine which forms a blind pouch at the junction with the small intestine

celiac disease dilatation of the small and large intestines

cell-mediated direct cellular response to antigens

cell membrane the structure which surrounds and encloses a cell

central situated at or related to a center

centrifuge a machine for the separation of heavier materials from lighter ones through the use of centrifugal force

centriole an organelle within the cell

cerebellum lower or back brain below the posterior portion of the cerebrum

cerebral pertaining to the cerebrum of the brain

cerebrospinal referring to the brain and spinal cord

cerebrospinal fluid the liquid that circulates within the meninges of the spinal cord and ventricles and meninges of the brain

cerebrovascular accident (CVA) a stroke; hemorrhage in the brain

cerebrum the largest part of the brain. It is divided into two hemispheres with four lobes in each hemisphere

cerumen waxlike brown secretion found in the external auditory canal; earwax

cervical pertaining to the neck portion of the spinal column; also to the entrance into the uterus

cervix the entrance into the uterus

cesarean surgical removal of an infant from the uterus through the abdomen

chain of custody a form submitted with a specimen for drug analysis verifying that proper precautions were used by all involved parties

chemical pertaining to chemistry

chemotherapy the use of chemical agents in the treatment of disease, usually associated with cancer therapy

Cheyne-Stokes a breathing pattern characterized by alternating periods of apnea and hyperventilation

chlamydia a sexually transmitted disease caused by the bacterium, *Chlamydia trachomatis*, which lives as an intracellular parasite

cholecystectomy surgical removal of the gallbladder

cholelithiasis stones in the gallbladder

cholenergic nerve fibers capable of secreting acetylcholine

cholera an acute, specific, infectious disease characterized by diarrhea, painful cramps of muscles, and a tendency to collapse

chorionic gonadotropin a hormone detectable in the urine of a pregnant female soon after conception

choroid the vascular coat of the eye between the sclera and the retina

chromosome structures within the cell's nucleus which store hereditary information

chronic continuing for a long time, returning; not acute

chronic obstructive pulmonary disease (COPD) a syndrome characterized by chronic bronchitis, asthma, and emphysema, or any combination of these conditions, resulting in dyspnea, frequent respiratory infections, and thoracic deformities from attempting to breathe

chyme the mixture of partially digested food and digestive secretions found in the stomach and small intestines during digestion of a meal

cilia hairlike projections from epithelial cells as in the bronchi

circulatory refers to the circulatory system. The process of blood flowing through the vessels to all the cells of the body

circumcision surgical removal of the foreskin of the penis

cirrhosis an interstitial inflammation with hardening of the tissues of an organ, especially the liver

clarity clearness, absence of cloudiness

claustrophobia an abnormal fear of being in enclosed or confined places

clavicle the collar bone, articulating with the sternum and scapula

CLIA see **Clinical Laboratory Improvement Amendments (1988)**

Clinical Laboratory Improvement Amendments 1988 (CLIA) legislation dealing with the operation of a clinical laboratory

clitoris an erectile organ located at the anterior junction of the labia minora

clone a genetically exact copy

coagulate to lessen the fluidity of a liquid substance; to clot or curdle

coccyx the tailbone; the last four bones of the spine

cochlea the snail-shaped portion of the inner ear

coitus sexual intercourse between a man and a woman

colitis inflammation of the colon

colon the large intestine

colorimeter an instrument used for measuring the amount of pigments and determining the amount of hemoglobin in the blood

colostomy incision of the colon for the purpose of making a more or less permanent opening

colposcopy a diagnostic examination to visualize the cervix through a colposcope

coma an abnormal deep stupor from which a person cannot be aroused by external stimuli

comminuted a crushed bone fracture with many fragments

common bile duct a duct carrying bile from the hepatic and cystic ducts to the duodenum

compatible able to be mixed or taken together without destructive changes (as in blood typing and cross-matching); matching; not opposed to

compensate to make amends; be equivalent to

complement a group of about 20 inactive enzyme proteins present in the blood

compliance consent; conformity to formal or official requirements

compound not simple, composed of two or more parts; with fractures, refers to bone fragments piercing the skin externally

computerize to store in a computer; to put in a form a computer can use; to bring computers into use to control an operation

computerized axial tomography (CAT) a series of X-ray views of the body used to construct a three-dimensional picture

conceal to hide, to keep secret, to withhold, as with information

conceive to become pregnant; the uniting of the sperm and ovum

conception the union of the sperm of a male and the egg of a female; fertilization

concise condensed, short

condenser part of a microscope substage that regulates the amount of light directed on a specimen

confidentiality to be held in confidence; a secret

confinement restriction within certain limits

conflict a clash of opinions or interests; a fight or struggle; an inner moral struggle; to come into opposition

congestive heart failure a complex condition of inadequate heart action with retention of tissue fluids; may be either right or left side failure, or both

conjunctiva a mucous membrane which lines the eyelids and covers the anterior sclera of the eyeball

connective that which connects or binds together; one of the five main tissues of the body

conscientious doing what one knows is right

consciousness awareness, full knowledge of what is in one's own mind, the state of being fully awake and alert

constipation a sluggish action of the bowel; usually refers to an excessively firm, hard stool which is difficult to expel, or lack of a bowel movement over a period of time

constrict to narrow; to become smaller due to contraction of a sphincter muscle

contact dermatitis inflammation and irritation of the skin due to contact with an irritating substance

contagious catching; able to be transmitted by physical or other contact

contaminate to place in contact with microorganisms

contraception against conception, methods for preventing conception

contractions the muscle action of the uterus during labor

contracture permanent shortening or contraction of a muscle

convulsion attack of involuntary muscular contractions often accompanied with unconsciousness

coordination a state of harmonious adjustment or function

COPD see **chronic obstructive pulmonary disease**

cornea the transparent extension of the sclera that lies in front of the pupil of the eye

coronal plane a line drawn through the side of the body from head to toe, making a front and back section

coronary referring to the arteries surrounding the heart muscle; also refers to a "heart attack" involving the coronary arteries

corpus luteum the yellow body that develops in the ruptured graafian follicle after the ovum has been discharged

cortex the outer portion of the kidney

corticosteroids hormones used to treat inflammation

countershock (in cardiology) a high intensity, short-duration, electric shock applied to the area of the heart, resulting in total cardiac depolarization

cramp a spasmodic, painful contraction of a muscle or muscles

cranial pertaining to the cranium or skull

cranium the skull; the eight bones of the head enclosing the brain; generally applied to the 28 bones of the head and face

crenated notched or scalloped, as the crenated condition of blood corpuscles

cretinism a congenital condition due to the lack of the hormone thyroxin

crisis the turning point of a disease; a very critical period; an emergency situation

Crohn's disease an inflammation of the GI tract with debilitating symptoms

cross-match a blood test used to ensure compatibility of the donor to the recipient when transfusing blood

cryosurgery the use of a substance at subfreezing temperature to destroy or remove tissue

cryptorchidism failure of the testicles to descend into the scrotum

current happening now, of the present time, the latest information; a stream of electricity

Cushing's syndrome a disorder resulting from the hypersecretion of glucocorticoids from the adrenal cortex

cyanosis   a bluish discoloration of the skin due to lack of oxygen

cyst   a bladder; any sac containing fluid

cystic   pertaining to a cyst; of disease, refers to a condition with multiple cysts

cystic fibrosis   a disease condition of fibrous tumors which have undergone cystic degeneration, accumulating fluid in the interspaces; also known as fibrocystic disease

cystitis   inflammation of the urinary bladder

cystoscope   an instrument for examining the interior of the urinary bladder

cytology   the study of cell life and cell formation

cytoplasm   cellular matter, not including the nucleus of a cell

cytotechnologist   a laboratory specialist who prepares and examines tissue cells to study cell formation

cytotoxic   capable of destroying cells

daltonism   color blindness involving red and green

D & C   see **dilatation and curettage**

DEA   see **Drug Enforcement Administration**

debilitated   weaken; impaired the strength of

debridement   to clean up or remove, as is done with damaged tissue around a wound

decibel   a unit for measuring the volume of sound

decline stage   becoming less intense, subsiding; a period when the symptoms of disease start to disappear

defecate   to pass stool or move the bowels

defibrillation   to cause fibrillation to end; restore to normal action

dehydration   withdrawal of water from the tissues either naturally or artificially

delirium tremens   a psychic disorder involving hallucinations, both visual and auditory, found in habitual users of alcohol

deltoid   the muscle of the shoulder

dendrite   an extension from a nerve cell

depressant   a drug which causes a slowing down of bodily function or nerve activity

depressed   a state of depression, a period of low spirits; referring to a fracture, usually a fracture of the skull where bone fragments are driven (depressed) inward

dermatitis   an inflammation of the skin, often the result of an irritant

dermis   true skin

descending   refers to the portion of the large intestine from the splenic flexure to the sigmoid

description   a word picture

desensitization   the process of making an individual less susceptible to allergens

detection   find out or discover

detrimental   harmful, injurious

deuteranopia   green color blindness, also difficulty with bluish reds and neutrals

devastate   to lay waste, plunder, destroy

dextrose   a simple sugar, also known as glucose

diabetes mellitus   a metabolic disease caused by the body's inability to utilize carbohydrates

diabetic   one afflicted with diabetes mellitus

diagnostic   referring to measures which assist in the recognition of diseases and disorders of the body

dialysis   removal of the products of urine from the blood by passage of the solutes through a membrane

diaphanography   a type of transillumination used to examine the breast, using selected wavelengths of light and special imaging equipment

diaphoresis   profuse sweating

diaphragm   the muscle of breathing which separates the thorax from the abdomen

diarrhea   frequent bowel movements, usually liquid or semisolid

diarthroses   a movable joint; another word for synovial

diastole   the relaxation phase of the heartbeat; the period of least pressure

dietician   one who is trained in dietetics, which includes nutrition, and in charge of the diet at an institution

differential   refers to determining the number of each type of leukocyte in a cubic millimeter of blood

diffuse   to scatter or spread

diffusion   a process whereby gas, liquid, or solid molecules distribute themselves evenly through a medium

digestion   the process by which food is broken down, mechanically and chemically, in the gastrointestinal tract and converted into absorbable forms

digestive   pertaining to digestion

digital   pertaining to or resembling a finger or toe, as an examination using a finger or fingers

dilatation and curettage (D & C)   dilation of the cervix and scraping of the interior lining of the uterus

dilate   to enlarge, expand in size; to increase the size of an opening

dimpling   a condition characterized by indentations in the skin

diphtheria   an acute infectious disease characterized by the formation of a false membrane on any mucous surface, usually in the air passages, interfering with breathing

disaster   an occurrence inflicting widespread destruction and distress

disciplinary   designed to correct or punish breaches of conduct

disclose   to uncover, reveal

discoid   a type of lupus erythematosus which is confined to the skin; also called cutaneous

discretion   the use of judgment, prudence

dislocate   the displacement of a part; usually refers to a bone temporarily out of its normal position in a joint

dispatch   to send off; to finish quickly or promptly

dispense   to distribute; to deal out in portions

displacement   the transfer of emotions about one person or situation to another person or situation

disposition   the act or manner of putting in a particular order; arrange

distal   farthest from the center, from the medial line, or from the trunk

distort   to misrepresent; to twist out of usual shape

diverticulitis   inflammation of the diverticula

diverticulum   a sac or pouch in the walls of a canal or organ, particularly the colon

documentation   factual recording of events

dominant   strongest; prevailing, the prime or main

dorsal   pertaining to the back

dorsalis pedis a pulse point palpable on the instep of the foot

douche an irrigation of the vagina

dowel a wooden peg or pin; a manufactured "stick"

dribbling uncontrolled leakage of urine from the bladder

drill disciplined repetitive exercises as a means of perfecting a skill or procedure

droplet a very small drop

Drug Enforcement Administration (DEA) a division of the federal government responsible for the enforcement of laws regulating the distribution and sale of drugs

duodenum the first segment of the small intestine

dura mater the outer membrane covering the brain and spinal cord

duration period for which a thing continues

dwarfism a condition caused by inadequate growth hormone during childhood

dysmenorrhea painful menstruation

dyspnea difficult or labored breathing

dystrophy progressive atrophy or weakening of a part, such as the muscles

dysuria painful urination; difficulty in urination

ECG/EKG see **electrocardiogram**

echocardiography ultrahigh-frequency sound waves directed toward the heart to evaluate function and structure of the organ

echoes reflections of sound

ectopic in an abnormal position; in pregnancy refers to the embryo or fetus being outside the uterus

eczema a noncontagious skin disease characterized by dry, red, itchy and scaly skin

edema a condition of body tissues containing abnormal amounts of fluid, usually intercellular; may be local or general

effacement the thinning out of the cervix during labor

ejaculation the expulsion of seminal fluid from the male urethra

ejaculatory duct the duct from the seminal vesicle to the urethra

elasticity ability to return to shape after being stretched

electrocardiogram (EKG, ECG) a graphic record of the electric currents generated by the heart; a tracing of the heart's action

electrocardiograph a machine for obtaining a graphic recording of the electrical activity of the heart

electrocautery an apparatus used to cauterize tissue with heat from a current of electricity

electrocoagulation coagulation of tissue by means of a high-frequency electric current

electrode an instrument with a point or a surface which transmits current to the patient's body

electroencephalogram a graphic record of the electric currents generated by the brain; a tracing of brain waves

electrolyte a substance, which in solution, conducts an electric current

electromagnet a soft iron core that temporarily becomes a magnet when an electric current flows through a coil surrounding it

electromagnetic radiation rays produced by the collision of a beam of electrons with a metal target in an X-ray tube

electromyography the insertion of needles into selected skeletal muscles for the purpose of recording nerve conduction time in relation to muscle contraction

electron a minute particle of matter charged with the smallest known amount of negative electricity; opposite of a proton

elements substances in their simplest form; the basic building blocks of all matter

elicit to draw out, to derive by logical process

eliminate to remove, get rid of, exclude; also to pass urine from the bladder or stool from the bowel

embolus a circulating mass in a blood vessel; foreign material which obstructs a blood vessel

embryo the initial eight weeks of development after fertilization

emesis to vomit

emetic medication that induces vomiting

emphysema a chronic lung disease characterized by overdistention of the alveolar sacs and inability to exchange oxygen and carbon dioxide

empyema exudate (pus) within the pleural space of the chest cavity

endocardium the serous membrane lining of the heart

endocervical pertaining to the endocervix, the lining of the cervical canal

endocrine a gland that secretes directly into the bloodstream

endocytosis a cellular process to bring large molecules of material into the cytoplasm of the cell

endometrium the mucous membrane lining of the uterus

endoplasmic reticulum an organelle within the cytoplasm of a cell

endoscope an instrument consisting of a tube and optical system for observing the inside of an organ or cavity

enema the instillation of fluid into the rectum and colon

enucleation surgical excision of the eyeball

enunciate to speak or pronounce clearly

enzyme a complex chemical substance produced by the body, found primarily in the digestive juices, which acts upon food substances to break them down for absorption

eosinophil a white blood cell or cellular structure that stains readily with the acid stain eosin; specifically an eosinophilic leukocyte

epidermis the outer layer of skin; literally *over the true skin*

epididymis a convoluted tube resting on the surface of the testicle, which carries sperm from the testicle to the vas deferens

epigastric pertaining to the area of the abdomen over the stomach

epiglottis a cartilagenous lid which closes over the larynx when swallowing

epilepsy a chronic disease of the nervous system characterized by convulsions and often unconsciousness

epinephrine a hormone produced by the adrenal medulla

epiphysis a portion of bone not yet ossified; the cartilagenous ends of the long bones which allow for growth

episiotomy an incision in the perineum to avoid tearing during childbirth

epistaxis nosebleed; hemorrhage from the nose

epithelial pertaining to a type of cell or tissue that forms the skin and mucous membranes of the body

erectile refers to tissue which is capable of erection, usually due to vasocongestion

erythema diffuse redness over the skin due to capillary congestion and dilation of the superficial capillaries

erythrocyte a red blood cell (RBC)

erythropoiesis the formation of red blood corpuscles

esophagus the collapsible tube from the pharynx to the stomach through which passes the food and water the body ingests

essential necessary; when referring to blood pressure, indicates an elevation without apparent cause

estrogen a female hormone produced by the ovaries

euphoria a feeling of well-being, elation

eustachian tube refers to the tube of the middle ear which connects to the pharynx

evacuate to empty, especially the bowels

evacuation withdrawal, to remove, to make empty

evaluation assessment; judgment concerning the worth, quality, significance, or value of a situation, person, or product

excretion the process of expelling material from the body

exemplify to show by example

exfoliate to scale off dead tissue

exhale to breathe out

exocrine a gland which secretes substances through a duct into the body

exocytosis a cellular process which moves materials within the cell to the outside

exogenous originating outside an organ or part

exophthalmia abnormal protrusion of the eyeball

expectorate to spit, to expel mucus or phlegm from the throat or lungs

expertise special knowledge or skill

expiration the expulsion of air from the lungs in breathing

explicit clearly and definitely expressed; unambiguous; leaving no room for question

express to utter; to make known in words or by action

expressed consent a written agreement for treatment

extensor the muscle of a muscle team which extends a part, allowing the joint to straighten

externship a supervised employment experience in a qualified health care facility as part of the educational curriculum

extinguish to put out; put an end to

extracellular outside the cell

extract a substance distilled or drawn out of another substance

extremity refers to the terminal parts of the body—the arms, legs

exudate pus; the collection of purulent material in a cavity

eyewash a device utilizing water to remove foreign material from the eyes, usually in emergency situations

facility a building; in medical situations, a building for the care and treatment of patients

facultative able to live under conditions of temperature or oxygen supply which vary; having the capability to adapt to more than one condition, as a facultative anerobe

fallopian tube the ovaduct; the passageway for the ova from the ovary to the uterus

fascia a fibrous membrane covering, supporting, and separating muscles; may also unite the skin with underlying tissue

fasting to abstain from food; without food or water

fatal causing death

febrile pertaining to a fever

fecal pertaining to feces

feces stool, bowel movement

femoral pertaining to the artery that lies adjacent to the femur

femur the thigh bone of the leg

fenestrated having a window or opening

fertilization impregnation of the ovum by the sperm; conception

fetal pertaining to a fetus, pregnancy beyond the third month

fetus an embryo after eight weeks of gestation

fibrillation the quivering of muscle fibers; ineffective, rapid but weak heart action

fibroid a tumor made up of fibrous and muscular tissue

fibula a long bone in the leg from the knee to the ankle

filtration the movement of solutes and water across a semi-permeable membrane as a result of a force, such as gravity or blood pressure

fissure an ulcer, split, crack, or tear in the tissue

fistula an abnormal tubelike passage from a normal cavity or an abscess to a free surface

flatulence the existence of flatus or intestinal gas

flatus intestinal gas

flexed bent, as at a joint

flexible easily bent, compliant, yielding to persuasion

flexor the muscle of a muscle team that bends a part

flora plant life as distinguished from animal life; plant life occurring or adapted for living in a specific environment, as flora in the intestines

flu an abbreviation for the word *influenza*; a respiratory or intestinal infection

fluoroscope a device consisting of a fluorescent screen in conjunction with an X-ray tube to make visible shadows of objects interposed between the screen and the tube

flush sudden reddish coloration of the skin

follicle a small excretory duct or sac or tubular gland; a hair follicle

folliculitis a staphlococcal infection of a hair follicle

foreign anything which is not normally found in the location; usually refers to dirt, splinters, etc

foreskin loose skin covering the end of the penis

formalin a colorless liquid form preservative, for tissue transport

fovea centralis a depression in the posterior surface of the retina which is the place of sharpest vision

fracture the sudden breaking of a bone

frenzy to make frantic; wild excitement

frequency the need to void urine often, though usually only a small amount at one time

friction resistance of one surface to the motion of another surface rubbing over it

frontal anterior; the forehead bone; refers to the plane drawn through the side of the body from the head to the foot

fundoscopy to look at the interior of the eye

fungus a vegetable, cellular organism that subsists on organic matter, such as bacteria or mold; a disease condition which causes growth of fungal lesions on the surface of the skin

furuncle the medical term for a boil

gait manner of walking

gallbladder a small sac suspended beneath the liver which concentrates and stores bile

galvanometer an instrument that measures current by electromagnetic action

gamete a germ cell; any reproductive body

ganglion a mass of nerve tissue which receives and sends out nerve impulses

gangrene a form of necrosis; the putrefaction of soft tissue

gastric pertaining to the stomach

gastrocnemius the large muscle in the calf of the leg

gastrointestinal (GI) pertaining to the stomach and intestines

gastroscopy examination of the stomach with a gastroscope

gauge the size of a needle bore; the smaller the number the larger the needle bore

gene a substance within the chromosome that dictates heredity

generic general; characteristic of a genus or group

genetic pertaining to the genes

genital herpes fluid-filled lesions on the external genitalia which are contagious upon direct contact

genitalia the external sexual organs

genogram a patient health history that covers at least three generations

genucubital pertaining to the elbows and knees; the knee-elbow position

genupectoral pertaining to the knees and the chest; the knee-chest position

gestation period of intrauterine fetal development

gigantism a condition resulting from the overproduction of growth hormone during childhood

glaucoma a disease of the eye characterized by increased intraocular pressure

glomerulonephritis inflammation of the glomerulus of the nephron of the kidney

glomerulus the microscopic cluster of capillaries within the Bowman's capsule of the nephron

glucose a colorless or yellow, thick, syrupy liquid obtained by the incomplete hydrolysis of starch; a simple sugar

gluteus maximus the large muscle of the buttocks

glycosuria sugar in the urine

goiter an enlargement of the thyroid gland

Golgi's apparatus an organelle within the cytoplasm of a cell

gonadotrophic related to stimulation of the gonads

gonads the sex glands, the ovaries in the female and the testicles in the male

gonorrhea a venereal disease of the reproductive organs which is highly contagious upon direct contact

graafian follicle the vesicle in which ova are matured and which releases them when ripened

graft a constructed part

gram-negative bacteria which take on a pink color with Gram's staining process

gram-positive bacteria which take on a purple color with Gram's staining process

greenstick an incomplete fracture, occurring in children

grillwork a bar-like device, usually constructed of heavy metal; an open grating for a door or window

groin the depression between the thigh and the trunk of the body; the inguinal region

gross anatomy refers to the study of those features that can be observed with the naked eye by inspection and dissection

guaiac a solution used to test for the presence of occult blood in the stool

GYN see **gynecology**

gynecologist a physician specializing in the care of diseases and disorders of women, particularly the genital organs

gynecology (GYN) the study of diseases of the female, particularly of the organs of reproduction

Haemophilus bacterial strains that grow best in hemoglobin

hallucinogen a substance which causes hallucinations

hamstring a group of muscles of the posterior thigh

hazardous dangerous; risky

HCFA Health Care Financing Administration

health a state of complete physical and mental or social well-being

heart block a condition in which impulses from the SA node fail to carry over to the AV node resulting in a slow heart rate and a different rate of contraction between the upper and lower heart chambers

heartburn a burning sensation beneath the breastbone, usually associated with indigestion

hematocrit an expression of the volume of red blood cells per unit of circulating blood

hematoma a tumor or swelling which contains blood

hematuria blood in the urine

hemodialysis a process whereby blood is passed through a thin membrane and exposed to a dialysate solution to remove waste products

hemoglobin the combination of a protein and iron pigment in the red blood cells that attracts and carries oxygen in the body

hemolysis dissolution; the breaking down of red blood cells

hemophilia a hereditary condition, transmitted through sex-linked chromosomes of female carriers; affects males only, causing inability to clot blood

hemorrhage abnormal discharge of blood either internally or externally from venous, arterial, or capillary vessels

hemorrhoidectomy surgical excision of hemorrhoidal tissue

hemorrhoids varicose veins of the anal canal

hemothorax blood within the pleural space of the chest cavity

heparin a substance formed in the liver which inhibits the coagulation of blood

hepatic pertaining to the liver

hepatitis inflammation of the liver

hernia a projection of a part from its normal location

herniorrhaphy the surgical repair of a hernia

herpes simplex the virus that causes fever blisters and an acute viral infection of the face, mouth, or nose

herpes zoster the virus that causes shingles—an acute viral infection of the dorsal root ganglia

hesitancy difficulty in starting a urine stream

heterosexual   sexual attraction toward the opposite sex

heterotrophs   microorganisms that feed on organic matter

HHS   Health and Human Services

hiatus   pertains to a herniation of the stomach through an opening, or hiatus

HIB/hib   *haemophilus influenzae* type B

hiccough   (also hiccup) a result of the spasmodic closing of the epiglottis and spasm of the diaphragm

hilum   the recessed area of the kidney where the ureter and blood vessels enter

hinge   a type of joint

histamine   a substance normally present in the body

histologist   (histotechnologist) a person engaged in the study of the microscopic structure of tissue

histology   the study of the microscopic structure of tissue

histoplasmosis   a fungal infection caused by an organism found in bird and bat droppings

holistic   considering the whole or entire scope of a situation

Holter monitor   a device that attaches electrodes to a patient's chest for the purpose of obtaining a 24-hour EKG tracing in an accessory tape recorder

homeostasis   maintenance of a constant or static condition of internal environment

homosexual   sexual attraction toward the same sex as oneself

horizontal   not vertical; flat and even; level; parallel to the plane of the horizon

hormone   a chemical substance secreted by an organ or gland

hostility   unfriendliness, enmity

hpf   high-power field; refers to microscope lens

humerus   the long bone of the upper arm

humoral   antibody-mediated immunity

hyaline membrane disease   a condition resulting from incomplete development of the respiratory system in premature infants

hydrocele   the accumulation of fluid in the scrotum

hydrochloric acid   a digestive juice found in the stomach

hygiene   the study of health and observance of health rules

hymen   a membranous fold partially or completely covering the vaginal opening

hyperglycemia   increase of blood sugar, as in diabetes

hyperopia   a defect of vision so that objects can only be seen when they are far away; farsightedness

hypersensitive   overly sensitive; abnormally sensitive to a stimulus of any kind

hypertension   elevated blood pressure

hyperthermia   higher than normal body temperature

hyperthyroidism   a condition caused by excessive secretion of the thyroid glands

hypertonic   having a higher concentration of salt than found in a red blood cell

hyperventilation   excessive deep and frequent breathing

hypoallergenic   unlikely to cause an allergic reaction

hypochondriac   pertaining to the upper outer regions of the abdomen below the thorax; also someone with a morbid fear of disease, resulting in abnormal concern about one's health

hypogastric   referring to an abdominal area in the middle lower third of the abdomen

hypoglycemia   deficiency of sugar in the blood

hypotension   abnormally low blood pressure

hypothalamus   a structure of the brain between the cerebrum and the midbrain; lies below the thalamus

hypothermia   below normal body temperature

hypothyroidism   a condition caused by a marked deficiency of thyroid secretion

hypotonic   having a lower concentration of salt than found in a red blood cell

hypoxia   a lack of oxygen

hysterectomy   surgical removal of the uterus

hysteroscopy   a procedure utilizing the hysteroscope to view the endometrium of the uterus

idiopathic   disease without recognizable cause

ileocecal   the valve between the end of the small intestine and the cecum

ileostomy   a surgical opening from the ileum onto the abdominal wall

ileum   the last section of the small intestine

iliac   the edge or crest of the pelvic bone

ilium   the hip bone

illicit   improper; unlawful; not sanctioned by custom or law; illegal

imaging   a representation or visual impression produced by a lens, mirror, etc.

immune   protected or exempt from a disease

immunization   becoming immune or the process of rendering a patient immune

immunodeficiency   lacking the components necessary to mount an immune response

immunoglobulin   a large protein molecule which assists in the immune response

immunological   pertaining to immunology

immunosuppressed   a condition wherein the immune system has been overpowered and cannot function adequately

impacted   refers to a fracture where the broken ends are jammed together

impaction   a collection of hardened feces in the rectum which cannot be expelled

impending   to be at hand or about to happen

implant   something implanted into tissue; a graft; artificial part

implement   a tool or instrument for doing something; to put into effect

implication   involvement, bringing into connection

implied agreements   when words or actions are considered to indicate a willingness to be treated

implied consent   when agreement to receive care or treatment is believed to have been given

impotence   inability of a male to obtain or maintain an erection

impulse   a charge transmitted through certain tissues, especially nerve fibers and muscles, resulting in physiological activity

inappropriate   not appropriate, out of place

incinerate   to burn, set afire

incision   cut

incision and drainage (I & D)   cutting into for the purpose of providing an exit for material, usually a collection of pus

incompetent   without adequate ability, knowledge; not legally qualified

incomprehensible   beyond belief, not to be grasped by the mind

incongruous   lacking harmony or agreement

incontinent   unable to control the bladder or bowel

incubation   the interval between exposure to infection and the appearance of the first symptom

incus   the anvil, the middle bone of the three in the middle ear

indigestion   difficulty in digesting food

inevitable   unavoidable, destined to occur

infarct   infiltration of foreign particles; material in a vessel causing coagulation and interference with circulation

infectious   capable of producing infection; denoting a disease in the body caused by the presence of germs; tending to spread to others

inferior   below, under

infertility   inability to achieve conception

infirmity   illness, disease

influenza   an acute illness characterized by fever, pain, coughing, and general upper respiratory symptoms

infrared   pertaining to those invisible rays just beyond the red end of the visible spectrum which have a penetrating heating effect

infusion   to instill; introduction of a substance into a vein

ingest   to eat

inguinal   referring to the region where the thigh joins the trunk of the body; the groin

inguinal canal   a passageway in the groin for the spermatic cord in the male

inguinal hernia   the presence of small intestine in the inguinal canal

inhale   to breathe in

initial   the first; beginning; the first letter of each of a person's names

inoculating loop   a laboratory instrument used to transfer organisms from one source to another

inorganic   not living; occurring in nature independently of living things

inseminate   to impregnate with semen

insertion   the place where a muscle is attached to the bone that it moves

insidious   hidden, not apparent

insignificant   unimportant; petty; of little or no value

inspection   the first part of a physical examination; close observation

inspiration   to breathe in, inhale

instill   to put in, drop by drop; to put in gradually

insulin   a hormone secreted by the islands (islets) of Langerhans in the pancreas

intact   unbroken, undamaged

intangible   that which cannot be touched, easily defined or grasped

integumentary   the skin; a covering

intellectualization   to employ reasoning to avoid confrontations or stressful situations

interaction   to act upon one another

intercede   to plead or make a request in behalf of another; to intervene for the purpose of producing agreement

intercostal   between the ribs

interference   confusion of desired signals due to undesired signals, as in artifacts on an EKG

interferon   a lymphokine that helps regulate the activities of macrophages and NK cells

interleukin   a substance which is a messenger between leukocytes

intermittent   stopping and starting again at intervals

intermuscular   within the muscle

interneurons   neurons connecting sensory to motor neurons

interpersonal   between persons

interpret   to explain, translate; to determine the meaning

intersect   to divide into two parts by passing through or across

interval   time between events; space

intervertebral   between the vertebrae

intestine   the alimentary canal extending from the pylorus of the stomach to the anus

intracellular   within the cell

intradermal   within the skin

intraocular   within the eyeball

intrauterine device (IUD)   an object inserted into the uterus to prevent pregnancy

intravenous   to insert into the vein

intravenous pyelography (IVP)   the insertion of a radio-paque material into the vein for the purpose of X raying the kidneys and ureters

intubate   to insert a tube

intuition   the immediate knowing or learning of something without the conscious use of reasoning

inunction   the process of administering drugs through the skin

invasive   diagnostic methods involving entry into living tissue

involuntary   independent of or even contrary to will or choice

iodine   a nonmetallic element belonging to the halogen group

iris   the colored, contractible tissue surrounding the pupil of the eye

irrigate   to flush with fluid

ischemia   temporary and localized anemia due to obstruction of the circulation to a part

ischium   posterior and inferior portion of the hip bone

Ishihara test   an eye test to determine color vision

islet of Langerhans   clusters of cells in the pancreas that produce insulin

isotonic   having the same concentration of salt as found in a red blood cell

I & D   see **incision and drainage**

IVP   see **intravenous pyelography**

Jaeger card   a system for measuring near vision acuity

jaundice   a yellowish discoloration of the sclera and skin due to the presence of bile pigments in the blood

jejunum   the middle segment of the small intestine, which measures approximately 8 feet in length

keloid   an overgrowth of new skin tissue; a scar

kidney   a bean-shaped organ that excretes urine and is located retroperitoneally, high in the back of the abdominal cavity

KUB   kidneys, ureters, and bladder; refers to a radiological study

kyphosis   a convex curvature of the spine; humpback

L & A   light and accommodation

labia majora   the two large folds of adipose tissue lying on each side of the vulva of the female; external genitalia

labia minora   the two mucocutaneous folds of membrane within the labia majora

laboratory   a room or building in which scientific tests or experiments are conducted

lacrimal   pertaining to tears; the glands and ducts which secrete and convey tears

laminectomy   the removal of a portion of the vertebral posterior arch

lancet   a sharp, pointed instrument used to pierce the skin to obtain a capillary blood sample

laryngeal   pertaining to the larynx

laryngectomy   surgical removal of the larynx or voice box

larynx   the voice box

lateral   pertaining to the side

latissimus dorsi   the large muscle of the back

lavage   washing out of a cavity; e.g., gastric lavage

laxative   a substance which induces the bowels to empty

legible   easy to read, readable

legionnaires' disease   an acute bronchopneumonia caused by *legionella pneumophila*

leisure   spare or free time, away from the pressure and responsibilities of work

lens   a part of the eye which bends or refracts images onto the retina

lesion   an injury or wound; a circumscribed area of pathologically altered tissue

lethal   deadly; capable of causing death

leukemia   a disease characterized by a great excess of white blood cells; it exists in a lymphatic and myelogenous form; it is often fatal, especially in adults

leukocyte   a white blood cell

liaison   intercommunication between two entities

license   a legal permit to engage in an activity

ligament   fibrous tissue which connects bone to bone

ligation   to tie off; the process of binding or tying

limbs   arms and legs

liter   a unit of measure; 1,000 mL or approximately 1 quart

liver   the largest gland in the body, located in the upper right quadrant of the abdomen beneath the diaphragm

lithotomy   an examination position wherein the patient lies upon the back with thighs flexed upon the abdomen and legs flexed upon the thighs

lithotripsy   destruction of stone; stonecrusher

LMP   last menstrual period

longitudinal fissure   the deep cleft between the two hemispheres of the cerebrum

lordosis   abnormal anterior curvature of the lumbar spine

lpf   low-power field; refers to microscope lens

lubb dupp   sounds made by the heart

lumbar   pertaining to the back, specifically to the five vertebrae above the sacrum

lumbar puncture   the insertion of a needle between the vertebrae in the lumbar area for the purpose of withdrawing spinal fluid

lumen   the space within an artery, vein, or capillary; the space within a tube

lung   the organ of respiration, located within the thoracic cavity

lupus erythematosus   a chronic autoimmune disease which causes changes in the immune system

luteinizing   a hormone effect which causes ovulation and progesterone in the female and sperm production and testosterone in the male

Lyme disease   a disease caused by the spirochete *Borrella burgdorferi*, which is carried by the deer tick

lymph   a body fluid formed within the tissue spaces and circulated throughout the body

lymphatic system   a network of transparent vessels carrying lymph fluid throughout the body

lymphocyte   a type of white blood cell

lymphokine   proteins produced by T cells

lysosomes   an organelle within the cytoplasm of the cell

macule   a discolored spot or patch on the skin neither elevated nor depressed

macrophage   a phagocytic cell that destroys antigens

magnetic   having the properties of a magnet, able to attract

magnetic resonance imaging (MRI)   a diagnostic test using magnetic waves to visualize internal body structures

magnify   to make something look larger than it really is

malaise   a feeling of discomfort or uneasiness

malignant   a cancerous growth; tumor

malinger   to pretend illness to escape dealing with a situation or obligation

malleus   the largest of the three bones of the middle ear, also called the hammer

mammary glands   the breasts

mammograph   an X ray of the breast

mandatory   required, receiving a command or order

manipulation therapy   any treatment or procedure involving the use of the hands; movement of a joint to determine its range of extension and flexion; additional manual skills utilized by osteopathic physicians

marginal   close to the lower limit of acceptability

marrow   the soft tissue in the hollow of long bones

mastectomy   surgical removal of a breast

maturation   refers to a stage of cellular development

maturity   a state of full development

measles   a highly contagious disease characterized by the presence of maculopustular eruptions

mechanical   pertaining to machinery

medial   pertaining to the middle or midline

medulla   the inner section of the kidney

medulla oblongata   enlarged portion of the spinal cord; the lower portion of the brain stem

melanin   a pigment which gives color to the skin, hair, and eyes

melanocyte   cells which produce the pigment of the skin, melanin

membrane   a thin, soft, pliable layer of tissue which lines a tube or cavity or covers an organ or structure

menarche   the first menstrual period

Meniere's disease   a disorder of the ear characterized by nausea, vomiting, tinnitus, and hearing loss

meninges   the membranes covering the brain and spinal cord

meningitis   inflammation of the meninges of the brain or spinal cord

meniscus   a concave level of fluid in a tube or cylinder

menopause   the permanent cessation of menstruation

menorrhagia   excessive menstrual flow, hemorrhage

menstruate   to periodically discharge bloody fluid from the uterus

mensuration   the process of measuring

mercury   a liquid metal used in measurement devices such as thermometers and sphygmomanometers; chemical symbol, Hg

merit   to deserve reward or praise; excellence

mesentery   a peritoneal fold connecting the intestine to the posterior abdominal wall

metabolism   the successive transformations to which a substance is subjected from the time it enters the body to the time it or its decomposition products are excreted, and by which nutrition is accomplished and energy and living substance are provided

metacarpals   the five bones of the hand between the wrist and the phalanges

metastasis   movement of cancer cells from one part of the body to another

metatarsals   the five bones of the feet between the instep and the phalanges

MI   see **myocardial infarction**

microbial   related to microbes

microorganism   a microscopic living body not perceivable by the naked eye

microscopic   visible only with a microscope

microscopic anatomy   an area of study that deals with features that can be seen only with a microscope

micturation   the passing of urine

midbrain   that portion of the brain connecting the pons and the cerebellum

midline   the middle

migraine   a severe headache with characteristic symptoms

minute   a measurement of time equal to 60 seconds; very small, tiny

misalignment   out of alignment; not straight

mitochondria   organelles within the cytoplasm of the cell

mitosis   the division of a cell

mitral   the valve in the heart between the chambers of the left side, also known as the bicuspid

monitor   to oversee or observe

monoclonal   a laboratory-produced hybrid cell which produces antibodies

monocular   possessing a single eyepiece as with a microscope

monocyte   single nucleated cells which leave the blood and enter into tissues to become macrophages

monogamous   being married or having only one mate at a time

monokine   protein produced by a monocyte

mons pubis   a pad of fatty tissue and coarse skin overlying the symphysis pubis in the female

moral   conforming to generally accepted ideas of what is right and just in human conduct

morphology   a branch of biology dealing with the form and structure of organisms

motor   refers to the nerves which permit the body to respond to stimuli

mouth   the oral cavity; can also refer to the opening to organs

MRI   see **magnetic resonance imaging**

mucosa   pertaining to mucous membrane

MUGA   see **multiple-gated acquisition scan**

multichannel   refers to the capability of ECG equipment of processing impulses from multiple leads

multiple-gated acquisition scan (MUGA)   a diagnostic test to evaluate the condition of the myocardium of the heart

mumps   an acute contagious disease characterized by inflammation of the parotid gland and other salivary glands

murmur   a soft blowing or rasping sound heard on auscultation of the heart

muscle   a type of tissue composed of contractile cells or fibers which effect movement of the body

muscle team   a pair of skeletal muscles, one which flexes and one which extends the joint

muscle tone   a state of muscle contraction in which a portion of the fibers are contracted while others are at rest

muscular   pertaining to muscles

musculoskeletal   pertaining to the muscular and skeletal systems

mutation   a change in an inheritable characteristic; cellular change due to an influence

myelin   a fatlike substance forming the principal component of the myelin sheath of nerve fibers

myelography   an X-ray examination of the spinal cord following an injection of a radiopaque material

myocardial infarction (MI)   blockage of a coronary artery which interrupts the flow of blood to the heart muscle

myocardium   the muscle layer of the heart

myometrium   the muscular structure of the uterus

myopia   a defect in vision so that objects can only be seen when very near; nearsightedness

myxedema   a condition resulting from the hypofunction of the thyroid gland

narcolepsy   overwhelming attacks of sleep which the victim cannot inhibit; paroxysmal sleep

narcotic   a drug capable of producing sleep and relieving pain or inducing unconsciousness and even death, depending upon the dosage

nasal   pertaining to the nose

nausea   an inclination to vomit

neoadjuvant   new attachment process; giving chemotherapy prior to surgery to shrink the tumor before removal

neonate   a newborn infant

neoplastic   new abnormal tissue formation; cancer-related

nephron   the structural and functional unit of the kidney

nephrotic syndrome   term applied to renal disease of whatever cause characterized by massive edema, proteinuria, and usually elevation of serum cholesterol and lipids

nerve   a group of nervous tissues bound together for the purpose of conducting nervous impulses

neurilemma   a thin membranous sheath enveloping a nerve fiber

neuron   a nerve cell

neutrophil   a granulated white blood cell

nicotine   a poisonous alkaloid extracted from tobacco leaves

nit   the egg of a louse or other parasitic insect

nocturia   having to void at night

node   a knot, knob, protuberance, or swelling

nomogram   representation by graphs, diagrams, or charts of the relationship between numerical variables

nonchalant   unconcerned, indifferent

noninvasive   a diagnostic method not requiring entry into body tissue

nonpathogen   an organism which does not produce a disease

nonspecific urethritis   inflammation of the urethra in males, vaginitis or cervicitis in females, due to bacteria or an allergy to substances used by a sexual partner

norepinephrine a hormone secreted by adrenal medulla in response to sympathetic stimulation

normal saline a solution with the same salt content as that found within a red blood cell

nuclear medicine the branch of medicine which utilizes radionuclides in the diagnosis and treatment of disease

nucleolus a structure found within the nucleus of the cell

nucleus the vital body in the protoplasm of a cell

nurse practitioner an RN with advanced clinical experience and education in a special branch of practice

nurture to care for, train, or educate

nutrition refers to edible material, food, things that nourish

objective the end toward which action is directed; of a disease symptom, perceptible to persons other than the one affected; on a microscope, a lens or series of lenses

obligate to bind legally or morally

obsolete out of use, discarded, no longer useful

obstetrical referring to obstetrics

obstetrics the branch of medicine dealing with women during pregnancy, childbirth, and postpartum

obturator anything that obstructs or closes a cavity or opening; refers to that internal portion of an examining instrument which facilitates the introduction of the instrument into the body and is then withdrawn permitting visualization of the internal area

occipital pertaining to the back part of the head, the posterior lobe of the cerebrum

occlude to close up, obstruct

occult obscure, hidden

O.D. oculus dexter; the right eye

ointment a salve; a fatty, soft substance having antiseptic or healing properties

olfactory pertaining to the sense of smell

oliguria scanty production of urine

oncogenes a gene in a tumor cell

ophthalmology the study of the eye and its diseases

opportunistic seizing the opportunity; taking advantage of the situation

optic pertaining to the eye or sight

optic disc the blind spot where the optic nerve exits from the retina of the eye

oral pertaining to the mouth

orbital refers to the cavity within the skull where the eye is located

organ a part of the body constructed of many types of tissue to perform a function

organ of Corti terminal acoustic apparatus in the cochlea of the inner ear

organelles functional structures within the cytoplasm of a cell

organic pertaining to or derived from animal or vegetable forms of life

origin the beginning or source of anything; of muscles, the anchor

orthopnea respiratory condition in which breathing is possible only in an erect sitting or standing position

os a mouth or opening

O.S. oculus sinister, the left eye

oscilloscope an instrument that displays a visual representation of electric variations on the fluorescent screen of a cathode-ray tube

OSHA Occupational Safety and Health Act

osmosis the process of diffusion of water or another solvent through a selected permeable membrane

osseous bonelike, concerning bones

osteoporosis a condition resulting from a decrease in the amount of calcium stored in the bone

otic pertaining to the ear

otitis inflammation of the ear; can be referenced to the external, middle, or internal ear

otosclerosis condition characterized by progressive deafness due to the fixation of the stapes of the middle ear

O.U. oculus uterque; each eye

ovary the female gonad which produces hormones causing the secondary sex characteristics to develop and be maintained

over the counter (OTC) referring to accessible, nonprescription drugs

ovulation the periodic ripening and rupture of a mature graafian follicle and the discharge of the ovum

ovum an egg, the female gamete or reproductive cell

oxalate a salt of oxalic acid

oxygen a colorless, odorless, tasteless gas found in the air; chemical symbol, O_2

oxygenate combine or supply with oxygen

pacemaker the SA node of the heart; also refers to an artificial device which initiates heartbeat

pallor lack of color, paleness

palpate to feel; to examine by touch

pancreas an organ which secretes insulin and pancreatic digestive juice

pancreatitis inflammation of the pancreas

Papanicolaou (Pap) smear a test to detect cancer cells in the mucus of an organ

papillae small protuberances or elevations, such as the taste buds of the tongue

papillary muscles muscular attachments to the undersides of the heart valves from the walls of the ventricles, which open the valves during the relaxation phase of the heartbeat

parabasal beside, near, an accessory to the base or lower part

paralytic ileus paralysis of the intestinal wall with symptoms of acute obstruction

parasite an organism that lives in or on another organism without rendering it any service in return

parasympathetic a division of the autonomic nervous system

parathyroid small endocrine glands located close to the thyroid gland

parenteral other than by mouth

parietal a central portion of the cerebrum located on each side of the brain

paroxysmal a sudden attack of a disease; fit of acute pain, passion, coughing, or laughter

patella the kneecap

pathogen any microorganism or substance capable of producing a disease

pathology the study of the nature and cause of disease

pathophysiology the study of mechanisms by which disease occurs, the responses of the body to the disease process, and the effects of both on normal function

PDR *Physician's Desk Reference*

pectoralis major   the principal muscle of the chest wall

pediculosis   the scientific name for lice infestation

pelvic   pertaining to the pelvis

penis   the male external sex organ

peptic   pertaining to digestion; can also refer to an ulcer of the upper digestive tract

percentage   rate or proportion of each hundred

percentile   any value in a series dividing the distribution of its members into 100 groups or equal frequency

perception   awareness through the senses; the receipt of impressions; consciousness

percussion   tapping the body lightly but sharply to determine the position, size, and consistency of an underlying structure

perfusion   passing of a fluid through spaces; the act of pouring over or through

pericarditis   inflammation of the pericardium, the covering of the heart

pericardium   the membranous sac that covers the heart

perinatal   refers to the period surrounding birth

perineum   the region between the vagina and anus of the female and the scrotum and anus of the male

periosteum   the fibrous membrane covering the bone except at the articulating surfaces

peripheral   pertaining to a portion of the nervous system; an item attached to a computer system

peristalsis   a progressive, wavelike muscular movement which occurs involuntarily in the urinary and digestive system

peritoneal   pertaining to the peritoneum

permeable   capable of being penetrated; allowing entrance

pernicious anemia   a severe anemia characterized by progressive decrease in the production of red blood cells

perplexing   troubling with doubt, puzzling

perspective   a view of things, or facts, in which they are in the right relations

pertinent   having to do with what is being considered; relevant or to the point

pertussis   an acute infectious disease characterized by a paroxysmal cough, ending in a whooping inspiration

petechiae   small, purplish, hemorrhagic spots on the skin

petty   small, having little value, mean, narrow-minded

pH   a measure of acidity or alkalinity

phagocyte   a white blood cell that engulfs and destroys antigens

phagocytosis   ingestion and digestion of bacteria and particles by phagocytes

phalanges   bones of the fingers and toes

phalanx   any one of the bones of the fingers or toes

phantom limb   an illusion following amputation of a limb that the limb still exists

pharmaceutical   concerning drugs or pharmacy

pharmacology   the study and practice of compounding and dispensing medical preparations

pharynx   the throat; that portion of the alimentary canal between the mouth and the esophagus

phenylalanine   an amino acid of a protein

phenylketonuria (PKU)   a genetic disorder resulting from the body's failure to oxidize the amino acid phenylalanine, perhaps because of a defective enzyme

phimosis   a narrowing of the opening of the foreskin of the penis

phlebitis   inflammation of a vein

photophobia   sensitive to light; avoiding light

physical   pertaining to the body; also used for the examination of the body

physiology   the study of the function of cells, tissues, and organs of the body

pia mater   innermost of the three meninges of the brain and spinal cord

pigment   any coloring matter

pineal body   a small endocrine gland attached to the posterior part of the third ventricle of the brain

pinocytosis   the process whereby a cell engulfs large amounts of liquid

pitch   the frequency of vibrations of sound which enable one to classify sound on a scale from high to low

pituitary   a small endocrine gland attached to the base of the brain; the "master" gland

PKU   see **phenylketonuria**

placenta   the structure through which the fetus obtains nourishment during pregnancy; the afterbirth

planes   a flat or relatively smooth surface; points of reference by which positions or parts of the body are indicated

plasma   the liquid part of the lymph and blood

platelet   a type of cell found in the blood which is required for clotting

pleura   a serous membrane which covers the lungs and lines the thoracic cavity

pleurisy   inflammation of the pleura

plexuses   a network of nerves

pneumoconiosis   a respiratory condition due to inhalation of dust particles from mining or stone cutting

pneumoencephalography   an X-ray examination of ventricles and subarachnoid spaces of brain following withdrawal of cerebrospinal fluid and injection of air or gas via a lumbar puncture

pneumonia   inflammation of the lung caused primarily by microbes, chemical irritants, vegetable dust, or allergy

pneumothorax   a collection of air or gas in the pleural cavity which displaces lung tissue, causing it to collapse

POL   physician's office laboratory

polio   (poliomyelitis) an acute, infectious, systemic disease which causes inflammation of the grey matter of the spinal cord

polycystic disease   a condition of multiple cysts

polycythemia   an excess of red blood cells

polyp   a tumor with a pedicle, especially on mucous membranes, such as in the nose, rectum, or intestines

polyuria   excessive secretion and discharge of urine

pons   a portion of the brain stem connecting the medulla oblongata and cerebellum with upper portions of the brain

portal   pertaining to the portal circulation of blood from impaired internal organs to the liver for processing before entering the inferior vena cava

positive   strongly affirmative

posterior   toward the rear or back or toward the caudal end

postoperative (post-op)   after or following a surgical procedure

postpartum   the period following delivery of a baby

potential   possible; ability to develop into actuality

precancerous   a state just prior to the development of cancer

precordial   pertaining to that area of the chest wall over the heart for the placement of EKG chest leads

pregnancy   the condition of having conceived

preliminary   coming before, leading up to

prenatal   before birth; the care of the pregnant woman during the period of gestation

preoperative (pre-op)   the preparatory period preceding surgery

presbycusis   impairment of acute hearing in old age

presbyopia   a defect of vision in advancing age involving loss of accommodation

prescribe   to lay down as a rule or direction; to order, advise, the use of

prescription   a written direction for the preparation of a medicine

primary   occurring first in time, development, or sequence; earliest

prioritize   to arrange in order of importance

priviledged communication   information provided in confidence to other health professionals regarding a patient's condition or treatment

proclivity   an inclination or predisposition toward something

proctology   the study of the rectum and anus and their diseases

proctoscope   an instrument for the inspection of the rectum

proctoscopy   instrumental inspection of the rectum

procurement   to obtain; acquire

professional's negligence   malpractice; an action or inaction different from what a similarly trained and competent person would do

proficient   well advanced in an art, occupation, skill, or branch of knowledge; unusually knowledgeable

progesterone   a hormone secreted by the graafian follicle following the expulsion of the ovum

progress notes   record of the continuing progress and treatment of a patient

project   to produce and send forth with clarity and distinctness

prolapse   dropping of an internal part of the body; usually refers to uterus or rectum

prone   a position, lying horizontal with the face down

prophylactic   warding off disease; preventive

prostaglandins   a group of chemical substances secreted by mast cells or basophils that constricts smooth muscles in some organs

prostate   a gland of the male reproductive system which surrounds the proximal portion of the urethra

prostatectomy   excision of part or all of the prostate gland

prosthesis   an artificial replacement of a missing body part

protanopia   partial color blindness

prothrombin   chemical substance existing in circulating blood which aids in the clotting process

protozoan   a single-celled animal

proximal   nearest the point of attachment

pruritus   severe itching

pruritus ani   itching about the anus

psoriasis   a chronic inflammatory disease characterized by scaly patches on the skin

psychedelics   hallucinogenic drugs

psychoneuroimmunology   a science studying the connection between the brain, behavior, and immunity

psychosis   mental disturbance of such magnitude that there is personality disintegration and loss of contact with reality

psychosomatic   pertaining to interrelationship between the mind or emotions and body

ptosis   a drooping or dropping of an organ or part, for example the eyelid or the kidney

puberty   the period of life at which one becomes functionally capable of reproduction

pubic   pertaining to the middle section of the lower third of the abdomen, also referred to as the hypogastric

pulmonary   concerning or involving the lungs

pulmonary edema   the presence of interstitial fluid in the lung tissue

pulmonary embolism   a blockage in the pulmonary artery or one of its branches

pulse   throbbing caused by the regular alternating contraction and expansion of an artery

pulse deficit   the difference between the pulse rate measured radially and apically

pulse pressure   difference between the systolic and diastolic measurements

puncture   a hole made by something pointed

pupil   the contractible opening in the center of the iris for the transmission of light

purkinje fibers   network of fibers found in the cardiac muscle which carries the electrical impulse resulting in the contraction of the ventricles

pustule   small elevation of the skin filled with lymph or pus

pyelonephritis   inflammation of the kidney, pelvis, and nephrons

pyloric   pertaining to the opening between the stomach and the duodenum

pyrogen   capable of producing fever

QNS   quantity not sufficient

quadrant   one of four regions, as of the abdomen, divided for identification purposes

quadriceps femoris   the large muscle on the anterior surface of the thigh which is composed of four separate muscles

radial   referring to the radial artery or pulse taken in the radial artery

radiation   the emission and diffusion of rays; a product of X ray and radium

radioactive   capable of emitting radiant energy

radiograph   a record produced on a photographic plate, film, or paper by the action of X rays or radium

radionuclides   a type of atom utilized in nuclear medicine for the diagnosis and treatment of disease

radiopaque   impenetrable to the X ray or other forms of radiation

radius   a long bone of the forearm

rales   an unusual sound heard in the bronchi on auscultation of respirations

random   by chance; without plan

range of motion (ROM)   refers to the degree of movement of the body's joints and extremities

rapport   relationship characterized by harmony and cooperation

rationalization   to explain on rational grounds, to devise plausible explanations for one's acts

Raynaud's phenomenon   a symptom of lupus erythematosus characterized by fingers which turn white or blue in the cold

reactivity   rate of nuclear disintegration in a reactor

reagent   a substance involved in a chemical reaction

receptor   peripheral nerve ending of a sensory nerve that responds to stimuli

rectal   referring to the rectum

rectocele   the protrusion of the posterior vaginal wall with anterior wall of rectum through the vagina

rectum   the lower part of the large intestine between the sigmoid and the anal canal

recumbent   lying down

recurrent   returning at intervals

reduce   to restore the ends of a fractured bone to their usual relationship

reference   a source of information or authority

reflex   an involuntary response to a stimulus

refractive   the degree to which a transparent body deflects a ray of light from a straight path

regimen   regulation of diet, sleep, exercise, and manner of living to improve or maintain health

regulate   control or direction

regulatory   to control according to a rule; to adjust so as to make work accurately

rejuvenate   to make young again; to give youthful qualities to

reliable   dependable, can be relied upon

reluctant   marked by unwillingness

remedy   anything that relieves or cures a disease

remission   a period that is disease- and symptom-free

renal   pertaining to the kidney

renal failure   loss of function of the kidneys' nephrons

renal threshold   the concentration at which a substance in the blood normally not excreted by the kidney begins to appear in the urine

repolarization   reestablishment of a polarized state in a muscle or nerve fiber following contraction or conduction of a nerve impulse

repression   to force painful ideas or impulses into the subconscious

reproductive   concerning reproduction

residual   pertaining to that which is left as a residue

residual barium   barium remaining in the intestinal tract following evacuation at the completion of X-ray studies

resistance   opposition, ability to oppose

resonance   quality of the sound heard on percussion of the chest; the intensification and prolongation of a sound by reflection or by vibration of a nearby object

resource   a source of support or supply

respiration   the taking in of oxygen and its utilization in the tissues and the giving off of carbon dioxide

respiratory   pertaining to respiration

respite   a temporary cessation of something that is painful or tiring; to delay, postpone

resuscitation   the act of bringing one back to dull consciousness

retardation   slowing, delay, lag; slow in development that is either mental or physical

retention   inability to void urine which is present in the bladder

reticuloendothelial   pertaining to that group of cells which

appear to aid in the making of new blood cells and the disintegration of old ones

retina   the innermost layer of the eye which receives the image formed by the lens

retinopathy   a degeneration of the retina due to a decrease in blood supply

retroflexed   refers to the body of the uterus being bent backward

retrograde   refers to an X-ray procedure in which a radiopaque material is instilled by catheter into the bladder, ureters, and kidneys

retroperitoneal   behind the peritoneum; posterior to the peritoneal lining of the abdominal cavity

retroverted   refers to the entire uterus being tilted backward

retrovirus   one with RNA genetic material

Rh factor   an antigenic substance in human blood similar to the A and B factors which determine blood groups; apparently present only in red blood cells

rhinitis   inflammation of the nasal mucosa

rhythm   a measured time or movement; regularity of occurrence

ribosome   an organelle within the cytoplasm of the cell

rickets   a disease of the bones primarily due to the deficiency of vitamin D

risk   chance; hazard; chance of loss or injury; degree of probability of loss

R/O   rule out

ROM   see **range of motion**

rotate   to move around; to turn on an axis

rubella   (German measles) a mild contagious viral disease which may cause severe damage to an unborn child

rubeola   (measles) an acute, highly contagious disease marked by a typical cutaneous eruption

sacrum   five fused vertebrae which lie between the coccyx and the lumbar vertebrae of the spinal column

sagittal   refers to a plane which is made by dividing the body down the center creating a right and left side

saliva   a digestive secretion of the salivary glands which empties into the mouth

salivary glands   three pairs of glands that secrete the saliva which begins the digestion of food, primarily the breakdown of starch or complex carbohydrates

salpingectomy   surgical removal of the fallopian tube or tubes

salpingo-oophorectomy   surgical excision of the ovary and fallopian tube

salve   an ointment

SA node   see **sinoatrial node**

sarcoma   malignant tumors of the connective, muscle, or bone tissue

sartorius   a long narrow muscle of the thigh; the longest muscle of the body

scan   to look over quickly but thoroughly

scapula   the shoulder blade

schedule   to arrange a timetable; to place in a list of things to be done

sciatica   inflammation and pain along the sciatic nerve felt at back of thigh running down the inside of the leg

sclera   the white or sclerotic outer coat of the eye

scoliosis lateral curvature of the spine

scrotum the double pouch containing the testes and part of the spermatic cord

scurvy a disease due to lack of fresh fruits, vegetables, and vitamin C in the diet

sebaceous an oily, fatty matter; glands secreting such matter

sebum oily secretion of the sebaceous glands of the skin

secondary one step removed from the first; not primary

secretion separation of certain materials from the blood by the activity of a gland

sedentary pertaining to sitting; inactivity

sedimentation formation or depositing of sediment; of blood, refers to the speed at which erythrocytes settle when an anticoagulant is added to blood

segment a part or section of an organ or a body

seizures a sudden attack of pain, or disease or of certain symptoms

semen the mixture of secretions from the various glands and organs of the reproductive system of the male, which is expelled at orgasm

semicircular canals structures located in the inner ear

semilunar the valves of the heart located between the ventricles and the pulmonary artery and aorta

senility feebleness of body or mind caused by old age

sensitivity abnormal susceptibility to a substance

sensorineural deafness a loss of hearing due to transmission failure of the nerves within the inner ear or the auditory nerve

sensory refers to the nerves which receive and transmit stimuli from the sense organs

septum a membranous wall dividing two cavities, as within the heart or the nose

series a group; a set of things in the same class coming one after another

sharps any object which can cut, prick, stab, or scrape the skin

sheath a covering structure of connective tissue such as the membrane covering a muscle

shock a condition in which the pulse becomes rapid and weak, the blood pressure drops, and the patient is pale and clammy

sickle cell anemia a blood disorder in which the red blood cells are shaped like sickles

sigmoid an S-shaped section of the large intestine between the descending colon and the rectum

sigmoidoscopy an inspection of the sigmoid with an instrument

simple referring to a bone fracture, one without involvement of the skin surface

simultaneous occurring at the same time

sinoatrial (SA) node the source of the nerve impulse which initiates the heartbeat; the pacemaker

sinusitis inflammation of the sinuses

skeletal pertaining to the skeleton or bony structure; also to the muscles attached to the skeleton to permit movement

slough to cast off, as dead tissue

smooth a type of involuntary muscle tissue found in internal organs

snap locks metal locking devices

Snellen chart the chart of alphabetic letters used to evaluate distant vision

somatic pertaining to the body as distinguished from the mind; physical

sonar a device that transmits high-frequency sound waves in water and registers the vibrations reflected back from an object

sonogram record obtained by ultrasound

spasm an involuntary sudden movement or convulsive muscular contraction

spastic colon spasmodic contractions of the large intestine

specimen a sample; a representative piece of the whole

sperm the male gamete or sex cell

spermatozoon a sperm cell

sphincter a circular muscle constricting an opening

sphygmomanometer a device that measures blood pressure; also called manometer

spina bifida a disorder characterized by a defect in the spinal vertebrae with or without protrusion of the spinal cord and meninges

spinal pertaining to the spinal column, canal, or cord

spinal fusion the surgical implanting of a bone fragment between the processes of two or more spinal vertebrae to render them immobile

spiral having a circular fashion

spirometer an apparatus which measures the volume of inhaled and exhaled air

spleen an oval, vascular, ductless gland below the diaphragm, in the upper left quadrant of the abdomen

spontaneous involuntary; produced of itself; unforced

spores hard capsules formed by certain bacteria which allow them to resist prolonged exposure to heat

sprain the forcible twisting of a joint with partial rupture or other injury of its attachments

sputum substance ejected from the mouth containing saliva and mucus; usually refers to material coughed up from the bronchi

standardization process of bringing into conformity with a standard; pertaining to EKG, a mark made at the beginning of each lead to establish a standard of reference

stapes one of the three bones of the middle ear, also called the stirrup

stasis ulcer an open lesion due to stagnant or inadequate blood supply to an area

STAT (statim) immediately

statistic facts or data of a numerical kind

stature height

stenosis narrowing or constriction of a passage or opening

sterile without any organisms

sterilization the process of destroying all microorganisms; a procedure which prohibits conception

sternocleidomastoid a muscle of the chest arising from the sternum and inner part of clavicle

sternum the breastbone

stethoscope an instrument used in auscultation to convey to the ear the sounds produced by the body

stimulant a substance which temporarily increases activity

stomach a dilated, saclike, distensible portion of the alimentary canal below the esophagus and before the small intestine

stool bowel movement, feces

strabismus an eye disorder caused by imbalance of the ocular muscles

strain   injury to muscles from tension due to overuse or misuse

stratagem   a trick or deception

stress   to put pressure on; emphasize; urgency; tension, strained exertion. Topical; causing strain or injury to the skin

striated   a type of muscle tissue marked with stripes or striae

stricture   the narrowing of an opening, tube, or canal, such as the urethra or esophagus

stylus   a pen; the EKG writer

subarachnoid   the space between the pia mater and the arachnoid containing cerebrospinal fluid

subcutaneous   beneath the skin

subdural   beneath the dura mater; the space between the arachnoid and the dura mater

subjective   relating to the person who is thinking, saying, or doing something; personal; of a disease symptom, felt by the individual but not perceptible to others

sublimation   to express certain impulses, especially sexual, in constructive, socially acceptable forms

sublingual   under the tongue

subsequent   coming after, following

suction   withdrawal by pressure; a sucking action

sudden infant death syndrome (SIDS)   the sudden, unexplainable death of an infant

superficial   on the surface

superior   above or higher than

supernatant   floating on the surface

supine   lying horizontally on the back

supplement   something added; an additional or extra section

suppository   a medicated conically or cylindrically shaped material which is inserted into the rectum or vagina

suppression   the shutdown of kidney function; the absence of urine excretion

suppressor   one that holds back or stops an action

suprapubic   above the pubic arch

surfactant   a fatty molecule on the respiratory membranes

susceptible   having little resistance to a disease or foreign protein

suture   to unite parts by stitching them together

symmetry   the state in which one part exactly corresponds to another in size, shape, and position

sympathetic   a portion of the autonomic nervous system

symphysis pubis   the junction of the pubic bones on the midline in front

symptom   any perceptible change in the body or its functions which indicates disease or the phase of a disease

synapse   the minute space between the axon of one neuron and the dendrite of another

syncope   fainting, a transient form of unconsciousness

syndrome   the combination of symptoms with a disease or disorder

synergism   something stimulating the action of another so that the effect of both is greater than the sum of the individual effects

synovial   a movable joint; also called diarthroses

syphilis   a communicable venereal disease spread by sexual contact

system   a group of organs working together to perform a function of the body

systematic   by a system or plan

systemic   pertaining to the whole body rather than its parts

systole   the contraction phase of the heart; the greatest amount of blood pressure

tachycardia   abnormal rapidity of heart action

tactful   possessing skill in saying or doing the right thing; thoughtfulness

tar   a sticky, brown or black carcinogenic substance produced by tobacco as it burns

tarry   referring to black, sticky stool associated with internal bleeding

tarsal   pertaining to the seven bones of the instep of the foot

taut   tightly drawn; tense

technical   relating to some particular art, science, or trade; also, requiring special skill or technique

temperature   degree of heat of a living body; degree of hotness or coldness of a substance; usually refers to an elevation of body heat

temporal   relating to the temporal bone on the skull

tendon   fibrous connective tissue serving to attach muscles to bones

tendonitis   inflammation of the tendon

tentative   experimental, provisional, temporary

terminal   final, end; a terminal illness, refers to a condition which cannot be reversed

testes   the male gonads of the scrotum which produce sperm

testosterone   a male hormone secreted by the testes which causes and maintains male secondary sex characteristics

tetanus   an acute infectious disease due to the toxins of the bacillus *Clostridium tetani*

tetany   intermittent tonic spasms resulting from inadequate parathyroid hormone

thalamus   a portion of the brain lying between the cerebrum and the midbrain

therapeutic   having medicinal or healing properties; pertaining to results obtained from treatment

thermal   characterized by heat; heat activated

thermography   a technique for sensing and recording on film, hot and cold areas of the body by means of an infrared detector that reacts to blood flow

thermometer   an instrument used to measure temperature

thoracic   pertaining to the thorax or chest

thorax   the chest; the body cavity enclosed by ribs and containing the heart and lungs

thready   term used to describe a weak pulse which may feel like a thread under the skin surface

thrombophlebitis   inflammation of a vein associated with the formation of a blood clot

thrombosis   the formation of a blood clot or thrombus

thymus   an unpaired organ located in the mediastinal cavity anterior to and above the heart

thyroid   an endocrine gland located anteriorly at the base of the neck

thyroidectomy   the surgical removal of the thyroid gland

TIA   see **transient ischemic attack**

tibia   a long bone in the leg from the knee to the ankle

tibialis anterior   a muscle of the leg

tinnitus   a ringing or tinkling sound in the ear which is heard only by the person affected

tissue   a collection of similar cells and fibers forming a structure in the body

tolerance the difference between the maximum and minimum; the amount of variation allowed from a standard

tongue the muscular organ of the mouth which assists in the production of speech, contains the taste buds, and provides the ability to swallow

tonometer instrument for measuring intraocular tension or pressure

topical pertaining to a specific area; local

torticollis stiff neck caused by spasmotic contraction of neck muscles drawing the head to one side with the chin pointing to the other; can be congenital or acquired

tourniquet any constrictor used on an extremity to produce pressure on an artery and control bleeding; also used to distend veins for the withdrawal of blood or the insertion of a needle to instill intravenous injections

toxin poisonous substance or compound of vegetable, animal, or bacterial origin

toxoid a toxin treated so as to destroy its toxicity, but still capable of inducing formation of antibodies on injection

trace the production of a sketch by means of a stylus passing over the paper as in electrocardiography; a very small amount

trachea a cartilaginous tube between the larynx and the main bronchus of the respiratory tree

tracheostomy a surgically made opening in the trachea through which a person will breathe

traction the process of pulling; with fractures, traction is applied in a straight line to stretch the contracted muscles and permit realignment of the bone fragments

transdermal through the skin

transducer a device that transforms power from one system to another in the same or different form

transfusion injection of the blood of one person into the blood vessels of another

transient ischemic attack (TIA) temporary interruption of blood flow in the brain due to small clots closing off blood vessels

transillumination inspection of a cavity or organ by passing a light through its walls

transition passing from one condition, place, or activity to another

transmitted sent from one person, thing, or place to another

transpose putting one in place of another, the accidental misplacing of words or letters

transurethral literally means through the urethra; refers to the removal of the prostate by going through the urethral wall

transverse lying across; the segment of large intestine which lies across the abdomen; a line drawn horizontally across the body or a structure

trapezius the large muscle of the back and neck

traumatic caused by or relating to an injury

traumatize to cause trauma or injury

treadmill an apparatus with a movable platform which permits walking or running in place

Trendelenburg's position a position with the head lower than the feet

triage to arrange in order; determine what needs to be taken care of first

triceps the posterior muscles of the arm which work as a team with the biceps; the triceps straighten the elbow

trichomoniasis infestation with the parasitic protozoa *Trichomonas*; usually refers to vaginal involvement

tricuspid a valve in the right side of the heart, between the chambers; literally means three cusps or leaflets

trimester divided into three sections; the third segment or period

tritanopia unable to distinguish the blue color

trivial of little value, insignificant

tuberculosis an infectious disease caused by the tubercle bacillus *Mycobaterium*; pulmonary tuberculosis is a specific inflammatory disease of the lungs which destroys lung tissue

tumor a swelling or enlargement; a neoplasm; often used to indicate a malignant growth

turbidity flaky or granular particles suspended in a clear liquid giving it a cloudy appearance; usually refers to cloudy urine

tympanic membrane the eardrum

typhoid an acute infectious disease acquired by ingesting contaminated food or water

ulcer an open lesion on the skin or mucous membrane of the body characterized by loss of tissue and the formation of a secretion

ulceration suppuration of the skin or mucous membrane; an open lesion

ulna a long bone in the forearm from the elbow to the wrist

ultrasonic scanning a process of scanning the body with sound waves to produce a picture on a screen of underlying internal structures

umbilical pertaining to the umbilicus or navel of the abdomen

universal relating to the universe, general or common to all

unobtrusive not forced upon others; not thrusted forward or pushed out

upper respiratory infection (URI) inflammatory process involving the nose and throat, may include the sinuses; refers to symptoms associated with the common cold

uremia a condition in which products normally found in the urine are found in the blood

ureter a tube carrying urine from the kidney to the urinary bladder

urethra a membranous canal for the external discharge of urine from the bladder

urgency the sudden need to expel urine or stool

URI see **upper respiratory infection**

urinalysis an analysis of the urine; a test performed on urine to determine its characteristics

urinary meatus the opening through which urine passes from the body

urinary tract infection (UTI) infection occurring within the kidneys, ureters, or urinary bladder or all three

urination the act of urinating or voiding of urine

urine fluid secreted from the blood by the kidneys, stored in the bladder, and discharged from the body by voiding

urology the study of the urine and diseases of the urinogenital organs

urticaria an inflammatory condition characterized by the eruption of wheals which are associated with severe itching; commonly called hives

uterus a muscular, hollow, pear-shaped organ of the female reproductive tract in which a fertilized ovum develops into a baby, the womb

UTI see **urinary tract infection**

vaccine any substance for prevention of a disease

vagina a musculomembranous tube which forms the passageway from the uterus to the exterior

vaginitis inflammation of the vagina

vagus the tenth cranial nerve which has both motor and sensory function, affecting the heart and stomach as well as other organs

valve any one of various structures for temporarily closing an opening or passageway, or for allowing movement of fluid in one direction only

varices enlarged, twisted veins

varicose pertaining to varices; distended, swollen veins, most commonly found in the legs

vas deferens the excretory duct of the testes

vasectomy the cutting out of a portion of the vas deferens

vein a blood vessel carrying blood toward the heart after receiving it from a venule

vena cava one of two large veins which empty into the right atrium of the heart

venipuncture the puncture of a vein; the insertion of a needle into a vein for the purpose of obtaining a blood sample or instilling a substance

venom the poison secreted by some snakes, spiders, and insects introduced into the victim by a bite or sting

venous pertaining to a vein

ventilatory that which ventilates, lets in fresh air

ventral pertaining to the anterior or front side of the body

ventricle one of the two lower chambers of the heart; also used in reference to cavities within the brain

venule a minute vein; a blood vessel which connects a capillary with a vein

veritable actual, genuine

vermiform appendix the appendix; a small tube attached to the cecum

verrucae warts; small, circumscribed elevations of the skin formed by hypertrophy of the papillae

vertebrae the bones in the spinal column

vertex the top of the head, the crown

vertical perpendicular to the plane of the horizon, upright

vesicle a small sac or bladder containing fluid; a small, blisterlike elevation on the skin containing serous fluid

viable capable of living

vial a small glass tube or bottle containing medication or a chemical

villi tiny projections from a surface; the villi of the small intestine which absorb nutrients during the process of digestion

villous adenoma a type of polyp which is invasive and malignant

virulent full of poison; deadly; malignant

virus a very simple, frequently pathogenic, microorganism capable of replicating within living cells

visceral pertaining to viscera, the internal organs, especially the abdomen

vital essential; pertaining to the preservation of life (the vital signs)

vital capacity the total volume of air exchanged from forced inspiration and forced expiration

vitreous humor the substance which fills the vitreous body of the eye behind the lens

void to pass urine from the urinary bladder; to make ineffective or invalid

volatile easily changed into a gas or tending to change into a vapor; usually considered potentially dangerous

voltage a measure of electromotive force

volume the amount of space occupied by an object as measured in cubic units

voluntary under one's control; done by one's own choice

vomit to expel the contents of the stomach through the mouth

voucher a document that serves as proof that terms of a transaction have been met

vulnerable liable to injury or hurt; capable of being wounded

vulva the female external genitalia, including the clitoris, the labia minora, and the labia majora

waiver to give up; forgo; waiving of a right or claim

warrant to justify, to give definite assurance as to the value of; to authorize

wart see **verrucae**

wheals more or less round and evanescent elevations of the skin, white in center with a pale red edge, accompanied by itching

whorl a type of fingerprint in which the central papillary ridges turn through at least one complete circle

wick a small piece of material inserted into an opening to which a solution is applied

womb nonmedical name for the uterus

writer the person who writes; the author

xiphoid a process which forms the tip of the sternum

Z-tract a method of injecting medication intramuscularly

zygote a cell produced by the union of an ovum and a sperm

Index

Page numbers in italics indicate figures; page numbers followed by t indicate tables.

AA (*See* Alcoholics Anonymous)
AAMA (*See* American Association of Medical Assistants)
Abandonment, 19, *20*
Abdomen, examination of, 325, *326*
Abdominal aneurysm, 170-171
Abdominal cavity, 74, *74*
Abdominal muscles, 134
Abdominal quadrants, 74, *75*
Abdominopelvic cavity, 74, *74*
Abduction, 132, *134*
Ablation, 258
Abortion, 14
  spontaneous (miscarriage), 255, 257
Absenteeism, 549-550
Absorption function of small intestine, 204, *205*
Abstinence, 256t
  as AIDS preventative, 189
AC interference, 439, *442*
Accelerator nerve, 158, *158*
Accessibility of medications, 510
Accidents:
  first aid care for, 526-533
  reports of, 68, *69*
Accommodation, 101, *101*
Acetabulum, 122, *125*
Acetylcholine, 45
Achilles tendon, 133
Achromatic vision, 345
Acids, 80, 81t
Acne vulgaris, 112
Acquaintances, job search and, 545
Acquired immunodeficiency syndrome (AIDS), 185-190, 188t-190t, 292, 370
  health care providers and, 187-188
  incidence of, 189t, 189-190, 190t
  transmission of, 187-188
  universal precautions and, 58, 60-61
Acquired torticollis, 139
ACTH (*See* Adrenocorticotropic hormone)
Action potential, 87
Activated helper T cell, 182
Active immunity, 185
Active transport, 78
Acute closed-angle glaucoma, 104
Acute glomerulonephritis (AGN), 222
Acute illnesses, documenting, 321
Acute renal failure, 224-225
Addiction:

  to drugs, 40
  to nicotine, 46
Adduction, 132, *134*
Adenitis, 163
Adenosine triphosphate (ATP), 78, 136
ADH (*See* Antidiuretic hormone)
Adrenal glands (suprarenal), 229t, 230, *231*
Adrenaline (epinephrine), 230, 428, 431-432, 511
Adrenocorticotropic hormone (ACTH), 97, 226, 232
Adverse reaction to intradermal test, 431
Aerobes, 55
Afebrile, 289
Afferent (sensory) nerves, 87
Afterbirth (*See* Placenta)
Agar, 420
Age of patient:
  pulse rate and, 302, 303t
  timing of physical examinations and, 329-330
Agglutination, 165
Agglutinogen, 165, *168*
AGN (*See* Acute glomerulonephritis)
Agranulocytes, 165, 182
AIDS (*See* Acquired immunodeficiency syndrome)
AIDS-related complex (ARC), 186
Al-Anon, 40
Al-Ateen, 40
Albino, 112
Alcohol:
  abuse of, 39-40
  cancer and, 194
  dependence on, 525
  urine specimens for analysis, 414-415
Alcoholic, 39
Alcoholics Anonymous (AA), 40
Aldosterone, 230
Alimentary canal, 197
Allergens, 178
Allergic reaction:
  testing for, 428-432, *429, 430*
  vaginitis and, 263
Allergic rhinitis, 108, 145-146
Allergies, *190*, 190-191
Allergy immunotherapy programs, 428
Allosteric protein, 381
Alopecia, 112
Alpha interferon (IFN-a), 183
ALS (*See* Amyotrophic lateral sclerosis)
Alveoli, 142, *143*

AMA (*See* American Medical Association)
Amblyopia (lazy eye), 102
Ambulatory ECG, 169
American Academy of Pediatrics, 506
American Association of Medical Assistants (AAMA), 9, 12, 13, 483
American Cancer Society, 113, 148, 193, 194, 241, 352, 456
American College of Radiologists, 255
American Diabetes Association, 497
American Heart Association, 519
American Medical Association (AMA), 12, 13, 23, 511
  standardized forms recommendations of, 18, *19*
Amniocentesis, 83
Amniotic fluid, 252
Amphetamines, 45, 525
Amphiarthrosis (cartilaginous) joint, 122
Ampule, 490-491
  withdrawing medication from, 494, *494*
Amputation, 125
Amyotrophic lateral sclerosis (ALS; Lou Gehrig's disease), 94-95
Anaerobes, 55
Anal canal, 205
Anaphylactic shock, 68, 191, 428, 490
  emergency kit for, 428
  first aid for, 519-520
Anaphylaxis, 191
Anatomical descriptors, 71-85
Anatomical directional terms, *73*, 73-74
Anatomy, 72
  anatomical descriptors and body structure, 71-85
  circulatory system, 152-177
  digestive system, 197-214, *198*
  endocrine system, 225-235
  immune system, 177-197
  integumentary system, 109-117
  muscular system, 130-139
  nervous system, 85, 87-99, *88*
  reproductive system, 236-264
  respiratory system, 139-152
  senses, 100-109
  skeletal system, 117-130, *119*
  urinary system, 215-225, *216*
Androgens, 230, *231*
Anemia, 170, 380
  sickle cell, 175-176
Aneroid dial of sphygmomanometer, 308, *309*

Anesthesia, local, 461
Anesthesiologist, 461
Anesthetization of eye, 341
Aneurysms, 169-171, *171*
Angina, 171
Angiograph (*See* Arteriography)
Angiography (*See* Arteriography)
Angioplasty, 173, *173*
Angle of injection, 491, *491*
Animal bites, 512, 524
Anorectal abscess, 208
Anorexia, 28
Antecubital space, 302, *302*
Anterior lobe of pituitary gland, 226-227, *228*, 229t
Anterior section, 73, *73*
Anti-HAV antibody, 211
Antibodies, 178, 182, 184, 428
Antibody-mediated immune response, 180, 182
Anticoagulant drugs, 175, 399
Antidiuretic hormone (ADH), 227-228
Antigen(s), 178, 428
Antigen-antibody complex, 179-180
Antihistamines, 68, 511
Antiseptic, 463
Antitoxins, 506
Anus, 205
    fissure of, 210
Anxiety, 38
Aorta, 153, *154*
Aortic aneurysm, 170
Apex, 304
Apgar scoring system, 254, 254t
Apical pulse, 304-305
    indications for, 305
    locating apex, 304-305, *305*
Apical-radial pulse, measuring, 305, *305*
Apnea, 306
Appendectomy, 205
Appendicitis, 205, 208
Appendicular skeleton, 118, *119*
Appendix, 205
Aqueous humor, 102, 104
Arachnoid layer, 92, *95*
Arachnoid villi, 92
Arbitration agreement procedures, 22
ARC (*See* AIDS-related complex)
Areata alopecia, 112
Areola, *249*, 250
Arm, sites for venipuncture, 396, *397*
Arrhythmias, 156-157, 171, 303
    Holter monitoring for, 446
Arterial bleeding, 517
Arteries, 153, 158-159, *160, 161*
Arteriography (angiography):
    cardiovascular, 169
    cerebral, 92
    pulmonary, 145
Arterioles, 158, *161*
Arteriosclerosis, 170, 171
Arteriovenous fistula, 219-220, *220*
Arteriovenous graft, 219-220, *220*
Arthritis, 126
Arthroscopy, 125
Articular processes, 120, *121*
Articulation, 122
Artifacts:
    from AC interference, 439, *442*
    in gallbladder problems, 455

muscle voltage, 438, *441*
Artificial immunity, 498
Artificial insemination, 14
Artificial kidney, 219, *219*
Artificial pacemaker, 157, *158*
Artificial veins, 220
Asbestosis, 150
Ascending colon, 205
Ascites, 208
Asepsis, 50-52
Asphyxiation, 68
Aspiration, preventing, 514
Assault, 15
Associative neurons, 87, *88*
Asthma, 146
    first aid for attack, 519
Astro-Clips, 436, *436*
Asymmetry of male genitals, 325
Ataxic cerebral palsy, 96
Atelectasis, 146
Atherosclerosis, 170, 171
Athetoid cerebral palsy, 96
Athletic heart syndrome, 171
ATP (*See* Adenosine triphosphate)
Atrial depolarization, 436
Atrioventricular (AV) node, 156, *157*, 436, *437*
Atrium, 154, *155*
Atrophy of muscle, 133
    in carpal tunnel syndrome, 126-127
Attendance at job, 549-550
Attenuated virus, 507
Attire:
    appropriate, 3
    for job interviews, 545, 547
    See also Personal appearance
Attitude, 3
Atypical cytology, 352, *353*
Audiometric devices, 349, *350*
Auditory acuity, measuring, 347-349, *349-351*
Auditory canal, 105, *105*
    measuring temperature in, 301
    obstruction of, 106
Auditory nerve:
    area of, 92, *94*
    damage to, 349
Augmented electrocardiograph leads, 437-438
Aural temperature, 299
Auscultation, 302, 321
Authorization forms (*See* Forms)
Autoclave, 510
Autoclaving, 62, *62-65*, 63t, *65*
    preparing articles for, 62, *63-65*, 65
Autolet, 377, *379*
Autologous bone marrow transplant, 192
Automated peritoneal dialysis, 221
Autonomic nervous system, 87, 89-90, 92
Autotrophs, 55
AV node (*See* Atrioventricular (AV) node)
Axial skeleton, 118, *119*
Axilla, 532
Axillary temperature, 295, *297*
    measuring, 297, 300
Axons, 87

B cells, 182
Baby (deciduous) teeth, 199, *200*
Bacteria, 52, *55*

Gram-positive and Gram-negative, 421-423, *424*, 426t
Bacterial smears and cultures, 419-423
    bacteriological smear, 420, *420*, 421
    culturing, *420*, 420-421, *421*
    gram staining, 421-423, *424*, 426t
Bacteriological smear, 420, *420*
    preparing, 421
Bandages, applying:
    arm sling, 532, *532*
    cravat to forehead, ear, or eyes, 531, *531*
    figure-eight to hand and wrist, 530, *530*
    in open or closed spiral, 529, *529*
    in recurrent turn, 527, *528*
    triangular to scalp, 531, *531*
Barbiturates, 40, 43, 525
Barium enema, 207, 454-455, *456*
Barium swallow, 207, 454, 455, *455*
Bartholin's glands, 248
Basal cell carcinoma, 112, 113
Base compounds, 80, 81t
Basic suture setup, 526
Basophils, 165, 178, 182
Battery, 15
BCDF (*See* Interleukins)
Behaviors:
    effect of mental and emotional status on, 48
    modification of, 46-49
    personal, 26-49
Bell's palsy, 95-96
Benign hypertension, 174
Benign prostatic hypertrophy, 243
Benign tumors, 191
Beriberi, 27
Beta interferon (IFN-b), 183
Bicuspid (mitral) valve, 154, *155*
Bigeminal rhythm, 157
Bile (bilirubin), 202
    in urine, 411
Bimanual palpation, 320, 355, *355*
Binocular microscope, 373, *375*
Biochemistry, 80
Biohazard (sharps) containers, 51, 62, *64*, 67, 370, *371*
Biohazardous items, 62
Biopsy, 191, 461
Birth, 254, 254t
Birth control pills, 256t
Bites, 524
    first aid for, 512
Black lung disease, 150
Bladder, 216
Bleeding from vein, 517
Bleeding time, 165
Blepharitis, 102
Blood, 163-169
    bleeding time, 164
    cell types, 164-165, *167*
    collecting sample, 381, *381*
    obtaining for PKU test, 378
    plasma, 164
    Rh factor, 166-169
    types of, 165-166, *168*
Blood cell count, 384, 389-390, *390, 392-393*
    differential count, 389, 390, 394, *395*, 395t
    erythrocytes (red blood cells), 386, 389
    leukocytes (white blood cells), 389
Blood pressure, 289, 307-314, *308*
    in children, 314

equipment (*See* Manometers)
maintaining, 307-308
measuring, 310, *313*, 313-314, 323
normal, 308, *309*
phases of, 308
pulse pressure and, 308
Blood smear, preparing slide, 390, 394, *396*
Blood tests:
capillary, 374-394
glucose screening, 232, 383-384, *388*, 389, *390*
patient education for, 378, 398
venous, 396-403
Blood tubes, preparing, 381, *387*
Blood vessels, 158-162, *159*
arteries, 158-159, *160, 161*
portal circulation, 161-162, *164*
systemic circulation, 160-161
veins, 159-161, *160, 162, 163*
Bloodborne pathogens, 370
Body cavities, organs and, 74, *74, 75*
Body fluids, spills of, 370, *371*
Body language, *3*, 3-4
Body mechanics in positioning patient, 332
Body scans, 457
Body surface area (BSA), 489
Boils (*See* Furuncles)
Bolus, 199
Bone(s):
fractures, 124-125, *127*, 516-517
healing process, 124-125, *128*
See also Skeletal system
Bone structure, 118, *120*
Boosters, 499
Bordetella pertussis, 52, 504
Bowman's capsule, 217, *217*
Brachial artery pulse point, 302, *302*
Bradycardia, 158, 171, 303
Bradypnea, 306
Brain, 90-92, *94*
Brain scan, 92
Breast(s):
cancer of, 194, 258-259
examination of, 325, *325*
Breast self-examination (BSE), 194, 259
explaining to patient, 354, *354*
Breathing pattern, alterations in, 144
Bronchi, 142, *142*
Bronchioles, 142
Bronchitis, 146
Bronchopneumonia, acute (Legionnaires' disease), 148-149
Bronchoscopy, 145
Brudzinski's sign, 97, *98*
Bruits, 321
BSA (*See* Body surface area)
BSE (*See* Breast self-examination)
Buccal administration of medicines, 483, 485-486
Buccal cavity, 74, *74*
Buffy coat, 381, *381*
Bulbourethral glands, 240, *242*
BUN (blood urea nitrogen), 222
Bundle of His, 156, *157*, 436, *437*
Burns, first aid for, *512*, 512-513, *513*
Bursa, 122, 134
Bursitis, 126, 138
Butterfly closures, 528

Callus in bone healing, 124-125, *128*
Calories, 28, 32t-33t
Calyx (calyces), 216
Cancer:
of breast, 194, 258-259
cervical, 259, 352
of colon, 452
detecting from sputum specimen, 417, *419*
diagnostic procedures for, 191-192
effect of race on survival rates, 195t
factors in development of, 193-194
immune system and, 191-194
of larynx, 148
of lung, 149, *149*
mutations and, 191
oral, 108-109, 213
ovarian, 259-260
prevention and early detection of, 193-194
of reproductive organs, 259-260
seven warning signals of, 193, 320t
of skin, 112-113, *114*
smoking and, 148, 149, *149*, 193
sun exposure and, 113, 193
treatment of, *192*, 192-193, *194, 195*
Cancer Facts and Figures—1993 (American Cancer Society), 193
Canes, 532, 535
Capillaries, 377
Capillary blood tests, 374-394
blood cell count, 384, 386, 389-390, *390*, 392-393, 394
blood glucose screening, 383-384, *388*
glucose tolerance test (GTT), 232, 384, 389, *390*
hemoglobin and hematocrit, 380-381, *381*, 382t, *386, 387*
laboratory classification and regulation of, 374-376, 375t
PKU test, 378-380, *380*
skin puncture for, 376-377, *379*
Capillary sphincters, 158
Capitis, 116
Carbohydrates, 199, 384
Carbon dioxide, 140, 143, 159
Carbon monoxide, 45
Carboxyhemoglobin, 45
Carbunculosis, 113, 115
Carcinoembryonic antigen (CEA), 191
Carcinogen, 191
Carcinogenesis, 191
Carcinomas, 191
Cardiac arrest, 171
Cardiac catheterization, 169
Cardiac muscle tissue, 84, *86*, 132, *132*
Cardiac notch, 144, *144*
Cardiac sphincter, 202, *202*
Cardinal signs (*See* Vital signs)
Cardiology, 434
Cardiology procedures, 433-434, *434-437*, 436-447
electrocardiograph leads, 437-438, *438, 439*
Holter monitoring, 444, *446*, 446-447, *447*
interference, 438-439, 441, *441, 442*
path of electrical impulses, 436, *437*
standardization of, 441-444, *442, 443*
stress tests, 444, *445, 446*
Cardiomegaly, 171
Cardiopulmonary resuscitation (CPR), 15, 513, 517, 519, 537
for infants and children, 523, *523*

procedures for, 521-522, *521-522*
Cardiovascular tests, 169-170
Carditis, 171-172
Career entry, 9-10
Career objective style resumé, 539, *540*
Carotid pulse point, 302, *302*
Carpal tunnel syndrome, 126-127
Carpals, 121, *124*
Cartilage, 121
Cartilaginous (amphiarthrosis) joint, 122
CAT scan (*See* Computerized axial tomography (CAT) scan)
Cataract, 102-103
Catarrhal stage of pertussis, 504
Catheterization, 409
cardiac, 169
urinary, 218, 221, 406, *409*
Catheterization kits, disposable, 409
Catheters, 169, 221
Caudal portion, *73*, 74
Caustic burns, 321
CDC (*See* Centers for Disease Control)
CEA (*See* Carcinoembryonic antigen)
Cecum, 202, 204-205
Cell(s), 74-77, *76*, 77t
origin of, 178, *179*
Cell markers, 178-179
Cell-mediated immune response, 180, 182
Cell membrane, 75, *76*
Cell membranes, 77-78, *78-80*, 80, 81t, *82*
Cellular division (*See* Mitosis)
Celsius thermometers, 301, *301*, 301t
Centers for Disease Control (CDC), 186, 188, 369, 399
universal precautions of, 60, 61, 67
Central nervous system (CNS), 87, 90-92
Centrifugal hematology system, 381, *386*
Centrifuge, *371*, 381, 399
determining hematocrit with, 382t, 383, *384, 385*
Centrioles, 75, *76*, 77
Cerebellum, 92, *94*
Cerebral aneurysm, 170
Cerebral angiography, 92
Cerebral palsy, 96
Cerebrospinal fluid (CSF), 92, 97
Cerebrovascular accident (CVA), 98, 172, 174
first aid for, 522
Cerebrum, 92, *94*
Certificate of waiver in laboratory testing, 375
Certified medical assistants (CMA), 553
Cerumen, 106, 338
Cervical cancer, 259, 352
Cervical erosion, 257
Cervicitis, 257, 262
Cervix, 247, *247*
Cesarean section, 254
CEUs (*See* Continuing education units)
CFS (*See* Chronic fatigue syndrome)
Chain of custody, in drug and alcohol analysis, 415
Chancre, 262
Chemical(s), office safety for, 510
Chemical burns, 513
Chemical urinalysis, 410-413, *412*
Chemotherapy, 192
Chest:
determining measurement of, 284-285
examination of, *324*, 324-325, *325*
procedure for measuring, 288, *288*

Chest: (Continued)
X rays of, 145, *453*, 454
Chest thrusts for respiratory emergencies, 518-519
CHF (*See* Congestive heart failure)
Chief complaint, 273
Child abuse, suspected cases of, 361
Children:
blood pressure in, 314
cardiopulmonary resuscitation (CPR) for, 523, *523*
developmental stages of, 361, *362*
examinations of, 358-365, *362*
immunizations for, 499
measuring visual acuity in, 340-342, *343*, 344t, *345*
rapport with, 361-362
warning signals of cancer in, 320t
See also Infants; Neonates
Chlamydia, 260-261
Choice in Dying, Inc., 15, *16*, *17*
Choice of treatment, 6
Choking, universal signal for, 518, *518*
Cholecystectomy, 203
Cholecystography, 206, 454, *454*
Cholelithiasis (gallstones), 203
Cholera, 507
Cholesterol Test Kit (in-home), 377
Cholinergic nerves, 45
Choroid, 101, *101*
Chromosomes, 76
Chronic fatigue syndrome (CFS), 195
Chronic glomerulonephritis, 222-223
Chronic illnesses, documenting, 321
Chronic leukemia, 174-175
Chronic obstructive pulmonary disease (COPD), 146-147
Chronic open-angle glaucoma, 104
Chronic renal failure, 225
Chronological resumé, 539, *540*, *541*
Chyme, 201-202, 209
Cilia, 140, *140*
Circulatory system, 152-177
blood, 163-169
blood vessels, 158-162, *159*
cardiovascular tests, 169-170
diseases and disorders of, 170-177
heart, *153*, 153-158
lymphatic system, 162-163
Circumcision, 241
Cirrhosis, 208-209
Civil law, 15
Civil Rights Act of 1964, Title VII of, 19
Classified advertisements, 542, *545*
Claustrophobia, MRI and, 450
Clavicle, 121, *123*
Cleaning services, 51
Clinical Laboratory Improvement Amendments of 1988 (CLIA-88), 375, 375t, 376
Clinitest tablet, urine testing with, *412*, 413, *415*
Clinitex 100 urine chemistry analyzer, 410, *412*
Clitoris, 237, *238*, 249, *249*
Clones, in immune response, 182
Closed fracture (*See* Simple fracture)
Closed spiral in applying bandages, 529, *529*
Clostridum tetani, 506
Closure materials for minor surgery, 471, *471*
Clotting process, 165

CMA (*See* Certified medical assistant)
Coagulation, 461
Cocaine, 45
Cochlea, *105*, 106, *106*
Code of Medical Ethics (AMA), 13
Coitus, 248
Cold treatment for sprains and strains, 520, 522, *524*
Colitis, 209
Collagenous fibers in dermis, 111
Colles fracture, 124, *127*
Colon, 204, 205, *206*
cancer of, 452
common conditions of, *215*
Colonoscopy, 207
Color blindness, 345-346
Color coding of test tubes, *398*, 398-399
Color vision, measuring with Ishihara method, 323, 345, 347, *348*
Colorectal examination, 194
Colostomy, 209
Colostrum, 252
Colposcopy, 255
Comminuted fracture, 124, *127*
Common bile duct, 203, *203*
Communicable diseases, 56, 59t-60t
Communication(s), 1-24
medical law and ethics, 10, 12-23
medical staff relationships, 7-10
with patients and families, 4-7, 279, 318
verbal and nonverbal, 2, 2-4
Community service, 543, 545, 547-548
Complement proteins, 178, 180, *182*, 182, 184
Complete stroke, 172
Complex reflex actions, 89, *92*
Compound fracture, 124, *127*
first aid for, 516-517
Compounds, 80
Computer(s), 510
Computerized axial tomography (CAT) scan, 92
Computerized axial tomography (CAT) scans, 191
Computerized-channel ECG machines, 441
Computerized electrocardiographs, 443
Computerized transaxial tomography (CTAT), 457
Conception (*See* Fertilization)
Condenser (of microscope), 374
Condoms, 256t, 325
Conductive hearing loss, 106
Confidentiality, 5-6, 18, 22
importance of, 315
of patient information, 269
Congenital hip dysplagia, 127
Congenital torticollis, 139
Congestive heart failure (CHF), 172-173, 223
Conjunctiva, 101, *101*, 103
Conjunctivitis (pinkeye), 103
Connecting neurons, 84, 87
Connective tissue, 83-84, *84*
Consent forms, 18, *19*, *20*, 460-461, *461*
for blood or urine tests, 414-415
for treatment, 18, *19*
See also Forms
Constipation, 205, 209, 363
Constriction of blood vessels in skin, 110
Contact dermatitis, 432
Continuing education units (CEUs), 12
Contraception, 255, 256t
Contractions, 254

Contrast-enhanced MRI, 449
Contrast media, 454
radiopaque, 455
Controlled Substances Act of 1970, 14, 480
Controlled substances schedule, 479t, 480-481, 483
Convolutions, 92, *94*
Convulsions, first aid for, 513-514
Coordination, testing, 327, *329*
COPD (*See* Chronic obstructive pulmonary disease)
Core body temperature, measuring, 299
Cornea, 101, *101*
Corneal abrasion, 103
Coronal plane, 73, *73*
Coronary arteries and veins, 153, *154*
Coronary artery disease, 173, *173*
Corpus luteum, 246
Cortex, of kidney, 216, *216*
Corynebacterium diphtheriae, 503
Coughing, 144
Countershock, 446
Courtesy, 2
Cover letter, in job search, 541-542, *544*
CPR (*See* Cardiopulmonary resuscitation)
Cramps, 131
Cranial portion, *73*, 74
Cranium, 92, *94*, 120, *123*
Cravat bandage, 530, *530*, 531, *531*
Creatinine, 222
Crenated red blood cells, 414
Cretinism, 232, *233*
Criminal law, 15
Crohn's disease, 209
ileostomy for, 212-213
Cross-eyed gaze, 105
Cross section, 74
Crowning, 254
Crutches, 532, 534, *534*
Crying, 144
Cryosurgery, 461
Cryptorchidism, 237
CSF (*See* Cerebrospinal fluid)
CTAT (*See* Computerized transaxial tomography)
Cul-de-sac (*See* Rectouterine pouch)
Culturing smears, *420*, 420-421, *421*
Cushing's syndrome, 232-233, *234*
CVA (*See* Cerebrovascular accident)
Cylindrical cage applicator, 530, 532, *533*
Cystic duct, 203, *203*
Cystitic (fibrocystic) breast disease, 257
Cystitis, 222
Cystocele, 257
Cystoscopy, 455
Cystourethroscopy, 221-222
Cytokines, 180, *182*, 183
Cytology, 72
report of results of, 355, *357*
request form, 353, *353*
specimens for, 326
Cytoplasm, 75, *76*
Cytotechnologists, 72
Cytotoxic (killer) T cells, 180

D & C (*See* Dilation and curettage)
Daltonism, 345
Database (*See* Patient database)
DEA (*See* Drug Enforcement Administration)
Debridement, 506

Decibels, 349, *349*
Deciduous (baby) teeth, 199, *200*
Decline stage of pertussis, 504
Deep vein thrombosis (DVT), 169, 170, 176
Defamation of character, 15, 22
Defecation, 205
Defense mechanisms, 47-48
    against disease, 56
Defibrillator, 157, 446-447, *447*
Dehydration, 83
Delirium tremens, 525
Deltoid muscle, 135
Dendrites, 87
Denial, 47
Deoxyribonucleic acid (DNA), 76-77
Deposition, 22
Depressants, 40, 43
Depressed fracture, 124, *127*
Depression, 38
Dermatitis, 113
Dermis, 110, *111*
Descending colon, 205
Desensitization in allergy treatment, 191, 428, *429*
Deuteranopia, 345
Developmental stages of children, 361, *362*
Diabetes mellitus, 231, 233-235
    factors contributing to, 233
    types of, 234
Diabetic coma, first aid for, 514, 514t
Diabetic patients, 68
    insulin injections for, 496, *500-501, 503*
Diabetic retinopathy, 104, 234
Diagnosis, 327, 329
Diagnostic procedures, 427-432, 447-452
    for allergens, 146
    for cancer, 191-192
    cardiovascular, 169-170
    of circulatory system, 169-170
    of digestive system, 206-208
    of endocrine system, 232
    of female reproductive system, 255
    Hemoccult Sensa tests, *451*, 451-452
    of integumentary system, 112
    magnetic resonance imaging, *449*, 449-450, *450*
    for neurological disorders, 92-94, *95-96*
    of pulmonary function, 145
    skin tests, 428-432, *429, 430*
    sonography, 448-449, *449*
    of urinary system, 221-222
    vital capacity tests, 447-448, *448*
    See also specific tests and procedures
Diagnostic related groups (DRGs), 14
Dialysate, 219
Dialysis, *219*, 219-221, *220*
    automated peritoneal, 221
    hemo-, 219
    peritoneal, 220, *220*
Diaphanography, 255, 449
Diaphragm, 74, *74*, 134, *135*
    for contraception, 256t
Diaphysis, 121
Diarrhea, 209-210
    in cirrhosis, 208
Diarthrosis (synovial) joint, 122, 124, *126*
Diastole, 153, 308
Diets:
    cancer and, 194
    for diabetes mellitus, 234

therapeutic, 28, 31
Differential blood cell count, 389, 390, 394, *395*, 395t
Diffusion, 78, *78*, 143
    process of, 87-88, *89, 90*
Digestive process, 197-199
Digestive system, 197-214, *198*
    diagnostic examinations of, 206-208
    disorders and diseases of, 208-214
    esophagus, 199
    large intestine, 204-206, *206*
    mouth, 199, *200, 201*
    small intestine, *202*, 202-204
    stomach, 200-202, *202*
Digital palpation, 320
Digital thermometers, 290, 291t, 300, *300*
Dilation and curettage (D & C), 257, 258
Dilation of blood vessels in skin, 110
Dimpling of breasts, 325
Diphtheria, 503-504
Direct pressure to wounds, 524, *524*
Disclosure of information forms, 23
Discoid lupus erythematosus, 196
Discretion in handling telephone calls, 268
Discrimination in hiring practices, 548
Diseases:
    autoimmune, 196
    of circulatory system, 170-177
    communicable, 56, 59t-60t
    of digestive system, 208-214
    of ear, 106-107
    of endocrine system, 232-235
    of eye, 102-105
    of female reproductive system, 255, 257-263
    of immune system, 185-197
    of integumentary system, 112-117, 117t
    of male reproductive system, 241-243
    mechanisms of transmission of, 52, 54-56, *55-58*
    of muscular system, 138-139
    of nervous system, 94-99
    prevention of, 56, 58, 59t-60t
    of respiratory system, 145-152
    sensory, 102-109
    sexually transmitted (*See* Sexually transmitted diseases)
    of skeletal system, 126-130
    transmission of, 52-58
    See also specific diseases
Disinfection, 56
Dislocations, 127, 514
Displacement, 47
Disposable syringes, 491, *493*
Disposable thermometers, 295-299, *297, 298*
    measuring oral temperature with, *297*, 298
    plastic, 290, 291t
    for rectal use, 298-299
Distal, 73, *73*
Distal convoluted tubule, 217, *217*
Distension in lower GI series, 454
Distortion in communication, 2
Distress, 37
Diversion Control Amendments of 1984, 480
Diverticulitis, 207
Diverticulosis, 210
DNA (*See* Deoxyribonucleic acid)
Doppler ultrasonography, 169, *169*
Dorsal recumbent position, 332, *332*

Dorsal section, 73, *73*
Dorsalis pedis pulse point, 302, *302*
Double barrel colostomy, 209
Douches, 256t, 326, 352, 489
Down syndrome, 83
DRGs (*See* Diagnostic related groups)
Dribbling, urinary, 219
Droplet infection, 52, 55
Drowning, artificial respiration for, 519
Drug(s):
    action of, 489
    approved by FDA, 476-477
    classifications of, 475t-476t
    urine specimens for analysis, 414-415
Drug abuse, 40, 41t-44t, 43-45, *45*
    indications of, 40, *45*
    stages of, 40
    treatment for, 45
Drug Enforcement Administration (DEA), 14, 480
    physician registration form, *478*, 480
Drug-induced lupus, 196
Dry heat oven, for sterilization, 63
Duchenne's muscular dystrophy, 138
Ductless glands (*See* Endocrine glands)
Duodenal peptic ulcer, 213
Duodenum, 202, *202*, 203, *203*
Dura mater, 92, *95*
Durable power of attorney for health care, 15, *17*
Duration, in percussion, 320-321
DVT (*See* Deep vein thrombosis)
Dysmenorrhea, 257
Dyspnea, 146, 306
Dysuria, 219

Ear(s), 105-107
    care of, 350
    diseases and disorders of, 106-107
    examination of, 323, *323*
    foreign bodies in, *515*, 515-516
Ear speculum, 337
ECG (*See* Electrocardiograph)
Echocardiography, 169, 448
Ectoderm layer, 252
Ectopic pregnancy, 247
Edema, 83
    pulmonary, 151
    of vocal cords, 519
EEG (*See* Electroencephalography)
Effacement, 254
Efferent (motor) nerves, 87
Ejaculation, 241, 250
Ejaculatory duct, 237, *238*, 240, *241*
Electrical burns, 513
Electrocardiogram, 434
    procedure for obtaining, *440*, 440-441, *443*
Electrocardiograph (ECG; EKG), 156, 157, 169, 517
    computerized, 443
    Holter monitoring, 444, *446*, 446-447, *447*
    interference in, 438-439, 441, *441, 442*
    operation of, 434, *434-437*, 436
    routine leads in, 437-438, *438, 439*
    standardization in, 441-444, *442, 443*
    stress tests, 444, *445, 446*
Electrocautery device, 461, *461*
Electrocoagulation, 461
Electrodes, 434, *435*, 436
    in electrocardiograph, 439, 441

Electroencephalography (EEG), 92
Electrolytes, 164, 436
Electromagnetic field, in MRI, 449-450
Electromagnetic radiation, 454
Electromyography, 93
Electron(s), 454
Electronic probe thermometers, 290, 291t, 300, *300*
    measuring oral temperature with, 299
Elements, 80
Elimination, 216
ELISA (*See* Enzyme-linked immunosorbent assay test)
Emancipated minor, 15
Embolism, 173-174
Embryo, 252, *253*
Emergency kit, for office laboratory, 68, *68*
Emergency medical identification cards, 511, *511*
Emergency procedures, for laboratories, 371-372, *372*
Emergency services, 371, *372*, 525-526, 537
Emetics, 68, 511
Emotional states, communicating, 48-49
Emphysema, 146
    effects on lung, 149, *149*
Employee evaluation, 10, *11*, 551, *551*, *552*
Employee qualities, desirable, 548-550
Employment, 538-553
    job search (*See* Job search)
    terminating, 552, *552*
Empyema, 150
Encephalitis, 96
Endocarditis, 172
Endocardium, 153, *155*
Endocervical brush, 354
Endocrine system, 204, 225-235
    adrenal glands (suprarenal), 230, *231*
    diagnostic examinations of, 232
    diseases and disorders of, 232-235
    gonads (testes and ovaries), 231-232
    pancreas, 231, *231*
    parathyroid glands, 230
    pineal body, 231
    pituitary gland, 226-228
    thymus, 231
    thyroid gland, 228, *228*, 230, *230*
Endocytosis, 77
Endoderm layer, 252
Endometriosis, 257-258
Endometritis, 262
Endometrium, 247
Endoplasmic reticulum, 75, *76*, 77
Endoscope, 365
Enemas, 321, 363, 365
    administration of, 366
Enzyme(s), 199
Enzyme-linked immunosorbent assay test (ELISA), 187
Eosinophil(s), 165, 178, 183
Eosinophil count, 432
Epicondylitis (tennis elbow), 127-128, 138
Epidermis, 110, *111*
Epididymis, 237, *238*, 239, *239, 241*
Epididymitis, 241-242
Epigastric region, 74, *75*
Epiglottis, 141, *142*
Epiglottitis, 502
Epilepsy, 68, 96-97
Epinephrine (adrenaline), 230, 428, 431-432, 511

Epiphyses, 121
Episiotomy, 249
Epistaxis (nosebleed), 107-108, 147, 518
Epithelial tissues, 83, *83*
Epitopes, 179
Epstein-Barr virus, 191
Erb's (juvenile) muscular dystrophy, 138
Erectile tissue, 241
Erection, 241
Ergonomics, 66
Erythema, 112
Erythrocyte(s) (red blood cells), 164, 178, 390, *395*
    in polycythemia, 380
Erythrocyte count, 386, 389
    manual, *390, 391, 395*
Erythrocyte sedimentation rate (ESR), 400, 403
    Wintrobe method for, 403, *405, 407*
Escherichia coli, 52, 222, 263
Esophageal varices, 210
Esophagus, 137, 199
Esophogastroduodenoscopy, 207
ESR (*See* Erythrocyte sedimentation rate)
Essential hypertension, 174, 308
Estradiol transdermal system, 488, *488*
Estrogen, 231-232
    cancer and, 194
ESWL (*See* Extra-corporeal shock-wave lithotripsy)
Ethics, medical law and, 10, 12-23
Euphoria, 40
Eustachian tube, *105*, 105-106
Eustress, 37
Evacuants, 363
Evacuation of bowel:
    before physical examination, 322
    before sigmoidoscopy, 365
Evacuation procedures, 66
    in case of fire, 510
Evaluation form for employee review, 551, *551*
Examination rooms:
    preparation of, 322, *322*
    safety and security in, 67, *67*
Excretion, 216
Exercise, 31, 33, *34-36*
    effects of stress and, 38
    nutrition, rest and, 26-33, *27*
    pulse rate and, 302
Exfoliated cells, Pap test and, 352
Exhalation, 305
Exocrine glands, 83, *83*
Exocytosis, 77
Exogenous obesity, 518
Exophthalmia, 230, *230*
Expectoration, 146
Expiration, 142
Express consent agreements, 18
Extensor muscles, 132, *133*
External oblique abdominal muscle, 134
External os, 247, *247*
External parasites, 54-55
External respiration, 142, *144*
Externships, 10
Extra-corporeal shock-wave lithotripsy (ESWL), 224
Extracellular fluid, 81
Extracellular invaders in immune response, 182
Extracts in allergy testing, 429
Extremities, 73, *73*

examination of, 327
Exudate (pus), 165, 323, 420
Eye(s), 100-102, *101, 102*
    diseases and disorders of, 102-105
    examination of, 323, 337-339
    foreign bodies in, 515, *515*
Eye contact, 3
Eyewash stations, 67, 371, *372*

Facial expression in communication, 3, *4*
Facultative parasites, 54
Fahrenheit thermometers, 291, *291*
Fainting (*See* Syncope)
Fallopian tubes, 237, *238, 244*, 246-257
Family history, 273
Fascia, 133
Fasting blood glucose range, 383-384
Fasting normal range for blood tests, 322
Fat(s), 199
Fat embolus, 125
FDA (*See* Food and Drug Administration)
Febrile, 289
Fecal impaction, 205-206
Fecal material, 365
Feces, 417
Federal Drug Administration, 14
Federal regulations on universal precautions, 61
Federal treatment facilities for drug abuse, 45
"Feeder questions," 48
Female reproductive system:
    contraception and, 255, 256t
    diagnostic tests of, 255
    diseases and disorders of, 255, 257-263
    fertilization, 250, 252, *252*
    organs of, 244-250
    pregnancy, 252-254, *253*
Female-to-male transsexuals, 264
Femoral pulse point, 302, *302*
Femur, *119*, 121
Fenestrated drape, 334, 462
Fertilization, 240, 247, *252*, 252
Fetal (pulse) monitor, 357, *361*
Fetus, 252, *253*, 253
Fevers, categories of, 290, 290t
Fibrillation, 157
Fibrin, 165
Fibrinogen, 164, 165
Fibrocystic (cystitic) breast disease, 257
Fibroids, 258
Fibromyositis, 138
Fibrous (synarthrosis) joint, 122
Fibula, *119*, 121
Figure-eight bandage, 530, *530*
Filtration, 78, *79*
Finger sweep, 519
Fingerprints, 110-111
Fire drills, 510
Fire extinguishers, 510
Fire prevention, 510
First aid, 512-524
    for accidents and injuries, 526-533
    bee, wasp, and hornet stings, 512
    bites, 512
    burns, *512*, 512-513, *513*
    convulsions, 513-514
    diabetic coma, 514, 514t
    dislocations, 514
    fainting, 515

foreign bodies, *515*, 515-516, *516*
fractures, 516-517
heart attack, 517
heat and cold exposure, 517
hemorrhage, 517-518
insulin shock, 514, 514t
poisoning, 518
respiratory emergencies, *518*, 518-519, *519*
shock, 519-520
sprains and strains, 520, 522, *524*
stroke, 522
wounds, 524, *524, 525*
First-degree burns, 512
First-degree heart block, 156
Fish hooks, removal of, 516, *516*
Fissures:
    of anus, 210
    in brain, 92, *94*
Fistulas, 208
    arteriovenous, 219-220, *220*
    examination for, 327
Flatulence, 365
Flatus, 209, 454
Flexibility exercises, 33, *36*
Flexor muscles, 132, *133*
Flu (*See* Influenza)
Fluoroscope, 454
Fluoroscopy, 222
Foley catheter, 409
Follicle-stimulating hormone (FSH), 227, 239, 246, 250
Follicular cysts, 260
Follicular infections, 113, 115
Follicular phase of menstruation, 250
Folliculitis, 113, 115
Follow-up letter after job interview, 548, *550*
Follow-up visits after minor surgery, 471
Fontanels, 120
Food and Drug Administration (FDA), 476
Food guide pyramid, 27, 27t, *28*, 28
Foramen, 120, *121*
Foreign bodies, first aid for, *515*, 515-516, *516*
Foreskin, 241
Formaldehyde, 367
Forms:
    consent (various), 18, *19*
    cytology request, 353, *353*
    disclosure of information, 23
    employee review, 551, *551*
    histology request, 466
    for immunizing minors, 492
    job application, 545, *546*, 547
    medical history, 272, 322-323, *323*
    medical insurance, 5, *15*
    request for sterilization, 18, *19*
    for specimen tests, 414-416, *417*
Fourth-degree burns, 513
Fovea centralis, 102
Fowler's position, 333, *333*
Fractures, 124-125, *127*
    complications of, 517
    first aid for, 516-517
Fraud, medical licensure requirements and, 12
French catheter, 409
Frontal lobe, 92, *94*
Frontal plane, 73, *73*
Frontalis muscle, 135
Frostbite, 517

FSH (*See* Follicle-stimulating hormone)
Functional type resumé, 541, *542*
Fundamental body structure, 71-85
Fungi, 54, *55*
Furuncles (boils), 113

G-CSF (*See* Granulocyte colony-stimulating factor)
Galactosemia, 81, 379
Gallbladder, 203, *203*, 455
    cholecystogram test, 454, *454*
Gallstones (*See* Cholelithiasis)
Galvanometer, 436
Gametes, 237
Gamma interferon (IFN-g), 183
Gastric glands, 201
Gastric ulcer, 201, 213
Gastroenteritis, 210
Gastrointestinal series (X ray), 207
Gastrointestinal (GI) tract, 197
Gastroscopy, 207
Gender, pulse rate and, 302-303
Genetic cellular change, 81, 83
Genetic predisposition to CFS, 195
Genital herpes, 261
Genitalia, 237, *238*
    examination of, 326-328
    female, 326-327
    male, 326-327, *327*
Genogram, 273, *278*
Genucubital position, 334
Genupectoral position, 333, *333*
German measles (*See* Rubella)
Gestation period, 357
Gestures in communication, 4
GH (*See* Growth hormone)
Glaucoma, 323
    chronic, 104, *104*
Glomerulonephritis, 222-223
Glomerulus, 217, *217*
Glossitis, 108
Glucometer, 383, *388*
Glucose, 383, 511
    in urine, 413
Glucose (blood sugar) level, screening, 232, 383-384, *388*, 389, *390*
Glucose level in diabetes mellitus, 234-235
Glucose tolerance test (GTT), 232, 384
    explaining to patient, 389, *390*
Gluteus maximus, 135
Glycogen, 131
Glycosuria, 231
GM-CSF (*See* Granulocyte-macrophage colony-stimulating factor)
Goiter, 228
Golgi apparatus, 75, *76*, 77
Gonadotropic hormones, 226-227
Gonads (testes and ovaries), 229t, 231-232
Gonorrhea, 261
Good Samaritan Act, 21-22
Gout (gouty arthritis), 128
Graafian follicles, 244, 246
Gram-negative bacteria, 421-423, *424*, 426t
Gram-positive bacteria, 421-423, *424*, 426t
Gram staining, 421-423, *424*, 426t
    preparing stain, *424*, 425
Granular lutein cysts, 260
Granulocyte(s), 165, 182-183
Granulocyte colony-stimulating factor (G-CSF), 183

Granulocyte-macrophage colony-stimulating factor (GM-CSF), 183
Graves' disease, 235, 346
Graves' ophthalmopathy, 346
Greenstick fracture, 124, *127*
Groin, 302
Gross anatomy, 72
Growth abnormalities, diagnosing:
    by chest measurement, 284-285
    by growth chart, 280
Growth chart:
    growth abnormalities and, 280
    recording height and weight on, 278, *278*, 280, *281-282*
Growth hormone (GH), 226, *228*
GTT (*See* Glucose tolerance test)
Guaiac test paper, 327, 451
Gunshot wounds, 524
Gynecological care, 352
Gynecological examination, 356, *358*
Gynecology, 249

Habits, 39
Haemophilus influenza type B immunization, 501-502, 502t
Haemophilus influenzae, 501
Hair follicles, 110
Hallucinogens, 43-44
Hallux valgus, 128
Hamstring group, 135
Handwashing, 51-53, *53-54*, 370
Hard connective tissue, 84, *84*
Hazardous medical waste:
    containers for, 370, *371*
    OSHA regulations on, 67
HBV (*See* Hepatitis B virus)
HCFA (*See* Health Care Financing Administration (HCFA))
HCG (*See* Human chorionic gonadotropin)
Head circumference, measuring, 284, 287, *288*
Headache, 97
Health and safety, promoting, 321
Health Care Financing Administration (HCFA), 376
Health care providers, AIDS and, 187-188
Health maintenance organization (HMO), 19
Healthcheck program for Medicaid patients, 363-364
Hearing loss, 106
Heart, *153*, 153-158, 436, *437*
    examination of, 325
    external structures of, 153, *154*
    internal structures of, 153-154, *155*
    pulmonary circulation, 154, *155*, 156-158
Heart attack, first aid for, 517
Heart block, 156
Heartburn, 363
Heat cramps, 517
Heat exhaustion, 517
Heat-fixing smears, 420, *420*
Heat treatment for sprains and strains, 520, 522, *524*
Heatstroke, 517
Height:
    measuring, 278, *278*, 286, *287*
    recording on growth charts, 280, *281-282*
Heimlich maneuver, 518, *519*

Helper T cells, 182, 184
Hematocrit, 377
    determining with centrifuge, 382t, 383, *384, 385*
    screening tests for, 380-381, *381*, 382t, *386, 387*
Hematoma, 397
Hematuria, 219, 410, 411
Hemiplegia, 98
Hemoccult Sensa tests, *451*, 451-452
Hemodialysis, 219
Hemoglobin, 164, 381, 386
    screening tests for, 380-381, *381*, 382t, *386, 387*
Hemoglobin count, 386, *388*
Hemoglobinometer, 381, *388*
    determining hemoglobin count with, 386, *388*
Hemophilia, 81, 461
    AIDS and, 188
Hemorrhage, 169
    first aid for, 517-518
Hemorrhoidectomy, 211
Hemorrhoids, 210-211
Hemothorax, 150
Heparin, 399
Hepatic duct, 203, *203*
Hepatitis, 211, 292
Hepatitis B immunization, 506
Hepatitis B virus (HBV), 60, 370, 506
Hernia:
    hiatal, 211-212, *212*
    inguinal, 212
Herniated disk (ruptured disk), 128
Herniorrhaphy, 212
Herpes, 261
Herpes simplex, 115
Herpes zoster (shingles), 97, 115
Heterotrophs, 55
HHS (*See* U.S. Department of Health and Human
    Services)
Hiatal hernia, 211-212, *212*
Hib (HIB) vaccine (*See* Haemophilus influenza
    type B)
Hiccoughs, 144
Hilum, 216, *216*
Hip dysplagia, congenital, 127
Hirsutism, 115
Histamine, 180, 428
Histology, 72
Histology request form, 466
Histoplasmosis, 147
Histotechnologists, 72
HIV (*See* Human immunodeficiency virus)
Hives (*See* Urticaria)
HMD (*See* Hyaline membrane disease)
HMO (*See* Health maintenance organization)
Holistic care, 7
Holter monitor, 169
Holter monitoring, 444, *446*, 446-447, *447*
Home pregnancy tests, 355
Homeostasis, 81
Homocystinuria, 379-380
Homosexuality, 185
Hordeolum (stye), 104
Horizontal recumbent position, 331, 332, *332*
Hormonal evaluation, 232, 354-355
Hormone therapy in transsexualism, 263, 264
Hospice movement, 7
Hospital, autoclaving services of, 62
Hostility, 6
Human bites, 512, 524

Human chorionic gonadotropin (HCG), 232, 252,
    255
Human immunodeficiency virus (HIV), 60, 186,
    370
    state regulations on test results, 18
Humoral immunity, 180
Humpback (*See* Kyphosis)
Hyaline membrane disease (HMD), 147
Hydrocele, 242
Hydrocephalus, 97
Hydrochloric acid, 201
Hyfrecator, 461, *461*
Hymen, 247-248, *249*
Hymenectomy, 248
Hyperglycemia, 231
Hyperopia, 102
Hyperparathyroidism, 230
Hypersensitive reaction, 428
Hypertension, 174, 308
Hyperthermia, 192
Hyperthyroidism, 228
Hypertonic solution, 78, *79*
Hyperventilation, 68, 306
Hypoallergenic tape, 468
Hypochondriac regions, 74, *75*
Hypodermics, *490*, 490-491
Hypogastric region, 74, *75*
Hypoglycemia, 97, 231
Hypoglycemic reactions, 68
Hypoparathyroidism, 230
Hypotension, 174, 308
"Hypothalamic thermostat," 290
Hypothalamus, 91-92
    control of body temperature by, 289-290
Hypothermia, 68
Hypothyroidism, 228, 380
Hypotonic solution, 78, *80*
Hypoxia, 150
Hysterectomy, 257, 258, *258*
Hysteroscopy, 255

I & D (*See* Incision and drainage)
ICP (*See* Intracranial pressure)
ICSH (*See* Interstitial cell-stimulating hormone)
Icteric stage of hepatitis B, 211
IDDM (*See* Insulin-dependent diabetes mellitus)
Idiopathic hypertension (*See* Essential hyperten-
    sion)
IFA (*See* Indirect immunofluorescent assay)
IFN-a (*See* Alpha interferon)
IFN-b (*See* Beta interferon)
IFN-g (*See* Gamma interferon)
IL (*See* Interleukin(s))
Ileocecal valve, 202
Ileostomy, 212-213
Ileum, 202
Iliac regions, 74, *75*
Ilium, 122, *125*
Illiteracy, 21
Immediate percussion, 321
Immune responses, *181*, 182-185, *186*, 428
Immune system, 177-197
    cell markers in, 178-179
    complement system, 181, *182*
    components of, 182-183
    cytokines, 181, 183
    diseases and disorders of, 185-197
    immunization, 185

lymphocytes, 179-180, *181*
    natural killer (NK) cells, 182
    organs of, 178, *180*
    origin of cells, 178, *179*
    responses of, *181*, 182-185, *186*
Immune therapy, 192
Immunization(s), 185, 497-507, 502t
    diphtheria, 503-504
    guidelines for, 505t, 506-507, *507*
    haemophilus influenza Type B, 501-502, 502t
    hepatitis B, 506
    influenza, 499
    measles, mumps, and rubella (MMR), 502-503,
        506
    pertussis, 504, 506
    pneumonia, 499, 501
    tetanus, 506
Immunization Alert, health information for travel-
    ers, 507
Immunization record, for patient, 507, *507*
Immunization schedule, 498, 502t, 505t, 507
Immunoglobulins, 179, 182, 190, 506
Immunosuppressed patients, 185
Immunotoxins, 192
Impacted fracture, 124, *127*
Impetigo, 115
Implied consent agreements, 18
Impotence, 242-243
In-service programs for medical office, 9
Incarceration in hiatal hernia, 212
Incineration, 62
Incision(s), 74, 524
Incision and drainage (I & D), 460
Incompetent valves, 335-336
Incontinence:
    of bladder, 219
    of feces, 205
Incubation period, 499
Incus, 105, *105*
Indirect immunofluorescent assay (IFA), 187
Indirect percussion, 321
Infants:
    cardiopulmonary resuscitation (CPR) for, 523,
        523
    procedure for measuring chest, 288, *288*
    screening for PKU, 378-380, *380*
    weighing, 283, *286*
    See also Children; Neonates
Infarction, 125
Infection cycle, 55-56, *57-58*
Infectious hepatitis, 211
Inferior portion, *73*, 74
Inferior vena cava, 159
Inflammatory bowel disease, 452
Influenza (flu), 147-148
    immunization against, 499
Information:
    conveying to patient, 279
    recording, 270, *271*
Informed consent, 18, *19*
Infrared thermometers, 290, 291t
Infusion systems, 489
Inguinal canal, 237, *239*
Inguinal hernia, 212, 237, *239*, 326
Inguinal region, 74, *75*
Inhalation, 305
    administration of medicines by, 483, 486
    poisoning by, 518

Injection(s), 490-492, *490-493*, 495-497
  angle of, 491, *491*
  intradermal, 492, 495, *496*
  intramuscular, 495-496, *499*
  intravenous, 496-497, *500-501, 503*
  poisoning by, 518
  subcutaneous, 495, *498*
Injection sites:
  for allergy immunotherapy, 428-429, *430*
  rotating, 496, *503*
Injuries:
  to face and head, preventing, 321
  first aid care for, 526-533
Inner ear, *105*, 106, *106*
Insertion point of muscle, 133
Insomnia, exercise and, 31
Inspection, in physical examination, 320
Inspiration, 142
Instillation, 338
  of eardrops, 342, *343*
  of eyedrops, 341, *343*
Instruments:
  care of, 61-63
  for minor office surgical procedures, 467, 468t
Insulin, 204, 231, 389
  injections of, 496, *500-501, 503*
Insulin-dependent diabetes mellitus (IDDM), 234
Insulin shock, first aid for, 514, 514t
Insurance companies, ethics issues and, 14
Intake-output measurement, 221
Integumentary system, 109-117
  color of skin, 112
  diseases and disorders of, 112-117, 117t
  functions of, 110, *110*
  skin as diagnostic testing site, 112
  structure of, 110-111, *111*
Intellectualization, 47
Interaction of medications, 489
Intercalated disks, 132
Intercostal muscles, 134
Interference, in electrocardiograph, 438-439, 441, *441, 442*
Interferons, 183, 192
Interleukins (BCDF; IL), 182-184, 192
Internal bleeding, 517-518
Internal oblique abdominal muscle, 134
Internal parasites, 54
Internal respiration, 78, 143, *144*
International Association of Laryngectomies, 148
Interneurons, 84, 89
Internuncial neurons, 87, *88*
Interstitial cell-stimulating hormone (ICSH), 227, 239
Interstitial fluid, 163
Intervertebral cartilage disks, 119, *120*
Intestinal mucosa, 366
Intestine, lesions of, 454
Intracellular fluid, 81
Intracellular invaders in immune response, 182
Intracranial pressure (ICP), 98
Intradermal injections, 492, 495, *496*
  procedure for, 497, *497*
Intradermal test, 430-432, *432*
Intramuscular injections, 495-496, *499*
  administration of, 504
Intraocular lens (IOL), 102-103
Intraoffice communication, 9
Intrauterine device (IUD), 256t

Intravenous injections, 496-497, *500-501, 503*
Intravenous pyelogram (IVP), 221, 455, *456*
Intubation, 141
Inunction, drug administration by, 110
Invasive procedures, 61
  contrast-enhanced MRI, 449
  for diagnostic tests of urinary system, 221-222
  minor surgical, 460, *461*
Involuntary muscle action, 84, *86*
Involuntary smoking, 46, 149
Iodine, 455
IOL (*See* Intraocular lens)
Ionizing radiation, cancer and, 193
Iris, 101, *101*
Iritis, 104
Irrigation (lavage), 338
  of ear, 339, *340*
  of eye, 338, *340*
Ischium, 122, *125*
Ishihara color plates, 323, 345, 347, *348*
Islets of Langerhans, 231, *231*
Isotonic solutions, 78, *80*
IUD (*See* Intrauterine device)
IVP (*See* Intravenous pyelogram)

Jackknife position, 336, *336*
Jaeger card, 323
Jaeger system, measuring visual acuity with, 343-345, *346*, 347
Jaundice, 203
Jejunum, 202
Job descriptions, 9, 548
Job search, 538-545
  application forms, 545, *546, 547*
  classified advertisements, 542
  cover letter in, 541-542, *544*
  interviewing, 547-548, *548-550*
  other contacts in, 543, 545
  private employment agencies, 543
  public employment agencies, 542-543
  resumé in, 539, *540-543*, 541
  variety in requirements, 553
Joints, 122, 124, *126*
Juvenile (insulin-dependent) diabetes mellitus (IDDM), 234
Juvenile (Erb's) muscular dystrophy, 138

Kaposi's sarcoma, 185-186
Keloids, 84, 115
Keratin, 111
Kernig's sign, 97, *98*
Ketone (acetone) bodies in urine, 411
Ketonuria, 411
Kidney(s), *216*, 216-218, *217*
  nephrons, 216-218
Kidney stones (*See* Renal calculi)
Kidney transplant, 221
Killer T cells, 182, 184
Klinefelter's syndrome, 81, 83
Knee-chest position, 333, *333*, 334
Koplik's spots, 502
KUB series (kidneys, ureters, bladder), 221, 455-456, *456*
Kyphosis (humpback, roundback), 128-129, *129*

L & A (*See* Light and accommodation)
Labia majora, 237, *238*, 248
Labia minora, 237, *238*, 248

Laboratory area, safety and security in, 67-68, *68, 69*
Laboratory procedures:
  capillary blood tests, 374-394
  instructing patients about, 372
  microscope, 372-374, *375*
  specimen collection and, 369-426
Laboratory request form for sputum specimens, 416, *417*
Laboratory safety, guidelines for, 370-372, *370-372*
Laboratory technicians, 384
Lacrimal glands, 101
Lamaze classes, 355
Laminectomy, 128
Laparoscopic surgery, for cholecystectomy, 203
Large intestine, 204-206, *206*
  ascending, transverse, and descending colon, 205
  cecum and appendix, 204-205
  sigmoid, rectum, and anal canal, 205-206
Laryngeal mirror, 323
Laryngectomy, 148, *148*
Laryngitis, 148
Larynx, 141, *142*
  cancer of, 148
Laser surgery:
  for glaucoma, 104
  for retinal detachment, 105
Lateral, 73, *73*
Latissimus dorsi, 134-135
Lavage (*See* Irrigation)
Law of agency, 21
Laxatives, 205-206, 321, 417
Lazy eye (*See* Amblyopia)
Left-sided heart failure, 172-173
Legal document, medical record as, 23
Legionnaires' disease, 148-149
Lens, 101, *101*
Lesions of intestine, diagnosing, 454
Letter of withdrawal by physician, 19, *20*
Leukemia, 174-175
Leukocyte(s) (white blood cells), 164-165, 178, 390, 395t
Leukocyte count, 389
  manual, 391, *395*
LH (*See* Luteinizing hormone)
Ligaments, 122
Light and accommodation (L & A), 323
Light path in eye, 102
Lipase, 201
Lithotomy position, 335, *335*, 336
  for gynecological exam, 354
Liver, 202-203, *203*
Living will, 7, *8*, 15, *16, 17*
Long bones, *119*, 121
Longitudinal fissure in brain, 92
Loop of Henle, 217, *217*
Lordosis, 129, *129*
"Lost Chord Club," 148
Lou Gehrig's disease (*See* Amyotrophic lateral sclerosis)
Low-power field (lpf) of microscope, 374
Lower extremity muscles, 135
Lower GI series, 207, 454-455, *456*
  preparation for, 455, *456*
LSD, 525
"Lubb dupp" sounds, 156
Lumbar myositis, 129
Lumbar puncture, 93, *95-96*

Lumbar regions, 74, *75*
Lumen, 365
Lumpectomy, 259
Lund-Browder chart, *513*
Lung:
    cancer of, 149, *149*
    pleura and, 143-144, *144*
Lung perfusion scan, 145
Lung ventilation scan, 145
Lupus erythematosus, 196
Luteal phase of menstruation, 250
Luteinizing hormone (LH), 227, 246, 250
Lyme disease, 115-116
Lymph, 162-163
Lymph nodes, examining, 162, 163, *324*, 327
Lymphatic system, 85, *86*, 153, 162-163
    lymph nodes, 162, 163
    lymph vessels, 163, *165, 166*
Lymphocytes, 178, 179-180, *181*, 182
    production of, 162, 163, 165
Lymphocytic leukemia, 174-175
Lymphokines, 180, 183, 184
Lysosomes, 75, *76*, 77

McBurney's point, 208
Macrophage(s), 178, 182
Macrophage colony-stimulating factor (M-CSF),
    183
Macule, 115
Magnetic resonance imaging (MRI), 93-94, 191,
    449, 449-450, *450*
Major histocompatibility complex (MHC), 178-180
Male-pattern baldness, 112
Male reproductive system:
    diseases of, 241-243
    organs of, 237, *239*, 239-241
Male-to-female transsexuals, 263-264
Malignant cells, 191
Malignant hypertension, 174
Malignant melanoma, 113, *114*
Malingering, 47
Malleus, 105, *105*
Malpractice, 21
    avoiding, 21-22
Mammary glands, *249*, 249-250, 252
Mammogram, 255
Mammography, *456*, 456-457, *457*
Manipulation, 321
Manometers, 308-310, *309-311, 313*
    augmenting sound and, 313, *313*
    auscultatory gap and, 313-314, *314*
    techniques for using, 310, *313*, 313-314
Marijuana, 43-44, 525
Marrow, 118
Masseter muscle, 135
Mast cells, 183
Mastectomy, 259
Maturation index (MI), 255, 354
M-CSF (*See* Macrophage colony-stimulating factor)
Measles, 502
    mumps, and rubella (MMR) vaccine, 502-503,
        506
Medial, 73, *73*
Medicaid patients, eligible for Healthcheck program, 363-364
Medical assistant rights, 19, 21

Medical Assistant's Code, 13
Medical Assistant's Creed, 13-14
Medical emergencies, 509-533
    first aid care for, 526-533
    office procedures for, 510-526, *511*
    office safety, 509-510
Medical history, 22, 270-273, 273
    format of form for, 322-323, *323*
    for obstetrics patients, 356, *359-360*
Medical insurance forms, 5, *5*
Medical law, ethics and, 10, 12-23
Medical records, 22-23
Medical staff relationships, 7-10
Medications, 473-508
    abbreviations and symbols for, 479t-480t, 483
    accessibility of, 510
    action of, 489
    injections and immunizations, 490-507
    math skills for evaluating, 482t, 483
    methods for administering, 483-489
    precautions in administering, 484
    prescription and nonprescription, 473-483
    recording, 479t-482t, 483
    storing, 475t-476t, 483
    weighing and measuring, 481t, 483
Medulla oblongata, 92, *94*
Medulla of kidney, 216, *216*
Melanin, 112
Melanocyte(s), 112
Melanocyte-stimulating hormone (MSH), 226
Membrane excitability, 87-89, *89, 90*
Memory cells, 182
Menarche, 250
Ménière's Disease, 106
Meninges, 90, 92, *94, 95*
Meningitis, 97, *98*, 502
Meningocele, spina bifida with, 98, 99, *99*
Meniscus, 398
Menopause, 250
Menorrhagia, 258
Menstruation, 244, 250, *251*
    phases of, 250
Mensurations, 273, 276, 278-285, 321
    chest measurement, 284-285
    head circumference, 284, *288*
    height and weight, 278, *278*, 280, *281-282, 284*
Mental retardation, 502
Mercury thermometers, 290, *291*, 291t
    cleaning and storing, *291*, 291-292, *292*
    measuring axillary temperature with, 297
    measuring oral temperature with, 295
    measuring rectal temperature with, *294*, 296
    reading and recording measurements, *291*, 291-292, *292*
Mesentery, 202
Metabolism, of phenylalanine, 378
Metacarpals, 121, *124*
Metal objects, MRI and, 449
Metallic implants, MRI and, 450
Metastasis, 163, 191
Metatarsals, 121, *124*
MHC (*See* Major histocompatibility complex)
MI (*See* Maturation index; Myocardial infarction)
Microbial accumulation, 463
Micronutrients, 27-28, 29t-33t
Microorganisms, 52
Microscope, 372-374, *375*
    binocular, 373, *375*

    examining urine sediment with, 414, *416*
    monocular, 373
    procedure for using, 373
Microscopic anatomy, 72
Midbrain, 92, *94*
Middle ear, 105-106
Midline, 73, *73*
Migraine headache, 97
Minerals, 27-28, 29t-33t, 199
Minor surgery:
    assisting with, 466-468, *467*, 468t
    preparing skin for, 462-463, *462-463*
Miscarriage, 255, 257
Mitochondria, 75, *76*, 77
Mitosis, 76, *76*, 80-81, *82*
Mitral (bicuspid) valve, 154, *155*
Mixed hiatal hernia, 211-212
Mixed muscular dystrophy, 138
MMR vaccine (*See* Measles, mumps, and rubella
        vaccine)
Monoclonal antibodies, *192*, 192-193
    radiolabeled, 193
Monocular microscope, 373
Monocytes, 165, 178, 182
Monogamous relationship as AIDS preventative,
    189
Monokines, 180, 182, 183
Mons pubis, 248
Morphology of bacteria, 52, 55
Motion sickness, 107
Motivation, patient compliance and, 6
Motor (efferent) nerves, 87
Motor neurons, 84, *85*, 87, *88*
Motor unit, 131
Mouth, 199, *200, 201*
    diseases and disorders of, 108-109
Mouth-to-mouth resuscitation, 60, 520
MRI (*See* Magnetic resonance imaging)
MS (*See* Multiple sclerosis)
MSH (*See* Melanocyte-stimulating hormone)
Mucus, 140
Mucus streaming, 140-141
MUGA scan, 169
Multiple sclerosis (MS), 97-98
Multistix 10 SG reagent strip test, 410, *412*
    testing urine with, 411
Mumps, 502
Murmur, 175, 325
Muscle(s):
    action of, 132, *133, 134*
    attachment of, 133
    of breathing, 144, *145*
    of expression, 135
    fuel for, 131
    functions of, 131
    growth of, 131
    major skeletal, 134-135, *135-137*
    strain and cramps, 135-137, 136-137
Muscle contraction (tension) headache, 97
Muscle recruitment, 131
Muscle sheaths, 133
Muscle team, 132, *134*
Muscle tissue, 84, *86*
    types of, 131-132, *132*
Muscle tone, 132-133
Muscle voltage artifacts, 438, *441*
Muscular dystrophy, 138-139
Muscular system, 130-139

disorders and diseases of, 138-139
Mutations, cancer and, 191
Myelogenous leukemia, 174-175
Myelography, 94-95
Myelomeningocele, spina bifida with, 98, 99, *99*
Myocardial infarction (MI), 170, 175
Myocarditis, 171
Myocardium, 153, *154*
Myometrium, 247
Myopia, 102
Myositis, lumbar, 129
Myxedema, 235, *235*

Narcolepsy, 45
Narcotics, 44-45, 477
Nasal cavity, 74, *74*
Nasal polyps, 108
Nasal smear, 432
Nasal speculum, 323
National AIDS Hotline, 190
National Board of Medical Examiners, 12
National Bureau of Standards, 309
National Center for Health Statistics (NCHS), 280
National Formulary, 477
National Kidney Foundation, 221
Natural immunity, 498
Natural killer (NK) cells, 182
Nausea, 202
    during blood tests, 395
NCHS (*See* National Center for Health Statistics)
Near vision, testing, 323
Needle(s):
    AIDS and, 188
    proper handling and disposal of, 492, 498
    sizes for venipuncture, 397
Needle and syringe method of venipuncture, 397, *397*, 401-402
Needle sticks, avoiding, 491, *492*
Negligence, 21-22
Neissera gonorrhoeae, 262
Neoadjuvant chemotherapy, 192
Neonates (newborns), 379
    screening for PKU, 378-380, *380*
    See also Children; Infants
Neoplasms, 191
Neoprobe, 193
Nephrons, 216-218
    filtration and reabsorption by, 217-218
    secretion function of, 218
    urinary output and, 218
Nephrotic syndrome (nephrosis), 223
Nerve tissue, 84, *85*
Nervous system, 85, 87-99, *88*
    central (CNS), 90-92
    diagnostic tests on, 92-94, *95-96*
    diseases and disorders of, 94-99
    membrane excitability, 87-89, *89, 90*
    peripheral and spinal cord, 89-90, *90-92*
Neuralgia, 98
Neuron(s), 81, 84, *85*
Neuron/spinal cord damage, 98
Neutral pH, 55
Neutrophils, 165, 178, 182
Nevi, 112
Newborns, AIDS and, 188
NGU (*See* Nongonococcal urethritis)
Nicotine, 45

overcoming addiction to, 46
Nicotine patches, 488
NIDDM (*See* Noninsulin-dependent diabetes mellitus)
Nissl bodies, *85*, 87
Nitrite in urine, 411-412
Nitroglycerin transdermal systems, 486, *486-487*, 488
NK cells (*See* Natural killer (NK) cells)
Nocturia, 219
Noduloulcerative lesions, 113
Nomogram, 489
Non compos mentis, 15
Nongonococcal urethritis (NGU), 261-262
Noninsulin-dependent diabetes mellitus (NIDDM), 234
Noninvasive procedures:
    for diagnostic tests of urinary system, 221
    magnetic resonance imaging, *449*, 449-450, *450*
Nonscarring alopecia, 112
Nonspecific urethritis (NSU), 261-262
Nonspecific vaginitis, 263
Norepinephrine, 45
Normal blood pressure, 308, *309*
Normal saline, 78
Nose, *107*, 107, *140*, 140-141
    diseases and disorders of, 107-108
    examination of, 323
Nosebleed (*See* Epistaxis)
Notice of employment termination, 552, *552*
NSU (*See* Nonspecific urethritis)
Nuclear medicine, 457
Nuclear medicine studies, 207-208
Nucleolus, 77
Nucleus, 75, 76, *76*
Nutrition, 27-31
    cancer and, 194
    exercise, rest and, 26-33, *27*

Obesity, MRI and, 450
Objective findings, 321
Objectives (microscope lenses), 374
Obligate parasite, 54
Obstetrics patients, examinations of, 355-358, *359-361*
Obturator, 365
Occipital lobe, 92, *94*
Occult blood, 327, 363, *451*, 451-452
    in stool specimens, 417
    testing for, 208
Occupational hazards, cancer and, 194
Occupational Safety and Health Administration (OSHA), 61, 67
    Hepatitis B immunization and, 506
    laboratory regulation by, 376
    laboratory safety standards of, 370
Office environmental control, 50-70
    AIDS and universal precautions, 58, 60-61
    asepsis, 50-52
    care of instruments, 61-63
    disease transmission, 52-58
    safety and security, 63-68
Office safety:
    general guidelines for, 509-510, 537
    procedures for medical emergencies, 510-526, *511*
    security and, 63-68
Office stress, 37

Ohio State University Medical Center, The, 193
Ointments, 486
Olfactory nerve area, 92, *94*
Oliguria, 219
On-site triage, 269
Oncogenes, 192
Oophoritis, 262
Open fracture (*See* Compound fracture)
Open spiral, in applying bandages, 529, *529*, 530
Ophthalmic medications, 341
Ophthalmoscope, 337
Opportunistic infections, 187
Optic disc, 102
Optic nerve fibers, 92, *94*
Oral cancer, 108-109, 213
Oral medication, obtaining and administering, *484, 485*, 485-486
Oral mucous membranes, examination of, 323-324, *324*
Oral temperature, measuring, 292-294, *294*, 299
    contraindications to, 293-294
    with disposable plastic thermometer, *297*, 298
    electronically, 299
    with mercury thermometer, 295
    sublingually, 292-293, *294*
Orbicularis oculi, 134, 135, *136*
Orbicularis oris, 134, 135, *136*
Orbital cavity, 74, *74*
Orchidectomy, 243
Orchitis, 242
Organ(s), 85
Organ donation, 14-15
Organ of Corti, *105*, 106, *106*
Organelles, 75-77, *76*, 77t
Origin of muscle attachment, 133
Orthopnea, 151
Os coxae, 122, *125*
Oscilloscope, 448
OSHA (*See* Occupational Safety and Health Administration)
Osmosis, 78, *79*
Osmotic pressure, 78
Osseous tissue, 84
Osteoarthritis, 126
Osteoporosis, 129
OTC medicines (*See* Over-the-counter medicines)
Otic medications, 342
Otitis externa, 107
Otitis media, 107
Otosclerosis, 107
Otoscope, 323, 337
Outer ear, 105, *105*
Ovarian cancer, 259-260
Ovarian cyst, 260
Ovaries, 229t, 231-232, 244, *244-246*, 246
Over-the-counter (OTC) medicines, 273, 477
Ovulation, 244, *246*, 250
Ovum, 237, 250, *252*
Oxygen, 139-140, 142-143, 150, 159
Oxygen debt, muscle fatigue and, 136-137
Oxygen tanks, 511-512
Oxytocin, 227

Pacemaker (SA node), 156, *157*
Pacemakers:
    artificial, 157, *158*
    magnetic resonance imaging and, 450
PACs (*See* Premature atrial contractions)

Pallor, 386
Palpation, 302, 320
Pancreas, 204, *204*, 229t, 231, *231*
Pancreatitis, 213
Papanicolaou's (Pap) smear, 194, 255, 352-355, *353-355, 357*
  assisting with, 356, *358*
Papillae, 108, *108*
Papillary muscles, 154, *155*
Paraesophageal (rolling) hiatal hernia, 211, 212
Paralytic ileus, 213
Paraplegia, 98
Parasites, 54-55, *56*
Parasympathetic nervous system, 90
Parathyroid glands, 229t, 230
Parenteral administration of medicines, 485
Parietal lobe, 92, *94*
Parietal pleura, 144
Parkinson's disease, 98
Paroxysmal nocturnal dyspnea (PND), 150
Paroxysmal stage of pertussis, 504
Passive immunity, 185
Passive smoking, 46, 149
Patch test, 432, *432*, 433
Patches, 486, *486-489*, 488
Patella, *119*, 121
Pathogens, 52
Pathophysiology, 72-73
Patient(s):
  assistance with ambulation, 510
  communication with, 318
  diabetic, 496, *500-501, 503*
  with disabilities, 267
  education of, 318
  explaining breast self-examination to, 354, *354*
  immunization record for, 507, *507*
  interacting with, 4-7
  interviewing for medical history form, 272
  positioning and draping for examinations, 330-336
  preparation of, 322
  in wheelchairs, 533, 536, *536*
Patient compliance, 6
Patient database, 266-315
  importance of accuracy in, 266
  managing triage, 267-270, *268, 269, 271*
  medical history, 270-273
  mensurations, 273, 276, 278-285
  vital signs, 285-314
Patient rights, 18-19, *20*
PDR (*See* Physician's Desk Reference)
Pectoralis major, 134
Pediatric examinations, 358-365, *362*
Pediatric urine collection bags, 408, *408*
Pediculosis, 116
Pediculosis corporis, 116
Pediculosis pubis (pubic lice), 116, 262
Peer review, 13
Pelli-Robson contrast sensitivity chart, 346-347, *348*
Pelvic cavity, 74, *74*
Pelvic girdle, 122, *125*
Pelvic inflammatory disease (PID), 262
Penile implants, 242-243
Penis, 237, *238*, 241
Penlight (otoscope), 323
Pepsin, 201
Peptic ulcer, 201, 213

Perception, 110
  in communication, 3
Percussion, 320
Percussion hammer, 327, *328*
Perfusion, 145, 516
Pericarditis, 171-172
Pericardium, 153, *154*
Perinatal transmission of HIV, 60
Perineum, 247, *249*, 249
Peripheral nervous system, 87, 89-90, *90-92*
  spinal cord and, 89-90, *90-92*
Peristalsis, 137-138, *138*, 199
Peritoneal dialysis, 220, *220*
Peritoneal membrane, 74
Permeability of blood vessels, 180
Personal appearance, 550
  for job interview, 545, 547
Personal behaviors, 26-49
Personal hygiene, 3, *3*
  job interview and, 547
Personal opinion notes, 272
  cautions about, 23
Personal protective equipment (PPE), 370, *370*
Personal/sociocultural history, 273
Personality types, 36
Pertussis, 504, 506
Pertussis vaccination, 504, 506
Petri dish, 421, *421*
Peyer's patches, 178, *180*
pH values, 80, *82*
  neutral, 55
  range for normal urine, 410, *412*
Phagocytes, 163, 178
Phagocytosis, 78, *80*
Phalanges, 121, *124*
Pharmaceutical references, 476-477
Pharmaceuticals (*See* Drug(s))
Pharmacist's Manual (DEA), 14
Pharmacology, 477
Pharmacopoeia Internationalis, 477
Pharmacopoeia of the United States of America (USP), 477
Pharynx, 141, *142*
Phenistix reagent strip for PKU testing, 412
Phenylalanine, 378
Phenylketonuria (PKU), 81, 378
  Phenistix reagent strip for testing, 412
  testing for, 378-380, *380*
Phimosis, 241
Phlebitis, 175
Phlebotomist, protection from needle injury, 399-400, *404*
Photophobia, 502
Physical condition, pulse rate and, 303
Physical examinations, 317-367
  complete, 319-330, 320t
  positioning and draping, 330-336
  procedures of eye and ear, 336-351
  specialty, 351-367
  timing of, 329, 330t
Physical reactions to stress, 37
Physical urinalysis, *409*, 409-410
Physician instructions, refusal to follow, 19
Physician rights, 18-19, *20*
Physician's Desk Reference (PDR), 473, 474
  using, 476-477
Physician's Desk Reference for Nonprescription Drugs, 473, 477

Physician's office laboratory (POL), classification and regulation of, 374-376, 375t
Physiology (*See* Anatomy)
Pia mater, 92, *95*
PID (*See* Pelvic inflammatory disease)
Pigment of hair shaft, 111
Pineal body, 229t, 231
Pinkeye (*See* Conjunctivitis)
Pinocytic vesicles, *76*, 77
Pinocytosis, 77, 80
Pitch, in percussion, 320-321
Pituitary gland, 226-228, 229t
  anterior lobe, 226-227, *228*
  posterior lobe, 227-228
PJCs (*See* Premature junctional contractions)
PKU (*See* Phenylketonuria)
Placenta (afterbirth), 252, 254
Plants, poisoning from, 518
Plasma, 158, 164
Plasma cell, 182
Platelets, 165, *168*
Pleura, lung and, 143-144, *144*
Pleural effusion, 150
Pleurisy, *146*, 149-150
Plexuses, 90
PMS (*See* Premenstrual syndrome)
PND (*See* Paroxysmal nocturnal dyspnea)
Pneumoconiosis, 150
Pneumocystis carinii, 185
Pneumoencephalograph, 94-95
Pneumonia, 150
  immunization against, 499, 501
Pneumothorax, 150-151
Poisoning, first aid for, 518
POL (*See* Physician's office laboratory)
Polio immunization, 507
Polycystic kidney disease, 223
Polycythemia, 380
Polyps, 207, 213-214, 260, 461
  nasal, 108
Polyuria, 219
POMR (*See* Problem-oriented medical record)
Pons, 92, *94*
Portal circulation, 161-162, *164*
Positioning patient, 330-336
Posterior lobe of pituitary gland, 227-228, 229t
Posterior section, 73, *73*
Postoperative care, educating patient about, 460, 471
Pouch of Douglas (*See* Rectouterine pouch)
Power table, 330, *331*, 332
PPE (*See* Personal protective equipment)
PR (*See* Prolactin)
Precordial electrocardiograph leads, 438, *439*
Pregnancy, 252-254, *253*
  assessing health status in, 355-358, *359-361*
  danger of rubella vaccination during, 503
  precautions about HIV during, 60
  Rh factor and, 167-168
  vaginal bleeding during, 518
Pregnancy testing, 232, 255
  urine specimen for, 413
Preicteric stage of hepatitis B, 211
Premature atrial contractions (PACs), 157
Premature contractions, arrhythmias and, 156-157
Premature junctional contractions (PJCs), 157
Premenstrual syndrome (PMS), 260
Prenatal care, 253-254

health assessment, 355
Preoperative care, educating patient about, 460
Presbycusis (senile deafness), 106, 107
Presbyopia, 104
Prescription blanks, 477, *477*
  security of, 525
Prescription medications, 474, 475t-476t
Prescription writing:
  physician registration for, *478*, 480-481
  prescription blanks, 477, *477*, 525
  schedule of controlled substances, 479t, 481, 483
Present illness, 273
Pressure points, 524, *525*
Primary series of immunizations, 499
Privacy, *5*, 5-6
Private employment agencies, 543
Privileged communication statutes, 18
Problem-oriented medical record (POMR), 321
Problem solving, 48
Procedures:
  administering disposable enema, 366
  administering injections, 497, *497*, 503-505, *505*
  answering office phone, 268
  applying arm sling, 532, *532*
  applying bandages, 527, *528-531*, 529-531
  applying patch tests, 433
  assisting patients to and from wheelchairs, 533, 536, *536*
  basic suture setup, 526
  cardiopulmonary resuscitation (CPR), 521-522, *521-522*
    for infants and children, 523, *523*
  catheterizing urinary bladder, 406, *409*
  cleaning and storing mercury thermometers, 293
  cleaning wound areas, 527
  collecting sputum specimen, 418
  collecting stool specimen, 418
  completing ESR using Wintrobe method, 403, *405, 407*
  completing medical history form, 272
  counting erythrocytes (RBCs) manually, *390*, 391, *395*
  counting leukocytes (WBCs) manually, 391, *395*
  determining glucose content of urine, *412*, 413, *415*
  determining hematocrit, 382t, 383, *384, 385*
  determining specific gravity using urinometer, 410
  gynecological examination and Pap test, 356, *358*
  handwashing, 53, *53-54*
  Hemoccult Sensa tests, 450
  hemoglobin determination, 386, *388*
  Holter monitoring, 444
  instillation, 341, 342, *343*
  irrigation, 338, 339, *340*
  Ishihara method of determining color vision, 347
  making blood smear, 395, *396*
  measuring blood pressure, 312
  measuring head circumference, 287, *288*
  measuring height, 286, *287*
  measuring infant's chest, 288, *288*
  measuring pulse, 303, 304
  measuring recumbent length of infant, 283, *287*
  measuring respiration, 307
  measuring temperature, *294*, 295-299, *297*
  microscope use, 373

  minor surgery, 466-468, *467*, 468t
  mouth-to-mouth resuscitation, 520
  obtaining and administering oral medication, 485, *485*
  obtaining blood for PKU test, 378
  obtaining standard 12-lead electrocardiogram, *440*, 440-441, *443*
  obtaining throat culture, 422, *423*
  obtaining urine sediment for microscopic examination, 414, *416*
  obtaining venous blood with sterile needle and syringe, *397*, 401-402
  obtaining venous blood with vacuum tube, 402, *405*, 405t
  performing scratch tests, 431
  positioning patients, 331, 333-336
  preparing bacteriological smear, 421
  preparing gram stain, *424*, 425
  preparing resumé, 539
  preparing skin for minor surgery, 462-463, *462-565*
  puncturing skin with Autolet, 377, *379*
  puncturing skin with sterile lancet, 376, *379*
  putting on sterile gloves, 464, *464-466*
  removing sutures, *469*, 469-470, *470*
  screening blood sugar (glucose) level, 389, *390*
  screening visual acuity, 344, *346*, 347
  sigmoidoscopy, 364
  testing urine with Multistix 10 SG, 411
  using canes, crutches, and walkers, 534, *534*, 535
  weighing infants, 283, *286*
  weighing patient on upright scale, 280, *285*
  withdrawing medication from ampule, 494, *494*
  withdrawing medication from vial, 495, *495*
  wrapping items for autoclave, 65, *65*
Proctological procedures, instruments used in, 367, *367*
Proctology tables, 366
Proctoscope, 208, *366*, 367
Proctoscopy, 208
Professional associations, job search and, 543
Progesterone, 232
Progress reports in patient chart, 322
Progressive stroke, 172
Projection, 47
Prolactin (PR), 227, 252
Prolapsed uterus, 247, *248*, 327
  postpartum, 333, *333*
Promptness, 547, 550
Prone position, 332, *332*, 333
Prophylactic substances for anaphylactic shock, 519
Prostaglandins, 190, *190*, 191
Prostate gland, 240, *242*
Prostatectomy, 243
Prostatic hypertrophy, 243, *243*
Prosthesis, 125
Protanopia, 345
Proteins, 199
Prothrombin time, 398
Protozoa, 54, *55*
Proximal, 73, *73*
Proximal convoluted tubule, 217, *217*
Pruritis ani, 214
Psoriasis, 116
Psychedelic drugs, 43-44
Psychological changes in pregnancy, 254

Psychological counseling in transsexualism, 263
Psychoneuroimmunology, 178
Psychopathic tendencies, LSD use and, 525
Psychoses, 38
Psychosomatic illness, 36, 38
Ptosis, 104-105, 216
Puberty, 227
Pubic lice (*See* Pediculosis pubis)
Pubic region, 74, *75*
Public employment services, 542-543
Public library, 543
Pulmonary angiography, 145
Pulmonary arteriography, 145
Pulmonary circulation, 154, *155*, 156-158
  artificial pacemaker for, 157, *158*
  controlling rate of, 158, *158*
  heart sounds, 156, *156*
  pacemaker in, 156, *157*
  rhythm disorders and, 156-157
Pulmonary edema, 151
Pulmonary embolism, 151
Pulmonary function tests, 145
Pulse, 289, *302*, 302-305
  apical, 304-305
  apical-radial, 305, *305*
  characteristics of, 303
  radial, 303-304, *304*
  rate of, 302-303, 303t
  rhythm of, 303
  volume of, 303
Pulse deficit, 305
Pulse oximeter, 145
Pulse points, 302, *302*
Pulse pressure, 308
Puncture wounds, 524
Pupil, 101, *101*
  examination of, 323
Purkinje fibers, 436, *437*
Pus (*See* Exudate)
Pustule, 115
Pyelonephritis, 223
Pyloric sphincter, 202, *202*
Pyloric stenosis, 214
Pyrogens, 290
Pytalin, 199

Quadriceps femoris, 135
Quadriplegia, 98
Quality assurance in health care, 375-376
Quick-weight-loss programs, 28

Race, cancer survival rates and, 195t
Radial pulse, measuring, 303-304, *304*
Radial pulse point, 302, *302*
Radiation, 191
Radioactive iodine uptake test, 232
Radioactive substances in uptake studies, 457
Radiographs of gallbladder, 455
Radiolabeled monoclonal antibodies, 193
Radiological studies, *453*, 454-457
  body scans, 457
  cholecystogram, 454, *454*
  intravenous pyelogram, 455, *456*
  kidney, ureters, bladder (KUB) series, 221, 455-456, *456*
  lower GI series (barium enema), 454-455, *456*
  mammography, *456*, 456-457, *457*

Radiological studies (Continued)
    upper GI series (barium swallow), 454, 455, *455*
Radiologist, 454
Radionuclides, 457
Radiopaque contrast medium, 455
Radius, *119*, 121
Rales, 306
Random urine specimens, 407-408
Range-of-motion (ROM) exercises, 33, *34-35*
Rapport, 63
    building, 4-5
    with children, 361-362
    with employer, 9
    with patients and families, 48, 266-267, 269-270, 279, 315
Rationalization, 47
Raynaud's phenomenon, lupus and, 196
RD (*See* Registered dietician)
RDS (*See* Respiratory distress syndrome)
Reagent strips, 383, 410
Recapping, 492, 493
Reception area:
    care and inspection of, 51
    play area for children in, 358
    safety and security in, *66*, 66-67
Receptors, 100, 110
Reciprocity in physician licensure, 12
Rectal examination:
    female, 327
    male, 327
    preparing patients for, 363
Rectal probe, of electronic probe thermometer, 300
Rectal temperature, *294*, 294-296
    measuring with mercury thermometer, *294*, 296
Rectocele, 260
Rectouterine pouch (cul-de-sac; pouch of Douglas), 247
Rectus abdominis, 134
Recurrent turns, in applying bandages, 528, *528*
Red blood cells (*See* Erythrocyte(s))
Red reflex, 323
Reflex actions, 89, *91, 92*
Reflexes, examination of, 327, *328*
Refraction error, 102, *103*
Registered dietician (RD), 28, 31
Regression, 48
Relaxation, 38
Release of information form, 5, *5*
Renal calculi (kidney stones), 218, 223-224
Renal failure, 224-225
Renal threshold, 410
Rennin, 201
Repolarization of ventricles, 436
Report of findings, 329, *329*, 399, *399*
Repression, 47
Reproductive system, 236-264
    birth process, 254, 254t
    contraception, 255, 256t
    diagnostic tests of, 255
    differentiation of organs, 237, *238*
    diseases and disorders of, 255, 257-263
    female organs, 244-250
    fertilization, 250, 252, *252*
    male organs, 237, *239*, 239-243
    pregnancy, 252-254, *253*
    transsexualism, 263-264
Request for sterilization forms, 18, *19*
Res ipsa loquitur, 21

Residual urine, 222
Resignation letters, 552, *552*
Resonance, in percussion, 320-321
Respiration, 142-143, *144*, 289, 305-307
    counting, *306*, 306-307
    quality of, 306, *306*
    rate of, 306
Respiratory distress syndrome (RDS), 143-144
Respiratory emergencies, first aid for, *518*, 518-519, *519*
Respiratory system, 139-152
    diagnostic examinations, 145, *146*
    disorders and diseases of, 145-152
    lung and pleura, 143-144, *144*
    muscles of breathing, 144, *145*
    oxygen pathway, *140*, 140-142, *141*
    respiration, 142-143, *144*
Respondeat superior, 21
Rest, nutrition, exercise and, 26-33, *27*
Resumé:
    in job search, 539, *540-543*, 541
    procedure for preparing, 539
Retina, 101, *101*, 102
Retinal detachment, 105
Retinopathy, 104
Retroflexed uterus, 247, *248*
Retrograde pyelogram, 455
Retrograde ureteropyelography, 222
Retroperineal, 74
Retroverted uterus, 247, *248*
Retrovirus, 186
Review of systems for patient's medical history, 273
Reye's syndrome, 98
Rh factor, 166-169
    compatibility of, 167-168
Rheumatoid arthritis, 126, 196-197
Rheumatoid factor, 196
Rh(D) immune human globulin, 168
Rhinitis, allergic, 108, 145-146
Rhythm disorders of pulmonary circulation, 146-157
Rhythm (contraception) method, 256t
Rib cage, 120-121, *123*
Ribonucleic acid (RNA), 77
Ribosomes, 75, *76*, 77
R.I.C.E. method for treating sprain, 130
Rickets, 27
Right-sided heart failure, 172-173
Right-to-die options, 15
Ringworm, 116
Rinne test, 106, 351
RNA (*See* Ribonucleic acid)
Roentgen rays, 454
Role model, 6
Rolling (paraesophageal) hiatal hernia, 211, 212
ROM (*See* Range-of-motion exercises)
Romberg balance test, 327
Roundback (*See* Kyphosis)
Route of administration of medications, 483-489
Rubella (German measles), 502-503, *506*
Rubeola, 502
Rugae, 200, *202*
Ruptured disk (herniated disk), 128

SA node (*See* Sinoatrial node)
Sabin vaccine, 485
Saf-T Clik needle adaptor, 399-400, *404*

Safe sex, 321
Safety:
    in laboratory, 370-372, *370-372*
    in office (*See* Office safety)
Sagittal plane, 73, *73*
Saliva, 199
Salivary glands, 199, *201*
Salpingitis, 262
Salpingo-oophorectomy, 257-258
Salves, 486
Sanitization, 56
Sarcomas, 191
Sartorius muscle, 135
Scabies, 116
Scanning tests of thyroid, 232
Scapula, 121, *123*
Scarring alopecia, 112
Schedule of controlled substances, 479t, 480-481, 483
Schick test for diphtheria immunity, 504
Schlemm's canal, 104
Sciatica, 98
Sclera, 101, *101*
Sclerosing basal cell carcinoma, 113
Scoliosis, *129*, 129-130
Scopolamine transdermal systems, 488, *489*
Scratch test, 429-430, *431, 432*
    procedure for performing, 431
Scrotum, 237, *238*
Scurvy, 27
Sebaceous (oil) glands, 111, *111*
Seborrhea of scalp (dandruff), 102
Sebum, 112
Second-degree burns, 512-513
Second-degree heart block, 156
"Second-hand" smoke, 46, 149
Second opinion, 6
Secondary hypertension, 174
Secondary sex characteristics:
    female, 244, *245*
    male, 239, *240*
Secretion, 216
Security procedures for reception area, 67
Sedentary life-style, 444
Semen, 240-241
Semi-Fowler's position, 335
Semicircular canals, *105*, 106, *106*
Semilunar valve, 154, *155*
Seminiferous tubules, 239, *240*
Senile deafness (*See* Presbycusis)
Senses, 100-109
    ear and sense of hearing, 105-107
    eye and sense of sight, 100-105, *101, 102*
    nose and sense of smell, *107*, 107-108
    skin and sense of touch, 109, *109*
    tongue and sense of taste, *108*, 108-109
Sensitivity to particular drugs, 490
Sensorineural hearing loss, 106
Sensory (afferent) nerves, 87
Sensory neurons, 84, 87
Sentinel pile, 210
Septum, 140, *140*, 153, *155*
Serotonin, 165
Serum albumin, 164
Serum globulin, 164
Serum hepatitis, 211
Seven warning signals of cancer, 193, 320t
Sexual harassment, 19, 21